Plasmid
Biopharmaceuticals

Plasmid Biopharmaceuticals

Basics, Applications, and Manufacturing

Duarte Miguel F. Prazeres

Instituto Superior Técnico
Lisbon, Portugal

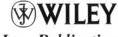

A John Wiley & Sons, Inc., Publication

Published by John Wiley & Sons, Inc., Hoboken, New Jersey
Published simultaneously in Canada

For general information on our other products and services or for technical support, please contact our Customer Care Department within the United States at 877-762-2974, outside the United States at 317-572-3993 or fax 317-572-4002.

Wiley also publishes its books in a variety of electronic formats. Some content that appears in print may not be available in electronic formats. For more information about Wiley products, visit our web site at www.wiley.com.

Library of Congress Cataloging-in-Publication Data:

Prazeres, Duarte Miguel F.
   Plasmid biopharmaceuticals : basics, applications, and manufacturing / Duarte Miguel F. Prazeres.
      p. ; cm.
   Includes bibliographical references and index.
   ISBN 978-0-470-23292-7 (cloth)
   1. Plasmids. 2. Biopharmaceutics. I. Title.
   [DNLM: 1. Plasmids–therapeutic use. 2. Biopharmaceutics–methods. 3. Drug Design.
4. Technology, Pharmaceutical–methods. QU 470]
   QH452.6.P73 2011
   615'.1–dc22

                                                                    2010033318

Printed in the United States of America

oBook ISBN: 978-0-470-93991-8
ePDF ISBN: 978-0-470-93987-1
ePub ISBN: 978-1-118-00225-4

10 9 8 7 6 5 4 3 2 1

Dedicated to my wife Ana, and to my young boys, João and Tiago

Contents

Preface

A few chance experiments performed in the early 1990s of the twentieth century showed that plasmid molecules injected in living mammalian hosts could reach the nucleus of cells. Furthermore, and to the surprise of many, the cell machinery of the transfected cells was able to express the genetic information hosted in the plasmid into a functionally active protein. The potential of the new technology soon became apparent—in principle, it was now possible to command a living organism into producing virtually any protein by supplying it with the appropriate genetic information carried in a plasmid molecule. Once expressed, the target protein could perform a number of functions, from replacing missing or defective proteins to eliciting an immune response against infectious agents or abnormal cells. The potential therapeutic and prophylactic applications of such plasmid-based gene transfer techniques fostered research efforts across the scientific community worldwide. As a consequence, a vast and multifaceted field emerged—plasmid biopharmaceuticals—whose ultimate goal is to provide society with a new range of medicinal agents.

The book *Plasmid Biopharmaceuticals: Basics, Applications, and Manufacturing* addresses the challenges faced by scientists and engineers involved in the development of plasmid biopharmaceuticals and of methods for their manufacture. The goal of the book is not to provide a very extensive coverage of the area nor to present a very detailed account of all of the scientific progress that has been made and described in the literature since the inception of the field. I rather set out to present and revisit fundamental issues and to discuss the most important ideas and relevant topics so as to provide both the beginner and the experienced researcher with an updated overview of the area. The book targets all those involved in the development and manufacturing of plasmid biopharmaceuticals, whether they come from academia or industry, but also the novice who knows nothing about the subject but nevertheless wishes to spend a modest portion of his/her time learning. The book is organized into three major parts: (1) Basics, (2) Applications, and (3) Manufacturing. The topics covered in the individual chapters within each part of the book were selected and laid down to provide a transversal overview of the plasmid biopharmaceutical area. Therefore, and although the scientific, engineering, and technological issues predominate, complementary issues like regulations, ethics, markets, and innovation are touched upon and discussed alongside. I expect this feature to make the book particularly useful.

The topics presented and discussed in the Basics part provide the necessary foundations for the understanding of plasmid action, but also for the design of plasmid products and processes. The starting chapter provides a historical perspective of the development of plasmid biopharmaceuticals. A special emphasis is put on the breakthrough discoveries and insights of gene therapy pioneers, plasmid scientists, and recombinant DNA technologists who opened the way for the succession of developments that ultimately led to the establishment of the field. Chapter 2 provides the rationale behind the medical uses of plasmids and organizes applications into two major types of clinical intervention: therapy and prophylaxis. The third chapter in this part discusses the major steps and peculiarities of the discovery, development, and commercialization processes that have to be undertaken to bring plasmid biopharmaceuticals to the market. The survey of the basic structural characteristics and properties of plasmids (Chapter 4) and of the analytical techniques most commonly used to analyze them and probe their structure (Chapter 5) is followed by a description of the most important methods used to deliver plasmid biopharmaceuticals *in vivo* (Chapter 6).

In the Applications part, the reader is first presented with the major safety and ethical issues surrounding the medical uses of plasmid biopharmaceuticals (Chapter 7) and is then guided through the potential market applications in the human and veterinary health segments (Chapter 8). The final chapters in this part of the book are devoted to the presentation of a set of case studies that deal with the development of plasmid biopharmaceuticals for the management of both human disease (Chapter 9)—pandemic influenza and critical limb ischemia, and veterinary disease (Chapter 10)—West Nile virus (condors), infectious hematopoietic necrosis (salmon), and melanoma (dogs). The major goals of these two chapters are to discuss specific issues associated with the development of the particular product under analysis, to highlight situations in which plasmid biopharmaceuticals are advantageous, and of course to describe those cases that have been blessed with regulatory approval.

The section on Manufacturing opens with a chapter devoted to good manufacturing practice (GMP) regulations and validation (Chapter 11), and is then followed by the presentation of the key specifications usually set forth for plasmid biopharmaceuticals, together with the analytical methodologies used to check compliance (Chapter 12). Chapter 13 is devoted to the production of plasmid DNA by *Escherichia coli* cultivation, focusing on specific topics like strain and clone selection, cell banking, growth media selection, inoculum preparation, and operational strategies. The remaining chapters in this part of the book deal with the purification part of manufacturing, that is, with downstream processing. In Chapter 14, the key starting points for the development of a plasmid biopharmaceutical downstream process, which include an adequate knowledge of the properties of the plasmid and associated *E. coli* impurities, an understanding of the major problems to be encountered, and a familiarity with the accumulated know-how and experience, are addressed. The three chapters that follow present an individual discussion of the different stages of the downstream processing: primary isolation (Chapter 15), intermediate recovery (Chapter 16), and final purification (Chapter 17). The information provided in those chapters is important not only to understand the different plasmid downstream processes that have been patented and published in the literature but also to suggest better combinations of the available unit operations. This process synthesis activity is the subject of Chapter 18, which presents a number of different plasmid manufacturing processes that have been described in the scientific and technical literature.

The major goal of the closing chapter is to look back, but also forward, in time, and to try to understand how this new category of medicinal agents—plasmid biopharmaceuticals—has evolved and will progress toward the future. More specifically, the dynamics of the innovation activity, which took place in the area during the last 30 years, is analyzed, and a side-by-side comparison of a specific class of plasmid biopharmaceuticals, DNA vaccines, with existing and proven conventional vaccines is made on the basis of the blue ocean business strategy.

Although the momentum gained by plasmid biopharmaceuticals can hardly be qualified as unstoppable, the investment made during the past 20 years enabled the accumulation of a substantial amount of scientific and technological knowledge. This body of information, together with some of the unique attributes of the products, is a strong indication that success is around the corner, at least for some prototypes. Still, many issues have to be resolved and clarified, the most important of which is clearly an annoying lack of efficacy. However, if this can be overcome, a bright future awaits plasmid biopharmaceuticals.

DUARTE MIGUEL F. PRAZERES

Acknowledgments

I would like to acknowledge Jonathan T. Rose, editor at Wiley, for the encouragement and support throughout this project. His never-ending patience, reassurance, and easygoing attitude contributed to ease the pressure that kept on building as a result of the succession of failed deadlines. I am grateful to all who have worked with me over the past 14 years in the laboratories of the Institute for Biotechnology and Bioengineering for their collaboration, ideas, and hard work on the field of plasmid biopharmaceuticals. Finally, I thank my wife Ana and my sons João and Tiago for their patience during the writing of this book.

Abbreviations

A	adenine
AAV	adeno-associated virus
ADA	adenosine deaminase
ADS	adsorption
AEX	anion exchange chromatography
AFM	atomic force microscopy
AIDS	acquired immune deficiency syndrome
AMC	Animal Medical Center
APCs	antigen-presenting cells
ATPS	aqueous two-phase systems
bp	base pair
BCA	bicinchoninic acid
BLA	biologics license application
BSE	bovine spongiform encephalopathy
cGMP	current good manufacturing practice
C	cytosine
CAD	coronary arterial diseases
CAGR	compound annual growth rate
CAT	chloramphenicol acetyltransferase
CBER	Centre for Biologics Evaluation Research
CDC	Centers for Disease Control
CFIA	Canadian Food Inspection Agency
CFTR	cystic fibrosis transmembrane regulator
CIP	cleaning in place
CLI	critical limb ischaemia

CMM	canine malignant melanoma
CPG	controlled pore glass
CpG	cytosine-phosphate-guanine
CTAB	cetyltrimethylammonium bromide
CTLs	cytotoxic T lymphocytes
D	diffusion coefficient
DCs	dendritic cells
DCW	dry cell weight
DHFR	dihydrofolate reductase
DMRIE	N-(2-hydroxyethyl)-N,N-dimethyl-2,3- *bis*(tetradecyloxy)-1-propanaminium bromide
DOPE	dioleoylphosphatidylethanolamine
DOTAP	1,2-dioleoyl-3-trimethylammonium propane
DOTMA	N-[1-(2,3-dioleyloxy)propyl]-N, N, N-trimethylammonium chloride
DTS	DNA targeting sequences
EC	endothelial cells
EDMA	ethylene dimethacrylate
EMA	European Medicines Agency
EMEA	European Medicinal Evaluation Agency
EPO	erythropoietin
EtOH	ethanol
EU	European Union
FDA	Food and Drug Administration
FGF	fibroblast growth factor
FISH	fluorescence *in situ* hybridization
FITC	fluorescein isothiocyanate
FP	final purification
gDNA	genomic DNA
G	guanine
GCP	good clinical practice
GDNF	glial cell line-derived neurotrophic factor
GHRH	growth hormone releasing hormone
GLP	good laboratory practice
GMA	glycidyl methacrylate
GM-CSF	granulocyte macrophage colony stimulating factor
GMO	genetically modified organism
GMP	good manufacturing practice
GRAS	generically regarded as safe
h	helical rise
hAAT	α1-antitrypsin
hGH	human growth hormone
HA	haemagglutinin
HBsAg	hepatitis B surface antigen
HEPA	high-efficiency particulate air

HGF	hepatocyte growth factor
HIC	hydrophobic interaction chromatography
HIF	hypoxia-inducible transcription factors
HIV	human immunodeficiency virus
HPLC	high performance liquid chromatography
HPV	human papilloma virus
HSV	herpes simplex virus
HSVtk	herpes simplex virus thymidine kinase
ICH	International Conference on Harmonisation
IFNγ	interferon γ
IHN	infectious hematopoietic necrosis
IHNV	infectious hematopoietic necrosis virus
IL	interleukin
IMPD	investigational medicinal product dossier
IND	investigational new drug
IPTG	isopropyl β-D-1-thiogalactopyranoside
IQ	installation qualification
IR	intermediate recovery
IRBs	institutional review boards
IS	insertion sequences
IsopOH	isopropanol
ISS	immunostimulatory DNA sequences
KAc	potassium acetate
L	superhelix axis
LAMP	lysosomal-associated membrane
LC	Langerhans cells
LIF	laser induced fluorescence
Lk	linking number
LPS	lipopolysaccharide
LRA	lipid removal agent
mRNA	messenger RNA
MCB	master cell bank
MDCK	Madin–Darby Canine Kidney
MHC	major histocompatibility complex
MSKCC	Memorial Sloan–Kettering Cancer Center
MW	molecular weight
NA	neuraminidase
NaOAc	sodium acetate
NCI	National Cancer Institute
NDA	new drug application
NeoR	neomycin phosphotransferase gene
NGF	nervous growth factor
NIAID	National Institute of Allergy and Infectious Diseases
NIH	National Institutes of Health
NLS	nuclear localization signals

NP	nucleoprotein
NPC	nuclear pore complex
oc	open circular
OQ	operational qualification
OTC	ornithine transcarbamylase
ppGpp	guanosine tetraphosphate
PAD	peripheral arterial disease
PAGE	polyacrylamide gel electrophoresis
PBS	phosphate buffered saline
PCR	polymerase chain reaction
PEG	poly ethylene glycol
PEI	poly ethyleneimine
PI	primary isolation
PLA	poly(DL-lactic acid)
PLGA	poly(DL-lactide-co-glycolide)
PMED	particle mediated epidermal delivery
PNA	peptide nucleic acid
POE	polyoxyethylene
POP	polyoxypropylene
PP	precipitation
PQ	performance qualification
PSA	prostate specific antigen
PTC	points to consider
QA	quality assurance
QC	quality control
r	superhelix radius
rRNA	ribossomal RNA
R	purine
RAC	Recombinant DNA Advisory Committee
R_G	radius of gyration
RNAi	RNA interference
RPC	reversed phase chromatography
RT	reverse transcriptase
shRNA	small hairpin RNA
siRNA	small interfering RNA
SARS	severe acute respiratory syndrome
SCID	severe combined immunodeficiency
SDS	sodium dodecyl sulphate
SEC	size exclusion chromatography
SFDA	State Food and Drug Administration
SIP	sterilization in place
SOP	standard operating procedure
tRNA	transfer RNA
T	temperature
T	thymine

TBAP	tetrabutyl ammonium phosphate
TEAA	triethyl amine acetate
TF	transcription factors
TFF	tangential flow filtration
T_h	T-helper cells
TIL	tumor-infiltrating lymphocytes
TK	thymidine kinase
TLR-9	toll-like receptor-9
TMP	transmembrane pressure
TNFα	tumor necrosis factor α
Tw	twist
UCLA	University of California at Los Angeles
UNICEF	United Nations Children's Fund
USDA	United States Department of Agriculture
UV	ultraviolet
VEGF	vascular endothelial growth factor
VLP	virus like particle
WADA	World Anti-Doping Agency
WCB	working cell bank
WHO	World Health Organization
WNV	West Nile virus
Wr	writhe
Y	pyrimidine

Part I

Basics

1

Historical Perspective

1.1 GENE THERAPY

1.1.1 Introduction

Humankind has been plagued with disease for centuries. From the most devastating pestilences such as the ancient black death and smallpox to the modern acquired immune deficiency syndrome (AIDS) epidemic, the suffering and death toll imposed on millions of human beings have continuously challenged medicine. The majority of those great killers of the past were associated with the ecological, nutritional and lifestyle changes brought about by human progress.[1] Although not so spectacular and abundant as infectious or acquired diseases, hereditary diseases have always attracted human curiosity. Perhaps this is associated to the tragedy of parents passing on a malady to their own children. Most certainly, medical and scientific communities have been lured by the fact that the origin of many of these hereditary diseases can be traced back to single molecular defects in genes (i.e., they conform to the Mendelian rules of inheritance).[2] As written by J. E. Seegmiller, an American pioneer in human genetics, "These disorders are experiments of nature that present unique opportunities for expanding our knowledge of many biological processes. Some of our fundamental concepts of the mechanism of gene action can be traced to basic studies of human hereditary diseases."[3]

Plasmid Biopharmaceuticals: Basics, Applications, and Manufacturing, First Edition.
Duarte Miguel F. Prazeres.
© 2011 John Wiley & Sons, Inc. Published 2011 by John Wiley & Sons, Inc.

Against this background, it is thus not surprising to realize that one of the holy grails of medicine e has been to cure hereditary abnormalities by eliminating or correcting the associated defective genes. This idea of "genetic correction" surfaced in the scientific literature shortly after Avery, MacLeod, and McCarty in 1944 described that genes could be transferred within nucleic acids,[4] and well before the advent of molecular biology. In an article entitled "Gene Therapy," and in what was probably one of the first times the two terms have been used together, Keeler realized that plant and animal breeding sometimes results in the permanent correction of hereditary diseases.[5] This correction, as he described it, is brought about by the crossing of the afflicted individual with a "normal one," becoming effective in their offspring and in generations thereafter. At the time, Keeler did not envisage the use of such "gene therapy" to cure human genetic diseases but concluded that the strategy could be applied to correct physical, physiological, and behaviorist gene-based deviations in plants and animals.[5] Nevertheless, the notion of correcting genetic defects through breeding could hardly be foreseen as an effective therapeutic technique to treat genetic diseases in man. And, although termed by the author as gene therapy, the process described in his article was very far from the deliberate transfer of specific genes into subjects, which is nowadays readily associated with the concept of gene therapy.

Foreign DNA and genes have been routinely introduced into humans by a number of well-established therapeutic and prophylactic procedures, although in a haphazard and unintentional way. Consider, for instance, Edward Jenner's smallpox vaccination, a technique developed in 1790 that involved the inoculation into recipients of the vaccinia virus, the agent responsible for cowpox, one of deadliest infectious diseases ever to affect humans.[6,7] As a consequence of this new procedure, patients were brought into contact with millions of viral particles, each of them harboring the 223 genes of the vaccinia virus genome. Jenner's pioneering work opened the way to the development of a steady stream of vaccines based on live or attenuated microorganisms. As a result, millions of people undergoing immunization against specific diseases are injected every year with foreign genes concealed inside bacteria, virus, and the like.[8] Although the majority of these genes are probably cleared by the recipient's immune system, their exact fate and whether they remain functional or not once inside the body is not completely clear.

Another procedure that involves the delivery of a genetic cargo into humans is the experimental use of bacteriophages to treat bacterial infections.[9,10] This type of therapy was originally developed by Felix d'Herelle in 1916, at the Pasteur Institute in Paris, and was further popularized by Georgian doctors in the former Soviet Union.[11] Again, the administration of bacteriophages in cases of infection with microbes like *Staphylococcus aureus* or *Pseudomona aeruginosa* requires patients to be loaded with phages and their genes, even though these are, in principle, expressed only in the invading bacteria and not in the cells of the human recipient.

Although genes are effectively administered to humans as a result of both traditional vaccination and bacteriophage therapy, neither procedure can be categorized as gene therapy. Rather, the conceptualization of human gene therapy as we know it today was fueled by the immense progress made in biochemistry and genetics in the 1950s and early 1960s, which included the discovery of basic concepts in bacteria and bacteriophage genetics, the elucidation of the DNA double helix structure, and the uncovering of the central dogma of molecular biology.

1.1.2 The Coming of Gene Therapy

Perhaps no other scientist contributed more to the initial development of gene therapy than Joshua Lederberg, the recipient of the Nobel Prize in Physiology in 1958 (Figure 1.1). His pioneering work and vision mark him out as one of the greatest in genetics and life sciences.[12] Lederberg is to be credited not only for his scientific discoveries in bacterial genetics and plasmid biology but also by his prescience in anticipating gene therapy. This is clear from the 1963 article "Biological Future of Man," a piece written at a time when, in his own words, molecular biology was unraveling the "mechanisms of heredity."[13] In this visionary article, and among other prospects, Lederberg discussed and hinted at the control, recognition, selection, and integration of genes in human chromosomes. The prediction of a therapy based on the "isolation or design, synthesis and introduction of new genes into defective cells or particular organs" was enunciated in more detail by Edward Tatum in 1966, who even went as far as to envision the concept of *ex vivo* gene therapy.[14] Lederberg and a number of authors elaborated further on the topic in the subsequent years, as described in two detailed accounts of the earliest writings on human

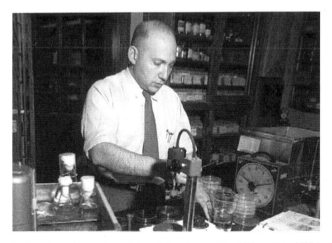

Figure 1.1 *Joshua Lederberg at work in a laboratory at the University of Wisconsin (1958). Downloaded from http://commons.wikimedia.org/wiki/File:Joshua_Lederberg_lab.jpg.*

gene therapy.[15,16] The excitement at the time was such that DNA was viewed by one of the early pioneers as "the ultimate drug."[17]

The first human gene therapy experiments, that is, those that involved the deliberate transfer of foreign genes into human recipients with a therapeutic purpose, were performed in 1970 by the American doctor Stanfield Rogers.[16,18] Earlier in 1968, and on the basis of experiments that involved the addition of polynucleotides to the RNA of tobacco mosaic virus, Rogers and his colleague Pfuderer anticipated that viruses could be potentially used as carriers of endogenous or added genetic information to control genetic deficiencies and other diseases such as cancer.[19] This belief was put to the test in a highly controversial human experiment, in which Rogers and coworkers attempted to treat three German siblings who had arginase deficiency by injecting them with the native Shope rabbit papilloma virus.[18] This attempt was based on previous studies that had apparently shown that the Shope virus codes for and induces arginase in rabbits and in man.[20] In the trial, however, and contrary to what was expected, arginase was not expressed from the gene carried by the virus, and the efforts to supplement the missing enzymatic activity failed. Although Rogers's experiments raised a number of ethical questions, no institutional or legal precepts were violated then since at the time, no specific regulations on gene therapy or institutional review boards (IRBs) existed.[21] In spite of the flawed design and consequent failure of this clinical trial, Rogers was one of the first scientists to anticipate the therapeutic potential of viruses as carriers of genetic information.[18] That such a gene therapy experiment was attempted before the establishment of recombinant DNA technology in 1973 (discussed ahead in Section 1.2.3) is a tribute to Rogers's vision.

Exactly a decade later, in July 1980, Martin Cline at the University of California, Los Angeles (UCLA) headed a human trial designed to treat two young women who were suffering from thalassemia. By that time, recombinant DNA technology had established itself as a powerful tool in the biological and biomedical sciences[22] (see Section 1.2.3), and a number of techniques for genetic modification of cultured mammalian cells had been crafted, including calcium phosphate transfection.[23] Cline's study was built upon experimental evidence which had shown that murine bone marrow cells could be transformed *in vitro* with plasmids harboring genes that coded for proteins like the herpes simplex virus thymidine kinase (HSVtk)[24] or dihydrofolate reductase (DHFR).[25] Once the modified cells were transplanted into recipient mice, those genes were found to be fully functional. This conferred a proliferative advantage to transformant cells when submitted to the pressure of a selective agent such as the anticancer drug methotrexate.[24] Recognizing that the techniques for inserting and selecting for expression of genes were as applicable to animals as they were to tissue culture cells, Cline and coworkers reasoned that "gene replacement" could be useful to treat patients with malignant diseases or hemoglobinopathies, such as sickle cell anemia and thalassemia.[24]

In what was judged by many as a bold leap, Cline then decided to apply these methodologies in a human study of β^0-thalassemia, a disease character-

ized by the inability of the patient cells to synthesize the β-chain of hemoglobin, as a result of mutations in the hemoglobin beta gene. The experiment
involved the removal of bone marrow cells from two patients, and their subsequent transformation *in vitro* with both the β-globin and the HSVtk genes.[26]
The genes were carried independently by plasmids, and the calcium phosphate
methodology was used to precipitate donor DNA and to transform the recipient cells. The higher efficiency of the HSVtk when compared with its human
counterpart was expected to provide a selective proliferative advantage to
marrow cells once these were transplanted back into the patients. Local irradiation was administered at the site of reinjection in order to provide space
for the transformed cells to settle in the bone marrow. However, neither signs
of gene (HSVtk or β-globin) expression nor improvements in the patient's
health were detected. Furthermore, and in what was probably the most significant outcome of the experiment, the National Institutes of Health (NIH) in
the United States ruled that Cline had broken federal regulations on human
experimentation, even though permission had been granted by the foreign
hospitals in Jerusalem and Naples, where the two experiments took place.[26]
Among the consequences suffered, Cline had to resign chairmanship of his
department at UCLA, lost a couple of grants, and had all of his grant applications in the subsequent 3 years accompanied with a report of the NIH investigations into his activities of 1979–1980.[27]

Although both Rogers's and Cline's trials were heavily criticized for scientific, procedural, and ethical reasons, their pioneering actions also contributed
to the establishment of ethic-scientific criteria and guidelines for prospective
human gene therapy experiments, and served as catalysts for the development
of the field.[15,28,29] Most notably, the Recombinant DNA Advisory Committee
(RAC) of the NIH in the United States intervened and created a new group in
1984, called the Human Gene Therapy Working Group (later the Human Gene
Therapy Subcommittee), specifically to deal with and regulate the human use
of molecular genetics.[29–31] From then on, "RAC approval" was mandatory for
any gene therapy clinical protocol sponsored by the NIH. The document *Points
to Consider in the Design and Submission of Human Somatic-Cell Gene
Therapy Protocols*, adopted by the RAC in 1986, constitutes one of the key
regulatory documents issued to provide guidance to researchers.[32] Later in
1991, the agency responsible for the regulation of pharmaceutical products in
the United States, the Food and Drug Administration (FDA), published its
own "Points to Consider in Human Somatic Cell Therapy and Gene Therapy,"
which focused on aspects like the safety, efficacy, manufacturing, and quality
control of gene therapy products.[33] In Europe, the European Medicines
Evaluation Agency (EMEA*) would eventually issue similar guidelines.[34]

---

* Since 2004, the EMEA changed its name to European Medicines Agency and started using the
acronym EMA. However, the old name and acronym is still found in documents/Web sites created
prior to December 2009 (A. Laka, Document and Information Services, EMA, pers. comm.). The
newest designation will be used in the text body of this book, even though the older name and
acronym might appear in specific documents on the reference list.

1.1.3 Early Clinical Trials

Once the regulatory framework was in place and some of the initial obstacles and ethical controversy had subsided, a number of human experiments ensued, many of which constitute milestones in the history of gene therapy (see Table 1.1) and served as nodes from which progress grew.[35] These include, for instance, the first federally approved (in the United States) human experiment in 1989/1990, which involved 10 patients with advanced melanoma.[36] In this trial, tumor-infiltrating lymphocytes (TILs) isolated from solid tumors were first marked with the *Escherichia coli* neomycin phosphotransferase gene (*NeoR*) using a retroviral vector and then were transferred back into the cancer patients.[36,37] Among other conclusions, the trial established that gene-modified TIL cells could be detected by polymerase chain reaction (PCR), either directly in tumor biopsies or after *in vitro* expansion of the tumor cells, and that the procedure did not harm patients.[38,39] Furthermore, transduced TILs were found in peripheral blood and tumor deposits 189 and 64 days after lymphocyte transfusion. Although the study involved the deliberate introduction of a foreign gene into human subjects, it qualifies better as a gene "transfer" rather than as a gene "therapy" trial. The NeoR/TIL trial was also the very first in a whole class of gene marking protocols designed to permanently mark specific cells so that their fate, distribution, and survival could be monitored during disease progression or in response to any form of conventional therapy.[39] An advantage of genetic over traditional physical marking methods, which typically use dyes or radiochemicals, relates to the fact that integration of the marker gene ensures that the "label" is not diluted out by cell division, thus allowing the long-term follow up of the cell progeny.[39]

Shortly after the NeoR/TIL gene marking trial, in September 1990, a gene therapy protocol was initiated to treat a 4-year-old girl afflicted with adenosine deaminase (ADA) deficiency, a rare but fatal disease.[39,40] A second, 9-year-old patient, was later enrolled in the same trial.[40] The lack of ADA, a key enzyme in the metabolism of purines, results in an accumulation of deoxyadenosine, especially in the patient's T lymphocytes, with the consequent impairment of the immune system. ADA patients are thus afflicted by a severe combined immunodeficiency (SCID), which makes them highly susceptible to common infectious agents.[40] The ADA gene therapy protocol involved the isolation of lymphocytes from the patient's blood, the *in vitro* cultivation and expansion of the T-lymphocyte subset, and the introduction of the ADA gene via a retroviral vector. Following expansion, the corrected cells were infused back intravenously.[41,42] This protocol not only confirmed the safety of the different procedures implicated in the therapy but also resulted in a positive response from both patients. Specifically, an increase in the amount of ADA in the T cells was detected and the number of modified lymphocytes remained nearly constant in between treatments.[39] Furthermore, the gene therapy intervention was accompanied by an improvement in antibody responses to *Hemophilus influenzae* B and tetanus toxoid vaccines, indicating at least some immune reconstitution. In spite of these biochemical and physiological changes, doubts

TABLE 1.1. Milestones in the Development of Human Gene Therapy

Year	Target Disease	Description
1970	Argininemia	In the first human gene therapy trial, three siblings were injected with the native Shope papilloma virus in an attempt to improve arginine levels.[16,18]
1980	Thalassemia	In the second human gene therapy trial, two young women in Israel and in Italy were reinfused with their own bone marrow cells, which had received *in vitro* the β-globin and the HSVtk genes via plasmid-mediated transformation.[26]
1984	–	The NIH created the Gene Therapy subcommittee of the RAC to deal with and to regulate the human use of molecular genetics.[29] The document "Points to Consider in the Design and Submission of Human Somatic-Cell Gene Therapy Protocols" was issued 2 years later.[32]
1990	Cancer	In the first federally approved gene marking study in humans, TIL cells isolated from tumors were marked with the *E. coli NeoR* gene using a retroviral vector and were transferred back into patients.[38]
1990	ADA-SCID	The first federally approved human gene therapy trial involved the removal of white blood cells, *in vitro* cell growth, insertion of the missing gene, and infusion of the modified blood cells back into the patient's bloodstream.[40–42]
1991	–	The FDA publishes the "Points to Consider in Human Somatic Cell Therapy and Gene Therapy."[33]
1991	Malignant melanoma	First federally approved human gene therapy trial to target a complex genetic disease. TIL cells isolated from tumors were transduced with the *TNF* gene using a retroviral vector and were transferred back into patients.[36]
1993	Cystic fibrosis	First human gene therapy trial with an adenovirus vector.[143]
1999	OTC deficiency	Death of patient due to a fulminant systemic inflammatory response syndrome developed in reaction to the recombinant adenovirus vector.[47–49]
2000	SCID-X1 syndrome	The immune dysfunction of two patients is apparently cured after the reinfusion of autologous cells transduced *ex vivo* with a retroviral vector hosting the γC gene.[52]
2003	SCID-X1 syndrome	Development of leukemia-like syndrome in recipients due to retrovirus integration and proto oncogene activation.[53]
2004	Head and neck carcinoma	The first human gene therapy product, Gendicine®, received approval from the Chinese FDA.[57]
2007	Arthritis	Death of patient after receiving two injections of an AAV hosting the *TNFR:Fc* gene. The death was attributed to a prior infection and not to gene therapy.[63,64]

ADA, adenosine deaminase; *NeoR*, neomycin phosphotransferase gene; OTC, ornithine transcarbamylase; RAC, Recombinant DNA Advisory Committee; SCID, severe combined immunodeficiency; TIL, tumor-infiltrating lymphocyte.

about the exact role played by gene therapy in this case were raised given that the patients underwent replacement treatment with a conjugate of polyethylene glycol and ADA prior to and after the gene therapy intervention.[40]

Although gene therapy was originally thought of as a strategy to treat classical Mendelian genetic diseases like thalassemia or ADA, it soon became apparent that the concept could be extended to manage multifactorial diseases like cancer, arthritis, or cardiovascular diseases. These diseases are not directly linked to single major genetic abnormalities but are often caused by a combination of environmental factors and genetic predisposition. In many cases, more than one gene may be involved in the onset and progression of the disease.[39,43] Infectious diseases such as hepatitis B, ebola, or AIDS constitute another whole category of targets for gene therapy, both from a therapeutic and prophylactic point of view. Whether in the case of multifactorial or infectious diseases, genes can be used as purveyors of any kind of genetic information that, once expressed *in vivo* as a protein, would provide cells with a new function that would contribute to treat, cure, or prevent the target disease (see Chapter 2 for more details on the specific roles of gene products).

Cancer was the first non-Mendelian target addressed by gene therapy. Previous studies on the therapeutic use of TIL in experimental animal models had shown that secretion of tumor necrosis factor (TNF), a powerful anticancer agent, plays an important role in the regression of established lung metastases.[44] A phase 1 safety trial (see Chapter 3 for a brief description of the clinical development of medicinal agents) was designed accordingly, which aimed to immunize patients with advanced malignant melanoma against their cancers. Briefly, a retroviral vector was used to introduce the gene coding for TNF into autologous TILs[36,45] (Table 1.1). The goal of the trial, which started in January 1991, was thus to make the TNF-expressing TIL more effective against the melanoma. Given the tendency of TIL to accumulate in tumor deposits, the promoters of the study were expecting to deliver high local concentrations of TNF that could destroy the tumor without exposing patients to the high systemic toxicity associated with intravenous injections of TNF alone. An objective response was ongoing in one of the 10 patients, 2 years after treatment.[36] Another approach to improve cancer immunotherapy relies not on adding a specific cytokine gene to TIL or tumor-specific T cells but to the tumor cells themselves, in order to make them more immunogenic.[35] In one of the earlier cancer gene therapy trials of the sort, five patients with advanced cancer were immunized with live autologous tumor cells that had been genetically modified *ex vivo* to secrete either TNF or interleukin 2 (IL-2). No evidence of viable tumor cells was found when the injection sites were surgically resected 3 weeks after the therapeutic intervention.[36]

1.1.4   Failures and Successes

The first serious setback faced by gene therapy came in 1999 when Jesse Gelsinger, a young man suffering from ornithine transcarbamylase (OTC) deficiency, an X-linked inborn error that affects urea synthesis, died after the administration of an adenovirus vector encoding OTC.[46–49] The first symptoms appeared 18h after the recombinant adenovirus was infused into the right hepatic artery at a dose of 6×10^{11} particles/kg. The cause of the subsequent patient's death, which occurred 98h after gene transfer, was attributed to a fulminant systemic inflammatory response syndrome developed in reaction to the adenovirus vector.[49] The effects of gene transfer in the other 17 patients who had enrolled in the trial were, on the contrary, limited to transient myalgias and fevers, and biochemical abnormalities. This seems to indicate that Gelsinger had predisposing factors to vector toxicity.[50] The direct consequences of this tragic event included the halting of several gene therapy trials by the FDA and the payment of fines amounting to more than 1 million dollars by the institutions concerned, the University of Pennsylvania, and the Children's National Medical Center in Washington, as ordered by the U.S. Department of Justice. Furthermore, the lead researchers of the study faced severe restrictions to their clinical research activities.[51]

The year 2000 saw gene therapy's first major success: a gene therapy protocol held in Paris was able to correct the phenotype of an X-linked severe combined immunodeficiency (SCID-X1) syndrome in two young patients. Specifically, the protocol involved the reinfusion of the patients with autologous CD34 bone marrow cells that had been transduced *ex vivo* with a retrovirus vector encoding the interleukin 2 receptor, gamma gene (γC).[52] These successes were later shadowed by the development of leukemia-like clonal lymphocyte proliferation in 4 of the 10 recipients of the treatment, as a consequence of the integration of the retrovirus vector in a number of sites located at or nearby genes such as *LMO2*, *BM1*, and *CCDN2*.[53,54] Although three of these four patients responded well to chemotherapy treatment, the fourth died in October 2004.[55] In spite of this unfortunate event, the follow-up of the trial clearly showed that the gene therapy procedure resulted in a direct benefit to patients, with a complete and stable restoration of the immunological phenotype extending for a number of years post-treatment.[54] A similar trial for SCID-X1 conducted in London recently yielded strikingly similar results: 1 of the 10 treated patients who had their immune dysfunction corrected was diagnosed with leukemia. Furthermore, the underlying mechanism of leukemogenesis was also associated with vector integration in a site nearby the proto-oncogene *LMO2*.[56]

In October 16, 2003, a recombinant adenovirus vector expressing the tumor suppressor gene p53 was approved by the State Food and Drug Administration (SFDA) of China for the treatment of head and neck squamous cell carcinoma.[57–59] Developed and manufactured by the Chinese firm Shenzen SiBiono GeneTech and trademarked under the name Gendicine, it became the first ever human gene therapy product to reach the market in April 2004.[57] According to SiBiono, as of October 2007, more than 400 hospitals in China had treated over 5000 patients with Gendicine, including some from several Western countries.[60] The skepticism of the international community over

Gendicine remains high, however, since accurate information regarding the design and outcome of the clinical trials that preceded approval is not available in non-Chinese, scientific journals.[55] China kept and reinforced its leading role in the development of commercial gene therapy when, in November 2005, the SFDA approved Oncorine®, a genetically modified adenovirus for head and neck cancer, which can selectively kill tumor cells with dysfunctional *p53* genes.[61,62]

In July 2007, a gene therapy patient undergoing treatment for arthritis died from massive organ failure after having her knee injected with an adeno-associated virus (AAV) vector. The vector contained the tumor necrosis factor receptor-immunoglobulin Fc fusion gene (TNFR:Fc), an anti-inflammatory protein that inhibits the cytokine tumor necrosis factor α (TNFα).[63,64] The trial, which had enrolled more than 100 patients, was put on clinical hold on cautionary grounds,* even though preliminary investigations associated the tragic outcome with a prior fungal infection. The hold was subsequently lifted after a detailed review by the RAC of the NIH ruled out the product of the transgene and its vector as the causative agent, and confirmed that the cause of death was disseminated histoplasmosis.[65]

In Europe, reference should be made to Cerepro®, an adenovirus-mediated gene-based medicine for brain cancer developed by Ark Therapeutics (Finland), which is currently being reviewed by the EMA for market authorization. The product combines the adenovirus-mediated local administration of the thymidine kinase from *herpes simplex* with the intravenous injection of the prodrug ganciclovir. The enzyme converts ganciclovir into a substance that specifically kills the dividing tumor cells without affecting the surrounding healthy cells[62] (see further details on this type of therapy in Chapter 2, Section 2.4.2.2). Although a previous request by Ark Therapeutics for marketing authorization had been refused by the EMA in 2007, on the grounds that the benefit–risk of Cerepro/ganciclovir had not been demonstrated then,[66] the expectation that the new set of phase 3 clinical data might convince the agency to turn Cerepro into the first gene therapy medicine to be marketed in the West is high.[62]

1.2   PLASMIDS

1.2.1   Introduction

The contributions of plasmids to molecular genetics and biology have been immense, as described in detail in a number of reviews by some of the most prominent scientists involved in the field.[67,68] In this section, a short summary of the most important discoveries and developments is provided, with a special emphasis on those that opened the way to the establishment of plasmid biopharmaceuticals.

* FDA Statement on Gene Therapy Clinical Trial, July 26, 2007.

1.2.2 Early Beginnings

Joshua Lederberg (Figure 1.1) devised the term plasmid in 1952[69] by joining the word cytoplasm with the Latin particle -id,[67] a suffix used to mean "a thing connected with or belonging to." According to the terminology used by Novick and coworkers in a nomenclature proposal made in 1976, "A plasmid is a replicon that is stably inherited (i.e., readily maintained without specific selection) in an extrachromosomal state."[70] Plasmid, which favorably contended with the earlier word plasmagene (see Lederberg[67] for further details), was thus intended to serve as a generic term for any genetic particle or element that is physically separated from the chromosome of the host cell and is able to be perpetuated in this condition.[69,71] From a functional point of view, the role of plasmids is to mediate gene flow within, and between bacterial species. They constitute a means of storing extra genetic information outside the genome of prokaryotes. Bacteria typically resort to this pool of cytoplasmic genes, which can be found dispersed across different populations, when faced with environmental changes or stresses that require adaptations for survival. The variety of plasmid-encoded genes found in nature is huge, ranging from genes that confer resistance to agents like antibiotics or heavy metals to genes that broaden the metabolic properties or confer pathogenicity to the host.[72] For instance, many of the genes that encode for restriction enzymes, the molecular tools that made recombinant DNA technology possible, are carried by antibiotic resistance plasmids. The recognition that the spread of antibiotic resistance among bacteria was frequently linked to plasmids further spurred the interest in their study.

Plasmid-mediated gene exchange among bacteria was originally described by microbial geneticists involved in the study of bacterial mating. This process was conceived for the first time as an unidirectional process involving a gene donor and a gene acceptor by Williams Hayes.[73] Soon after, the transmissible factor F (for fertility), "an ambulatory or infective hereditary factor," became one of the first plasmids to be identified and studied,[74,75] even though its exact physical and molecular nature was not readily recognized at the time. The demonstration that plasmids are made up of DNA was first presented by Marmur and coworkers in 1961 while studying the transfer of the F-factor from *E. coli* to *Serratia marcescens*.[76] This discovery was confirmed shortly after with further evidence gathered from the study of the transmission of colicinogenic factors by Silver and Ozeki.[77] The next important contribution to the understanding of the nature of plasmids was provided by Campbell, who conceptualized that episomes, a type of DNA molecule that, like plasmids, traffics in and out of cells but, unlike them, interacts with chromosomes, must exist with a circular structure.[78] This was an important departure from the established notion of DNA molecules as long, linear biopolymers. The first confirmation of Campbell's hypothesis was provided by Fiers and Sinsheimer, who demonstrated that the double-stranded DNA from the phage phi-X174 is circular.[79] Additional insights into the molecular structure of plasmids came from the study of the circular DNA molecule of the polyomavirus. An important contribution was made in 1965 by Vinograd and coworkers, who described the presence of a "twisted circular structure" containing left-hand tertiary turns in polyoma DNA. They further demonstrated that this structure could be converted to a less compact, open circular duplex by introducing a single strand break.[80] Shortly after, Hickson et al. reported that electronic microscopic preparations of an isolated bacterial sex factor (i.e., a plasmid) showed a circular DNA molecule that similarly contained the tightly twisted and the open circular forms. The electron micrographs in Hickson's paper probably constitute the first visual record of supercoiled plasmid DNA molecules.[81] As we will see next, another report published in the same year, which would have far-reaching implications for all those involved in DNA and plasmid research, described that the intercalating agent ethidium bromide emitted an intense orange-red fluorescence when bound to DNA.[82]

1.2.3 Recombinant DNA

Three proximal scientific discoveries were at the heart of the invention and development of cloning, a pivotal technology that would radically change molecular biology and have a huge impact in the development of gene therapies. The first of these discoveries was the demonstration that bacteria treated with calcium chloride were able to uptake plasmids, and that such "transformed" bacteria could stably generate a progeny that contained replicas of the original plasmid.[83] Furthermore, the presence of antibiotic resistance genes in the plasmids made it possible to select transformed from nontransformed cells using media supplemented with the corresponding antibiotic. The combination of agarose gel electrophoresis with low concentrations of ethidium bromide was another important contribution that revolutionized the analysis of DNA fragments, which had hitherto relied on the lengthy staining and destaining of autoradiographs.[84] The third breakthrough was the isolation of the EcoRI restriction enzyme from an antibiotic resistant strain of *E. coli* and the discovery that the double-stranded DNA cut by it had cohesive termini.[85,86] This set the stage for the advent of recombinant DNA technology, as succinctly described next.

In 1973, Cohen and coworkers ingeniously combined the discoveries described above and performed the first cloning experiments.[22] In the first step of the process, a plasmid (pSC101) that contained the gene for tetracycline resistance was cut at a single site with the EcoRI restriction enzyme. Donor DNA was also treated with EcoRI, yielding multiple fragments. When these fragments were mixed with the open pSC101, complementary base pairing took place between the cohesive ends of the plasmid and of the individual fragments of the donor DNA. Subsequent ligation with DNA ligase thus generated recombined or "recombinant" DNA molecules of pSC101 with inserted DNA fragments. In the next step, these replicons were inserted into *E. coli* cells by using the calcium chloride transformation procedure.[83] Cells transformed with the plasmids were then selected by cultivation in a medium containing tetracycline. This prevented the growth of nontransformed cells but fostered the proliferation of the transformed ones. An agarose gel electrophoresis/ethidium bromide analysis of the recombinant plasmid isolated from these selected clones then showed that they contained "genetic properties and DNA nucleotide sequences of both parent molecular species."[22] Reports soon appeared demonstrating that genes derived from totally unrelated bacterial (e.g., *S. aureus*[87]) and eukaryotic (e.g., *Xenopus laevis*,[88] mouse[89]) species could be replicated in *E. coli* cells. Furthermore, those genes could be expressed in the bacterium, yielding biologically active "recombinant" proteins like somatostatin[90] or insulin.[91] Once the ability to clone virtually any gene into a plasmid and subsequently to express it in a bacterial host was mastered, researchers looked into the possibility of delivering functional genes via plasmid vectors to cultured mammalian cells. Methods were rapidly developed that combined cellular transfection techniques such as calcium phosphate,[23] diethyl aminoethyl (DEAE)-dextran,[92] and liposomes with plasmids encoding genes under the control of mammalian promoters (see Scangos and Ruddle[93] for an earlier review on the mechanisms and applications of DNA-mediated gene transfer in mammalian cells).

The crafting of recombinant DNA technology represented in many aspects a turning point for molecular biology. With the new technique and its basic tools (restriction enzymes, plasmids, and *E. coli*), scientists could now manipulate DNA and genes at will. Many consider also that the multibillion dollar biotechnology industry was born with recombinant DNA. One of the reasons for this is related to the fact that the 1984 "Cohen and Boyer patent" that protected the new discovery and granted exclusive rights to Stanford University[94] would ultimately realize around 300 million dollars in licensing deals with companies like Amgen, Eli Lilly, or Genentech. More importantly, the new technology would eventually make it possible to produce unlimited amounts of medically and industrially relevant proteins from any organism in bacteria. For example, recombinant insulin, which was marketed in 1982, became the first of a stream of commercially successful protein biopharmaceuticals that radically altered the pharmaceutical business.

1.3 PLASMID BIOPHARMACEUTICALS

1.3.1 Introduction

The majority of the earlier gene transfer and gene therapy experiments involving humans and animals resorted to viral vectors as carriers of the therapeutic genes, essentially by using cell-mediated *ex vivo* approaches. However, the ability of viral vectors to recombine, interact with endogenous viruses, and integrate raised safety concerns right from the time the first gene therapy experiments were attempted.[35] The fact that all of the severe adverse events of gene therapy reported so far have resulted from trials in which recombinant viruses were used as vectors underscores these concerns. The use of nonviral gene carriers like plasmids, on the other hand, has been always regarded as a potentially safer alternative.[95] Plasmids had already played a prominent role in the first human experiment that resorted to recombinant DNA technologies, the thalassemia experiment headed by Martin Cline.[25,26] As seen in Section 1.1.2, the genes that were transferred *ex vivo* to the patient's bone marrow cells were hosted in a plasmid, the notorious pBR322 vector. In this case, however, plasmids were used as a tool for the genetic transfection of cells, which then constituted the therapeutic agent themselves. In the following pages, some of the milestones that marked the development of plasmid biopharmaceuticals (also shown in Table 1.2) are briefly described.

TABLE 1.2. Milestones in the Development of Plasmid Biopharmaceuticals

Year	Comments
1983	*In vivo* expression of a gene (rat preproinsulin) harbored in a plasmid is demonstrated for the first time after intravenous injection of carrier liposomes in mice.[96]
1983	The concept of targeted gene expression is demonstrated by the *in vivo* injection of plasmids complexed with liposomes carrying ligands toward cell surface receptors.[99]
1985	The uptake of a plasmid DNA vector in a phosphate buffered saline by mouse liver cells was demonstrated after *in vivo* intravenous injection in mice.[100]
1989	Integration of reporter genes into the host genome is demonstrated after the *in vivo* intravenous injection of plasmid-carrier complexes in mice.[144]
1990	Direct intramuscular injection of "naked" plasmid DNA in mice is taken up by muscle cells, and the encoded reporter gene is expressed *in vivo*.[98]
1990	Genes encoded in plasmid are delivered *in vivo* to the liver, muscle, and skin tissues of rats and mice by particle bombardment.[104]
1991	The possibility of eliciting an immune response against a foreign protein by the introduction of the corresponding gene directly into the skin of mice is demonstrated for the first time.[114]
1991	Skin cells of mice are transformed by plasmid DNA with the aid of *in vivo* electroporation.[129]
1993	The direct administration of naked plasmid DNA encoding a pathogen's (influenza virus) antigen in mice elicits a cell-mediated response and confers protection against a subsequent challenge with the pathogen.[115]
1994	In the first human gene therapy clinical protocol to use plasmid vectors, the gene encoding for the MHC protein HLA-B7 is introduced into advanced melanoma patients to improve tumor immunogenicity.[117]
1994	The name DNA vaccine is selected among others to designate plasmid-based vaccination technology.
1996	The stimulation of the immune system by CpG motifs cloned in plasmids is demonstrated.[120]
1996	Alphavirus replicon elements are added to plasmid vectors to increase the number of copies of mRNA.[127]

TABLE 1.2. *Continued*

Year	Comments
1997	Encapsulation of plasmid DNA in PLG microparticles is described. This mode of delivery protects plasmids against degradation after administration and facilitates uptake, expression, and antigen presentation.[130]
1997	Compaction of single plasmid DNA molecules into minimally sized nanoparticles is described. The complexes can efficiently transfer and express the DNA information both *in vitro* and *in vivo*.[131]
2002	Plasmids are used to direct the intracellular synthesis of siRNA transcripts in mammalian cells, with the concomitant downregulation of the genes targeted for knockdown.[132]
2003	Californian condors become the first animals immunized with a DNA vaccine to be deliberately released into the environment in an attempt to save a local population from WNV infection.[134]
2005	Prophylactic vaccines that protect horses against WNV and farm-raised salmon against infectious hematopoietic necrosis virus become the first ever DNA vaccines to receive marketing approval.[135,137]
2007	The first therapeutic DNA vaccine is conditionally approved to treat melanoma in dogs.[138]
2008	A plasmid encoding for the growth hormone releasing hormone is approved in Australia to decrease offspring morbidity and mortality in pigs.[140]

PLG, poly(DL-lactide-co-glycolide); siRNA, small interfering RNA; WNV, West Nile virus.

1.3.2 The Initial Experiments

One of the first scientific accounts of an experiment in which a plasmid DNA molecule harboring a gene was administered directly into a live animal appeared in 1983[96] (Table 1.2). In their studies, Nicolau and coworkers used liposomes made up of phospholipids and cholesterol to encapsulate a recombinant plasmid encoding the preproinsulin gene.[96] This gene had been isolated from rat and comprised, among others, a putative promoter site for the initiation of transcription.[97] Following intravenous injection of the plasmid-loaded liposomes into rats, the authors found that blood glucose and insulin were respectively lower and higher when compared with the corresponding parameters in control animals. Further experimental evidence confirmed that the injected liposomes had been taken up essentially by the spleens and livers of the animals. These results led to the unambiguous conclusion that the insulin gene had been expressed *in vivo*, under the control of the referred putative promoter.[96] Interestingly, the researchers also described a control experiment in which free, nonencapsulated plasmid DNA solubilized in a tris(hydroxymethyl aminomethane) hydrochloride (tris–HCl)/NaCl buffer was injected intravenously in mice. In this case, however, the levels of insulin and blood glucose remained unchanged. To the best of my knowledge, this was the first time ever that plain (i.e., "naked," as it would be later referred to) plasmid DNA was injected *in vivo*.[96] Seven years would have to pass before *in vivo* expression from naked plasmid DNA was described by Wolff and colleagues.[98]

Nicolau's group also attempted to increase the uptake of the preproinsulin gene by hepatocytes, by incorporating a glycolipid terminated with a β-galactose residue in the carrier liposomes. The hypothesis that β-galactosyl receptors on the surface of hepatocytes would increase the uptake of the liposomes and plasmid was confirmed, albeit this was also observed with endothelial cells, which lacked the aforementioned receptor.[99] Controls in which free plasmid was injected were also performed, but no signs of uptake were detected. Shortly after, attempts aimed at elucidating the *in vivo* intracellular fate of liposome–plasmid complexes injected intravenously in mice were reported. In these experiments, Cudd and Nicolau injected a radiolabeled pBR322 plasmid vector encapsulated in phospholipids/cholesterol liposomes in the tail vein of mice and then used electron microscope autoradiography to analyze liver tissue samples.[100] At that time, they concluded that liposome–plasmid DNA is selectively transported among organelles in the liver cells, mainly to the lysosomes, the mitochondria, and the nuclei. Again, a control experiment in which free plasmid DNA in phosphate buffered saline (PBS) was injected intravenously was described. In this case, the majority of the DNA that was taken up by the liver was found associated with the endoplasmatic reticulum and degraded 5 min after injection. Even though the model plasmid did not carry any transgene, plasmid uptake was unequivocally demonstrated for the first time after *in vivo* injection of naked plasmid DNA.[100]

Shortly after, Dubensky et al. prepared a calcium phosphate-precipitated plasmid DNA vector harboring the DNA from polyomavirus and injected it directly into the liver and spleen of mice.[101] They concluded that plasmid DNA was not stable after transfection due to degradation in the target organs. Benvenisty and Reshef also evaluated the potential of calcium phosphate to mediate the *in vivo* introduction of genes into rats. The selected chloramphenicol acetyltransferase (CAT), hepatitis B surface antigen (HBsAg), and human growth and preproinsulin genes were harbored in plasmids, precipitated with calcium phosphate, and injected intraperitoneally into newborn rats. All genes were expressed by the animal tissues, albeit transiently and with large variations among individuals. Additionally, they concluded that the injection method used favored the distribution of the genetic material in the liver and spleen.[102]

Although the calcium phosphate methodology was widely used at the time, alternative ways of delivering plasmids to target cells gradually emerged. Building up on the previous liposome work,[96,99] Felgner described the synthesis of a cationic lipid, N-[1-(2,3-dioleyloxy)propyl]-N, N, N-trimethylammonium chloride (DOTMA), the spontaneous formation of plasmid–DOTMA complexes, and their use in the transfection of cells *in vitro*.[103] The effectiveness of the technique was attributed to the formation of positively charged complexes that completely neutralize and entrap the DNA and facilitate fusion with the negatively charged surface of cells. When compared with calcium phosphate or DEAE transfection, the process was found to be from 5- to > 100-fold more effective. The process was termed "lipofection" by the authors, a word that has since entered the vocabulary of gene therapy.[103]

Particle bombardment, a technique that would radically alter the way in which plasmids were being administered into animals was developed roughly at the same time.[104] The method was originally developed to deliver nucleic acids to plant cells in calluses and leaves[105] but was soon extended to animal cells cultured *in vitro*.[106] It relies on the coating of plasmids onto fine metallic particles of tungsten or gold, with diameters typically in the 0.1- to 5.0-μm range. The use of a device that accelerates the particles to high velocity then allows penetration of target tissues or organs. The method was used in live animals for the first time in 1990 by Yang and coworkers, who demonstrated that the *in vivo* bombardment of liver, muscle, and skin tissues of rat and mice enabled the transient expression of the reporter genes *CAT* and β-galactosidase.[104] Ever since, handheld biolistic systems or "gene guns" have been one of the favorite methods of plasmid DNA delivery. Although in the original report a gunpowder charge was used to propel the particles,[105] high-voltage electric discharge devices[104] and pressurized gases such as helium[107] can also be used for the same purpose.

1.3.3 Naked Plasmid DNA

In 1990, Wolff and coworkers pushed the boundary further and injected plain saline solutions of plasmids containing genes for CAT, luciferase, and β-galactosidase into skeletal muscle of live mice.[98] They found out that such a naked plasmid DNA molecule, devoid of any kind of adjuvant, could be taken up by the mice's cells and that the encoded reporter transgenes were expressed within the muscle cells. In the case of luciferase, substantial activity could be detected in the muscle for at least 2 months. The experimental data suggested that this persistence of activity was not related to the stability of luciferase or of its RNA transcript, but rather to the extrachromosomal lingering of the injected plasmid DNA inside the muscle cells. Nevertheless, the possibility of chromosomal integration of plasmid DNA was not excluded. The high uptake of plasmid DNA and expression levels of the reporter proteins in the muscle were attributed to structural features of this type of tissue, including its multinucleated cells, sarcoplasmic reticulum, and transverse tubule system. The expression of transgenes hosted in plasmids following their direct intramuscular injection was shortly after demonstrated to occur also in species as varied as fish,[108] chicken,[109] and cattle.[110] And transfection by direct injection of naked DNA was soon found in tissues other than the skeletal muscle, like heart,[111] liver,[112] and brain.[113]

1.3.4 DNA Vaccines

In concluding their seminal paper, Wolff and his colleagues envisaged the use of the method of direct transfer of genes via naked plasmids and into human muscle, as a means of (1) improving the effects of genetic diseases of muscle and (2) expressing genes encoding antigens to provide alternative approaches to vaccine development.[98] The experimental demonstration of this last possibility was left to Tang, DeVit, and Johnston, who showed in 1992 that it was possible to elicit an immune response against a foreign protein by introducing the corresponding gene directly into the skin of mice.[114] The experiment involved the use of a gene gun to inoculate gold microprojectiles coated with plasmids containing the human growth hormone (hGH) or human α1-antitrypsin (hAAT) genes in the ears of mice. In either case, antibodies to both proteins were detected in the sera of the genetically immunized mice. Furthermore, secondary and tertiary inoculations of the immunized mice with the same plasmids showed conclusively that the primary response could be augmented by those subsequent DNA boosts. Overall, the data gathered led the authors to speculate that genetic vaccination of animals against pathogenic infections could be achieved by using plasmids with genes encoding for specific antigens. Natural infections could thus be mimicked by a gene-based process that involved the production of the foreign antigens in the host cells. This approach constituted a radical departure from the established immunization methodologies that required the external production and purification of the vaccinating antigens prior to their administration. The fact that the corresponding immunological response could be different in terms of antibody production and T-cell response when compared with conventional immunization did not escape the authors' attention either.[114]

The use of plasmids as carriers of antigen information for immunization purposes was validated shortly after by Ulmer and coworkers, with the quantum leap discovery that mice could generate cytotoxic T lymphocytes (CTLs) in response to the direct administration of naked plasmid DNA encoding the influenza A virus nucleoprotein (NP).[115] Following immunization by intramuscular injection, a series of assays enabled the detection of NP expression, NP-specific antibodies, and NP-specific CTLs. Although high titers of anti-NP immunoglobulin G were detected, these antibodies did not confer protection to the mice. The specificity of CLTs and their ability to detect the epitopes generated naturally were confirmed in an experiment, which showed that CTLs isolated from the immunized animals were able to recognize and lyse target cells infected with the influenza A virus. Furthermore, the cell-mediated immune response was found to be functionally significant since the immunized mice were protected from a subsequent challenge with a heterologous strain of influenza A virus, as measured by increased survival, inhibition of mass loss, and decreased viral lung titers. In the concluding remarks of their paper, the authors speculated that plasmid-based vaccination should not be restricted to the prophylaxis of infectious diseases but that it could eventually be used to elicit an immune response against tumors, given the importance of CTL response in cancer processes.[115] The findings reported by Ulmer et al. were highly relevant since the generation of CTLs *in vivo* usually requires endogenous expression of antigens and presentation of peptides processed thereof to major histocompatibility complex (MHC) class I molecules (see Chapter 2, Section 2.5.1). And, for the first time, protection against a pathogenic infection had been obtained by plasmid immunization.

Still in 1993, and concurrently with Ulmer's paper, a number of reports described the development of "gene vaccines" as a means to generate immune responses against infectious agents such as influenza, human immunodeficiency virus (HIV), and bovine herpes virus. The first study was focused on the effect of the route of inoculation on the ability of plasmid vaccines expressing influenza virus hemagglutinin glycoproteins to raise protective immunity both in mice and in chicken.[109] Experiments were set up in which DNA was inoculated via the intramuscular, intranasal, intradermal, intravenous, subcutaneous, and intraperitoneal routes. The results showed that by bombarding plasmid-coated gold particles to the epidermis of the test animals with a gene gun, 250–2500 times less DNA was required to obtain protection when compared with direct injection in saline. Though less effective, the mucosal, intravenous, and intramuscular routes could also be used to raise protective immunity. An important conclusion was that the higher efficiency of transfection obtained with intramuscular injections did not necessarily correlate with a higher efficiency of vaccination.[109] The second study, by Wang and coworkers, was the first of many to come in the subsequent years, which attempted to develop vaccine prototypes based on the use of HIV genes hosted in plasmids. The experimental evidence accumulated in this report proved that direct injection of a plasmid DNA construct harboring the HIV-1 gp160 envelope protein in mice muscle could elicit both cellular and immune responses.[116] Serological responses of mice and cattle immunized with plasmids encoding bovine herpes virus-1 glycoproteins were also detected following intramuscular injection.[110]

Besides conferring protection against a plethora of phatogens, the immune system contributes to the surveillance and destruction of neoplastic cells. However, the fact that most tumor cells escape normal defenses in immunocompetent hosts suggests that an appropriate stimulation is required to augment the response of the immune system. As described in Section 1.1.3, the delivery of specific genes via viral vectors had already been attempted in humans by a cell-mediated *ex vivo* approach with the objective of obtaining an immune therapeutic effect against malignancy.[36] In the early 1990s, Gary Nabel's group rather focused on the direct use of plasmids encapsulated in liposomes as carriers of MHC genes to tumor cells.[117,118] In what was probably the first human gene therapy clinical protocol to use plasmid vectors, the gene encoding for the MHC protein HLA-B7 was introduced into advanced melanoma patients, with the expectation that expression of HLA-B7 would stimulate the local release of cytokines, thus inducing a T-cell response against the tumor.[117,118] Lactated Ringer's solution containing the plasmid/HLA-B7 constructs complexed with liposomes were typically injected directly into the patient's melanoma nodules. Both plasmid DNA and HLA-B7 protein were detected in tumors biopsies. Most importantly, immune responses to HLA-B7 and tumor were detected and tumor regression was even observed in one of the five patients enrolled.[117] This study provided the first evidence on the safety and effectiveness of intratumoral gene transfer in cancer.

The immunization experiments reported in 1992 and 1993 gave birth to a new generation of vaccines. On a meeting convened by the World Health Organization (WHO) in May 1994, the name DNA vaccine was selected among others (genetic immunization, gene vaccines, and polynucleotide vaccines) to designate the new technology.

1.3.5   Further Developments

The few experiments carried out in the decade that run from 1983 to 1993 and described above (Table 1.2) constituted the seeding ground from which a whole new class of medicinal products, plasmid biopharmaceuticals, would emerge. Researchers worldwide swiftly built upon the findings, hints, and speculations of the pioneers, and as a consequence, the research devoted to the potential application of plasmids as biopharmaceuticals for gene therapy or vaccination virtually exploded. Entrepreneurs and investors were also lured by the potential of plasmids as therapeutic and prophylactic agents, and not surprisingly, a significant number of research publications and clinical trials involving plasmids have been sponsored by commercial ventures and companies. The growth is exemplified, for instance, in Figure 1.2, which shows the cumulative number of scientific articles published between 1994 and 2009 that had the words DNA vaccine in the title. The evolution of the number of gene therapy clinical trials in which the target genes were carried by naked plasmid

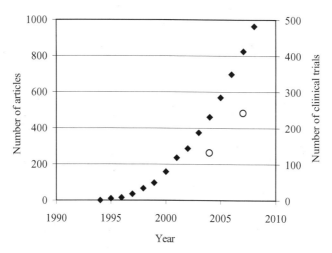

Figure 1.2 *Evolution of the number of DNA vaccine scientific publications (♦) and human clinical trials, which used naked plasmid DNA as a gene delivery vector (○). The number of publications (reviews, articles, and proceeding papers) with the words "DNA vaccine" in the title was obtained from the ISI Web of knowledge (http://isiwebofknowledge.com, accessed February 18, 2010). Clinical trial data were extracted from Edelstein et al.[55,142]*

DNA is also shown in the figure. The popularity of plasmids among the cohort of gene therapy vectors available can be attributed to a number of tangible and perceived characteristics, which include the short time and simplicity associated with their manipulation, production, and purification, and their potential safety, as justified by the lack of severe adverse reactions and events observed so far.

Some events, scientific breakthroughs, and a few papers among the huge numbers that have been published in the last 15 years deserve to be mentioned due to their incremental contributions to the development of plasmid biopharmaceuticals (see Table 1.2). This includes, for instance, the use of cytosine–phosphate–guanine (CpG) motifs, either cloned in the plasmids themselves or added as adjuvants to DNA vaccine formulations, as a means to stimulate the immune system. The search for ways to improve the immunogenicity of DNA vaccines was prompted by the recognition that expression of an antigen hosted in a DNA vaccine does not always and necessarily translate into an immune response. Building upon the finding that bacterial DNA and synthetic oligodeoxynucleotides containing unmethylated CpG dinucleotides activate the immune system,[119] Sato and colleagues included CpG dinucleotides in precise locations of a plasmid backbone.[120] Their subsequent experiments showed that human monocytes transfected with plasmid DNA containing those short immunostimulatory DNA sequences (ISSs) transcribed large amounts of cytokines like interferon-alpha, interferon-beta, and interleukin 12 (IL-12).[120] Other ways to manipulate the immunogenicity of DNA vaccines have been devised, which include, for example, the fusion of specific targeting or signal sequences to antigens. According to the sequence that is added, different pathways can be used by the host cells to process the antigen, and thus the concomitant recognition by the immune system can be modulated and controlled to some extent[121] (see Chapter 2, Section 2.5.2 for further details).

Further realization of the potential of DNA vaccines came with the discovery that the immune response generated by DNA vaccination could be manipulated through the coexpression of immunologically relevant proteins such as cytokines. One of the first experiments was reported by Xiang and Ertl, who showed that coimmunization of mice with a plasmid coding for the G protein of the rabies virus and with a plasmid expressing the granulocyte macrophage colony-stimulating factor (GM-CSF), a hematopoietic growth factor that enhances the antigen-presenting capacity of dendritic cells, clearly improves T-helper and B-cell responses.[122] On the contrary, coinoculation of a plasmid expressing interferon γ (IFNγ), a cytokine that regulates responses by upregulating the expression of MHC determinants in different cells, led to a slight decrease in the T-helper and B-cell response.[122] Subsequently, several laboratories published reports describing the effects of codelivering other cytokine genes such as *IL-2*[123] or *IL-12*.[124] In many cases, plasmid DNA vaccines are only capable of eliciting weak immune responses. The so-called prime-boost vaccination has been developed to take advantage of this characteristic. The strategy consists in priming with a first DNA vaccine inoculation and then boosting the immune system with either recombinant antigen or with attenuated recombinant viral vectors. This leads to a more effective recognition of antigens and thus to an augmentation of immune responses (e.g., antibody titers) to pathogens.[125,126] The incorporation of alphavirus replicons in plasmids was a further contribution in the struggle to ameliorate the efficacy of DNA vaccines and plasmid vectors.[127] The approach relies on putting the transgenes under the control of replicase genes used by members of the alphavirus genes, such as the Sinbis virus. Once the plasmid DNA reaches the cell nucleus, the encoded replicase complex is expressed and an antisense RNA is synthesized. This self-amplifying RNA, which encodes the transgene of interest, is then directly replicated in the cytoplasm by the replicase complex, resulting in high-level expression of the transgene.[128]

The development of novel and more efficient delivery strategies has always been at the forefront of research on nonviral gene therapy. For instance, in 1991, Titomirov and colleagues injected plasmid DNA sub-cutaneously in mice and then used a special device to deliver two high-voltage pulses in opposite polarities to the corresponding skin area.[129] These experiments showed that this type of *in vivo* electroporation was a feasible method to transform cells. Subsequent efforts have developed the *in vivo* electroporation technology up to a point where it is probably one of the most effective ways to deliver plasmid DNA. The encapsulation of plasmid DNA in poly(DL-lactide-co-glycolide) (PLG) microparticles, a methodology first described in 1996, constitutes another example of an incremental innovation in the delivery area. Key features of the technology are the ability of the particles to protect plasmid DNA against degradation after administration, and to promote uptake, expression and antigen presentation in appropriate cells in such a way as to elicit both systemic and mucosal antibody responses.[130] A third milestone in plasmid delivery was reached in 1997 with the description of a process to compact single molecules of DNA into unimolecular nanoparticles with sizes small enough to enable nuclear pore entry.[131]

The range of applications of plasmid biopharmaceuticals was further expanded in 2002 with the description that plasmids can direct the intracellular synthesis of small interfering RNA (siRNA) transcripts in mammalian cells, with the concomitant downregulation of the genes targeted for knockdown.[132] This constituted a credible alternative to the specific suppression of gene expression by RNA interference, which until then was typically accomplished by the direct administration of synthetic siRNAs.

At the same time that progress was being made in the area of plasmid biopharmaceuticals, governmental agencies in the United States, Europe, and elsewhere started intervening in an attempt to regulate the experimentation performed with human subjects. Relevant documents issued earlier by the FDA include the Points to Consider (PTC) documents "Points to Consider in Human Somatic Cell Therapy and Gene Therapy" of 1991[33] and "Points to Consider on Plasmid DNA Vaccines for Preventive Infectious Disease Indications" of 1996.[133] These have since then been superseded by guidance to industry documents (see Chapter 11 for more information on regulatory issues).

1.3.6   The Road to the Market

One of the ultimate goals of the scientific and technological advances described in the previous pages has been to introduce safe and efficacious plasmid bio-pharmaceuticals in the market for the benefit of society. Although this goal remains elusive, a number of successes can be described that are contributing to the paving of a road to the market. In 2003, condors were the first animals immunized with a DNA vaccine to be deliberately released into the environment. The high risk faced by a small colony of California condors in face of the West Nile virus (WNV) epidemic, which reached New York City in 1999 and subsequently spread westward, prompted the U.S. Centers for Disease Control and Prevention (CDC) to expedite the inoculation of the entire population of the endangered animal, both in captivity and in the wild, with a DNA vaccine containing genes coding for WNV proteins. This prospective vaccination is believed to have saved the endangered population of condors from subsequent infections with the natural WNV, which circulated during the 2004 season.[134] The immunization of the Californian condor with DNA vaccines is one of the veterinary case studies described in more detail in Chapter 10.

The year 2005 was marked by two historical events, the full licensing of two veterinary DNA vaccines. The first vaccine, licensed by the Center for Veterinary Biologics of the United States Department of Agriculture (USDA) to Fort Dodge Animal Health (Fort Dodge, Iowa), a division of Pfizer Animal Health (New York), became the first DNA vaccine for any species to be registered with a governmental regulatory body.[135] The vaccine was designed and developed jointly by the CDC and Fort Dodge to protect horses against WNV, and was the predecessor of the WNV vaccine used experimentally in condors referred above and described in detail in Chapter 10. Although the license was issued in 2005, Fort Dodge only launched the vaccine in December 2008, under the trade name West Nile-Innovator® DNA.[136] The second DNA vaccine licensed in 2005 was developed by Aqua Health, Ltd., an affiliate of Novartis Animal Health (Victoria, Canada), to protect farm-raised salmon against infectious hematopoietic necrosis virus.[137] Commercialized under the trade name Apex®-IHN, the DNA vaccine is supplied in sterile saline with the recommendation to be administered intramuscularly into anesthetized fish (Apex-IHN information, Novartis Animal Health Canada, Inc.—Aqua Health Business). The circumstances surrounding the development of the Apex-IHN DNA vaccine, together with the underlying rationale and the major findings regarding efficacy and safety, are described in detail in Chapter 10.

More recently, in early 2007, the USDA conditionally approved a therapeutic DNA vaccine to treat melanoma in dogs.[138] The vaccine was designed to deliver an MHC gene to dog tumors on the basis of the underlying principle developed in the early 1990s by Nabel and coworkers.[139] This case study is also examined in more detail in Chapter 10. Finally, in 2008, the Australian Pesticides and Veterinary Medicines Authority approved the market entrance of an injectable plasmid DNA encoding for porcine growth hormone releasing hormone (GHRH), a protein that plays an important role in the growth and development of mammals.[140] Manufactured and sold by VGX Animal Health, Inc. (The Woodlands, Texas) under the trade name LifeTide™ SW 5, this veterinary product is used with the specific goal of decreasing perinatal mortality and morbidity in pigs, and therefore improving sow productivity.[140] According to the company's description, the plasmid is delivered to muscle cells by intramuscular injection followed by electroporation with the portable electrokinetic device, cellectra™. The GHRH, which is produced by the transfected cells, then induces the production and secretion of the endogenous growth hormone. The net result is a decrease in offspring morbidity and mortality and an increase in body weight.[141] LifeTide SW 5 thus became the first plasmid biopharmaceutical approved for the gene therapy of animals produced with the intent of supplying the human food chain.

The events described in the last paragraphs constitute a remarkable record if one considers that only 13–16 years had gone by since an immune response was demonstrated following the injection of an antigen encoded in a plasmid.[114] This extraordinary speed in bringing a product from a totally new class to the marketplace, together with the large number of plasmid biopharmaceuticals undergoing preclinical development and clinical trials (more than 300), suggests that other products are likely to hit the market in the near future. At the current stage of development, it is very hard to anticipate the potential value of the plasmid biopharmaceutical market (see Chapter 8). The number of disease targets (infectious diseases, cancer, cardiovascular disease, etc.) and potential consumers (humans and domestic and farm-raised animals) is certainly huge (see Chapters 2 and 8). However, the field is in much need of a commercial success in the human arena, which, once arrived, could provide the necessary momentum for further progress.

1.4 CONCLUSIONS

Major developments have taken place in the past 30 years, which have contributed significantly to the establishment of plasmid biopharmaceuticals as a whole new category of medicinal agents. The profound progress made in this area owes much to the breakthrough discoveries and insights of gene therapy pioneers like Joshua Lederberg and Stanley Rogers, and plasmid scientists like Stanley Cohen, Jon Wolff, and Gary Nabel, but also to the incremental advances described by so many researchers. Now that this collective effort is on the verge of producing tangible benefits for society, it is only fit to recall how it all started and progressed. Although this has been the major purpose of this introductory chapter, I am aware that the brief account given in the preceding pages may have missed influential discoveries and scientists. I hope nevertheless that I have provided the reader with a factually correct and stimulating historical perspective of the development of the plasmid biopharmaceuticals field.

REFERENCES

1. Kiple K. *Plague, pox and pestilence*. London: Weidenfeld & Nicolson, 1997.

2. Steward RE, MacArthur MW, Laskowski RA, Thornton JM. Molecular basis of inherited diseases: A structural perspective. *Trends in Genetics*. 2003;19:505–513.

3. Seegmiller JE. Genetic and molecular basis of human hereditary diseases. *Clinical Chemistry*. 1967;13:554–564.

4. Avery OT, MacLeod CM, McCarty M. Studies on the chemical nature of the substance inducing transformation of pneumococcal types. *The Journal of Experimental Medicine*. 1944;79:137–158.

5. Keeler CE. Gene therapy. *The Journal of Heredity*. 1947;38:294–298.

6. Mullin D. Prometheus in Gloucestershire: Edward Jenner, 1749-1823. *The Journal of Allergy and Clinical Immunology*. 2003;112:810–814.

7. Stern AM, Markel H. The history of vaccines and immunization: Familiar patterns, new challenges. *Health Affairs (Project Hope)*. 2005;24:611–621.

8. Andre FE. Vaccinology: Past achievements, present roadblocks and future promises. *Vaccine*. 2003;21:593–595.

9. Boyd JSK, Portnoy B. Bacteriophage therapy in bacillary dysentery. *Transactions of the Royal Society of Tropical Medicine and Hygiene*. 1944;37:243–262.

10. Barrow PA, Soothill JS. Bacteriophage therapy and prophylaxis: Rediscovery and renewed assessment of potential. *Trends in Microbiology*. 1997;5:268–271.

11. Stone R. Bacteriophage therapy. Stalin's forgotten cure. *Science*. 2002;298:728–731.

12. Crow JF. Joshua lederberg: 1925-2008. *Nature Genetics*. 2008;40:486.

13. Lederberg J. Biological future of man. In: Wolstenholme G, ed. *Man and his future*. London: J & A Churchill, 1963:263–273.

14. Tatum EL. Molecular biology, nucleic acids, and the future of medicine. *Perspectives in Biology and Medicine*. 1966;10:19–32.

15. Wolff JA, Lederberg J. An early history of gene transfer and therapy. *Human Gene Therapy*. 1994;5:469–480.

16. Anderson WF. Human gene therapy: The initial concepts. In: Brigham KL, ed. *Lung biology in health and disease*, Vol. 104. New York: Marcel Dekker, 1997:3–16.

17. Aposhian HV. The use of DNA for gene therapy-the need, experimental approach, and implications. *Perspectives in Biology and Medicine*. 1970;14:98–108.

18. Friedmann T. Stanfield Rogers: Insights into virus vectors and failure of an early gene therapy model. *Molecular Therapy*. 2001;4:285–288.

19. Rogers S, Pfuderer P. Use of viruses as carriers of added genetic information. *Nature*. 1968;219:749–751.

20. Rogers S. Shope papilloma virus: A passenger in man and its significance to the potential control of the host genome. *Nature*. 1966;212:1220–1222.

21. United States, US Congress, Office of Technology Assessment. *Human gene therapy—A background paper (OTA-BP-BA-32)*. Washington, DC: US Government Printing Office, 1984.

22. Cohen SN, Chang AC, Boyer HW, Helling RB. Construction of biologically functional bacterial plasmids *in vitro*. *Proceedings of the National Academy of Sciences of the United States of America*. 1973;70:3240–3244.

23. Graham FL, van der Eb AJ. A new technique for the assay of infectivity of human adenovirus 5 DNA. *Virology*. 1973;52:456–467.

24. Mercola KE, Stang HD, Browne J, Salser W, Cline MJ. Insertion of a new gene of viral origin into bone marrow cells of mice. *Science*. 1980;208:1033–1035.

25. Cline MJ, Stang H, Mercola K, et al. Gene transfer in intact animals. *Nature*. 1980;284:422–425.

26. Wade N. UCLA gene therapy racked by friendly fire. *Science*. 1980;210:509–511.

27. Coutts M. Human gene therapy [bibliography]. *Kennedy Institute of Ethics Journal*. 1994;4:63–83.

28. Friedmann T, Roblin R. Gene therapy for human genetic disease? *Science*. 1972;175:949–955.

29. Friedmann T. A brief history of gene therapy. *Nature Genetics*. 1992;2:93–98.

30. Walters L. Ethical issues in human gene therapy. *The Journal of Clinical Ethics*. 1991;2:267–274. Discussion 274-268.

31. Walters L. Human gene therapy: Ethics and public policy. *Human Gene Therapy*. 1991;2:115–122.

32. United States National Institutes of Health—Human Gene Therapy Subcommittee. *Points to consider in the design and submission of Human somatic-cell gene therapy protocols*. Bethesda, MD: FDA, 1986.

33. United States Food and Drug Administration. Points to consider in human somatic cell therapy and gene therapy. *Human Gene Therapy*. 1991;2:251–256.

34. European Medicines Evaluation Agency. Note for guidance on quality, pre-clinical and clinical aspects of gene transfer medicinal products (Doc. Ref. CPMP/BWP/3088/99). London, April 24, 2001.

35. Anderson WF. Human gene therapy. *Science*. 1992;256:808–813.

36. Rosenberg SA, Anderson WF, Blaese M, et al. The development of gene therapy for the treatment of cancer. *Annals of Surgery*. 1993;218:455–463. Discussion 463-454.

37. Anonymous. The N2-TIL human gene transfer clinical protocol. *Human Gene Therapy*. 1990;1:73–92.

38. Rosenberg SA, Aebersold P, Cornetta K, et al. Gene transfer into humans-immunotherapy of patients with advanced melanoma, using tumor-infiltrating lymphocytes modified by retroviral gene transduction. *The New England Journal of Medicine*. 1990;323:570–578.

39. Morgan RA, Anderson WF. Human gene therapy. *Annual Review of Biochemistry*. 1993;62:191–217.

40. Blaese RM, Culver KW, Miller AD, et al. T lymphocyte-directed gene therapy for ADA- SCID: Initial trial results after 4 years. *Science*. 1995;270:475–480.

41. Anonymous. The ADA human gene therapy clinical protocol. *Human Gene Therapy*. 1990;1:327–362.

42. Culver KW, Anderson WF, Blaese RM. Lymphocyte gene therapy. *Human Gene Therapy*. 1991;2:107–109.

43. Friedmann T. Gene therapy-a new kind of medicine. *Trends in Biotechnology*. 1993;11:156–159.

44. Barth RJ, Jr., Mule JJ, Spiess PJ, Rosenberg SA. Interferon gamma and tumor necrosis factor have a role in tumor regressions mediated by murine CD8+ tumor-infiltrating lymphocytes. *The Journal of Experimental Medicine*. 1991;173: 647–658.

45. Anonymous. TNF/TIL human gene therapy clinical protocol. *Human Gene Therapy*. 1990;1:441–480.

46. Lehrman S. Virus treatment questioned after gene therapy death. *Nature*. 1999;401:517–518.

47. Somia N, Verma IM. Gene therapy: Trials and tribulations. *Nature Reviews. Genetics*. 2000;1:91–99.

48. Zallen DT. US gene therapy in crisis. *Trends in Genetics*. 2000;16:272–275.

49. Raper SE, Chirmule N, Lee FS, et al. Fatal systemic inflammatory response syndrome in a ornithine transcarbamylase deficient patient following adenoviral gene transfer. *Molecular Genetics and Metabolism*. 2003;80:148–158.

50. Raper SE, Yudkoff M, Chirmule N, et al. A pilot study of *in vivo* liver-directed gene transfer with an adenoviral vector in partial ornithine transcarbamylase deficiency. *Human Gene Therapy*. 2002;13:163–175.

51. Couzin J, Kaiser J. Gene therapy. As Gelsinger case ends, gene therapy suffers another blow. *Science*. 2005;307:1028.

52. Cavazzana-Calvo M, Hacein-Bey S, de Saint Basile G, et al. Gene therapy of human severe combined immunodeficiency (SCID)-X1 disease. *Science*. 2000;288:669–672.

53. Hacein-Bey-Abina S, Von Kalle C, Schmidt M, et al. LMO2-associated clonal T cell proliferation in two patients after gene therapy for SCID-X1. *Science*. 2003; 302:415–419.

54. Cavazzana-Calvo M. Gene therapy for SCID-X1. *Human Gene Therapy*. 2007;18:944.

55. Edelstein ML, Abedi MR, Wixon J. Gene therapy clinical trials worldwide to 2007-an update. *The Journal of Gene Medicine*. 2007;9:833–842.

56. Board of the European Society for Gene and Cell Therapy. Case of leukaemia associated with X-linked severe combined immunodeficiency gene therapy trial in London. *Human Gene Therapy*. 2008;19:3–4.

57. Peng Z. Current status of Gendicine in China: Recombinant human Ad-p53 agent for treatment of cancers. *Human Gene Therapy*. 2005;16:1016–1027.

58. Rolland A. Gene medicines: The end of the beginning? *Advanced Drug Delivery Reviews*. 2005;57:669–673.

59. Surendran A. News in brief: China approves world's first gene therapy drug. *Nature Medicine*. 2004;10:9.

60. Peng Z. Current status of gene therapy in China. *Human Gene Therapy*. 2007; 18:942.

61. Jia H. Gene dreams troubled by market realities. *Chemistry World*. 2007;4.

62. Räty JK, Pikkarainen JT, Wirth T, Ylä-Herttuala S. Gene therapy: The first approved gene-based medicines, molecular mechanisms and clinical indications. *Current Molecular Pharmacology.* 2008;1:13–23.

63. Kaiser J. Gene therapy. Questions remain on cause of death in arthritis trial. *Science.* 2007;317:1665.

64. Wadman M. Gene therapy might not have caused patient's death. *Nature.* 2007;449:270.

65. Wilson JM. Adverse events in gene transfer trials and an agenda for the New Year. *Human Gene Therapy.* 2008;19:1–2.

66. European Medicines Agency. CHMP-Committee for Medicinal Products for Human Use. Withdrawal assessment report for Cerepro (Doc.Ref.: EMEA/203243/2008). London 26 April 2007.

67. Lederberg J. Plasmid (1952-1997). *Plasmid.* 1998;39:1–9.

68. Cohen SN. Bacterial plasmids: Their extraordinary contribution to molecular genetics. *Gene.* 1993;135:67–76.

69. Lederberg J. Cell genetics and hereditary symbiosis. *Physiology Reviews.* 1952;32:403–430.

70. Novick RP, Clowes RC, Cohen SN, Curtiss R, Datta N, Falkow S. Uniform nomenclature for bacterial plasmids: A proposal. *Bacteriology Reviews.* 1976;40:168–189.

71. Clowes RC. Molecular structure of bacterial plasmids. *Bacteriology Reviews.* 1972;36:361–405.

72. Summers DK. *The biology of plasmids.* Oxford: Blackwell Science, 1996.

73. Hayes W. Recombination in *Bact. coli* K 12; unidirectional transfer of genetic material. *Nature.* 1952;169:118–119.

74. Lederberg J, Cavalli LL, Lederberg EM. Sex compatibility in *Escherichia coli.* *Genetics.* 1952;37:720–730.

75. Hayes W. Observations on a transmissible agent determining sexual differentiation in *Bacterium coli.* *Journal of General Microbiology.* 1953;8:72–88.

76. Marmur J, Rownd R, Falkow S, Baron LS, Schildkraut C, Doty P. The nature of intergeneric episomal infection. *Proceedings of the National Academy of Sciences of the United States of America.* 1961;47:972–979.

77. Silver S, Ozeki H. Transfer of deoxyribonucleic acid accompanying the transmission of colicinogenic properties by cell mating. *Nature.* 1962;195:873–874.

78. Campbell A. Episomes. *Advances in Genetics.* 1962;11:101–145.

79. Fiers W, Sinsheimer RL. The structure of the DNA of bacteriophage phi-X174. III. Ultracentrifugal evidence for a ring structure. *Journal of Molecular Biology.* 1962;5:424–434.

80. Vinograd J, Lebowitz J, Radloff R, Watson R, Laipis P. The twisted circular form of polyoma viral DNA. *Proceedings of the National Academy of Sciences of the United States of America.* 1965;53:1104–1111.

81. Hickson FT, Roth TF, Helinski DR. Circular DNA forms of a bacterial sex factor. *Proceedings of the National Academy of Sciences of the United States of America.* 1967;58:1731–1738.

82. LePecq JB, Paoletti C. A fluorescent complex between ethidium bromide and nucleic acids. Physical-chemical characterization. *Journal of Molecular Biology.* 1967;27:87–106.

83. Cohen SN, Chang AC, Hsu L. Nonchromosomal antibiotic resistance in bacteria: Genetic transformation of *Escherichia coli* by R-factor DNA. *Proceedings of the National Academy of Sciences of the United States of America.* 1972; 69:2110–2114.

84. Sharp PA, Sugden B, Sambrook J. Detection of two restriction endonuclease activities in *Haemophilus parainfluenzae* using analytical agarose-ethidium bromide electrophoresis. *Biochemistry.* 1973;12:3055–3063.

85. Mertz JE, Davis RW. Cleavage of DNA by R 1 restriction endonuclease generates cohesive ends. *Proceedings of the National Academy of Sciences of the United States of America.* 1972;69:3370–3374.

86. Sgaramella V. Enzymatic oligomerization of bacteriophage P22 DNA and of linear Simian virus 40 DNA. *Proceedings of the National Academy of Sciences of the United States of America.* 1972;69:3389–3393.

87. Chang AC, Cohen SN. Genome construction between bacterial species *in vitro*: Replication and expression of *Staphylococcus* plasmid genes in *Escherichia coli*. *Proceedings of the National Academy of Sciences of the United States of America.* 1974;71:1030–1034.

88. Morrow JF, Cohen SN, Chang AC, Boyer HW, Goodman HM, Helling RB. Replication and transcription of eukaryotic DNA in *Escherichia coli*. *Proceedings of the National Academy of Sciences of the United States of America.* 1974; 71:1743–1747.

89. Chang AC, Nunberg JH, Kaufman RJ, Erlich HA, Schimke RT, Cohen SN. Phenotypic expression in *E. coli* of a DNA sequence coding for mouse dihydro-folate reductase. *Nature.* 1978;275:617–624.

90. Itakura K, Hirose T, Crea R, et al. Expression in *Escherichia coli* of a chemically synthesized gene for the hormone somatostatin. *Science.* 1977;198:1056–1063.

91. Goeddel DV, Kleid DG, Bolivar F, et al. Expression in *Escherichia coli* of chemically synthesized genes for human insulin. *Proceedings of the National Academy of Sciences of the United States of America.* 1979;76:106–110.

92. Vaheri A, Pagano JS. Infectious poliovirus RNA: A sensitive method of assay. *Virology.* 1965;27:434–436.

93. Scangos G, Ruddle FH. Mechanisms and applications of DNA-mediated gene transfer in mammalian cells—a review. *Gene.* 1981;14:1–10.

94. Cohen SN, Boyer HW, inventors; Board of Trustees of the Leland Stanford Jr. University, assignee. Process for producing biologically functional molecular chimeras. U.S. patent 4,237,224, December 2, 1980.

95. Ledley FD. Nonviral gene therapy: The promise of genes as pharmaceutical products. *Human Gene Therapy.* 1995;6:1129–1144.

96. Nicolau C, Le Pape A, Soriano P, Fargette F, Juhel MF. *In vivo* expression of rat insulin after intravenous administration of the liposome-entrapped gene for rat insulin I. *Proceedings of the National Academy of Sciences of the United States of America.* 1983;80:1068–1072.

97. Cordell B, Bell G, Tischer E, et al. Isolation and characterization of a cloned rat insulin gene. *Cell.* 1979;18:533–543.

98. Wolff JA, Malone RW, Williams P, et al. Direct gene transfer into mouse muscle *in vivo. Science.* 1990;247:1465–1468.

99. Soriano P, Dijkstra J, Legrand A, et al. Targeted and nontargeted liposomes for *in vivo* transfer to rat liver cells of a plasmid containing the preproinsulin I gene. *Proceedings of the National Academy of Sciences of the United States of America.* 1983;80:7128–7131.

100. Cudd A, Nicolau C. Intracellular fate of liposome-encapsulated DNA in mouse liver. Analysis using electron microscope autoradiography and subcellular fractionation. *Biochimica et Biophysica Acta.* 1985;845:477–491.

101. Dubensky TW, Campbell BA, Villarreal LP. Direct transfection of viral and plasmid DNA into the liver or spleen of mice. *Proceedings of the National Academy of Sciences of the United States of America.* 1984;81:7529–7533.

102. Benvenisty N, Reshef L. Direct introduction of genes into rats and expression of the genes. *Proceedings of the National Academy of Sciences of the United States of America.* 1986;83:9551–9555.

103. Felgner PL, Gadek TR, Holm M, et al. Lipofection: A highly efficient, lipid-mediated DNA-transfection procedure. *Proceedings of the National Academy of Sciences of the United States of America.* 1987;84:7413–7417.

104. Yang NS, Burkholder J, Roberts B, Martinell B, McCabe D. *In vivo* and *in vitro* gene transfer to mammalian somatic cells by particle bombardment. *Proceedings of the National Academy of Sciences of the United States of America.* 1990;87:9568–9572.

105. Klein TM, Wolf ED, Wu R, Sanford JC. High-velocity microprojectiles for delivering nucleic acids into living cells. *Nature.* 1987;327:70–73.

106. Zelenin AV, Titomirov AV, Kolesnikov VA. Genetic transformation of mouse cultured cells with the help of high-velocity mechanical DNA injection. *FEBS Letters.* 1989;244:65–67.

107. Williams RS, Johnston SA, Riedy M, DeVit MJ, McElligott SG, Sanford JC. Introduction of foreign genes into tissues of living mice by DNA-coated microprojectiles. *Proceedings of the National Academy of Sciences of the United States of America.* 1991;88:2726–2730.

108. Hansen E, Fernandes K, Goldspink G, Butterworth P, Umeda PK, Chang KC. Strong expression of foreign genes following direct injection into fish muscle. *FEBS Letters.* 1991;290:73–76.

109. Fynan EF, Webster RG, Fuller DH, Haynes JR, Santoro JC, Robinson HL. DNA vaccines: Protective immunizations by parenteral, mucosal, and gene-gun inoculations. *Proceedings of the National Academy of Sciences of the United States of America.* 1993;90:11478–11482.

110. Cox GJ, Zamb TJ, Babiuk LA. Bovine herpesvirus 1: Immune responses in mice and cattle injected with plasmid DNA. *Journal of Virology.* 1993;67:5664–5667.

111. Ardehali A, Fyfe A, Laks H, Drinkwater DC, Qiao J-H, Lusis AJ. Direct gene transfer into donor hearts at the time of harvest. *The Journal of Thoracic and Cardiovascular Surgery.* 1995;109:716–720.

112. Hickman MA, Malone RW, Lehmann-Bruinsma K, et al. Gene expression following direct injection of DNA into liver. *Human Gene Therapy.* 1994;5:1477–1483.

113. Schwartz B, Benoist C, Abdallah B, et al. Gene transfer by naked DNA into adult mouse brain. *Gene Therapy.* 1996;3:405–411.

114. Tang DC, DeVit M, Johnston SA. Genetic immunization is a simple method for eliciting an immune response. *Nature.* 1992;356:152–154.

115. Ulmer JB, Donnelly JJ, Parker SE, et al. Heterologous protection against influenza by injection of DNA encoding a viral protein. *Science.* 1993;259:1745–1749.

116. Wang B, Ugen KE, Srikantan V, et al. Gene inoculation generates immune responses against human immunodeficiency virus type 1. *Proceedings of the National Academy of Sciences of the United States of America.* 1993;90: 4156–4160.

117. Nabel GJ, Nabel EG, Yang ZY, et al. Direct gene transfer with DNA-liposome complexes in melanoma: Expression, biologic activity, and lack of toxicity in humans. *Proceedings of the National Academy of Sciences of the United States of America.* 1993;90:11307–11311.

118. Nabel GJ, Chang AE, Nabel EG, et al. Immunotherapy for cancer by direct gene transfer into tumors. *Human Gene Therapy.* 1994;5:57–77.

119. Krieg AM, Yi AK, Matson S, et al. CpG motifs in bacterial DNA trigger direct B-cell activation. *Nature.* 1995;374:546–549.

120. Sato Y, Roman M, Tighe H, et al. Immunostimulatory DNA sequences necessary for effective intradermal gene immunization. *Science.* 1996;273:352–354.

121. Ciernik IF, Berzofsky JA, Carbone DP. Induction of cytotoxic T lymphocytes and antitumor immunity with DNA vaccines expressing single T cell epitopes. *Journal of Immunology.* 1996;156:2369–2375.

122. Xiang Z, Ertl HC. Manipulation of the immune response to a plasmid-encoded viral antigen by coinoculation with plasmids expressing cytokines. *Immunity.* 1995;2:129–135.

123. Chow YH, Huang WL, Chi WK, Chu YD, Tao MH. Improvement of hepatitis B virus DNA vaccines by plasmids coexpressing hepatitis B surface antigen and interleukin-2. *Journal of Virology.* 1997;71:169–178.

124. Kim JJ, Ayyavoo V, Bagarazzi ML, et al. *In vivo* engineering of a cellular immune response by coadministration of IL-12 expression vector with a DNA immunogen. *Journal of Immunology.* 1997;158:816–826.

125. Davies HL, Mancini M, Michel M-L, Whalen RG. DNA-mediated immunization to hepatitis B surface antigen: Longevity of primary response and effect of boost. *Vaccine.* 1996;14:910–915.

126. Richmond JF, Mustafa F, Lu S, et al. Screening of HIV-1 Env glycoproteins for the ability to raise neutralizing antibody using DNA immunization and recombinant vaccinia virus boosting. *Virology.* 1997;230:265–274.

127. Dubensky TW, Jr., Driver DA, Polo JM, et al. Sindbis virus DNA-based expression vectors: Utility for *in vitro* and *in vivo* gene transfer. *Journal of Virology.* 1996;70:508–519.

128. Herweijer H, Latendresse JS, Williams P, et al. A plasmid-based self-amplifying Sindbis virus vector. *Human Gene Therapy.* 1995;6:1161–1167.

129. Titomirov AV, Sukharev S, Kistanova E. *In vivo* electroporation and stable transformation of skin cells of newborn mice by plasmid DNA. *Biochimica et Biophysica Acta.* 1991;1088:131–134.

130. Jones DH, Corris S, McDonald S, Clegg JCS, Farrar GH. Poly(DL-lactide-co-glycolide)-encapsulated plasmid DNA elicits systemic and mucosal antibody resphses to encoded protein after oral administration. *Vaccine.* 1997;15: 814–817.

131. Perales JC, Grossmann GA, Molas M, et al. Biochemical and functional characterization of DNA complexes capable of targeting genes to hepatocytes via the asialoglycoprotein receptor. *The Journal of Biological Chemistry.* 1997;272: 7398–7407.

132. Brummelkamp TR, Bernards R, Agami R. A system for stable expression of short interfering RNAs in mammalian cells. *Science.* 1991;296:550–553.

133. United States Food and Drug Administration. *Points to consider on plasmid DNA vaccines for preventive infectious disease indications.* Rockville, MD: FDA, 1996.

134. Chang GJ, Davis BS, Stringfield C, Lutz C. Prospective immunization of the endangered California condors (*Gymnogyps californianus*) protects this species from lethal West Nile virus infection. *Vaccine.* 2007;25:2325–2330.

135. Powell K. DNA vaccines-back in the saddle again? *Nature Biotechnology.* 2004;22:799–801.

136. Anonymous. *West Nile-Innovator DNA—The first USDA approved DNA vaccine.* Fort Dodge: Fort Dodge Animal Health, 2008.

137. Novartis. *Novel Novartis vaccine to protect Canadian salmon farms from devastating viral disease.* Basel: Novartis Animal Health, 2005.

138. Merial. *USDA grants conditional approval for first therapeutic vaccine to treat cancer.* Duluth, GA: Merial Limited, 2007.

139. Plautz GE, Yang ZY, Wu BY, Gao X, Huang L, Nabel GJ. Immunotherapy of malignancy by *in vivo* gene transfer into tumors. *Proceedings of the National Academy of Sciences of the United States of America.* 1993;90:4645–4649.

140. Person R, Bodles-Brakhop AM, Pope MA, Brown PA, Khan AS, Draghia-Akli R. Growth hormone-releasing hormone plasmid treatment by electroporation decreases offspring mortality over three pregnancies. *Molecular Therapy.* 2008;16:1891–1897.

141. Draghia-Akli R, Fiorotto ML, Hill LA, Malone PB, Deaver DR, Schwartz RJ. Myogenic expression of an injectable protease-resistant growth hormone-releasing hormone augments long-term growth in pigs. *Nature Biotechnology.* 1999; 17:1179–1183.

142. Edelstein ML, Abedi MR, Wixon J, Edelstein RM. Gene therapy clinical trials worldwide 1989-2004-an overview. *The Journal of Gene Medicine.* 2004;6: 597–602.

143. Zabner J, Couture LA, Gregory RJ, Graham SM, Smith AE, Welsh MJ. Adenovirus-mediated gene transfer transiently corrects the chloride transport defect in nasal epithelia of patients with cystic fibrosis. *Cell.* 1993;75:207–216.

144. Wu CH, Wilson JM, Wu GY. Targeting genes: Delivery and persistent expression of a foreign gene driven by mammalian regulatory elements *in vivo. The Journal of Biological Chemistry.* 1989;264:16985–16987.

2

Gene Transfer with Plasmid Biopharmaceuticals

2.1 INTRODUCTION

In spite of the disappointing results and setbacks encountered during many clinical trials, the field of gene therapy has grown immensely since the early 1990s in the twentieth century. The explosion of research and development on the subject can be judged by analyzing the cumulative number of clinical trials conducted in the last two decades (Figure 2.1). As of September 2007, more than 220 genes had been introduced in humans in the context of more than 1340 gene therapy clinical trials (either completed, ongoing, or approved).[1] The number of scientific articles published in the 1990–2009 period that had the words gene therapy in the title (more than 7000) is also a good indication of both the interest spurred and the progress made in the area (Figure 2.1). Together with this, the original gene therapy concept also evolved to include the development of a diversity of therapeutic "molecular" strategies, which focus on the use of genes and nucleic acids as agents and targets for disease management. Most noteworthy among the newest strategies are those that, rather than using whole genes, rely on the administration of RNA interference (RNAi) molecules,[2] antisense oligoribonucleotides,[3] and deoxyoligonucleotides (e.g., triplex-forming oligonucleotides[2-4]). As illustrated by these last few examples, the broadening of the field has been such that a redefinition of what can, or should be, called gene therapy is probably timely. First, the two words

Plasmid Biopharmaceuticals: Basics, Applications, and Manufacturing, First Edition.
Duarte Miguel F. Prazeres.
© 2011 John Wiley & Sons, Inc. Published 2011 by John Wiley & Sons, Inc.

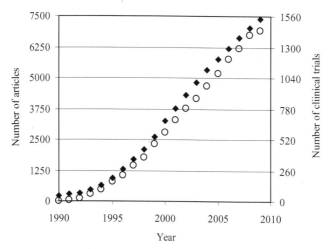

Figure 2.1 *Evolution of the number of gene therapy scientific publications (◆) and human clinical trials (○). The number of publications (reviews, articles, and proceeding papers) with the words "gene therapy" in the title was obtained from the ISI Web of knowledge (http:// isiwebofknowledge.com). Clinical trial data were extracted from* The Journal of Gene Medicine Gene Therapy Clinical Trials Worldwide *Web site at http://www.wiley.co.uk/genmed/clinical (accessed February 18, 2010).*

in "gene therapy" readily convey the idea of using genes to treat a disease or disorder by restoring the normal functions of the body. In a broader sense, however, gene therapy may also include prophylactic strategies like immunization with DNA vaccines, whose primary goal is to prepare the immune system to fight future episodes of disease. Moreover, in other cases, the administration of genes to humans is solely used as a means to tag specific cells or tissues. The purpose of this latter approach, which is known as gene marking, is to monitor the fate, distribution, and survival of the marked cells during disease progression or in response to any form of conventional therapy.[5]

An ample definition of gene therapy is provided by Meager in the preface of the book *Gene Therapy Technologies, Applications and Regulations: From Laboratory to Clinic.*[6] The author wrote that gene therapy

> encompasses a set of procedures deliberately aimed at the efficient transfer of genetic material into the somatic cells of individual patients in order that the expression or other function, of the part(s) of the genetic material designed to elicit preventive, therapeutic or diagnostic activity is fully functional and effective for its intended purpose.

Clearly, a wide range of products (recombinant viral vectors, plasmids, and oligonucleotides) and procedures (gene replacement, gene addition, DNA vaccination, and gene marking) fit within this very comprehensive definition. Given this diversity of purposes, "gene transfer" is probably the most appropriate designation for the ensemble of interventions described above, since it does not make any distinction between what is therapy, prophylaxis, or diagnostics. Since this book focuses essentially on the role played by plasmids as transporters of genes and on their emergence as a whole new class of medicinal agents (i.e., plasmid biopharmaceuticals), I will narrow the scope of gene therapy/gene transfer and use it to refer to a strategy in which genes are intentionally introduced in animals or humans with the purpose of expressing the encoded information *in vivo* and thus to contribute to the management of health and disease.

Apart from being more precise, the use of the wording gene transfer suggested earlier may also be advantageous from a communication point of view, when compared with the alternative and more widely used gene therapy. This better adequacy of gene transfer has been pointed out by some authors, who suggested that an inadequate use of terminology in the media and in guidance documents may be partially responsible for the exaggerated expectations and misconceptions currently surrounding gene therapy.[7] According to their reasoning, the word "therapy" would mislead the general public into believing that those individuals involved in clinical trials will be undergoing a treatment that will contribute to minimize the consequences of their underlying condition. But in fact, the reality is that no particular treatment involving the transfer of genes into humans has yet been fully proven,[7] despite the promising results that have been obtained in a number of cases (see Chapter 1, Section 1.1.4). Until that happens, it should be very clear to everyone that clinical trials are about performing research on a specific intervention using humans, and the term gene transfer should thus be preferred to gene therapy. The term "patient," which is also commonly used by specialists and nonspecialists alike when discussing human gene transfer clinical trials, has also been identified as inappropriate and misleading. Rather, those who volunteer to participate in gene transfer trials should be regarded and denominated as "subjects."[7] This designation should emphasize the fact that the individuals involved are not being treated but instead are merely participating in controlled research experiments. Despite this, the use of the terms gene therapy and patient when describing clinical trials is firmly entrenched in the scientific community and is usual among laymen and media. Rather than a problem of semantics, this concern with the terminology used in the context of gene therapy interventions and research is especially important, since one of the issues usually debated within the ethical context is how to convey accurate information to those directly involved in clinical trials and also to the general public (Chapter 7).

This chapter gives an overview of the different types of gene transfer interventions that are being pursued nowadays with the goal of managing disease in humans and animals, especially those involving the use of plasmids. The specific role that is expected from the transgene products *in vivo* and the rationale behind their functioning is first discussed. In the second part of the chapter, the disease management applications targeted by plasmid biopharmaceuticals are organized into two broad categories—therapy and prophylaxis. In therapeutic applications, the discussion focuses into the specific classes of diseases that are addressed by plasmids (genetic disorders, cancer, and cardiovascular and neurological diseases). In prophylactic applications, the mechanisms underlying the action of DNA vaccines as well as their current limitations are the main focus.

2.2 GENE TRANSFER WITH PLASMIDS

2.2.1 Plasmids versus Viral Vectors

The success of the medicinal use of genes depends, first, on (1) the efficiency of the DNA delivery method used and (2) the expression of the administered gene in the target cells. The word delivery is used here to signify the processes used to facilitate and mediate the transport of the target DNA sequences from the outside of the body of the research subject/patient into the nucleus of the end cells. Such a delivery of DNA *in vivo* is difficult to achieve due to the existence of a series of defense barriers and mechanisms that act together to clear the organism from the extraneous DNA molecule. In order to overcome these barriers, a carrier vehicle, that is, a vector, must first be selected to harbor the transgene. This can be done by integrating that transgene in the genome of recombinant viruses or alternatively by cloning it into a plasmid molecule (Figure 2.2). Recombinant viral vectors take advantage of the natural ability

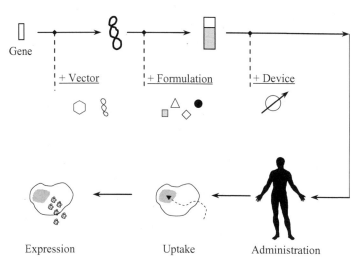

Figure 2.2 *Plasmid biopharmaceuticals: from* in vitro *genes to* in vivo *proteins. Once chosen and constructed, gene therapy plasmid vectors are formulated with buffers, stabilizers, and inorganic or organic matrices, and are used in conjunction with devices specifically designed for delivery. Following administration, plasmids progress through a series of steps (tissue distribution, cell recognition and internalization, intracellular trafficking, and nuclear entry) to reach the target nucleus where they are transcribed into mRNA, which is subsequently translated into the target therapeutic protein.*

acquired by different viruses (retroviruses, adenoviruses, adeno-associated viruses, etc.) over the course of evolution to infect cells. The superior aptitude of viruses to avoid the different defense barriers of the invaded organisms and cells when compared to plasmids has made them the most popular vectors for gene transfer. Furthermore, many recombinant viruses retain the ability to integrate within the genome of host cells and thus potentially provide for a long-lived expression of transgenes. It is thus not surprising to find that more than 60% of the clinical trials of gene therapy registered as of May 2010 were using viral vectors (adenoviruses, retroviruses, adeno-associated viruses, etc.) as gene carriers (Figure 2.3). In spite of this dominance, the incidents and serious adverse events that have been recorded during a number of clinical trials have stressed the safety concerns that were always associated with the use of viral vectors (see Chapter 1, Section 1.1.4). Fortunately, and despite their lower efficiency, plasmids have managed to remain competitive due to their better safety profile (see Chapter 7). Consequently, plasmid vectors have progressively gained some ground in recent years, and as a result, close to 20% of the gene therapy clinical trials recorded up to 2007 had used plasmid DNA as carriers of the therapeutic/prophylactic transgenes.[1] An important caveat of plasmid biopharmaceuticals in many applications has to do with the fact that expression of the transgene is transient. In order to circumvent this limitation, plasmids with integrating systems have been designed to promote the insertion of the target gene in the host genome.[8] Although this strategy could offer advantages in a number of cases, it would nevertheless carry with it the concerns of insertional mutagenesis that are normally (and justifiably, one might argue) associated with recombinant viral vectors.

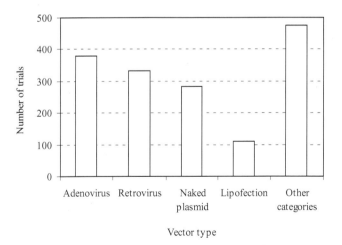

Figure 2.3 *Breakdown of the clinical trials of gene therapy registered as of May 2010 according to the type of vector used to deliver the transgene. Data were extracted from* The Journal of Gene Medicine *Gene Therapy Clinical Trials Worldwide Web site at http://www.wiley.co.uk/genmed/clinical (accessed May 9, 2010).*

2.2.2 Administration, Delivery, Uptake, and Expression

A substantial amount of data shows that in order for one naked plasmid DNA molecule to ultimately reach the cell nucleus, thousands have to be present at the site of intramuscular injection. This means that doses of a plasmid biopharmaceutical have to be at least two orders of magnitude larger when compared with the amount that is effectively transcribed. Such a poor efficiency of plasmid vectors, when it comes to transferring genes to the nucleus of cells, owes a lot to a series of barriers that DNA molecules encounter during their journey across the entry route, capillaries, interstitial spaces, tissues, body fluids, membranes, and cell cytoplasm. These barriers might include mononuclear phagocytes, blood components, harsh environmental conditions (e.g., low pH), plasma and cellular endonucleases that relentlessly cleave plasmid DNA, cellular membranes that do not favor plasmid uptake, and degradation and entrapment in endosomes and lysosomes.[9] In order to overcome these hurdles and to improve the efficiency of nonviral vectors, delivery systems are used to protect plasmids and bypass many of the barriers encountered. Thus, and once they are chosen and constructed, plasmid vectors used for gene transfer are typically formulated with buffers, stabilizers, and inorganic or organic matrices (Figure 2.2). These formulated plasmids are then used in conjunction with a device that is specifically designed for administration (Figure 2.2). The delivery systems and the exact route used to introduce plasmid biopharmaceuticals in a recipient's body are usually selected by taking into consideration the nature of the disease and of the target cells. For example, DNA vaccines for the prevention of infectious diseases are typically administered via muscular or skin tissues; intratumoral administration is used in the treatment of solid tumors, and the airways are usually preferred when addressing diseases that affect the lungs (e.g., cystic fibrosis). Furthermore, the route of administration and delivery system also determines which barriers are encountered along the way.[9] For example, although serum proteins and/or blood cells may constitute a problem in the case of intravascular delivery, this barrier is irrelevant when resorting to intramuscular injection.[9] Although some administration routes predominate (e.g., muscle and skin), virtually all organs and tissues in the human body have been used as entry points for plasmids (Figure 2.4). As for the delivery methodologies, the options are vast, and range from the simple needle injection of naked DNA formulated in a saline buffer to the more sophisticated electroporation and gene gun strategies. Since administration and delivery are one of the keys for the success of plasmid biopharmaceuticals, this topic will be dealt with in more detail later on in Chapter 6.

Once administered, plasmids have to progress through a series of steps to reach the target nucleus: (1) tissue distribution, (2) cell recognition and internalization, (3) intracellular trafficking, and (4) nuclear entry.[10] Depending on the exact delivery system used, some of these steps may be bypassed, whereas the exact mechanisms regulating others may be different. If a plasmid succeeds in arriving at the nucleus, it must then be transcribed and the resulting mRNA

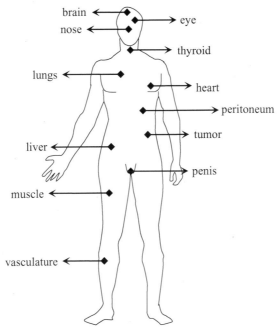

Figure 2.4 *Routes of administration of plasmid biopharmaceuticals. Although some routes predominate (e.g., muscle and skin), virtually all organs and tissues in the human body have been used as entry points for plasmids.*

translated into amounts of the target protein sufficient to obtain a therapeutic effect (Figure 2.2). The efficiency of transcription and translation can vary substantially, and will depend on a range of factors, from the size and type of gene to the exact nature of the different elements that form the plasmid vector backbone and of the recipient cells. Concomitantly, problems with low levels of expression can be tackled by manipulating the structure of plasmids in order to select the promoters, enhancers, or polyadenylation signals best adapted to the target cells and expression needs.[11] Clearly, only by understanding the different mechanisms involved in plasmid trafficking, uptake, and expression can we expect to perfect gene delivery systems and thus improve the efficiency of plasmid vectors.

2.3 THE ROLE OF PLASMID-BORNE GENE PRODUCTS

Once expressed, the products encoded by the plasmid-borne transgenes can act in different ways in the recipient organism, depending on the strategy designed to tackle and resolve the specific disease and clinical condition under study (Figure 2.5). The variety of gene transfer approaches explored has been such that it is difficult to systematize the different roles and possible functions

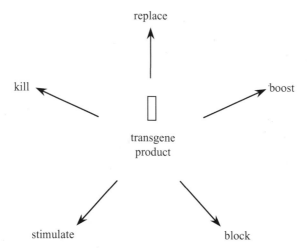

Figure 2.5 *Overview of the major roles of products encoded in plasmid-borne genes when used in the context of disease management.*

of transgene products. In many cases, more than one function is present at the same time. Nevertheless, and in order to provide a first, bird's eye view of therapeutic and prophylactic gene transfer, it is useful to recognize and group those different functions of transgene products into a few number of categories. The description that follows and the possibilities listed in Table 2.1 intend to cover most of the situations studied and described in the literature. A limited number of examples are presented alongside solely for illustrative purposes.

2.3.1 Boosting

The increase in the expression of a specific gene product is typically used when we wish to augment the intensity of a given physiological response. Many times, the endogenous responses generated by our bodies when challenged by disease or abnormal events may be insufficient or too slow to restore the normal status. The underlying objective of gene transfer in this case is thus to stimulate and accelerate the expression of key proteins, whose level is otherwise normal, by adding more copies of the key coding genes. The possible outcomes of this response can be as diverse as (1) an increase in the vascularization of ischemic tissue in patients with arterial disease[12] (see Chapter 9); (2) an increase in the production of endogenous growth hormone in pigs;[13] or (3) an increase in the levels of proteins like erythropoietin, insulin-like growth factor 1, or growth hormone in the context of physical enhancement strategies,[14] just to state a few examples. Whichever the setting, plasmids offer a convenient way to boost the expression of a particular protein by orders of magnitude in the tenth to the ten thousandth range.

TABLE 2.1. Functions Played by Products Encoded in Plasmid Biopharmaceuticals

Function	Some Examples
Boosting Goal: Increase physiological response.	(1) The expression of the vascular endothelial growth factor (VEGF) promotes the formation of new capillary blood vessels in coronary and peripheral arterial diseases.[12] (2) The expression of the hepatocyte growth factor (HGF) reduces the death and enhances the function of dopaminergic neurons associated with Parkinson's disease.[59] (3) The expression of the porcine growth hormone releasing hormone induces the production and secretion of the endogenous growth hormone and contributes to decreased offspring morbidity and mortality and increased body weight in pigs.[13] (4) The overexpression of proteins like erythropoietin, insulin-like growth factor 1, or growth hormone can be used in the context of physical enhancement strategies[14]
Replacement Goal: Replace defective proteins.	(1) The expression of the gene product replaces proteins that are abnormal or inexistent due to the single-gene defects, which are characteristic of diseases like antitrypsin deficiency, cystic fibrosis,[15] or Duchenne muscular dystrophy.[16] (2) The declining levels of a protein that result from the deterioration of a physiological response can be restored by the expression of the corresponding genes. Examples are insulin in type 1 diabetes patients[100] and erythropoietin in anemia[18]
Immune stimulation Goal: Stimulate the immune system.	(1) The local expression of cytokines increases tumor immunogenicity and drives clearance of cancer cells by the host immune system. (2) Tumor-specific genes that code for cell surface markers are delivered as a means to increase tumor immunogenicity and to drive clearance of cancer cells by the host immune system.[55] (3) The expression of antigens from microorganisms that cause diseases like AIDS,[19] malaria,[20] tuberculosis,[21] influenza[22], or anthrax[101] prepares the immune system for future infections.
Cytotoxicity Goal: Kill specific host cells.	(1) The restoration of normal expression levels from tumor suppressor genes like p53 arrests growth of cancer cells and renders them more sensitive to chemo- and radiotherapies.[39,40] (2) Suicide gene therapy relies on the expression of a foreign enzyme in a tumor that converts a coadministered prodrug into an active cytotoxic agent that kills tumor cells.[44,45] (3) Specific antiangiogenic genes (e.g., sFLT1[47]) are delivered to the affected tissues in order to inhibit the proliferation of blood vessels that supply nutrients and oxygen to tumor cells
Blocking Goal: Block the expression of host genes.	(1) RNA molecules encoded in a plasmid can block the expression of endogenous genes by interfering at the mRNA level.[23]

2.3.2   Replacement

Another possible function of the transgene product is to replace a protein that is defective or inactive in the host. This function is typically explored in the management of disorders like cystic fibrosis[15] or Duchnenne muscular dystrophy,[16] where a hereditary defect in a single gene prevents the body from producing regular levels of a normal protein. This function is also explored if one wishes to counteract the deterioration of previously normal levels of a given protein, as a consequence of physiological alterations. For example, the levels of insulin in type 1 diabetes patients that results from the loss of pancreatic beta islet cells can be restored in theory by the administration of a plasmid carrying the genes that encode insulin or proinsulin.[17] Likewise, the decline in the levels of erythropoietin, a protein that is a central regulator of red blood cell production, in patients who develop anemia can be increased by delivering plasmid constructs containing the corresponding gene.[18] Replacement can be used also in the context of conditions other than single-gene diseases, which are nevertheless characterized by a deficient expression of a given gene. For example, many cancer cells lack p53, a protein that controls cell death and growth (see Section 2.4.2.2). The replacement of this protein in cancer cells via the delivery of the *p53* gene is thus a potentially useful therapeutic strategy for cancer management.

2.3.3   Immune Stimulation

One of the best ways to manage disease is via the manipulation and stimulation of immune responses. The pharmaceutical products that mediate these responses are generically termed vaccines due to the fact that their action is directed toward the immune system. Although plasmid biopharmaceuticals in this category are collectively called DNA vaccines, two important subcategories have to be distinguished—prophylactic and therapeutic vaccines. The first class includes those vaccines that are administered to healthy people and animals with the goal of preventing future episodes of the target disease (see Section 2.5). The typical DNA vaccine in this category carries the gene that codes for a specific antigen of the causative infectious agent, be it a virus, a parasite, or a bacteria. DNA vaccines for AIDS,[19] malaria,[20] tuberculosis,[21] and influenza[22] would fit in this class. One of the key differences of DNA vaccines when compared with traditional protein-based vaccines has to do with the fact that the vaccinating antigens are synthesized endogenously. This means that in some cases, the process of antigen presentation that ensues may mimic natural infection more closely. Although we traditionally associate a preventive role to vaccines, those medicinal products that motivate the immune system to fight an underlying condition (usually cancer) have also become known as vaccines. For example, some of the therapeutic vaccines in this second class have been developed on the basis of genes that code for products that increase tumor immunogenicity, and thus more effectively mobilize cells from the immune system to control cancer (see Section 2.4.2.2).

2.3.4   Cytotoxicity

Gene transfer can be used as a means to kill malignant cells. The role of the gene product in the process is usually an indirect one; that is, the product typically plays an intermediate function in a larger, more complex network of events that ultimately results in the death of the target cells. The variety of gene transfer approaches explored in this context has been such that it is difficult to systematize the different strategies pursued, but the function of the gene product could range from replacing a missing key protein, stimulating the immune system into recognizing harmful cells (as described in the previous section) or introducing a new functionality that contributes to kill cells (more details are given in Section 2.4.2.2).

2.3.5   Blocking

The genetic information in a plasmid can also code for a product that blocks or inhibits the expression of a specific host gene that is relevant in the context of a given pathology. This blocking or silencing of a specific gene can potentially alter the course of some diseases. A number of approaches have been tested in order to accomplish such gene knockdown *in vivo*. For example, triplex-forming or antisense oligonucleotides can be delivered that hybridize to specific regions in the gene or corresponding mRNA transcript, respectively. This relies on the design and chemical synthesis of complementary oligonucleotides that, once delivered, bind to their complementary target, blocking transcription and translation. Another strategy explores RNAi, a sequence-specific gene-silencing phenomenon mediated by double-stranded RNA. Although synthetic, small interfering RNAs (siRNAs) or small hairpin RNAs (shRNAs) can be directly introduced in cells to silence the gene of interest, plasmids can also be used to deliver the genetic information required to direct the intracellular synthesis of the RNA transcripts.[23] Once expressed, such nonprotein coding transcripts will then participate in the RNAi pathway, silencing the target gene.

2.3.6   Conclusions

Although the description of plasmid biopharmaceuticals according to the function or action displayed by the product that is encoded in the transgene is elucidatory, this classification makes it difficult to grasp the full scope of disease management applications where plasmid biopharmaceuticals may play a role. For this purpose, it is rather more useful to organize applications according to the type of clinical intervention, separating them into two categories: therapy and prophylaxis (see Table 2.2). In the first case, the product of the gene that is carried by the plasmid is expected to trigger or play a therapeutic action. In the second case, the gene product will stimulate the immune system of the host, preparing it for a potential future encounter with the disease. The two types of intervention are described in the following sections in more detail.

TABLE 2.2. Examples of Human Diseases Addressed by Plasmid Biopharmaceuticals and Illustrative References

Therapy	Prophylaxis
Alzheimer's[102]	AIDS[103]
Anemia[18]	Amebiasis[104]
Arthritis[62]	Anthrax[101]
Coronary and arterial diseases	Chagas's disease[105]
Critical limb ischemia[106,107]	Dengue[108]
Myocardial infarct[109]	Ebola[110]
Cancer	Hantavirus[111]
Melanoma[53,54]	Hepatitis B[112]
Breast[41]	Hepatitis C[113]
Ovarian[114]	Herpes simplex[115]
Lymphoma[116]	Human papillomavirus[117]
Dental caries[64]	Influenza[22,118]
Diabetes[17]	Japanese encephalitis[119]
Genetic disorders	La Crosse virus[120]
Duchenne muscular dystrophy[16]	Leishmania[121]
Cystic fibrosis[15]	Malaria[122,123]
Hemophilia[124]	Rabies[125,126]
Glaucoma[65]	Schistosomiasis[127,128]
Lupus[66]	Severe acute respiratory syndrome (SARS)[129]
Parkinson's[59]	Sleeping sickness[130]
Sepsis[67]	Smallpox[131]
Spinal cord injury[68]	Toxoplasmosis[132]
Wound healing[69]	Tuberculosis[133,134]
	West Nile[135]

The diseases are separated according to the type of clinical intervention, that is, therapy versus prophylaxis.

2.4 PLASMIDS FOR THERAPY

As described in Chapter 1, gene therapy was originally contemplated as a strategy to treat single-gene disorders, which conform to the Mendelian rules of inheritance (i.e., Mendelian or classical genetic diseases). However, researchers soon realized that they could take advantage of the ability to express a given protein within a specific locus of the human body, to manage multifactorial diseases like cancer, arthritis, hypertension, or other cardiovascular diseases. These diseases are not directly linked to single major genetic abnormalities but are often caused by a combination of environmental factors and genetic predisposition. In many cases, more than one gene may be involved in the onset and progression of the disease.[5,24] Whichever is the exact nature of the disease in question, what the literature shows is that the use of plasmid biopharmaceuticals has been advocated as a means to treat both genetic disorders and multifactorial diseases (see examples listed in Table 2.2), as will be explained next.

2.4.1 Genetic Disorders

Congenital disorders are characterized by deficiencies at the single-gene level, which either originate defective proteins or hamper their synthesis altogether.

As a result, afflicted individuals display a series of symptoms whose severity may vary widely. Although in many cases it is possible to manage the disease, normalizing both life expectancy and quality of life, for example, by resorting to protein replacement therapies or appropriate dietary regimens, other disorders are severe and life threatening. While some single-gene disorders are extremely rare, others affect considerable numbers of individuals. Additionally, the incidence of such diseases can vary widely across populations, racial groups, and genders. Gene therapy has long promised to cure and treat such disorders. The rationale underlying this expectation is that the administration of the correct genes to the patients, via viral or plasmid vectors, results in the restoration of normal levels of the encoded protein. The course of the disease could thus be halted. A major drawback of plasmids when used in this context is related to the fact that in most cases, the added genetic material remains extrachromosomal. Since the plasmid material is typically cleared by the cell machinery after a certain amount of time has elapsed, the expression of the correct gene product is thus essentially transient. Although the use of transient expression might be preferred from a safety point of view, it is clear that the management of a genetic disorder using this approach will rely on the chronic administration of the plasmid biopharmaceutical. This may carry with itself other concerns, namely, the possibility of the development of autoimmune responses (see Chapter 7, Section 7.3.3).

In most cases, the gene transfer procedure is carried out at a time when individuals already exhibit symptoms of the genetic disease. This may be too late to alter the course of the disease, since often, irreversible damage has already occurred. Thus, the point has been made that the full benefits of a gene therapy approach in the case of genetic disorders can only be obtained if the treatment is initiated with presymptomatic individuals.[25] This means that diagnostic methods should be available to determine as soon as possible (i.e., in newborns) if a given individual is a candidate for a gene transfer. A set of criteria have been proposed to decide whether a given genetic disorder is an appropriate target for gene therapy. Apart from ethical criteria, which should always be considered when pondering the use of gene transfer in humans (this will be discussed later on in Chapter 7, Section 7.2), the following scientific criteria should be met: (1) The disorder should be inherited as a Mendelian trait; (2) a human mRNA clone should be available to correct the gene defect; and (3) the length of the mRNA should be compatible with available vectors.

Favorite targets for gene therapy of genetic disorders are, among others, (1) hemophilia, a coagulation disorder characterized by uncontrolled hemorrhagic episodes due to defects in factor VIII (hemophilia A) and factor IX (hemophilia B)[26]; (2) cystic fibrosis, a multiorgan disease caused by an abnormal cystic fibrosis transmembrane regulator (CFTR) gene[27]; (3) severe combined immunodeficiencies (SCIDs), a genetically heterogeneous group of conditions (e.g., ADA, X-linked SCID) characterized by a profound reduction or absence of T-lymphocyte production[28]; (4) lysosomal storage disorders, a group of ~50 diseases (e.g., Gaucher's disease) whose symptoms are linked to the abnormal functioning of lysosomal hydrolytic enzymes, and that prevent the organism from disposing of specific metabolites;[29] and (5) Duchene muscular dystrophy, a neuromuscular disorder associated with abnormalities in the dystrophin gene, which leads to progressive muscle wasting.[30] The number of people affected by monogenic diseases shies away in comparison with the millions that are affected by cancer and cardiovascular disease (see Chapter 8, Section 8.3.2). Nevertheless, in the near future, gene therapy is expected to have an impact on the treatment of those diseases. Around 20 different monogenic diseases have been studied at the clinical trial level, with cystic fibrosis and immune deficiencies accounting for one-third and one-fifth, respectively, of the total number of trials registered during 1989–2007.[1]

2.4.2 Multifactorial Diseases

Gene transfer via plasmid molecules has been studied as a possibility to treat many diseases that are caused by a combination of environmental factors and genetic predisposition. Once expressed in the target cells or tissues of the diseased organism, the product of the gene carried by the plasmid may play different roles. In the following sections, multifactorial diseases are subdivided into three major groups: cardiovascular diseases, cancer, and neurological disorders.

2.4.2.1 Cardiovascular Diseases

Cardiovascular diseases are the leading cause of death in the world (see Chapter 8, Section 8.3.2). Together, the different types of heart disease (rheumatic, hypertensive, ischemic, and inflammatory) plus cerebrovascular diseases killed more than 17 million people worldwide in 2004.[31] Vascular dysfunctions caused by underlying conditions like atherosclerosis, high blood pressure, or thrombosis are usually at the basis of cardiovascular diseases.[32] The majority of the problems of the vasculature are typically caused by a blockage (e.g., due to the buildup of fatty deposits on the inner walls of the blood vessels) that reduces or prevents blood flow. This usually results in a defective functioning of the heart and of the brain, eventually leading to events like myocardial infarction and stroke, respectively. A malfunctioning of the heart can also be linked to infection of the muscle and valves by streptococcal bacteria (rheumatic heart disease) or to birth malformations of the heart structure (congenital heart disease). The dislodgment of blood clots from the leg veins and into the heart and lungs causes deep vein thrombosis and pulmonary embolism. Although cardiovascular diseases affect mostly the heart and the brain, the arms and the legs can also be affected by poor blood supply, a condition known as peripheral arterial disease (PAD).

A number of risk factors contribute to the emergence of cardiovascular diseases. Chief among these are tobacco use, lack of physical exercise, and unhealthy diet. Poverty and stress have also been implicated in the onset of cardiovascular diseases. Apart from these risk factors, there is also strong evidence pointing to the existence of a heritable component to cardiovascular diseases.[33] In some cases, disorders at the single-gene level are sufficient to cause disease, even though these constitute a minority of cases. Examples of such monogenic cardiovascular diseases include familial hypercholesterolemia, Gitelman's syndrome, or hypertrophic cardiomyopathy.[33] In the case of the more complex cardiovascular diseases, however, it has been more difficult to pinpoint the exact genes and genetic variants implicated.

Preventive and therapeutic actions can be taken to reduce the burden imposed by the epidemic of cardiovascular diseases in the world. For once, it is consensual that substantial numbers of premature deaths could be averted by changes in lifestyle. If nevertheless disease sets in, a range of therapeutic strategies are currently available to control and treat cardiovascular diseases, including medication (e.g., aspirin and statins), medical devices (e.g., pacemakers, prosthetic valves, and stents), and medical interventions (e.g., coronary bypass, heart transplantation, valve repair). Still, alternatives like cell and gene therapy are actively being sought to complement these more traditional approaches and to reduce the impact of cardiovascular diseases.

A number of cardiovascular diseases have been addressed by gene therapy, including hypertension, thrombosis, heart failure, angina, and coronary arterial disease (CAD) and PAD.[1,34] Among these, CAD and PAD have mobilized most efforts. The progressive occlusion of arteries in patients with CAD and PAD, for instance, as a result of atherosclerosis, results in a restriction of the blood supply (i.e., ischemia), which ultimately leads to tissue damage due to lack of nutrients and oxygen.[35,36] Although the human body attempts to compensate for this deficiency by producing new conduits for blood flow (neovascularization), the efficiency of this response is usually poor. One of the three processes by which neovascularization can occur is angiogenesis—the formation of new capillary blood vessels from existent microvessels.[36] This complex process relies on an adequate balance of angiogenic and antiangiogenic agents (e.g., cytokines and metalloproteinases) that usually function in a cascade mode. The induction of neovascularization via the administration of specific angiogenic agents has thus emerged as a possible solution to improve blood flow to ischemic tissues in CAD and PAD patients. Although therapeutic angiogenesis can be carried out by direct administration of the recombinant angiogenic agent, gene transfer could offer advantages like prolonged local exposure and the potential for single-dose regimens.[35,36] The basic strategy relies on delivering key genes like the fibroblast growth factor (*FGF*), the vascular endothelial growth factor (*VEGF*), or the hepatocyte growth factor (*HGF*) that, once expressed, will stimulate the formation of new blood vessels and thus increase blood flow to the affected ischemic tissues (the myocardium and limbs in CAD and PAD). Other cardiovascular diseases that have been addressed by gene therapy include atherosclerosis, thrombosis, and hypertension. Although significant progress has been made in recent years (see the critical limb ischemia case study in Chapter 9, Section 9.3), major obstacles for a successful treatment of cardiovascular disease by gene therapy include the identification of the best candidate gene and delivery option.

2.4.2.2 Cancer

Cancer is one of the clinical domains in which plasmid biopharmaceuticals are most likely to have the largest impact.[37] Several facts attest to this, namely, the large number of clinical trials with plasmids targeting oncological diseases and the large body of scientific literature devoted to the subject. A number of distinct therapeutic strategies based on genes can be devised to kill cancer cells, which involve (1) the induction of cell apoptosis (tumor suppression), (2) the activation of prodrugs via gene products (suicide gene therapy), (3) the blocking of the formation of vessels in the tumor vicinity (antiangiogenesis), or (4) the stimulation of immune cells (cancer vaccination). A brief description of each of these strategies is given next.

Tumor Suppressor Genes One of the best ways to drive cancer cells to commit suicide is to deliver a tumor suppressor gene that is missing or defective in the tumor cells.[38] The approach is perfectly illustrated with *p53*, a gene that plays a key role in pathways such as DNA repair, control of cell cycle, and apoptosis. Mutations in *p53* lead to the malfunctioning of these critical cell pathways and have been associated with the genesis of tumors in a large proportion of human cancers.[39] Additionally, the presence of mutations in *p53* correlates with poor prognosis in many cancers. In line with these observations, the delivery of the wild-type *p53* gene to cancer cells and the concomitant re-establishment of normal levels of the p53 protein is expected to normalize the control of cell growth and to render cells more sensitive to the induction of apoptosis by conventional chemotherapy and radiotherapy treatments, among other functions.[39] Additionally, the apoptotic effect of the p53 product can also extend to neighbor, nontransfected tumor cells, a phenomenon known as the "bystander effect." As for normal cells, these are not detrimentally affected if transfected with the tumor suppressor gene, since this is constitutively present. Although *p53* has been delivered mostly by viral vectors, a number of studies have investigated the use of plasmids to this end.[39–42]

Enzyme–Prodrug Suicide Therapy Another stratagem to treat cancer is suicide gene therapy, a two-step approach that allies gene transfer with conventional therapeutics.[43] Here, plasmid-encoded proteins act synergistically with so-called prodrugs to fight cancer cells. The first step in the treatment consists in the administration and delivery of a gene that codes for a foreign enzyme to the tumor mass. Once this gene is expressed in the target cancer cells, a prodrug with no pharmacological action is administered. The enzyme then acts upon this prodrug, converting it into an active, cytotoxic agent that kills the tumor cells. This cytotoxic mechanism is not limited to those cells that have expressed the enzyme, since the active drug can diffuse to neighboring cells. This so-called bystander effect is important to extend the cytotoxicity to nontransfected cells. Among other factors, the success of such suicide gene therapy will depend on a correct matching of the expression levels of the transgene and prodrug concentrations, and on maximizing expression in tumor cells, as opposed to normal cells.[43] The combinations of the herpes simplex virus (HSV) thymidine kinase (TK) gene with the antiviral drug ganciclovir[44] and of the cytosine deaminase gene with the prodrug 5-fluorocytosine[45] are two of the reference enzyme–prodrug systems among the many that have been investigated. Although proof-of-concept studies providing the worth of the approach have been produced, a more intensive clinical development needs to follow.

Antiangiogenesis The growth and proliferation of tumors from a few isolated cells to a larger mass depends on an adequate supply of nutrients and oxygen. This means that in many cases, the formation of a network of blood vessels in the vicinity of cancer cells is essential for tumor survival. This angiogenesis process is induced by the tumors themselves that stimulate the host endothelial cells to produce new vessels by interfering with angiogenic and antiangiogenic factors.[46] A logical inference that surfaced when these observations were confirmed was that the inhibition of angiogenesis could potentially constitute a means to treat cancer. The exploration of this approach in a gene therapy context relies on the delivery of specific antiangiogenic genes to the affected tissues.[36] The fact that no specific side effects or cancer resistance has been associated with antiangiogenic gene therapy constitutes two advantages of the approach in a clinical setting. An example of an antiangiogenic gene studied in the laboratory and in the clinic is the one that codes for the soluble splice variant of the VEGF receptor (sFLT1).[47] Certain cytokines like interleukin 12 (IL-12), for example, are also known to display strong antiangiogenic properties alongside their more readily recognized immunomodulatory properties[48](see below).

Therapeutic Vaccines DNA vaccines that promote the expression of cytokines or cell surface markers as a means to increase tumor immunogenicity and to drive clearance of cancer cells by the host immune system are being actively developed for cancer therapy. In the first case, the goal is to explore the regulatory role of interleukins, interferons, tumor necrosis factors (TNFs), and colony-stimulating factors in the pathogenesis of cancer, as a means of generating potent antitumor responses.[49,50] Examples of cytokines used in the gene-based immunotherapy of cancer include interferon γ (IFNγ), granulocyte macrophage colony-stimulating factor (GM-CSF), interleukin 2 (IL-2), IL-12, and IL-15.[49] The results obtained with IL-12, either alone or in combination with other cytokines and costimulatory molecules, have been especially promising.[48,51,52] This cytokine combines both immunomodulatory features like the ability to induce the proliferation of T lymphocytes and natural killer cells, with antiangiogenic properties such as a strong inhibition of VEGF that can be exploited to control tumor growth as well. Although recombinant adenovirus vectors are the best choice when it comes to the efficient transfer of the IL-12 gene, beneficial and promising effects have also been obtained with plasmid vectors in phase 1 clinical trials.[53,54]

Cancer DNA vaccines that code for cell surface markers, that is, proteins that are specifically expressed in certain tumor cells, have also been used to foster systemic immunity against cancer. Examples of such tumor-associated antigens are, for example, Her-2/neu in breast cancer, prostate-specific antigen (PSA) in prostate cancer, and gp75/tyrosinase-related proteins (see Chapter 10, Section 10.4) in melanoma.[55] By delivering the corresponding gene to the cytoplasm of the correct cells, these antigenic markers are expressed endogenously and are adequately processed into antigenic peptides (see Section 2.5). These peptides are then brought to and displayed in the surface of the tumor cells by major histocompatibility complex (MHC) molecules. The subsequent recognition of the presented antigen by cytotoxic T lymphocyte (CTLs) eventually leads to the killing of the neoplastic cells.[56] Although this strategy has been particularly successful in mice models, human clinical trials have essentially demonstrated that it is hard for such DNA vaccines to elicit robust immune responses.[55] Major reasons for this include, for example, a difficulty to break the tolerance against the vaccinating self-antigen, which is characteristic of oncogenic processes, the shielding of the tumor cells from the immune system due to the secretion of immunosuppressive cytokines, and the proliferation of tumor cells with downregulated surface antigens.[55]

2.4.2.3 Neurological Disorders

Neurological diseases are characterized by the malfunctioning of the brain, the spinal cord, or the nerves in one's body. Although the severity of this type of disorder may vary across the spectrum of the more than 600 conditions known, the typical outcome is usually some type of restriction, impairment, or degeneration of body functions like locomotion, movement, speech, breathing, sensing, memory, or learning. Social behavior is also affected in many cases. Many of the diseases that affect the nervous system can also be categorized in one of the categories discussed in the previous sections. For example, diseases like Huntington's syndrome or muscular dystrophy are the result of mutations in single genes, whereas others, like stroke, are directly related to problems in the vasculature that supports brain function. Additionally, cancers and benign tumors can also affect our brains. Those diseases that lead to a progressive, but relentless, loss of function of the nervous system, like Alzheimer's, Parkinson's, or multiple sclerosis, are among the ones that have the most impact, not only in the patients themselves but also on their close relatives.

A number of gene therapy approaches, including the use of plasmid vectors, have been studied as an alternative to deal with such diseases.[57,58] Consider, for example, the case of Parkinson's disease, a neurodegenerative condition that is clinically characterized by resting tremors, loss of balance, and slowness. These symptoms are directly linked to the progressive loss of dopamine-producing (i.e., dopaminergic) neurons, which is thought to result from the accumulation of deposits of fibrous proteins in the cytoplasm.[57,59] One of the key strategies to handle the disease relies on the replacement of dopamine in the brain so as to restore motor. Alternatively, factors like the glial cell line-derived neurotrophic factor (GDNF) and the HGF that reduce the death and enhance the function of dopaminergic neurons could, in principle, be used to halt the progression of the disease.[59] With a gene therapy strategy, the genes coding for those neutrotrophic factors should be shuttled to specific locations in the brain using an appropriate vector. A recent study with a rat model of Parkinson's disease has demonstrated that the naked plasmid-mediated trans-fer of HGF is able to protect dopaminergic neurons and thus prevent the onset of the disease.[59] In this specific case, the expressed HGF acted not only as a neutrotrophic factor but also as an angiogenic factor, stimulating local blood flow.[59] Another gene that could be used in the context of gene therapy is the one that codes for tyrosine hydroxylase, the enzyme that converts tyrosine into L-3, 4-dihydroxyphenylalanine (L-DOPA).[57]

Attempts have also been described to use gene therapy to mitigate the debilitating effects of Alzheimer's disease, a common human neurodegenera-tive disorder that is characterized by the death and loss of function of cholin-ergic neurons in the hippocampal and association area of the neocortex.[57,60] Like in the case of Parkinsons' disease, the underlying strategy relies on the delivery of genes that code for factors that stimulate the function of neurons and prevent their death. For example, in a phase 1 trial, skin fibroblasts from Alzheimer's disease subjects were transfected *ex vivo* with retroviral vectors that express the nervous growth factor (NGF) and were reimplanted back in degenerating regions of the brain.[61] The follow-up revealed no adverse events, a response of the degenerating neurons to NGF and a potential (though not conclusive) slowing of cognitive decline. Although here a retroviral vector was used to deliver the gene, in principle, a similar strategy could be used with a plasmid vector.[61] Despite these advances, the results obtained on the gene therapy of neurological disorders at the clinical level are still very scarce.

2.4.2.4 Other
The diseases described in the previous sections have been the favorite targets for gene therapy, essentially due to the large impact they have on human health. Still, the possibility of using gene therapy to mitigate the effects of a vast array of other less-impacting diseases has been actively explored by researchers. Examples of additional diseases and conditions in which plasmid vectors have been specifically used to deliver the therapeutic genes include anemia,[18] arthritis,[62] burn wounds,[63] dental caries,[64] diabetes,[17] glaucoma,[65] lupus,[66] sepsis,[67] spinal cord injury,[68] and wound healing[69] (Table 2.2).

2.5 PLASMIDS FOR PROPHYLAXIS

Infectious diseases have scourged humankind for centuries, decimating entire civilizations, altering the course of wars and history, and imposing huge eco-nomical burden to societies.[70] This impact of infectious diseases, however, has been greatly diminished over the last two centuries with the advent, development, and dissemination of immunization practices. Still, there are numerous infectious diseases nowadays for which effective vaccines have yet to be developed (see Chapter 8, Section 8.3.1). Against this background, the immunization of humans and animals against infectious diseases is precisely one of the most appealing applications of plasmid biopharmaceuticals. In principle, DNA vaccines can be designed to confer protection against an enormous range of human and veterinary infectious diseases, as judged by the number of examples listed in the right-hand column of Table 2.2. The causative agents of these diseases include bacteria, viruses, fungi, and protozoans.

2.5.1 Immunization Mechanisms

Many studies performed with animal models have demonstrated that DNA vaccines can provide protection against infectious agents via the activation of the innate immune system and the induction of CTLs, T-helper (T_h) cells, and neutralizing (i.e., protective) antibodies, which are antigen specific.[71] While much is known today about the ability of DNA vaccines to mobilize both the cellular and humoral arms of the immune system, the full scope and interconnection of the mechanisms underlying these immune responses has yet to be fully understood. Still, a brief overview of what is known is given next since familiarity with the basic facts is important to fully understand the material presented in some of the coming chapters.

Although the specific type of immune response depends on the specific route of delivery, adjuvant, and DNA vaccine used, it is obvious that after plasmid delivery, some types of cells (e.g., myocytes, fibroblasts, keratinocytes, and specialized antigen-presenting cells [APCs]) must be transfected (see Figure 2.6). For example, transfection of muscle cells and keratinocytes is to be expected after plasmid administration by intramuscular injection and particle-mediated epidermal delivery[72] of plasmid DNA, respectively. Apart from non-APCs, experimental evidence shows that resident professional APCs, including macrophages, B cells, and dendritic cells (DCs), can sometimes be transfected *in situ*.[73] Among them, DCs are especially important, given their prominent role as activators of naive T cells.[74]

After the antigen-coding gene finds its way into the nucleus and is transcribed into mRNA, a certain amount of the antigen is synthesized. From here on, the antigen can follow essentially one of two routes. It can be targeted to the endoplasmic reticulum of the transfected cell where it is partially degraded by proteases (i.e., processed) into smaller peptides (9–24 amino acids). This antigen uptake process promotes the migration of the transfected APCs to regional lymph nodes where they initiate an immune response by interacting with naive T cells, the ultimate controllers of the immune response.[75,76] In this case, the antigen is said to be endogenous[77] (Figure 2.6a). Alternatively, the antigen is secreted from the transfected cell into the extracellular medium, where it will linger on until it is eventually taken up by resident APCs via the

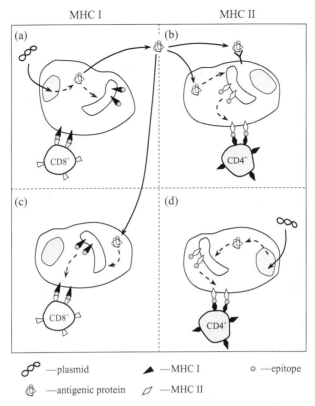

MHC I   MHC II

—plasmid   ▲ —MHC I   ○ —epitope

—antigenic protein   ▱ —MHC II

Figure 2.6 *The presentation of plasmid-encoded antigens to T cells. Transfected cells origi-nate antigens that are either (1) processed in the endoplasmic reticulum of the cell (endogenous antigens) or (2) secreted to the extracellular medium, engulfed by APCs and processed in the endoplasmic reticulum (exogenous antigens). Following processing, antigenic peptides are presented to CD8⁺ T cells via the MHC I (a,c) or to CD4⁺ T_h cells via the MHC II pathways (b,d). As a rule, CD8⁺ T cells recognize endogenous antigens that are presented via the MHC I pathway (a), and CD4⁺ T cells recognize exogenous antigens that are presented via the MHC II pathway (b). As exceptions, CD8⁺ T cells may recognize exogenous antigens engulfed by some APCs and presented by the MHC I (c), and CD4⁺ T_h cells may recognize endogenous antigens presented by the MHC II (d).*

lysosomal/endosomal pathway (Figure 2.6b). In this case, the antigen is said to be exogenous.[77] Secreted antigens may also be recognized by membrane-bound antibodies on the surface of B cells, a subtype of APCs that specialize on the secretion of neutralizing antibodies to the serum. Whichever the case is, that is, engulfment via endocytosis or antibody recognition, the cells will in turn process the antigen in the endoplasmic reticulum, generating antigenic peptides for presentation to T cells in the lymph nodes.

The antigen presentation that ensues after endogenous or exogenous anti-gens are processed in the endoplasmic reticulum is a key step in the develop-ment of immune responses. There are two pathways by which antigens are presented to T cells, one that involves the binding of the antigenic peptides (i.e., epitopes) to host glycoproteins of the class I MHC and subsequent recognition by CD8+ T cells (Figure 2.6a,c), and another that involves binding to class II MHC and recognition by CD4+ T cells* (Figure 2.6b,d). In either case, and once the binding grooves of the MHC molecules are filled, the complex is delivered to the cell surface, thus rendering the antigenic peptides "visible" either to CD8+ or CD4+ T cells. Another important distinction between the two pathways resides in the fact that MHC class I molecules are expressed across the majority of somatic cells (including APCs) and mostly present epitopes derived from endogenous antigens[77] (as schematized in Figure 2.6a). On the contrary, MHC class II molecules are expressed mostly by specialized APCs and essentially present epitopes that are derived from exogenous antigens (as shown in Figure 2.6b). This means that as a general rule, CD8+ T cells are able to recognize any transfected somatic cell that expresses the antigen, whereas CD4+ T cells, on the contrary, will only recognize epitopes generated from exogenous antigens.[77] There are, however, some exceptions to these norms. First, some APCs are able to engulf antigens from the extracellular space and process them via the MHC I pathway, a process termed cross-presentation or cross-priming (see Figure 2.6c). This mechanism is relevant in the context of intramuscular injection of DNA vaccines—in this case, and although muscle cells are poorly effective antigen presenters, cross-priming provides a way for transferring the expressed antigen to APCs and for priming T cells.[75] Another deviation to the norm is related to the fact that APCs are able to constitutively express both MHC I and MHC II. This means that APCs are able to process antigens synthesized endogenously via the MHC II pathway (Figure 2.6d), as well as via the canonical MHC I pathway (see Figure 2.6a).

Once activated by MHC I APCs, the CD8+ T cells proliferate into cytotoxic clones that will ultimately destroy cells that present the same antigen, for example, by releasing cytotoxic compounds.[74] Unlike CD8+ T cells, the CD4+ cells recruited by MHC II antigen presentation are not able to kill infected cells or pathogens. Rather, their key role is to secrete cytokines and thus provide help to B cells and CD8+ T cells, and also autostimulation. These so-called CD4+ T_h cells are usually categorized into the T_h1 class if they produce cytokines like IL-2, IL-12, TNF, and IFNγ, or into the T_h2 class if they produce cytokines such as IL-4, IL-5, and IL-10.[77] The release of cytokines like IL-2 and IFNγ alongside IgG2a antibodies by T_h1 cells produces proinflammatory responses that stimulate CD8+ T cells recruited by MHC I antigen presentation to destroy and further search for infected cells. In excess, T_h1 responses can lead to tissue damage and autoimmune responses. The impact of these negative effects is curtailed by the anti-inflammatory nature of the cytokines and IgG1 antibodies released by T_h2 cells. An important effect of the secretion of cytokines by T_h2 cells is to encourage those B cells that activated them in

---

* T cells are termed CD4+ or CD8+ depending on whether they express the cell surface protein CD4 or CD8, respectively.

the first place, to differentiate into antibody-secreting plasma cells and memory cells. The exact type of T_h response induced by a DNA vaccine depends on a number of factors, which include the nature of the target antigen, the presence of immune stimulators, the delivery methodology, and the nature of the species being immunized.[77] This means that, in principle, the vaccine and immunization procedure can be manipulated so as to bias the immune response to a T_h1 or T_h2 pattern according to the needs posed by the specific disease being investigated. For example, much experimental evidence shows that particle-mediated epidermal delivery usually polarizes responses toward the T_h2 arm, whereas intramuscular injection polarizes responses toward the T_h1 arm.[72] However, this cannot be taken as a rule since in other situations, similar delivery strategies yield more balanced T_h responses.[72]

2.5.2 Overcoming Limitations

Although strong CD8[+] T-cell responses can be obtainable in mice and in other murine models, DNA vaccines have largely remained ineffective in humans (and also in large animals) due to an inability to elicit potent and durable cellular immunity. Several strategies have been devised to counteract this critical limitation, as reviewed in a number articles (Table 2.3).[71,75,76,78–80] For once, the plasmid DNA backbone that supports the antigen gene can be modified (e.g., deleted, replaced, and mutated) so that higher levels of expression are attained *in vivo*. Examples of specific regions in a plasmid that could be targeted for modification include promoters and terminators,[81] polyadenylation sequences,[82,83] and enhancers. Additionally, the codons in the foreign antigen gene can be optimized to improve the efficiency of usage by the target organism.[84] In principle, the increases in the amount of expressed antigen brought about by these modifications will translate into a higher immunogenicity, even though what ultimately determines the magnitude of T-cell response is the amount of epitope/MHC that is presented at the cell surface.[77] As an alternative or complement to these modifications, genes that code for immune-stimulatory functions like cytokines and costimulatory factors can also be

---

TABLE 2.3. Examples of Strategies Used to Improve the Immunogenicity of DNA Vaccines

(1) Modify plasmid DNA vaccine backbone to increase antigen expression and to optimize codons in the antigen gene.

(2) Coadminister genes coding for immunostimulatory functions (e.g., cytokines and chemokines) either in the antigen-expressing plasmid or in a separate plasmid.

(3) Use plasmid backbones that harbor CpG motifs.

(4) Formulate vaccines with recombinant cytokines and chemokines and CpG motifs.

(5) Fuse the antigen with sequences that target specific MHC pathways and T_h cell responses.

(6) Design heterologous prime/boost immunization modalities.

(7) Improve formulations (delivery agents and adjuvants) and delivery methodologies.

coadministered (see Table 2.3).[71] These genes can be cloned either in the antigen-expressing plasmid, in which case there is a guarantee that both the antigen and the immune-stimulatory protein are expressed in the same cell, or in another separate plasmid.[76] The rationale behind this approach is that those genetic coadjuvants will contribute to boost or even tailor the immune response, for instance, by activating and recruiting professional APCs.[71] Numerous studies can be found in the literature where the ability of cytokines like IL-2, IL-12, and IL-15 to drive T_h1 responses, of IL-4 and IL-10 to drive T_h2 responses, and of GM-CSF to recruit DCs and macrophages has been tested as a means to improve immune responses to DNA vaccination in a number of animal species.[76] Costimulatory molecules like chemokines (e.g., macrophage inflammatory protein 1, monocyte chemotactic protein 1[85]) may also offer a means to enhance stronger immune responses or bias immunity to a specific pattern.[76] While the use of the immunostimulatory action of cytokines and chemokines described above relies on the insertion of the coding genes into plasmid DNA molecules, the molecules may also be added to DNA vaccines as recombinant proteins. A different outcome, however, should be expected in this case.

Unmethylated cytosine–phosphate–guanine (CpG) motifs constitute another type of genetic coadjuvant molecules that may contribute to boost DNA vaccine immunogenicity[86] (see Table 2.3). These motifs are known to interact with the host toll-like receptor 9 (TLR-9), activating B cells and plasmacytoid DCs, and promoting the proliferation of T cells, macrophages, monocytes, and natural killer cells.[86] These in turn trigger the production of chemokines, cytokines, and antibodies such as IgM, and the generation of inflammatory responses.[87,88] In view of these properties, unmethylated CpG motifs are often cloned into the antigen-expressing plasmid or simply coadministered as an adjuvant to step up and improve specific antibody responses.[86,89]

As described in the previous section, the process by which the expressed antigens are presented to T cells is one of the key steps for the development of effective immune responses.[75,76] A number of ways to improve the presentation of the antigens encoded in DNA vaccines and hence to increase their visibility to T cells have been devised, which rely on the coupling of specific sequences to the target gene so as to direct the expressed antigen to different locations and subcellular compartments, including the cytosol, the endoplasmic reticulum, the cell surface, and the exterior[77] (see Table 2.3). The exact type of trafficking that is engineered into the plasmid vector affects both processing and presentation, and hence the immunogenicity of the DNA vaccine.[90] For example, when fused to the antigen gene, the adenovirus E3 leader sequence will improve its transport and release into the endoplasmic reticulum. This means that larger amounts of antigen can be processed in the endoplasmic reticulum and loaded onto MHC class I molecules, and thus presentation of endogenous antigens to $CD8^+$ T cells increases (Figure 2.6a).[91] The MHC II pathway can also be targeted in a number of ways. For example, specific signals can be fused to the antigens in order to improve secretion to the extracellular milieu and thus to induce $CD4^+$ T_h responses more effectively (Figure 2.6b). Another sequence that can be fused to antigens to target and enhance MHC II presentation is the one that codes for the lysosomal-associated membrane protein (LAMP).[77]

One of the best ways to augment T-cell responses in humans and animals is to resort to heterologous prime-boost immunization regimens where the same antigen is delivered sequentially with two different vectors[92] (see Table 2.3). When used specifically with DNA vaccines, the strategy involves the priming of the immune system with a DNA vaccine and then the boosting of the response with a recombinant virus (e.g., modified vaccinia virus Ankara, fowlpox, and adenovirus) that also encodes the target antigen.[92,93] Alternatively, the boost can be made by immunizing with a recombinant antigen or with a conventional vaccine. The ability of this strategy to induce humoral and T-cell responses that are significantly higher when compared with DNA vaccines alone has been demonstrated in a number of situations (e.g., see the case of malaria DNA vaccines described by Sedegah et al.[94] and Vuola et al.[92]). The downside to this approach, however, is that the boosting vaccine must be developed alongside the priming DNA vaccine, increasing the complexity and costs of development, and ultimately the price of the final immunization scheme.

As described in the previous section, the immunogenicity of DNA vaccines can also be improved and manipulated by changing the delivery methodology used (see Table 2.3). For example, gene guns and electroporation devices are able to induce stronger immune responses of the T_h2 type with smaller amounts of plasmid DNA when compared with intramuscular injection, which usually requires larger doses and tends to bias responses toward T_h1. Another means of improving and manipulating DNA vaccine immunogenicity that is directly related to the delivery methodology used involves the use of specific delivery agents. For example, DNA vaccines may be combined with cationic lipids to form liposomes,[95] with poly(lactide-co-glycolide) to yield polymer-based microparticles[96] or with poly(N-isopropylacrylamide) to form stimuli-responsive complexes.[97] These formulations may protect DNA from degradation, improve its uptake, or allow for a more effective escape from endosomes/lyssomes, thus increasing the amount of antigen expressed.[71] A number of chemical compounds can also be incorporated in a DNA vaccine formulation to increase antibody titers and to enhance T_h and CTL responses.[71] Examples of such adjuvants include levamisole,[98,99] bupivacaine,[98] cardiotoxin, and saponins.[99]

2.5.3 The Development of DNA Vaccines

The second column in Table 2.2 gives a short sample of the diseases for which DNA vaccines are currently being studied at the different levels of the development pathway (see Chapter 3). Among the examples listed, one can find diseases that impose a significant burden to our societies, like malaria, tuberculosis, or AIDS. The usefulness of DNA vaccines in the context of sudden outbreaks of diseases, whether brought about by natural causes (e.g., pandemic influenza and ebola) or by human action (e.g., anthrax), is also being intensely explored (see the case study on pandemic influenza described in Chapter 9, Section 9.2). In spite of these efforts, finding a human DNA vaccine with an adequate potency and efficacy has proven to be a very difficult task. Although the technology has yet to prove itself in terms of efficiency, a major problem that will have to be faced by the first human DNA vaccines has to do with safety. It is true that all possible adverse reactions traditionally associated with plasmid biopharmaceuticals (e.g., integration and autoimmunity) have been addressed conveniently in the course of many preclinical and clinical studies and have been discarded as unlikely events (see Chapter 7, Section 7.3). Nevertheless, since the management of infectious diseases via immunization relies on administering vaccines to whole communities of healthy individuals, it may be too daring to start immunizing huge numbers of individuals without fully understanding the consequences of delivering exogenous DNA. Only in a crisis situation will people be willing to sacrifice the caution that should be mandatory once the first human DNA vaccines hit the market. There are a number of specific characteristics associated with DNA vaccine technology that will facilitate the dissemination of DNA vaccines, once safe and effective products have been developed. For once, the methodologies used to construct and produce DNA vaccines are much simpler and cheaper when compared, for example, with cell-based vaccines. The inherently higher stability of DNA when compared with proteins is another interesting characteristic, particularly if use in subtropical countries is envisaged. Further discussion on this topic is presented in Chapter 19 (Section 19.3).

2.6 CONCLUSIONS

The number of situations in which genes can be used to manage health and disease is virtually unlimited. Although the effectiveness of gene transfer is superior with recombinant viruses, plasmids constitute a very interesting and complementary alternative to viral gene transfer. The most distinctive characteristic of plasmids when compared with recombinant viruses is probably safety, though features like speed of development, potential for generic and affordable manufacturing, and stability are also important drivers of development and progress. Whether used in a therapeutic or prophylactic context, plasmid biopharmaceuticals have been proposed as a solution for a whole range of diseases including major killers like malaria, cancer, or cardiovascular disease. Given the current stage of development, only the future will tell if the promises made by scientists, research institutions, and companies will be fulfilled one day. What is very clear, however, is that the global resources and efforts that have to be devoted to the development of plasmid biopharmaceuticals are tremendous. The peculiarities of this development process are discussed in some detail in the following chapter.

REFERENCES

1. Edelstein ML, Abedi MR, Wixon J. Gene therapy clinical trials worldwide to 2007—An update. *The Journal of Gene Medicine.* 2007;9:833–842.

2. Dykxhoorn DM, Palliser D, Lieberman J. The silent treatment: siRNAs as small molecule drugs. *Gene Therapy.* 2006;13:541–552.

3. Akhtar S, Hughes MD, Khan A, et al. The delivery of antisense therapeutics. *Advanced Drug Delivery Reviews.* 2000;44:3–21.

4. Buchini S, Leumann CJ. Recent improvements in antigene technology. *Current Opinion in Chemical Biology.* 2003;7:717–726.

5. Morgan RA, Anderson WF. Human gene therapy. *Annual Review of Biochemistry.* 1993;62:191–217.

6. Meager A, ed. *Gene therapy technologies, applications and regulations: From laboratory to clinic.* Chichester: John Wiley & Sons, 1999.

7. King NMP. Rewriting the "Points to Consider": The ethical impact of guidance document language. *Human Gene Therapy.* 1999;10:133–139.

8. Hackett PB. Integrating DNA vectors for gene therapy. *Molecular Therapy.* 2007;15:10–12.

9. Nishikawa M, Huang L. Nonviral vectors in the new millennium: Delivery barriers in gene transfer. *Human Gene Therapy.* 2001;12:861–870.

10. Zhou R, Geiger RC, Dean DA. Intracellular trafficking of nucleic acids. *Expert Opinion on Drug Delivery.* 2004;1:127–140.

11. Mairhofer J, Grabherr R. Rational vector design for efficient non-viral gene delivery: Challenges facing the use of plasmid DNA. *Molecular Biotechnology.* 2008; 39:97–104.

12. Zhong J, Eliceiri B, Stupack D, et al. Neovascularization of ischemic tissues by gene delivery of the extracellular matrix protein Del-1. *The Journal of Clinical Investigation.* 2003;112:30–41.

13. Draghia-Akli R, Fiorotto ML, Hill LA, Malone PB, Deaver DR, Schwartz RJ. Myogenic expression of an injectable protease-resistant growth hormone-releasing hormone augments long-term growth in pigs. *Nature Biotechnology.* 1999;17: 1179–1183.

14. Kiuru M, Crystal RG. Progress and prospects: Gene therapy for performance and appearance enhancement. *Gene Therapy.* 2008;15:329–337.

15. Alton EW, Stern M, Farley R, et al. Cationic lipid-mediated CFTR gene transfer to the lungs and nose of patients with cystic fibrosis: A double-blind placebo-controlled trial. *Lancet.* 1999;353:947–954.

16. Romero NB, Braun S, Benveniste O, et al. Phase I study of dystrophin plasmid-based gene therapy in Duchenne/Becker muscular dystrophy. *Human Gene Therapy.* 2004;15:1065–1076.

17. Croze F, Prud'homme GJ. Gene therapy of streptozotocin-induced diabetes by intramuscular delivery of modified preproinsulin genes. *The Journal of Gene Medicine.* 2003;5:425–437.

18. Sebestyén MG, Hegge JO, Noble MA, Lewis DL, Herweijer H, Wolff JA. Progress toward a nonviral gene therapy protocol for the treatment of anemia. *Human Gene Therapy.* 2007;18:269–285.

19. Giri M, Ugen KE, Weiner DB. DNA vaccines against human immunodeficiency virus type 1 in the past decade. *Clinical Microbiology Reviews.* 2004;17:370–389.

20. Rainczuk A, Scorza T, Spithill TW, Smooker PM. A bicistronic DNA vaccine containing apical membrane antigen 1 and merozoite surface protein 4/5 can prime humoral and cellular immune responses and partially protect mice against virulent *Plasmodium chabaudi adami* DS malaria. *Infection and Immunity.* 2004;72:5565–5573.

21. Haile M, Kallenius G. Recent developments in tuberculosis vaccines. *Current Opinion in Infectious Diseases.* 2005;18:211–215.

22. Drape RJ, Macklin MD, Barr LJ, Jones S, Haynes JR, Dean HJ. Epidermal DNA vaccine for influenza is immunogenic in humans. *Vaccine.* 2006;24:4475–4481.

23. Kaykas A, Moon RT. A plasmid-based system for expressing small interfering RNA libraries in mammalian cells. *BMC Cell Biology.* 2004;5:16.

24. Friedmann T. Gene therapy-a new kind of medicine. *Trends in Biotechnology.* 1993;11:156–159.

25. Pindolia KR, Wolf B. Candidate disorders for gene therapy: Newborn screening facilitates ascertainment of presymptomatic individuals. *Human Gene Therapy.* 2008;19:213–216.

26. Hoeben RC, Schagen FHE, Van der Eb MM, Fallaux FJ, Van der Eb AJ, Hormondt HV. Gene therapy for haemophilia. In: Meager A, ed. *Gene therapy technologies, applications and regulations.* Chichester: John Wiley & Sons, 1999:195–206.

27. Caplen N. Cystic fibrosis: Gene therapy approaches. In: Meager A, ed. *Gene therapy technologies, applications and regulations.* Chichester: John Wiley & Sons, 1999:207–226.

28. Thrasher AJ, Gaspar HB, Kinnon C. Gene therapy for severe combined immunodeficiency. In: Meager A, ed. *Gene therapy technologies, applications and regulations.* Chichester: John Wiley & Sons, 1999:179–193.

29. Lashford LS, Fairbairn LJ, Wraith JE. Lysosomal storage disorders. In: Meager A, ed. *Gene therapy technologies, applications and regulations.* Chichester: John Wiley & Sons, 1999:267–290.

30. Murphy S, Dickson G. Gene therapy approaches to Duchenne muscular dystrophy. In: Meager A, ed. *Gene therapy technologies, applications and regulations.* Chichester: John Wiley & Sons, 1999:243–266.

31. World Health Organization. *The global burden of disease: 2004 update.* Geneva: WHO, 2008.

32. Basson M. Cardiovascular disease. *Nature.* 2008;451:908.

33. Nabel EG. Cardiovascular disease. *The New England Journal of Medicine.* 2003;349:60–73.

34. Dishart KL, Work LM, Denby L, Baker AH. Gene therapy for cardiovascular disease. *Journal of Biomedicine & Biotechnology.* 2003;2003:138–148.

35. Khan TA, Sellke FW, Laham RJ. Gene therapy progress and prospects: Therapeutic angiogenesis for limb and myocardial ischemia. *Gene Therapy.* 2003;10:285–291.

36. Malecki M, Kolsut P, Proczka R. Angiogenic and antiangiogenic gene therapy. *Gene Therapy.* 2005;12(Suppl 1):S159–S169.

37. Shekelle PG, Ortiz E, Newberry SJ, et al. Identifying potential health care innovations for the future elderly. *Health Affairs (Project Hope).* 2005;24(Suppl 2): W5R67–W5R76.

38. McCormick F. *Cancer* gene therapy: Fringe or cutting edge? *Nature Reviews. Cancer.* 2001;1:130–141.

39. Xu L, Pirollo KF, Chang EH. Tumor-targeted p53-gene therapy enhances the efficacy of conventional chemo/radiotherapy. *Journal of Controlled Release.* 2001;74:115–128.

40. Kim CK, Choi EJ, Choi SH, Park JS, Haider KH, Ahn WS. Enhanced p53 gene transfer to human ovarian cancer cells using the cationic nonviral vector, DDC. *Gynecological Oncology.* 2003;90:265–272.

41. Lesoon-Wood LA, Kim WH, Kleinman HK, Weintraub BD, Mixson AJ. Systemic gene therapy with p53 reduces growth and metastases of a malignant human breast cancer in nude mice. *Human Gene Therapy.* 1995;6:395–405.

42. Xu L, Huang CC, Huang W, et al. Systemic tumor-targeted gene delivery by anti-transferrin receptor scFv-immunoliposomes. *Molecular Cancer Therapeutics.* 2002;1:337–346.

43. Kirn D, Niculescu-Duvaz I, Hallden G, Springer CJ. The emerging fields of suicide gene therapy and virotherapy. *Trends in Molecular Medicine.* 2002;8:S68–S73.

44. Maruyama-Tabata H, Harada Y, Matsumura T, et al. Effective suicide gene therapy *in vivo* by EBV-based plasmid vector coupled with polyamidoamine dendrimer. *Gene Therapy.* 2000;7:53–60.

45. Bil J, Wlodarski P, Winiarska M, et al. Photodynamic therapy-driven induction of suicide cytosine deaminase gene. *Cancer Letters.* 2010;290:216–222.

46. Carmeliet P, Jain RK. Angiogenesis in cancer and other diseases. *Nature.* 2000;407:249–257.

47. Kendall RL, Thomas KA. Inhibition of vascular endothelial cell growth factor activity by an endogenously encoded soluble receptor. *Proceedings of the National Academy of Sciences of the United States of America.* 1993;90:10705–10709.

48. Fewell JG, Matar MM, Rice JS, et al. Treatment of disseminated ovarian cancer using nonviral interleukin-12 gene therapy delivered intraperitoneally. *The Journal of Gene Medicine.* 2009;11:718–728.

49. Jinushi M, Tahara H. Cytokine gene-mediated immunotherapy: Current status and future perspectives. *Cancer Science.* 2009;100:1389–1396.

50. Minuzzo S, Moserle L, Indraccolo S, Amadori A. Angiogenesis meets immunology: Cytokine gene therapy of cancer. *Molecular Aspects of Medicine.* 2007;28:59–86.

51. Maheshwari A, Mahato RI, McGregor J, et al. Soluble biodegradable polymer-based cytokine gene delivery for cancer treatment. *Molecular Therapy.* 2000;2:121–130.

52. Melero I, Mazzolini G, Narvaiza I, Qian C, Chen L, Prieto J. IL-12 gene therapy for cancer: In synergy with other immunotherapies. *Trends in Immunology.* 2001;22:113–115.

53. Daud AI, DeConti RC, Andrews S, et al. Phase I trial of interleukin-12 plasmid electroporation in patients with metastatic melanoma. *Journal of Clinical Oncology.* 2008;26:5896–5903.

54. Heinzerling L, Burg G, Dummer R, et al. Intratumoral injection of DNA encoding human interleukin 12 into patients with metastatic melanoma: Clinical efficacy. *Human Gene Therapy.* 2005;16:35–48.

55. Lowe DB, Shearer MH, Kennedy RC. DNA vaccines: Successes and limitations in cancer and infectious disease. *Journal of Cellular Biochemistry.* 2006;98:235–242.

56. Condon C, Watkins SC, Celluzzi CM, Thompson K, Falo LD. DNA-based immunization by *in vivo* transfection of dendritic cells. *Nature Medicine.* 1996;2: 1122–1128.

57. Shastry BS. Parkinson's disease: Etiology, pathogenesis and future of gene therapy. *Neuroscience Research.* 2001;41:5–12.

58. Wang L, Muramatsu S, Lu Y, Ikeguchi K, Fujimoto K, Okada T. Delayed delivery of AAV-GDNF prevents nigral neurodegeneration and promotes functional recovery in a rat model of Parkinson's disease. *Gene Therapy.* 2002;9:381–399.

59. Koike H, Ishida A, Shimamura M, et al. Prevention of onset of Parkinson's disease by *in vivo* gene transfer of human hepatocyte growth factor in rodent model: A model of gene therapy for Parkinson's disease. *Gene Therapy.* 2006;13:1639–1644.

60. Various authors. Progress and prospects: Gene therapy clinical trials (Part 2). *Gene Therapy.* 2007;14:1555–1563.

61. Tuszynski MH, Thal L, Pay M, et al. A phase 1 clinical trial of nerve growth factor gene therapy for Alzheimer's disease. *Nature Medicine.* 2005;11:551–555.

62. Fernandes JC, Wang H, Jreyssaty C, et al. Bone-protective effects of nonviral gene therapy with folate-chitosan DNA nanoparticle containing interleukin-1 receptor antagonist gene in rats with adjuvant-induced arthritis. *Molecular Therapy.* 2008; 16:1243–1251.

63. Steinstraesser L, Hirsch T, Beller J, et al. Transient non-viral cutaneous gene delivery in burn wounds. *The Journal of Gene Medicine.* 2007;9:949–955.

64. Liu C, Fan M, Bian Z, Chen Z, Li Y. Effects of targeted fusion anti-caries DNA vaccine pGJA-P/VAX in rats with caries. *Vaccine.* 2008;26:6685–6689.

65. Ishikawa H, Takano M, Matsumoto N, Sawada H, Ide C, Mimura O. Effect of GDNF gene transfer into axotomized retinal ganglion cells using *in vivo* electroporation with a contact lens-type electrode. *Gene Therapy.* 2005;12:289–298.

66. Hayashi T, Hasegawa K, Sasaki Y, Mori T, Adachi C, Maeda K. Systemic administration of interleukin-4 expressing plasmid DNA delays the development of glomerulonephritis and prolongs survival in lupus-prone female NZB x NZW F1 mice. *Nephrology, Dialysis, Transplantation.* 2007;22:3131–3138.

67. Tohyama S, Onodera S, Tohyama H, et al. A novel DNA vaccine-targeting macrophage migration inhibitory factor improves the survival of mice with sepsis. *Gene Therapy.* 2008;15:1513–1522.

68. De Laporte L, Yang Y, Zelivyanskaya ML, Cummings BJ, Anderson AJ, Shea LD. Plasmid releasing multiple channel bridges for transgene expression after spinal cord injury. *Molecular Therapy.* 2009;17:318–326.

69. Ferraro B, Cruz YL, Coppola D, Heller R. Intradermal delivery of plasmid VEGF(165) by electroporation promotes wound healing. *Molecular Therapy.* 2009;17:651–657.

70. Kiple K. *Plague, pox and pestilence.* London: Weidenfeld & Nicolson, 1997.

71. Laddy DJ, Weiner DB. From plasmids to protection: A review of DNA vaccines against infectious diseases. *International Reviews of Immunology.* 2006;25: 99–123.

72. Dean HJ, Haynes J, Schmaljohn C. The role of particle-mediated DNA vaccines in biodefense preparedness. *Advanced Drug Delivery Reviews.* 2005;57: 1315–1342.

73. Porgador A, Irvine KR, Iwasaki A, Barber BH, Restifo NP, Germain RN. Predominant role for directly transfected dendritic cells in antigen presentation to CD8$^+$ T cells after gene gun immunization. *The Journal of Experimental Medicine*. 1998;188:1075–1082.

74. Little SR, Langer R. Nonviral delivery of cancer genetic vaccines. *Advances in Biochemical Engineering/Biotechnology*. 2005;99:93–118.

75. Liu MA, Wahren B, Hedestam GBK. DNA vaccines: Recent developments and future possibilities. *Human Gene Therapy*. 2006;17:1051–1061.

76. Babiuk S, Babiuk LA, van Drunen Littel-van den Hurk S. DNA vaccination: A simple concept with challenges regarding implementation. *International Reviews of Immunology*. 2006;25:51–81.

77. Leifert JA, Rodriguez-Carreno MP, Rodriguez F, Whitton JL. Targeting plasmid-encoded proteins to the antigen presentation pathways. *Immunology Reviews*. 2004;199:40–53.

78. Ulmer JB, Donnelly JJ, Liu MA. Toward the development of DNA vaccines. *Current Opinion in Biotechnology*. 1996;7:653–658.

79. Donnelly J, Berry K, Ulmer JB. Technical and regulatory hurdles for DNA vaccines. *International Journal for Parasitology*. 2003;33:457–467.

80. Donnelly JJ, Wahren B, Liu MA. DNA vaccines: Progress and challenges. *Journal of Immunology*. 2005;175:633–639.

81. Galvin TA, Muller J, Khan AS. Effect of different promoters on immune responses elicited by HIV-1 gag/env multigenic DNA vaccine in *Macaca mulatta* and *Macaca nemestrina*. *Vaccine*. 2000;18:2566–2583.

82. Ribeiro SC, Monteiro GA, Prazeres DMF. The role of polyadenylation signal secondary structures on the resistance of plasmid vectors to nucleases. *The Journal of Gene Medicine*. 2004;6:565–573.

83. Azzoni AR, Ribeiro SC, Monteiro GA, Prazeres DM. The impact of polyadenylation signals on plasmid nuclease-resistance and transgene expression. *The Journal of Gene Medicine*. 2007;9:392–402.

84. Uchijima M, Yoshida A, Nagata T, Koide Y. Optimization of codon usage of plasmid DNA vaccine is required for the effective MHC class I-restricted T cell responses against intracellular bacterium. *Journal of Immunology*. 1998;161:5594–5599.

85. Eo SK, Lee S, Chun S, Rouse BT. Modulation of immunity against herpes simplex virus infection via mucosal genetic transfer of plasmid DNA encoding chemokines. *Journal of Virology*. 2001;75:569–578.

86. Yew NS, Cheng SH. Reducing the immunostimulatory activity of CpG-containing plasmid DNA vectors for non-viral gene therapy. *Expert Opinion on Drug Delivery*. 2004;1:115–125.

87. Mor G, Singla M, Steinberg AD, Hoffman SL, Okuda K, Klinman DM. Do DNA vaccines induce autoimmune disease? *Human Gene Therapy*. 1997;8:293–300.

88. Mor G, Eliza M. Plasmid DNA vaccines. Immunology, tolerance, and autoimmunity. *Molecular Biotechnology*. 2001;19:245–250.

89. Zhao H, Hemmi H, Akira S, Cheng SH, Scheule RK, Yew NS. Contribution of toll-like receptor 9 signaling to the acute inflammatory response to nonviral vectors. *Molecular Therapy*. 2004;9:241–248.

90. Reimann J, Kwissa M, Schirmbeck R. Genetic vaccination with plasmid vectors. In: Schleef M, ed. *Plasmids for therapy and vaccination*. Weinheim: Wiley-VCH, 2001.

91. Ciernik IF, Berzofsky JA, Carbone DP. Induction of cytotoxic T lymphocytes and antitumor immunity with DNA vaccines expressing single T cell epitopes. *Journal of Immunology*. 1996;156:2369–2375.

92. Vuola JM, Keating S, Webster DP, et al. Differential immunogenicity of various heterologous prime-boost vaccine regimens using DNA and viral vectors in healthy volunteers. *Journal of Immunology*. 2005;174:449–455.

93. Schneider J, Gilbert SC, Hannan CM, et al. Induction of CD8$^+$ T cells using heterologous prime-boost immunisation strategies. *Immunology Reviews*. 1999; 170:29–38.

94. Sedegah M, Weiss W, Sacci JJB, et al. Improving protective immunity induced by DNA-based immunisation: Priming with antigen and GM-CSF encoding plasmid DNA and boosting with antigen expressing recombinant poxvirus. *Journal of Immunology*. 2000;164:5905–5912.

95. Liu D, Ren T, Gao X. Cationic transfection lipids. *Current Medicinal Chemistry*. 2003;10:1307–1315.

96. Singh M, Briones M, Ott G, O'Hagan D. Cationic microparticles: A potent delivery system for DNA vaccines. *Proceedings of the National Academy of Sciences of the United States of America*. 2000;97:811–816.

97. Dinçer S, Türk M, Piskin E. Intelligent polymers as nonviral vectors. *Gene Therapy*. 2005;12:S139–S145.

98. Jin H, Li Y, Ma Z, et al. Effect of chemical adjuvants on DNA vaccination. *Vaccine*. 2004;22:2925–2935.

99. Sasaki S, Sumino K, Hamajima K, et al. Induction of systemic and mucosal immune responses to human immunodeficiency virus type 1 by a DNA vaccine formulated with QS-21 saponin adjuvant via intramuscular and intranasal routes. *Journal of Virology*. 1998;72:4931–4939.

100. Kumar M, Hunag Y, Glinka Y, Prud'homme GJ, Wang Q. Gene therapy of diabetes using a novel GLP-1/IgG1-Fc fusion construct normalizes glucose levels in db/db mice. *Gene Therapy*. 2007;14:162–172.

101. Luxembourg A, Hannaman D, Nolan E, et al. Potentiation of an anthrax DNA vaccine with electroporation. *Vaccine*. 2008;26:5216–5222.

102. Qu B, Rosenberg RN, Li L, Boyer PJ, Johnston SA. Gene vaccination to bias the immune response to amyloid-beta peptide as therapy for Alzheimer's disease. *Archives of Neurology*. 2004;61:1859–1864.

103. Singh DK, Liu Z, Sheffer D, et al. A noninfectious simian/human immunodeficiency virus DNA vaccine that protects macaques against AIDS. *Journal of Virology*. 2005;79:3419–3428.

104. Martinez MB, Rodriguez MA, Garcia-Rivera G, et al. A pcDNA-Ehcpadh vaccine against *Entamoeba histolytica* elicits a protective Th1-like response in hamster liver. *Vaccine*. 2009;27:4176–4186.

105. Vasconcelos JR, Hiyane MI, Marinho CR, et al. Protective immunity against *Trypanosoma cruzi* infection in a highly susceptible mouse strain after vaccination with genes encoding the amastigote surface protein-2 and trans-sialidase. *Human Gene Therapy*. 2004;15:878–886.

106. Makinen K, Manninen H, Hedman M, et al. Increased vascularity detected by digital subtraction angiography after VEGF gene transfer to human lower limb artery: A randomized, placebo-controlled, double-blinded phase II study. *Molecular Therapy*. 2002;6:127–133.

107. Nikol S, Baumgartner I, Van Belle E, et al. Therapeutic angiogenesis with intramuscular NV1FGF improves amputation-free survival in patients with critical limb ischemia. *Molecular Therapy*. 2008;16:972–978.

108. Imoto J, Konishi E. Dengue tetravalent DNA vaccine increases its immunogenicity in mice when mixed with a dengue type 2 subunit vaccine or an inactivated Japanese encephalitis vaccine. *Vaccine*. 2007;25:1076–1084.

109. Vera Janavel G, Crottogini A, Cabeza Meckert P, et al. Plasmid-mediated VEGF gene transfer induces cardiomyogenesis and reduces myocardial infarct size in sheep. *Gene Therapy*. 2006;13:1133–1142.

110. Sullivan NJ, Sanchez A, Rollin PE, Yang ZY, Nabel GJ. Development of a preventive vaccine for Ebola virus infection in primates. *Nature*. 2000;408:605–609.

111. Zheng LY, Mou L, Lin S, Lu RM, Luo EJ. Enhancing DNA vaccine potency against hantavirus by co-administration of interleukin-12 expression vector as a genetic adjuvant. *Chinese Medicine Journal (Engl)*. 2005;118:313–319.

112. Roberts LK, Barr LJ, Fuller DH, McMahon CW, Leese PT, Jones S. Clinical safety and efficacy of a powdered hepatitis B nucleic acid vaccine delivered to the epidermis by a commercial prototype device. *Vaccine*. 2005;23:4867–4878.

113. Alvarez-Lajonchere L, Shoukry NH, Gra B, et al. Immunogenicity of CIGB-230, a therapeutic DNA vaccine preparation, in HCV-chronically infected individuals in a phase I clinical trial. *Journal of Viral Hepatitis*. 2009;16:156–167.

114. Mizrahi A, Czerniak A, Levy T, et al. Development of targeted therapy for ovarian cancer mediated by a plasmid expressing diphtheria toxin under the control of H19 regulatory sequences. *Journal of Translational Medicine*. 2009;7:69.

115. Kim TW, Hung CF, Kim JW, et al. Vaccination with a DNA vaccine encoding herpes simplex virus type 1 VP22 linked to antigen generates long-term antigen-specific CD8-positive memory T cells and protective immunity. *Human Gene Therapy*. 2004;15:167–177.

116. Timmerman JM, Singh G, Hermanson G, et al. Immunogenicity of a plasmid DNA vaccine encoding chimeric idiotype in patients with B-cell lymphoma. *Cancer Research*. 2002;62:5845–5852.

117. Peng S, Ji H, Trimble C, et al. Development of a DNA vaccine targeting human papillomavirus type 16 oncoprotein E6. *Journal of Virology*. 2004;78:8468–8476.

118. Zheng L, Wang F, Yang Z, Chen J, Chang H, Chen Z. A single immunization with HA DNA vaccine by electroporation induces early protection against H5N1 avian influenza virus challenge in mice. *BMC Infectious Diseases*. 2009;9:17.

119. Zhai YZ, Li XM, Zhou Y, Ma L, Feng GH. Intramuscular immunization with a plasmid DNA vaccine encoding prM-E protein from Japanese encephalitis virus: Enhanced immunogenicity by co-administration of GM-CSF gene and genetic fusions of prM-E protein and GM-CSF. *Intervirology*. 2009;52:152–163.

120. Pavlovic J, Schultz J, Hefti HP, Schuh T, Molling K. DNA vaccination against La Crosse virus. *Intervirology*. 2000;43:312–321.

121. Ahmed SB, Touihri L, Chtourou Y, Dellagi K, Bahloul C. DNA based vaccination with a cocktail of plasmids encoding immunodominant *Leishmania* (Leishmania) *major* antigens confers full protection in BALB/c mice. *Vaccine.* 2009;27:99–106.

122. Wang R, Doolan DL, Le TP, et al. Induction of antigen-specific cytotoxic T lymphocytes in humans by a malaria DNA vaccine. *Science.* 1998;282:476–480.

123. Epstein JE, Gorak EJ, Charoenvit Y, et al. Safety, tolerability, and lack of antibody responses after administration of a PfCSP DNA malaria vaccine via needle or needle-free jet injection, and comparison of intramuscular and combination intramuscular/intradermal routes. *Human Gene Therapy.* 2002;13:1551–1560.

124. Fewell JG, MacLaughlin F, Mehta V, et al. *Gene therapy* for the treatment of hemophilia B using PINC-formulated plasmid delivered to muscle with electroporation. *Molecular Therapy.* 2001;3:574–583.

125. Cruz ET, Romero IAF, Mendoza JGL, et al. Efficient post-exposure prophylaxis against rabies by applying a four-dose DNA vaccine intranasally. *Vaccine.* 2008;26:6936–6944.

126. Perrin P, Jacob Y, Aguilar-Setien A, et al. Immunization of dogs with a DNA vaccine induces protection against rabies virus. *Vaccine.* 1999;18:479–486.

127. Siddiqui AA, Phillips T, Charest H, et al. Induction of protective immunity against *Schistosoma mansoni* via DNA priming and boosting with the large subunit of calpain (Sm-p80): Adjuvant effects of granulocyte-macrophage colony-stimulating factor and interleukin-4. *Infection and Immunity.* 2003;71:3844–3851.

128. Da'dara AA, Li YS, Xiong T, et al. DNA-based vaccines protect against zoonotic schistosomiasis in water buffalo. *Vaccine.* 2008;26:3617–3625.

129. Yang ZY, Kong WP, Huang Y, et al. A DNA vaccine induces SARS coronavirus neutralization and protective immunity in mice. *Nature.* 2004;428:561–564.

130. Silva MS, Prazeres DM, Lanca A, Atouguia J, Monteiro GA. Trans-sialidase from *Trypanosoma brucei* as a potential target for DNA vaccine development against African trypanosomiasis. *Parasitology Research.* 2009;105:1223–1229.

131. Golden JW, Hooper JW. Heterogeneity in the A33 protein impacts the cross-protective efficacy of a candidate smallpox DNA vaccine. *Virology.* 2008;377: 19–29.

132. Cong H, Gu QM, Yin HE, et al. Multi-epitope DNA vaccine linked to the A2/B subunit of cholera toxin protect mice against *Toxoplasma gondii*. *Vaccine.* 2008;26:3913–3921.

133. Wang QM, Kang L, Wang XH. Improved cellular immune response elicited by a ubiquitin-fused ESAT-6 DNA vaccine against *Mycobacterium tuberculosis*. *Microbiology and Immunology.* 2009;53:384–390.

134. Mir FA, Kaufmann SH, Eddine AN. A multicistronic DNA vaccine induces significant protection against tuberculosis in mice and offers flexibility in the expressed antigen repertoire. *Clinical and Vaccine Immunology.* 2009;16: 1467–1475.

135. Martin JE, Pierson TC, Hubka S, et al. A West Nile virus DNA vaccine induces neutralizing antibody in healthy adults during a phase 1 clinical trial. *The Journal of Infectious Diseases.* 2007;196:1732–1740.

3

Product and Process Development

3.1 OVERVIEW

The discovery, development, and commercialization of a drug or biologic is a long, multistage process, which can take from 10 to 15 years (Figure 3.1). It is also an extremely costly enterprise, with expenses ranging anywhere from US$300 to US$1 billion, depending on the product.[1,2] The succession of events shown in Figure 3.1 is often called a value chain since the successful completion of a given step in the sequence adds value to the product, which is under development. The starting point in the overall process, which is usually one of the keys to success, is the gathering and generation of knowledge about the disease being tackled. In principle, the choice of this disease as the target is supported by a prospective and sound market scanning. Such a market analysis attempts to anticipate whether revenues associated with a hypothetical product, once it reaches the market, are worth the risks taken and investment made during its development. If the prospects are good, an adequate biological target must then be discovered and identified, which will drive and direct the selection of potential therapeutics (whether drugs or biologics).[1] The decision to proceed with the development of a particular candidate product for that disease is then taken, usually on the basis of solid scientific evidence accumulated during basic research studies. This research/discovery stage is followed by a series of activities that includes preclinical testing and clinical trials, and

Plasmid Biopharmaceuticals: Basics, Applications, and Manufacturing, First Edition.
Duarte Miguel F. Prazeres.

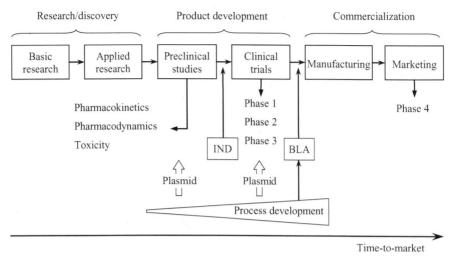

Figure 3.1 *The discovery, development, and commercialization of medicinal products for therapeutic use in humans. IND, investigational new drug; BLA, biologics license application.*

that together constitute what is known as product development. The development of the manufacturing process is an activity that is parallel to the product development. It is a key not only to generate material for trials but also to establish the manufacturing process, which will ultimately produce the product for sale. Once a product receives marketing approval from the competent regulatory authorities, it can then be manufactured on a routine basis and sold to the public.

3.2 PRODUCT DEVELOPMENT

The ultimate goal of product development is to gain approval to market the target product. This development proceeds through a sequence of studies with the candidate product in animals (preclinical trials) and humans (clinical trials), which have specific objectives on their own and involve different resources and volunteers (Table 3.1).

3.2.1 Preclinical Trials

The goal of preclinical trials is to determine in advance the potential safety risks that could be faced by the subjects involved in the subsequent human clinical trials. At this stage, every reasonable precaution should be explored to anticipate a toxicity that may eventually harm human volunteers. Preclinical studies are done by performing laboratory tests *in vitro* (cell/tissue cultures) and by resorting to adequate animal models of the disease (e.g., mice, rats, and

TABLE 3.1. Developing a Biopharmaceutical: The Preclinical and Clinical Trials

Stage	Goal	Cost ($US Million)	Subjects (Number)	Duration (Years)
Preclinical	Safety	5		2.0–5.0
Clinical phase 1	Safety	10	10–100	0.5
Clinical phase 2	Safety Efficacy	20	50–500	1.0–2.0
Clinical phase 3	Confirm efficacy Set dosage, frequency, and duration	80–100	Hundreds to thousands	3.0–5.0
Clinical phase 4	Monitor adverse events, effectiveness, economic benefit, and quality of life	Variable	Variable	Variable

Figures are rough estimates drawn from the literature.[1]

primates). A set of rules known as good laboratory practice (GLP) has been written specifically to ensure the quality, integrity, and reliability of the nonclinical study data gathered during these preclinical trials (see Chapter 11, Section 11.2 for further details).[3] Preclinical evaluation of a therapeutic usually involves pharmacodynamic, pharmacokinetic, and toxicity studies.[1] Pharmacodynamic experiments are conducted to investigate the interaction of the therapeutic with its target, whereas the object of pharmacokinetics is the study of the absorption, distribution, metabolism, and excretion of the therapeutic agent. In the case of a plasmid biopharmaceutical, such a pharmacokinetic study will typically evaluate the fate of the plasmid (blood half-life and tissue distribution), as well as the potential expression of the encoded protein(s) in mice at selected time points post administration.[4] Toxicological tests are designed to determine if the therapeutic is safe or if it presents some kind of toxicity, carcinogenicity, or genotoxicity. In the case of plasmids, and apart from looking into the effect of the administration of escalating doses on clinical chemistry, hematology, or organ pathology,[5] it is also important to look into issues like the potential integration of plasmid DNA into the host genomic DNA[5] and the generation of anti-DNA antibodies[6] (see Chapter 7, Section 7.3 for further details). Preclinical trials constitute one of the pivotal points of development, since the identification of a safety risk at this moment in time will lead to the failure of the candidate therapeutic. The probability of success at the onset of preclinical development is around 10%, whereas successful completion of the study increases probabilities up to 20%.[7] Preclinical testing has been estimated to take 1–3 years, costing up to US$5 million.[1]

3.2.2 Clinical Trials

If by the end of the preclinical studies it is possible to conclude that a certain therapeutic candidate has an acceptable safety profile, it can then be moved into clinical trials. First, the institution (research center, company) that is pushing the development, that is, the sponsor, prepares a trial protocol, which is submitted to a local institutional review board (IRB) or ethics committee.[8] This document includes information on aspects like the number of subjects to include, informed consent and confidentiality statements, statistical methods to be used for data analysis and evaluation of results, means for protecting the subject during the trial, and so on.[8,9] Following approval of the trial protocol, and in order to move the process forward, all the data gathered during preclinical development are collected together with a description of the planned human trials and are submitted to the Food and Drug Administration (FDA) as an investigational new drug (IND) application[7,8] (Figure 3.1). In the European Union (EU), the sponsor has to file an equivalent document known as investigational medicinal product dossier (IMPD).[8] If these documents are approved by the corresponding regulatory agency, then the trials can begin.

Clinical trials use the therapeutic in human volunteers to examine its effects (safety and efficacy) and to determine whether it should be approved for wider use in the general population. The subjects are usually separated randomly into test and control groups so that on completing the study, any differences observed can be attributed to the experimental product.[10,11] Strict eligibility criteria must be used to select the test subjects, and written informed consent is mandatory. The rights, safety, and well-being of the trial subjects are safeguarded by a set of good clinical practice (GCP) regulations that contain ethical and scientific quality requirements, which must be observed by the responsible investigators throughout the trial process (see Chapter 11, Section 11.2 for more details). The monitoring of subjects and recording of information during the trials is crucial, since part of it will eventually be submitted to regulatory agencies.

Clinical trials are carried out as a series of three phases. The first studies are termed phase 1 trials and typically involve 10–100 healthy volunteers (Table 3.1). This is the first time the product is tested in humans, and the major objectives are to determine dosing, to analyze how the product is metabolized and excreted, and to identify severe side effects. Phase 1 clinical testing can be separated into two studies. For instance, in the case of a DNA vaccine toward hepatitis B virus, which is administered by particle-mediated epidermal delivery (PMED), the first study (phase 1a) focused on the local skin reaction and tolerability of the vaccine as a function of device pressure, whereas the second study (phase 1b) was designed as a dose escalation study in terms of particle dose, DNA dose, and number of administration sites.[12] Phase 1 trials can cost up to US$10 million and may be completed in half a year.[1] A successful conclusion of studies at this stage has been estimated to step up the probabilities of success up to 30%.[7] Although many safety concerns can be ruled out by phase 1 results, efficacy is still an unknown that must be addressed in the subsequent phases.

Phase 2 trials use subjects that are affected by the target disease or at risk of contracting it (in the case of vaccines) to further determine safety and gather preliminary evidence on the effectiveness of the medicinal agent[10] (Table 3.1). Comparative studies are usually performed in which the candidate therapeutic is evaluated side by side with an alternative medicine or with a placebo. The patients are randomly separated into treatment and control groups and are kept ignorant of the group they are in (single-blinding). The clinical investigators may also be kept unaware of the allocation of patients to either group (double-blinding). Phase 2 trials may involve from 50 to 500 patients during 1–2 years. A cost of more than US$20 million has been esti-mated for phase 2 trials.[1] A successful conclusion of this trial phase is a crucial event, which improves the probability of success to 60%.[7]

At the end of phase 2, it should be possible to evaluate if the candidate therapeutic is potentially effective and whether the risks associated with its use are acceptable in the face of the severity of the disease.[10] In the affirmative case, the therapeutic then moves to phase 3 trials. A large number of people with the disease (1000–3000) are used as test subjects in this phase so that in the end, any results can be considered statistically significant. The trials will often involve multiple geographic locations. During the study, the effectiveness is further tested and side effects are carefully monitored. Given that more patients are involved, side effects that were not apparent in phase 2 may be revealed.[10] The larger number of patients involved typically drives costs of phase 3 studies to US$100 million and more.[1] The ultimate success or failure of the product will be decided at the end of this phase. In the United States, the successful completion of phase 3 will lead to the submission of a biologics license application (BLA) to the Center for Biologics Evaluation Research (CBER) at the FDA (Figure 3.1). In Europe, an equivalent application is submitted to the European Medicines Agency (EMA) under the Centralised Procedure.[1] The information contained in a BLA or equivalent dossier includes an analysis of all animal and human data and also information on how the medicinal product is manufactured. With this application, the sponsor of the product is formally requesting approval for the marketing of the new biologic or drug. The regulatory authority then reviews all the information the sponsor has collected on the product safety and effectiveness, inspects the facilities where the product is manufactured, and finally decides whether the applica-tion is "approvable" or "not approvable."[1]

The monitoring of the safety and efficacy of a medicinal product does not end upon marketing approval and commercialization. Even though the con-trolled clinical trials performed during phases 1–3 offer a substantial degree of assurance that a product is safe and efficacious, the truth is that the number of volunteers involved in those studies may be too small to enable the detec-tion of rare but nevertheless important adverse effects. Only after a product has been marketed and widely distributed may these events become apparent. Furthermore, there is always the possibility that some adverse events may occur in specific groups that had not been enrolled in the previous clinical trials, or that other reactions might appear only late after administration.[13] For these reasons, companies usually design phase 4 trials to keep a track record of their product, collecting information on issues like adverse events, but also on the effectiveness of the product in comparison with competitors, its economic benefits, and its impact on the quality of life of the recipients[1] (Table 3.1). Some phase 4 studies can also be designed to look into subpopulations of patients or further optimize dosage.[7] Such a careful postmarketing monitoring and scrutiny will be even more important in the specific case of the first plasmid biopharmaceuticals since this will be the first time such products will be administered in humans in a nonclinical trial context. This will enable the rapid detection and thorough investigation of any new adverse event, and hence the adoption of adequate measures that in the limit can include the withdrawal of the product.

3.3 PROCESS DEVELOPMENT

3.3.1 Introduction

Small amounts of the target product are produced from an early stage to support much of the proof-of-concept studies of the early phases of research and preliminary preclinical tests. This material is typically produced in research and development laboratories with non-optimized, small-scale protocols. In the case of plasmid biopharmaceuticals, this typically means producing less than 1 mg of material per batch. This demand can be met by resorting to some plasmid isolation "mega kits" as the ones commercialized by the Germany-based company QIAGEN (Hilden, Germany).[14] Serious thinking about developing a process to manufacture the target product starts when preclinical and clinical trials are on the horizon (Figure 3.1). The material used in these animal and human experiments, and especially in phase 2 and phase 3 trials, should be produced by a process as close to the one that will produce material for market approval as possible. This is particularly justified if the medicinal product is a biologic, since in this case it has been widely recognized and accepted that the quality, safety, and effectiveness of the product is intimately linked to the process used to produce it (i.e., the product *is* the process). Also, as seen in the previous section, the BLA that is submitted after the successful completion of phase 3 must already contain detailed information about the process used to manufacture the product at the full scale.

The ultimate goal of process development is thus to come up with a reliable manufacturing operation capable of delivering the amounts of the medicinal product required for trials and commercialization with an adequate quality and at an acceptable cost. Given the nature of the product development steps described above, the money invested in process development should be ramped up according to the progress the product is making through the trial phases.[15] Thus, investment should be kept low while the probability of success is low (during the preclinical and phase 1 stages) and increase progressively with the decrease of the risk of failure, which is brought about by a successful

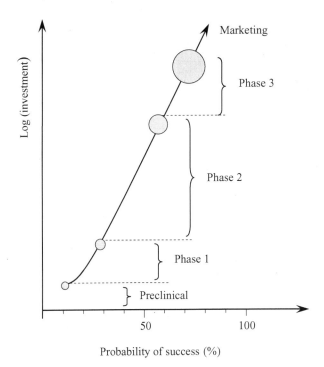

Figure 3.2 *Balancing the investment in process development with the increasing probability of success through product development. The figure is essentially qualitative. The circles are positioned according to the probability of product success after the completion of the corresponding phase. These numbers (R&D:10%, preclinical: 20%, phase 1: 29%, phase 2: 61%, and phase 3: 74%) have been taken from Figure 2.20 in Northrup.[7] The increasing area of each circle qualitatively represents the increased amounts of product that were required at each phase.*

completion of phase 2 and phase 3 trials (Figure 3.2). For preclinical and phase 1 studies, the larger amounts of material required are typically produced in a GLP-compliant laboratory.[15] Specially adapted, small-scale production facilities, operating in the context of research centers, can be used for this purpose. For instance, a recent report describes the establishment of a process that allows the manufacture of pilot to phase 1-scale amounts of 200 mg of clinical-grade plasmid DNA in a 96 ft² facility.[16] Features of this facility are discussed in more detail in Chapter 11 (Section 11.7). Alternatively, a number of firms have specialized in manufacturing plasmid DNA for preclinical and clinical experiments under contract (see Chapter 8, Section 8.5). The materials for phases 2 and 3 are produced by an equivalent process at pilot scale, in facilities that operate under good manufacturing practice (GMP; see Section 3.3.3 and also Chapter 11, Section 11.3). Manufacturing of the product for marketing is finally implemented at full scale with a process that is essentially the same than the one used to produce material for phase 2 and phase 3 trials.[15]

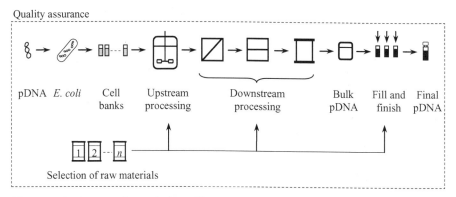

Figure 3.3 *An overview of the different activities and steps involved in plasmid manufacturing.*

The process used to manufacture a plasmid biopharmaceutical product will consist of a string of activities (Figure 3.3) that are set up and implemented with the goal of producing a certain amount (measured as mass or biological activity) of the target product at an acceptable cost and quality. As we have seen before, two major aspects of this quality attribute within the context of manufacturing medicinal products are safety and efficacy. At the forefront of the activities mentioned, we find the preparation of cell banks and the selection and testing of raw materials. Upstream and downstream processing unit operations are then selected, arranged, designed, and operated to manufacture bulk (i.e., unformulated) plasmid DNA. Subsequently, this purified bulk product has to be adequately formulated, a task that requires consideration of aspects like the method of delivery, the final product form, ingredients (excipients, adjuvants, and stabilizers), dosage details, packaging, and so on.[17] After "filling and finishing," as this stage is usually known, the product can be shipped, distributed, and marketed (Figure 3.3). This set of activities has to be carefully selected and planned in order that the final goal is met once a routine operation is established.

Designing and developing a process for the manufacturing of a medicinal biological product for commercialization is more than just (bio)engineering. Such undertaking requires an awareness of a number of key issues that, to a large extent, constrain and frame the design space available to the bioprocess engineer or scientist (Figure 3.4). An adequate knowledge of the specific intellectual property landscape is also an important aspect. Like in many other engineering systems, additional important attributes of the manufacturing process to be considered include flexibility, resilience, sustainability, and energy consumption. To have an overall and integrated view of all these circumstances is important for the successful implementation of plasmid manufacturing (Figure 3.4).

A number of the elements identified in Figures 3.3 and 3.4 will be dealt with in detail in the forthcoming chapters, namely, GMPs and validation

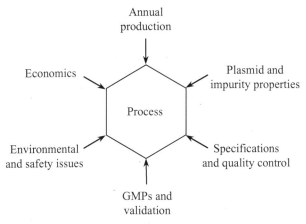

Figure 3.4 *Key aspects in the design of processes for the manufacturing of plasmid biopharmaceuticals.*

(Chapter 11), product specifications and quality control (Chapter 12), available options for the upstream (Chapter 13) and downstream (Chapters 14–17) processing, and process synthesis solutions (Chapter 18). A tentative analysis of the market size will also be made in Part II (Chapter 8). As for plasmid properties, these will be examined in some detail in Chapter 4, whereas properties of some of the usual and most important impurities are discussed in the context of Chapter 12 (product specifications and quality control) and Chapter 14 (overview of downstream processing). In the remaining sections of this chapter, I wish to provide only a short introduction to some of these aspects while simultaneously providing the reader with a bird's eye view of the network of activities and issues surrounding plasmid manufacturing.

3.3.2 Annual Production

A key decision in process development is that of scale. It is important to have at least a rough idea of the annual production (e.g., mass of plasmid DNA) in advance. This will depend of course on the exact size of the target market and on the anticipated market share. In other words, we need to know how many individuals are affected by the disease being tackled and what percentage of these is likely to use the product. Additionally, it is also critical to know the mass of plasmid DNA per dose and the number of administrations of the plasmid biopharmaceutical product per patient and per year. In this context, the potency or biological activity of the plasmid product being developed is of course extremely important since it will ultimately determine the mass of plasmid per dose. The biological and clinical data that are available in the literature indicate that the potency of a plasmid biopharmaceutical depends strongly on the delivery technique used. At present, it is clear that there are delivery platforms that are superior in terms of the efficacy of the plasmid being delivered when compared with others (see Chapter 6). These aspects are briefly illustrated next by considering the case of a hypothetical seasonal influenza DNA vaccine.

Currently, around 300 million doses of trivalent vaccine are produced every year for seasonal influenza.[18] Let us assume for the sake of argument that a successful trivalent DNA vaccine will capture 1% of this market. If a single dose is sufficient for a successful immunization, this translates into 3 million doses of vaccine per year. This number in itself says nothing about the annual amount of plasmid DNA that must be manufactured. In order to have an idea of this figure, we need to know the exact amount of plasmid in a DNA vaccine dose. In one case reported in the literature, the use of PMED technology (see Chapter 6 for further details on this type of delivery) has shown that it is possible to obtain an immune response against flu using a single dose with 4 μg of plasmid.[19] In another case, a clinical trial (identifier: NCT00408109, www.clinicaltrials.gov) sponsored by the U.S. National Institute of Allergy and Infectious Diseases (NIAID) is using a needle-free injection system to administer three 1000 μg doses of a monovalent plasmid DNA vaccine. Although at this stage the data are preliminary, if we presume that those plasmid amounts per dose will be kept in successful products, trivalent flu DNA vaccines would contain 3×4 μg and 3×1000 μg of plasmid DNA per dose, in the case of the PMED and needle-free injection systems referred to earlier, respectively. This means that an annual production of 36 g of plasmid will be required in the first case in comparison with 9000 g of plasmid in the second case. The magnitude of the manufacturing challenge is clearly different in both cases, and the final process solution adopted may well be different, notwithstanding the fact that the disease and market are exactly the same. Anyway, many times, a decision will have to be made regarding the production scale well before the real demand is known.

3.3.3 Regulation

Plasmid biopharmaceuticals, like all medicines designed to be administered to humans or animals, must be manufactured in a way that ensures that the product (1) is fit for its intended use, (2) complies with the requirements of the marketing authorization, and (3) does not place patients at risk due to inadequate quality (safety or efficacy). In order to meet these goals, and thus to receive regulatory approval for new products, the holder of a manufacturing authorization must implement a quality assurance (QA) system that incorporates a set of rules known as current good manufacturing practices (cGMP).[20,21] cGMP regulations cover all aspects of the production, from choosing and testing raw materials to utilities, packaging, shipping, and transferring final products to the clinic (see Chapter 11, Section 11.3). If these items are not in conformity with cGMPs, the product is deemed to be adulterated and cannot be legally approved.[22] One of the cornerstone provisions of cGMPs is validation (see Chapter 11, Section 11.4). This concept has been introduced to assure product consistency from production batch to production batch.[23] The validation of a product, process, activity, procedure, system, equipment, or software used in the control and manufacturing of a biopharmaceutical requires the generation of documentary evidence that provides a high degree of assurance that the item in question performs or meets its predetermined specifications.[23] For instance, downstream processing operations, especially those where a high degree of variability is expected to occur, must be validated to prove that they are capable of consistently removing impurities such as host cell components, process-related materials, and adventitious agents down to an acceptable level.[22] Additionally, acceptance limits and operating ranges for each step must be determined. Another extremely important aspect that needs to be validated is the cleaning of individual equipment items.[23] Validation studies usually lead to optimized processes with reduced variability and, as a consequence, to a decrease in the number of failed batches. Accordingly, the development of a bioprocess (and associated facility) with validation in mind not only helps to improve QA and accelerate approval but usually leads to a reduction of costs.[24,25]

3.3.4 Plasmid Properties, Specifications, and Quality Control

The setup of the bioprocess should always take into consideration the properties of the target molecule and associated impurities. This knowledge is particularly important for the design of the downstream processing, the stage where plasmids are purified by successively removing impurities until the final purity degree is met, since the separation operations involved explore differences in the properties of plasmids and impurities like RNA, genomic DNA, proteins, and lipopolysaccharides (see Chapter 14, Section 14.3). The most important physical-chemical properties and characteristics of the typical plasmid used in a biopharmaceutical will be reviewed in detail in Chapter 4 but can be enumerated in a short sentence: Plasmids are large (2000–10,000 bp, 1320–6600 kDa, micron sized), covalently closed, double-stranded DNA molecules, which are mostly found as a tightly twisted, supercoiled topoisomer. Other features of plasmids are directly inferred from this description: Being made from DNA means that they are polyanionic and have a relatively high thermal stability, whereas their large size translates directly into very small diffusion coefficients. From a downstream processing point of view, the prevailing notion is that plasmids behave pretty much alike and independently of their base composition and size. However, more attention should be given to the presence of subtle plasmid-to-plasmid differences like the presence of local, unusual secondary conformations (e.g., cruciforms, triple helixes, and denaturation bubbles), since these may alter molecule stability and binding behavior.[26] The separation challenges faced during the downstream processing owe as much to the awkward structure of plasmids, as to the fact that most *Escherichia coli*-derived impurities share a number of properties with them: (1) RNA and genomic DNA are also nucleic acids (hence polyanionic); (2)

some RNA species and genomic DNA fragments that arise during the course of processing have comparable molecular weights; and (3) lipopolysaccharides are similar in size and are also positively charged.

The bulk and formulated plasmid DNA obtained at the end of the downstream processing, and fill and finish steps (Figure 3.3), respectively, should be adequately tested to confirm that they meet a set of pre-established specifications. These critical quality standards are proposed by the manufacturer and pertain to parameters like identity, efficacy, safety, potency, and purity (see Chapter 12, Section 12.2). Some of them will depend on the intended therapeutic use and are thus defined during the course of product development,[27] whereas others can be established in advance on the basis of guidelines and quality standards recommended by regulatory agencies. If adequate and approved by regulatory authorities, the specifications proposed by the manufacturer will constitute conditions of approval or rejection of specific production lots. In order to conform to a particular specification, plasmid DNA products must meet certain acceptance criteria when tested according to predetermined analytical procedures. This requires the development and setup of a range of "validatable" analytical methodologies (see Chapter 12, Section 12.3). Some of these analytical techniques are also used to characterize and control the performance of the manufacturing. This control is extremely important, given the focus of cGMP regulations on product and process consistency.

3.3.5 Environmental, Economic, and Safety Issues

Environmental and economic sustainability are as important goals in process development as are achieving maximum yield and purity, ensuring adequate product stability or complying with cGMP regulations. An early evaluation of those two aspects is important since the more advanced the product development stage is, the lower is the freedom to make alterations in the process, given that these might change the attributes of the product being tested in the clinic. The "ecological footprint" of a bioprocess is a concept that is likely to become more and more important in the context of future societies. Bioprocess engineers should consider issues like the amount of waste generated, how it is treated or disposed of, recycling options, and safety, not only due to the increasing strictness of regulations but also because this may well result in a reduction of costs and may contribute to a favorable image of the manufacturing company. A good design will target waste minimization, recycling, or downcycling of materials and will favor the use of environmentally friendly and safe materials.[2,28,29] This means, for instance, avoiding environmentally unfriendly unit operations such as those that produce large amounts of hazardous materials and solvents that are costly to dispose off. Assessment methods can be used early on during development to identify the process steps and materials that cause the most environmental burdens in a process.[30,31] Cost-effectiveness is another specific goal of the bioprocess developer. Options that reduce costs without compromising performance, safety, and quality should always be considered. A correct economic assessment of a process involves an analysis of costs (capital and operating) and profitability. These estimates should be used as one of the key elements in the final decision on which process to select. Finally, processes should also be designed in such a way that the working environment is as safe as possible.[15] Unit operations that require unusual safety precautions like explosion proof tanks, blow-out walls, emission containment, personnel protection, and so on, to operate should also be carefully considered since these requirements can dramatically increase the cost of equipment, building design, and construction.[32] Overall, environmental and safety issues require an intimate knowledge of the process technology solutions available.

3.3.6 Heuristics and Process Synthesis

Bioprocess development is all about making choices.[15] Basically, one has to consider the options available (e.g., unit operations and corresponding operating variables), experiment and evaluate them individually or in combination, and in the end string them together as a full, reliable, and cost-effective process for the production, recovery, and purification of the target product. The know-how accumulated over the years with similar biomolecules is important to narrow down the array of combinations available. Some attempts have been made to crystallize this bioprocessing experience into a number of heuristics[28,33] or rules of thumb. Many times, these can serve as general guidelines for the design and initial drafting of a couple of process alternatives, and for this reason, it is important to be acquainted with them (see Chapter 14 for further details). On top of this guidance, further details of the flow sheet can be established on the basis of the accumulated experience with that product or with closely related ones. In the specific case of plasmids, for instance, the specificities of their purification have been extensively addressed by molecular biologists in their search for methodologies that could rapidly yield vectors with a quality adequate for cloning. These scientists have perfected the "art of plasmid purification" and have developed a range of efficient laboratory-scale protocols, many of which are still used today in their entirety or as part of more sophisticated purification kits.[34] Unfortunately, many of these protocols cannot be easily scaled up beyond the milligram amount nor use reagents that are acceptable for the manufacturing of a biological pharmaceutical. It is nevertheless interesting to realize that many of the process solutions that are currently used to manufacture plasmid biopharmaceuticals integrate modifications or adaptations of steps from these laboratory protocols. Obviously, bioprocess scientists and engineers can find a significant value associated to the skills and practice of molecular biologists. The advent of plasmid-based gene therapy and DNA vaccination has pushed academicians and industrialists into the research and development of methods for plasmid manufacturing. As a result of these efforts, highly valuable information can nowadays be found in an increasing number of articles that deal with the challenge of producing and purifying plasmids for therapeutic applications. Patents and patent applications are also becoming more abundant, and access to them is straightforward in most cases. Clearly, the old "art" of laboratory-scale plasmid purification has evolved into the "science" of large-scale plasmid manufacturing.

3.4 CONCLUSIONS

Bringing a biopharmaceutical to the market, which adds value to patients and the society as a whole, is not an easy undertaking. It involves time, qualified human resources, and capital (i.e., "month, men, and money"). The stakeholders are diverse: companies, patients, doctors, regulatory and other governmental agencies, nongovernmental organizations, pharmacies, and so on. The complexity of the task and the interaction between the different players is even more intricate in the case of innovative products like plasmid biopharmaceuticals, which belong to a whole new class of medicinal agents, and represent a whole new way of treating and preventing disease, that is, gene transfer. Many steps have to be taken along the road, which include testing in animals and humans and getting regulatory approval. Another aspect that is critical to the success of plasmid biopharmaceuticals is the development of manufacturing processes. Apart from the engineering involved, this requires an awareness of issues like GMPs, validation, quality control, safety, environmental impact, and so on, which, to a large extent, constrain and limit the available bioprocessing options.

REFERENCES

1. Rosin LJ. Product development: From aha! to saving lives. *BioProcess International.* 2006;4:6–14.

2. Heinzle E, Biwer A, Cooney C. Development of bioprocesses. In: Heinzle E, Biwer A, Cooney C, eds. *Development of sustainable bioprocesses*. West Sussex: John Wiley & Sons, 2006:11–59.

3. Sheperd AJ. Good laboratory practice in the research and development laboratory. In: Meager A, ed. *Gene therapy technologies, applications and regulations.* Chichester: John Wiley & Sons, 1999:375–381.

4. Lew D, Parker SE, Latimer T, et al. Cancer gene therapy using plasmid DNA: Pharmacokinetic study of DNA following injection in mice. *Human Gene Therapy.* 1995;6:553–564.

5. Parker SE, Vahlsing HL, Serfilippi LM, et al. Cancer gene therapy using plasmid DNA: Safety evaluation in rodents and non-human primates. *Human Gene Therapy.* 1995;6:575–590.

6. Isaguliants MG, Iakimtchouk K, Petrakova NV, et al. Gene immunization may induce secondary antibodies reacting with DNA. *Vaccine.* 2004;22:1576–1585.

7. Northrup J. The pharmaceutical sector. In: Burns LR, ed. *The business of healthcare innovation*. Cambridge: Cambridge University Press, 2005:27–102.

8. Rosin LJ. Regulatory affairs: If you didn't write it down, it didn't happen. *BioProcess International*. 2006;4:16–23.

9. Nabel GJ, Chang AE, Nabel EG, et al. Immunotherapy for cancer by direct gene transfer into tumors. *Human Gene Therapy*. 1994;5:57–77.

10. Rados C. Inside clinical trials: Testing medical products in people. *FDA Consumer Magazine*. 2003;37:30–35.

11. Bren L. The advancement of controlled clinical trials. *FDA Consumer Magazine*. 2007;41:23–30.

12. Swain WF, Fuller DH, Wu MS, et al. Tolerability and immune responses in humans to a PowderJect DNA vaccine for hepatitis B. In: Brown F, Cichutek K, Robertson J, eds. *Development and clinical progress of DNA vaccines*, Vol. 104. Basel: Karger, 2000:115–119.

13. Global Advisory Committee on Vaccine Safety (GACVS). Global safety of vaccines: Strengthening systems for monitoring, management and the role of GACVS. *Expert Review of Vaccines*. 2009;8:705–716.

14. QIAGEN. *QIAGEN plasmid purification handbook*, 3rd ed. Hilden: QIAGEN GmbH, 2005.

15. Scott C. Process development: Turning science into technology. *BioProcess International*. 2006;4:24–41.

16. Przybylowski M, Bartido S, Borquez-Ojeda O, Sadelain M, Riviere I. Production of clinical-grade plasmid DNA for human phase I clinical trials and large animal clinical studies. *Vaccine*. 2007;25:5013–5024.

17. Scott C. Formulation development: Making the medicine. *BioProcess International*. 2006;4:42–57.

18. Ulmer JB, Valley U, Rappuoli R. Vaccine manufacturing: Challenges and solutions. *Nature Biotechnology*. 2006;24:1377–1383.

19. Drape RJ, Macklin MD, Barr LJ, Jones S, Haynes JR, Dean HJ. Epidermal DNA vaccine for influenza is immunogenic in humans. *Vaccine*. 2006;24:4475–4481.

20. European Union, Drug Review Agency. Good manufacturing practices. In: *The rules governing medicinal products in the European Union*, Vol. 4. Luxembourg: Office for Official Publications of the European Communities, 1998.

21. Kanarek AD. *A guide to good manufacturing practice*. Westborough, MA: D&MD, 2001.

22. Doblhoff-Dier O, Bliem R. Quality control and assurance from the development to the production of biopharmaceuticals. *Trends in Biotechnology*. 1999;17: 266–270.

23. Sofer G. Validation of biotechnology products and processes. *Current Opinion in Biotechnology*. 1995;6:230–234.

24. Akers J, McEntire J, Sofer G. Biotechnology product validation, part 2: A logical plan. *Pharmaceutical Technology Europe*. 1994;6:230–234.

25. Tolbert W, Merchant B, Taylor J, Pergolizzi R. Designing an initial gene therapy manufacturing facility. *BioPharm*. 1996;November:32–40.

26. Wells RD. Non-B DNA conformations, mutagenesis and disease. *Trends in Biochemical Sciences*. 2007;32:271–278.

27. Prazeres DMF, Ferreira GNM, Monteiro GA, Cooney CL, Cabral JMS. Large-scale production of pharmaceutical-grade plasmid DNA for gene therapy: Problems and bottlenecks. *Trends in Biotechnology.* 1999;17:169–174.

28. Petrides D. Bioprocess design. In: Harrison RG, Todd PW, Rudge SR, Petrides D, eds. *Bioseparations science and engineering.* Oxford: Oxford University Press, 2003:319–372.

29. Petrides DP, Koulouris A, Lagonikos PT. The role of process simulation in pharmaceutical processes development and product commercialization. *Pharmaceutical Engineering.* 2002;22:1–8.

30. Biwer A, Heinzle E. Environmental assessment in early process development. *Journal of Chemical Technology and Biotechnology.* 2004;79:597–609.

31. Heinzle E, Biwer A, Cooney C. Sustainability assessment. In: Heinzle E, Biwer A, Cooney C, eds. *Development of sustainable bioprocesses.* West Sussex: John Wiley & Sons, 2006:81–117.

32. Marquet M, Horn NA, Meek JA. Process development for the manufacture of plasmid DNA vectors for use in gene therapy. *BioPharm.* 1995;September:26–37.

33. Wheelwright SM. Designing downstream processes for large-scale protein purification. *Bio/technology.* 1987;5:789–793.

34. Sambrook J, Fritsch EF, Maniatis T. *Molecular cloning: A laboratory handbook.* Cold Spring Harbor, NY: CSH Press, 1989.

4

Structure

4.1 INTRODUCTION

The structure of a biological molecule determines its function. Accordingly, it is obvious that the rational development of a biopharmaceutical must rest on a profound knowledge of the structural features of the biomolecule in question. Some of the key worries of those concerned with the development of plasmid biopharmaceuticals are thus inherently associated with structural aspects. For instance, what is the structural form of a plasmid molecule that best serves its biological activity? Additionally, how do we separate this form from other plasmid variants, and which structural properties can we explore for this purpose? Which environmental factors affect the stability of plasmids and why? And how does the structure of a plasmid change when it is combined with a given delivery agent? Some of the most important and striking structural properties and characteristics of plasmids were described in the 1960s, as explained in Chapter 1: Marmur demonstrated that plasmids are made up of DNA;[1] Campbell introduced the notion of circular, covalently closed DNA molecules;[2] and Vinograd described supercoiling.[3] In the subsequent years, studies on the topic expanded, and the subject moved and developed substantially. In this chapter, I review several matters related to plasmid structure. The detailed description and discussion of issues such as plasmid topology, dynamics, and alternate DNA structures are intended to

Plasmid Biopharmaceuticals: Basics, Applications, and Manufacturing, First Edition.
Duarte Miguel F. Prazeres.
© 2011 John Wiley & Sons, Inc. Published 2011 by John Wiley & Sons, Inc.

provide a support for many of the topics that will be presented in upcoming chapters.

4.2 BASIC STRUCTURAL FEATURES

4.2.1 Geometry

The majority of plasmid vectors used in gene therapy and DNA vaccination are covalently closed, double-stranded DNA molecules.[4] The DNA strands are linear polymers of deoxyribonucleotides, each composed of a phosphate group, a pentose (2′-deoxyribose) and a heterocyclic nitrogenous base. The polymeric strands are formed by linking the 3′- and 5′-hydroxyl groups of adjacent pentose molecules in nucleotides via 3′–5′ phosphodiester bonds. The genetic message encoded in the DNA molecule is given by its primary structure, that is, by the exact sequence of the four universal bases: adenine (A), guanine (G), thymine (T), and cytosine (C). These bases can be grouped into the purine (R) class (A and G) and into the pyrimidine (Y) class (T and C). The winding of the two antiparallel DNA strands around each other and around a common axis originates the classical right-handed double helix, a structure first proposed more than 50 years ago by Watson and Crick.[5] The two strands in this double helix are kept together by hydrogen bonds (~2–3 kcal/mol H-bond),[4] which link adenine to thymine and guanine to cytosine, forming the so-called Watson–Crick base pairs (bp) (Figure 4.1). The interior of the double helix is highly hydrophobic due to the aromatic nature of the nitrogenous bases, whereas the external sugar–phosphate backbone is hydrophilic. Since the average molecular weight (MW) of A•T and C•G base pairs is around 660 Da, the average molecular weight, MW, of any double-stranded DNA molecule (hence of any plasmid), which is composed of N base pairs, can be calculated according to the following equation:

$$MW = 660N. \tag{4.1}$$

Although base pairing has always been thought to contribute to the stabilization of the double helix, recent findings indicate that A•T pairing is in fact destabilizing and that G•C adds no stabilizing effect.[6] The current view is that the determinant role in stabilizing and maintaining the two complementary strands together as a double helix is almost exclusively played by base stacking along the helix axis, a net phenomenon that involves van der Waals forces and electrostatic and hydrophobic interactions.[6] According to this new paradigm, the well-known linear relationship between the GC content of DNA and its melting temperature is not exclusively due to the fact that G•C pairs are kept together with three hydrogens bonds instead of two, as in A•T pairs. Instead, 50% of the dependence of DNA stability on GC content can be attributed to the stronger stacking contribution of G•C-containing contacts when com-

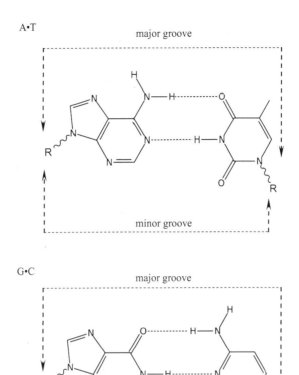

Figure 4.1   *The canonic Watson–Crick base pairs between adenine (A) and thymine (T), and cytosine (C) and guanine (G). Each base is linked to a deoxyribose sugar (represented by the letter R) through the so-called glycosidic bond. The hydrogen bonds are indicated by the dashed lines. The edges of the base pairs, which give rise to the minor and major grooves in double-stranded B-DNA, are indicated.*

pared with A•T-containing contacts.[6] In spite of their stability, the complementary DNA strands in the double helix can be separated by disrupting hydrogen bonds and stacking interactions through the use of elevated temperatures or pH extremes. The effect of temperature on the stability of DNA is fully determined by the effect that that parameter has on base stacking. Thus, since stacking free energies of A•T- and G•C-containing contacts increase (i.e., stacking becomes less stable) gradually with increasing temperature, DNA is more stable at low temperatures.[6]

Double-stranded DNA molecules can adopt a variety of conformations, of which the A-, B-, and Z-forms are probably the most relevant.[7] The existence of these different DNA alloforms is intimately linked to (1) the two alternative conformations that can be adopted by the deoxyribose sugar and (2) the ability of the bases to rotate around the glycosyl bond that links them to the sugar moiety.[4] This leads to differences in the spatial arrangement of the different components of the DNA, and hence to double helices that have different key structural features and geometric parameters. In B-DNA, the most common DNA polymorph one can find inside cells, the base pairs are closely packed and are almost perpendicular to the helix axis. The axial or helical rise, that is, the distance between consecutive base pairs, is approximately equal to $3.4\,\text{Å}$.[8] The total length of a DNA molecule, P (angstrom), is thus readily estimated by multiplying the number of base pairs, N, times the helical rise:

$$P = 3.4N. \qquad (4.2)$$

Since each base pair in a B-DNA molecule is rotated, on average, $34.3°*$ from the preceding, the helical repeat (also known as the helical pitch, h), that is, the number of base pairs required to complete a full 360° helical turn of B-DNA, is around $360°/34.3° \approx 10.5\,\text{bp}$.[4] A distinctive characteristic of B-DNA is the presence of longitudinal grooves, which run along the edges of the double helix. Since the two sugar residues in a base pair are closer to each other from one edge of the base pair when compared with the other (see Figure 4.1), one of the grooves (i.e., the minor groove) is smaller than the other (i.e., the major groove). The bases and their functional groups can be accessed through these grooves and engaged into different types of interactions (e.g., hydrogen bonding, intercalation, and π interactions) with a range of extraneous molecules (e.g., drugs, proteins, and nucleic acids).[4]

When compared with a B-DNA helix, the helix of an A-DNA molecule is broader but shorter along the axis. The mean twist angle between consecutive base pairs is 31°, and thus the number of base pairs required to complete a full 360° helical turn is around 12. Furthermore, the bases in A-DNA are displaced from the helix axis in such a way that the major and minor grooves are deeper and shallower, respectively, when compared with the grooves in B-DNA.[7] Alternating purine–pyrimidine sequences (e.g., multiple CG inserts) may lead to the formation of a specific type of double-stranded DNA known as Z-DNA, which has the particularity of being left-handed. Alongside this change in the handedness of the double helix, Z-DNA is characterized by a smaller geometric diameter of approximately $18\,\text{Å}$ and a larger helical pitch of around $12\,\text{bp}$.[4] The sugar–phosphate backbone follows a characteristic zigzag pattern (hence the name Z-DNA), with every other phosphate group closer to another phosphate when compared with B-DNA.[9] Such a structure is made possible because every other base is rotated around the glycosyl bonds so that *anti* and *syn* conformations alternate along the chain.[10]

---

* Individual twist angles between consecutive base pairs in B-DNA may range from 24° to 51°.[6]

4.2.2 Electrostatics

The phosphate groups in the backbone of DNA molecules are negatively charged at pH values higher than 4. Plasmids are thus polyanionic molecules with an overall net charge, z, which is equal to the total number of nucleotides in the molecule:

$$z = +2N. \tag{4.3}$$

Due to this polyelectrolyte character, the structure and stability of nucleic acids in general is profoundly affected by electrostatic interactions. For example, the screening of the phosphate groups by positive counterions such as Na^+ at high salt concentrations allows the complementary chains in the double helix to come into closer contact. At low salt, on the other hand, the chains are kept further apart by repulsive forces between phosphate groups.[11] The tightening of the double helix as the salt concentration increases is accompanied by a decrease in the helical repeat and an increase in the twist. For instance, changing the Na^+ concentration from 10 to 200 mM has been reported to decrease the helical repeat by about 0.04 bp/turn.[12] This situation can be illustrated with data from the theoretical predictions made by Stigter in his pioneering work,[13] which shows the dependence of the effective diameter of the DNA double helix as a function of sodium salt concentration (Figure 4.2). The figure shows that the diameter of DNA decreases sharply from 223 to 44 Å as the sodium-ion concentration increases from 0.05 to 0.2 M, gradually approaching the geometric value of 20 Å for higher concentrations.[4] These

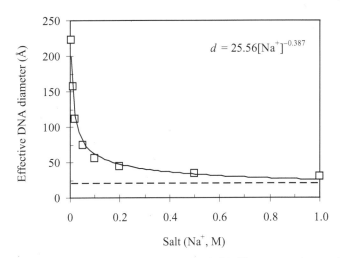

Figure 4.2 Theoretical predictions of the effect of salt (NaCl) concentration on the effective diameter of the DNA double helix. Data points were obtained from the calculations presented by Stigter.[13] The solid line corresponds to a fit of the data obtained with the power function shown.

predictions agree extremely well with experimental determinations (as given in Figure 7 of the paper authored by Vologodskii and Cozzarelli[14]).

The ability of DNA double helices to resist temperature-induced melting is reinforced in the presence of increased salt (e.g., NaCl) concentration. This effect is essentially attributed to the higher stacking free energies (i.e., lower stability) of A•T- and G•C-containing contacts at low salt, since base pairing is virtually independent of the salt concentration. The exact mechanisms underlying this dependence of base stacking on the ambient ionic strength are still unclear, but both the electrostatic component of base stacking interaction (substantial or not) and interactions between highly negatively charged DNA backbones are thought to be involved.[6]

Although the simplest view of DNA in a polyelectrolyte solution assumes that cations distribute evenly around the molecules in a sequence-independent manner, shielding the individual phosphate groups, a substantial body of experimental evidence suggests that cations may preferentially partition into specific sites in the molecule.[15] Such uneven cation distribution may cause a deformation of the nucleic acid both at the global (axial bending) and local (groove-width variation) levels, through a mechanism known as "electrostatic collapse." For instance, monovalent cations such as ammonium have been shown to partition preferentially into the minor groove of AT tracts. This accumulation of cations in a specific locus changes the local charge density and produces the sequence-directed axial bends, which are typical of AT tracts.[16] In solution, divalent cations will compete with monovalent cations, although not necessarily for the same binding sites in the molecule. Furthermore, and although it is more or less consensual that cations stabilize DNA duplexes, it has been proposed that, in some instances, the Mg^{2+} cations located in the minor groove of B-DNA may engage in noncovalent cation-π interactions, pulling out bases like cytosine from the helical stack.[17] Such a cation-π induced base displacement could explain the magnesium-dependent protein recognition of DNA, which is so often observed.

4.2.3 Hydration

The conformations, interactions, and recognition properties of nucleic acids are strongly influenced by the surrounding water molecules. For example, the main DNA alloform, B-DNA, requires the substantial amount of more than 20 water molecules per base pair to maintain its structure. Dehydration past this figure will lead to the reconfiguration of a B-DNA structure into an A-DNA conformation. Structural techniques have revealed that a fraction of the water molecules that are associated with DNA forms well-defined and relatively ordered networks that are usually found in close proximity to the double helix.[18] These water molecules interact specifically with the DNA by establishing hydrogen bonds with several of the hydrogen bond donors and acceptor groups, which are characteristic of the bases and backbone of DNA (Figure 4.1). In the case of the phosphate groups, hydration is concentrated in six well-defined regions and involves the two partially charged and free phosphate oxygens.[19] Consecutive phosphate groups can thus be bridged by water molecules via hydrogen bonding with these free oxygen atoms. The number of potential donors, or acceptors of hydrogen bonds in G•C and A•T base pairs, is six and five, respectively (see Figure 4.1). In the case of purines, for example, two major hydration sites are found in the major groove and one in the minor groove, whereas for pyrimidines, one such site is found in each groove.[18] These sites participate actively in hydration networks, which run alongside the minor and major grooves of DNA. These so-called hydration spines are made of "first shell" water molecules, which bind directly to the bases via hydrogen bonds, and of "second shell" water molecules, which bridge first shell waters.[18] Additional contacts with the sugar moieties are also possible. In some cases, the hydration sites may be partially occupied by ions like sodium.[18]

The hydrogen-bonded hydration spines described above can be considered to a certain extent an integral part of the helix.[20] Other waters of hydration, on the other hand, appear not to have a specific localization in the double helix and are rather more loosely associated with the DNA. Nevertheless, they play an important role in stabilizing the helix conformation statically.[20] According to this view, the removal of hydration water from the helix and its vicinity inevitably leads to an alteration in the DNA conformation. The dehydration of a B-DNA molecule, for instance, may lead to the reconfiguration of the structure into an A-DNA conformation. This ability to change the conformation of nucleic acids by manipulating the hydration water is important, for example, in the context of plasmid DNA purification. An excellent illustration of this is given by unit operations such as salt precipitation (see Chapter 16, Section 16.3.3) and hydrophobic interaction chromatography (see Chapter 17, Section 17.2.6), which rely on the addition of high amounts of so-called chaotropic salts, a process known as salting out. The preferential hydration of the corresponding ions effectively removes hydration waters from plasmid DNA and nucleic acid impurities, promoting a change in configuration, which may result in self-aggregation or binding to a hydrophobic surface. The addition of alcohols to a plasmid-containing solution is another way to perturb the hydration shells and to foster changes in conformation and aggregation (see Chapter 16, Section 16.3.2).

4.2.4 Dynamics

Double-stranded DNA is very stiff at the local level as a result of the strong hydrogen bonding and stacking interactions of the base pairs. Consequently, fragments of duplex DNA that are shorter than a quantity known as the persistent length do not bend easily and rather behave as stiff rods, with small, almost imperceptible fluctuations of individual chemical residues.[21] This persistence length, which is a classical measure of the distance over which the direction of a polymer chain is maintained, is about 500–680 Å (~150–200 bp) in the case of double-stranded DNA.[4] As the length of a given double-stranded

DNA tract increases past this persistent length, DNA fragments in solution start behaving like random coils, adopting a whole range of three-dimensional, bent, or curved spatial arrangements. Bending may also be induced by the association of DNA with specific proteins involved in gene regulation, DNA repair, and DNA replication.[4] The complementary DNA strands are also flexible enough to twist about the double helix axis. This torsional flexibility causes variations in the helical repeat, which have important consequences for the three-dimensional structure of plasmids.[12]

4.3 TOPOLOGY

4.3.1 Introduction

The discovery that the helix axis of the DNA double helix can also be coiled in space, forming a higher-order structure named supercoiling, was made by Vinograd and coworkers in 1965 while they were studying different circular duplex DNA forms isolated from the polyomavirus. On the basis of experimental results that included the analysis of sedimentation coefficients and electron micrographs, the authors identified a "twisted circular structure" containing left-handed tertiary turns. Furthermore, these structures could be converted to a less compact, open circular (oc) duplex by introducing a single break in one of the DNA strands.[3] The "supercoiling" of polyoma DNA described by Vinograd and coworkers was soon observed in plasmids by Hickson et al., who reported on the basis of electron microscopy that an isolated bacterial sex factor was a circular DNA molecule, which similarly contained the tightly twisted and the oc form. The electron micrographs in Hickson's paper probably constitute the first visual record of supercoiled plasmid DNA molecules.[22] Further understanding of DNA supercoiling was subsequently developed by a number of authors who combined mathematics with experimentation.[23] Notable achievements include the definition and application of the linking number concept to DNA,[24] the application of the concepts of writhe and twist to DNA by Fuller,[25] a clarification of these concepts by Crick,[26] and the first description of a DNA topoisomerase by Wang.[27]

4.3.2 Biologic Role and Types of Supercoiling

Supercoiling arises from constraints imposed on the rotation of DNA molecules. The considerable compaction of DNA, which is brought about by supercoiling, provides prokaryotic and eukaryotic cells with a convenient way to store large amounts of DNA. Supercoiling also plays an important role in cell physiology, influencing key regulatory processes such as DNA replication, recombination, and transcription,[28] which require DNA to adopt favorable configurational, dynamic, and energetic states. Events like the transient melting of the double helix, the close juxtaposition and alignment of sites that are

(a)   (b)

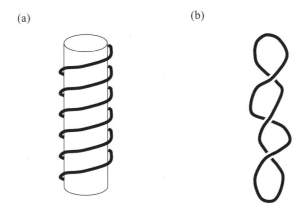

Figure 4.3 *The spatial higher-order coiling of the DNA coil. (a) Solenoidal or toroidal supercoiling: in individual eukaryotic nucleosomes, the DNA is constrained to wrap helically in a left-hand manner around a cylindrical core of eight histones. (b) Plectonemic or interwound supercoiling: in plasmids and in portions of prokaryote DNA, two DNA duplexes wind helically up and down around each other and about a superhelix axis.*

separated by many base pairs along the DNA molecule, or the binding of regulatory proteins are all facilitated by supercoiling.[14,29,30]

There are two major ways in which the DNA helix can itself be spatially coiled. In individual eukaryotic nucleosomes, the DNA is constrained to wrap helically in a left-hand manner around a cylindrical core of eight histones. This so-called solenoidal or toroidal supercoiling is found in the vast majority of eukaryotic DNA (Figure 4.3a). A different type of higher-order coiling is found in plasmids and in a large portion of prokaryote DNA, which is called plectonemic or interwound supercoiling (Figure 4.3b). Here, two DNA duplexes wind helically up and down around each other and about a superhelix axis.[23] Solenoidal supercoiling provides a more effective way of DNA packaging. Thus, and not surprisingly, it predominates in differentiated eukaryotic cells, where, typically, only 5–10% of the genome is being transcribed at a given instant. Plectonemic supercoiling, on the other hand, is more adapted to DNA that is used more actively. For this reason, it is largely found in prokaryotes, where a large fraction of the genome is undergoing transcription and replication.[30] Likewise, plectonemic supercoiling is also a key characteristic of extrachromosomal elements such as plasmids.

Plasmids can be supercoiled to different degrees. In other words, the existence of different plasmid isomers is possible. Since the distinctive feature among such plasmid species is their particular three-dimensional conformation, they are best known as topoisomers. The quantitative description of DNA supercoiling is usually made using geometric and topological parameters. Geometric properties of a given plasmid, like the superhelix axis length or the radius of gyration, may change under deformation of the backbone. The topological properties of the molecule, on the other hand, remain unaltered as long as the continuity of the DNA backbone is maintained. Some of these properties will be described in the subsequent sections.

4.3.3 Linking Number

The linking number, Lk, is a topological property of closed DNA, which captures the complexity of the winding of the two complementary strands of DNA around each other into a single number.[23] Lk is defined as the number of times one strand crosses the other when the DNA lies flat on a plane, and therefore must be an integer.[4] By convention, the Lk of right-handed DNA is taken to be positive.[14] If the free ends of a linear segment of double-stranded DNA of N base pairs are ligated without introducing torsion into the molecule, the number of helical turns is equal to N/h, where h is the number of base pairs per helical turn, that is, the helical pitch.[31] In most cases, N/h is not an integer since the strand ends of a linear DNA will normally require some slight twisting to match precisely.[12] The linking number, Lk, of the ligated DNA molecule described above can then be estimated as the closest integer to N/h:[12]

$$Lk = Lk_o \approx \frac{N}{h}. \tag{4.4}$$

The subscript "o" in Lk in the equation above refers to the fact that the circular DNA molecule is in a "relaxed," torsion-free state. When dealing with plasmids, this particular topoisomer, which has a linking number Lk_o, is known as a relaxed or open circular (oc) plasmid DNA (Figures 4.4a and 4.5). Although

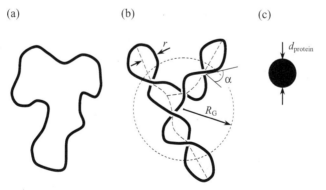

(a)   (b)   (c)

Figure 4.4 *Schematic representations of covalently closed plasmid DNA molecules. (a) A relaxed or open circular plasmid topoisomer is obtained by ligating the free ends of a linear DNA segment without introducing torsion into the molecule. The thick line represents the DNA double helix. (b) A negatively supercoiled plasmid topoisomer is formed if helical turns are removed prior to the circularization of the DNA. The torsional tension created in such underwound DNA helix is alleviated by the formation of supercoils and branches. The scheme assumes a 1050-bp plasmid with $\sigma = -0.06$ (~6 supercoils). The superhelix axis, $L = 1464 \text{Å}$ (Equation 4.15), represented by the dashed line and the radius of gyration, $R_G = 388 \text{Å}$ (Equation 4.17), are drawn roughly at scale. (c) The black circle represents a globular protein equivalent to the 1050-bp plasmid (MW = 693 kDa) in (b) and is drawn at scale ($R_{protein} = 82 \text{Å}$; Equation 4.21).*

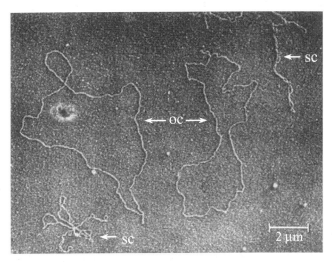

Figure 4.5 *Electron microscopy of supercoiled and open circular (oc) molecules of plasmid R-1 isolated from Escherichia coli. oc and supercoiled (sc) plasmid molecules are seen at the center and at the corners of the photograph, respectively. Reprinted by permission from Macmillan Publishers Ltd.: Nature, 224, Cohen SN, Miller CA. Multiple molecular species of circular R-factor DNA isolated from Escherichia coli, 1273-1277, Copyright 1969.[93]*

h is a function of base composition and of conditions of the surrounding environment like temperature and ionic strength. DNA molecules in solution typically adopt the B-DNA conformation, which has an average helical pitch of 10.5 bp/helical turn[4] (Section 4.2.1). Thus, if we take the case of a 5000-bp-long, relaxed, oc plasmid, for instance, its Lk_o will be equal to 476 ($\approx$5000/10.5; see Table 4.1). This linking number will remain unchanged as long as the phosphodiester backbone in the two strands remains intact, no matter which deformation is imposed onto the molecule. On the other hand, if helical turns are removed or added by applying torsion to the double helix prior to the circularization and closing of the DNA molecule, the linking number becomes different from Lk_o. In the first situation, that is, when helical turns are removed, the DNA is said to be underwound, and $Lk < Lk_o$, whereas in the second case, that is, when helical turns are added, the DNA is overwound, and $Lk > Lk_o$. In either situation, we can define a linking number difference, ΔLk, according to

$$\Delta Lk = Lk - Lk_o = Lk - \frac{N}{h}. \qquad (4.5)$$

The removal or the addition of helical turns changes the average rotation per residue and the helical pitch in the DNA molecule from the standard 34.3° and 10.5 bp, respectively. This creates a torsional tension in the helix, which is associated with an unfavorable Gibbs free energy. In order to compensate for this and to relieve a fraction of the tension, plasmid molecules fold and form supercoils and branches (Figures 4.4b and 4.5), yielding a configuration of minimum energy.[32] This returns the helical pitch and the average rotation per

TABLE 4.1. Quantitative Descriptors of Negatively Supercoiled Plasmid Molecules and Their Corresponding Equations

Parameter	Equation	Number	Example
Molecular weight, MW (Da)	$MW = 660N$	(4.1)	3,300,000 Da
Total DNA length, P (Å)	$P = 3.4N$	(4.2)	17,200
Charge, z	$Z = +2N$	(4.3)	+10,000
Linking number, Lk_o	$Lk_o \approx \dfrac{N}{h}$	(4.4)	476
Linking number difference, ΔLk	$\Delta Lk = Lk - Lk_o = Lk - \dfrac{N}{h}$	(4.5)	−28.6
Superhelix density, σ	$\sigma = \dfrac{\Delta Lk}{Lk_o} = \dfrac{h\Delta Lk}{N}$	(4.7)	−0.06*
Number of supercoils, n	$n = -0.89\Delta Lk$	(4.6)	~25
Writhe, Wr	$Wr = 0.72\Delta Lk$	(4.12)	−20.6
Twist, ΔTw	$\Delta Tw = 0.28\Delta Lk$	(4.14)	−8
Superhelix axis, L (Å)	$L = 1.394N$	(4.15)	6,970
Superhelix radius, r (Å)	$\dfrac{1}{r} = 0.00153 - 0.2689\sigma$	(4.16)	53
Radius of gyration, R_G (Å)	$R_G = 0.1247N + 257.18^†$	(4.17)	881
	$R_G = 0.0895L + 257.18^†$	(4.20)	
	$R_{Goc} \approx 1.4R_G$	(4.18)	1,233
	$R_{Gl} \approx 2.0R_G$	(4.19)	1,762
Area, A (Å²)	$A = \dfrac{\pi}{2}rL$	(4.22)	0.6×10^6
Diffusion coefficient, D (cm²/s)	$D = \dfrac{AT}{\mu}\,bp^{-2/3}$	(4.24)	3.37×10^{-8}

The value taken up by each of the parameters shown is exemplified for the case of a plasmid molecule with $N = 5000\,bp$ and $\sigma = -0.06$.
*Supercoiled plasmids from prokaryotes have σ values between −0.07 and −0.05.
†These equations were obtained by fitting lines to the experimental data shown in Figure 4.7.

residue to the preferred 10.5 bp and 34.3°, respectively. Although this topological reconfiguration partially decreases the unfavorable free energy associated with the linking deficit or excess, the resulting molecule still contains a certain amount of tension. Thus, supercoiled plasmids are thermodynamically less stable when compared with their relaxed counterparts.[33]

If there is a deficiency in Lk, ΔLk is negative and right-handed supercoils or supertwists are introduced—the molecule is said to be negatively supercoiled.[12] If there is an excess in Lk, the ΔLk is positive and left-handed supercoils or supertwists are introduced—the molecule is said to be positively supercoiled. In a way, the structural distortions in supercoiled DNA are equivalent to the tertiary folding of helical segments, which is observable in proteins. The value of ΔLk of a given supercoiled plasmid can be measured reliably using well-established experimental methodologies (see Chapter 5, Section 5.3).

On the basis of site-specific recombination experiments, Boles and cowork-ers[30] have found that the number of right-handed supercoils in a plasmid molecule, n, is approximately equal to 89% of the linking deficit; that is,

$$n = -0.89\Delta Lk. \tag{4.6}$$

The degree of supercoiling is usually expressed in terms of a length-independent parameter, the specific linking number difference or superhelix density, σ, which is given by

$$\sigma = \frac{\Delta Lk}{Lk_o} = \frac{h\Delta Lk}{N}. \tag{4.7}$$

Substitution of this relation into Equation 4.6 yields

$$n = -0.89\sigma Lk_o. \tag{4.8}$$

Plasmid topoisomers isolated from prokaryotes like *E. coli* are negatively supercoiled, typically following a Boltzmann–Gaussian distribution centered at an average value of σ, which falls between -0.07 and -0.05.[4] The heteroge-neity in the superhelix density of plasmids in these populations results from thermally induced fluctuations in the DNA double helix that exists at the time of ring closure.[34] At the average super helix densities mentioned above, a 5000-bp plasmid is characterized by Lk between 442.7 and 452.2 (Equation 4.7), whereas the number of supercoils will vary between 21 and 30 (Equation 4.8, Table 4.1). Electron microscopy images have shown that plasmid molecules with this degree of supercoiling are long and thin, with a characteristic branched shape,[30] as illustrated in Figures 4.4b and 4.5. Such structures are highly dynamic, oscillating between different energy minima, with branches forming and retracting rapidly.[30,32] The size and number of branches are variable, increase linearly with the molecule length, and are affected by the ionic conditions.[30]

The formation of supercoiling requires the deformation of the helix axis and of the turns of the double helix. Such deformations demand energy, and hence supercoiling is associated with an increase in free energy. The free energy of supercoiled DNA, ΔG_s (joule per mole), which is essentially the sum of the energies associated with these deformations, is proportional to the square of the linking number difference, ΔLk, according to

$$\Delta G_s = \frac{1050RT}{N}\Delta Lk^2, \tag{4.9}$$

where R is the gas constant and T is the absolute temperature. This equation indicates that less energy is required to introduce a given linking difference in larger plasmids. Furthermore, any process that somehow favors the reduction of the superhelical stress (i.e., that decreases ΔLk) results in a molecule that has an overall lower free energy (i.e., that is more stable).

4.3.4 Twist and Writhe

The linking number, Lk, can be decomposed into two geometric contributions, the twist, Tw, and the writhe, Wr, according to the well-known White's equation:

$$Lk = Tw + Wr. \tag{4.10}$$

The twist, Tw, is a geometrical property that essentially measures the helical winding of the two DNA strands around each other, while Wr describes and measures the supercoiling of the DNA axis in space. In solution, a given plasmid molecule is constantly changing its conformation (see Section 4.5.1). This means that values of Wr and Tw ascribed to a plasmid molecule are not the property of a unique conformation but rather are average values that reflect the full distribution of conformations that the molecule can adopt.[14] The writhe of a negatively supercoiled plasmid can be related to the number of supercoils, n, in the molecule and to the pitch angle of the superhelix, α, by the following equation:

$$Wr = -n\sin\alpha. \tag{4.11}$$

The superhelix pitch angle α, which is illustrated in Figure 4.4b, has been shown to be nearly constant, with a limiting value equal to 54° for plasmid molecules with values of superhelical density within the typical range.[30] Using this value in Equation 4.11 together with the relation between n and ΔLk expressed by Equation 4.6, it then follows that Wr can be estimated from experimental measurements of the linking deficit:

$$Wr = 0.72\Delta Lk. \tag{4.12}$$

In order to change the Lk of a plasmid, the phosphate backbone must be cleaved by physical (e.g., shear stress and elevated temperature), chemical, or enzymatic processes. In the first two cases, and in the case of enzymes like single-stranded nucleases, once a break or "nick" is introduced, the plasmid molecule spontaneously reacquires the preferred helical twist, that is, $h = 10.5\,\text{bp}$. In the case of specialized enzymes like topoisomerases, on the other hand, supercoils can be added or removed in a more controlled way before the phosphate diester bond is reformed. In any case, Wr and Tw change alongside with Lk. However, the number of helical turns in DNA (i.e., Tw) and the number of supercoils (i.e., Wr) can, and do change, even when Lk is kept constant, since in solution the shape of the double helix and of super-coiled plasmids is not fixed. However, such changes are interdependent as described by White's equation; that is, a change in Tw is always accompanied by a symmetric change in Wr.[12] In the case of relaxed plasmid molecules, no supercoils are present ($Wr = 0$) and White's equation reduces to $Lk_0 = Tw$; that is, the twist is equal to the linking number. In the case of the 5000-bp-long, relaxed, oc plasmid described in the previous section, $Lk_o = Tw = 476$. Suppose that this molecule is linearized and that a number of helical turns, say 7, are removed by untwisting the helix before rejoining the strands' extremities. The linking number difference associated with this change is thus $\Delta Lk = -7$ and hence $Lk = 469$. This change in the linking number will manifest itself geometrically as a change in the twist and/or the writhe; that is,

$$\Delta Lk = \Delta Tw + Wr.^* \tag{4.13}$$

This equation basically states that the linking difference introduced (ΔLk) freely partitions between twist, Tw, and writhe, Wr, provided that the algebraic sum of both parameters remains constant. As we have seen before, the tension introduced in the plasmid is partially relieved via the supercoiling of the molecule. Since Wr can be estimated on the basis of ΔLk, ΔTw is obtained simply by combining Equations 4.12 and 4.13:

$$\Delta Tw = 0.28 \Delta Lk. \tag{4.14}$$

In the case of the 5000-bp plasmid with $\Delta Lk = -7$ described earlier, it follows from Equations 4.6, 4.11, and 4.14 that $n \approx 6$, $Wr \approx -5$, and $\Delta Tw \approx -2$, respectively. For a more detailed description of these two complex geometric quantities (Wr and Tw), the reader should consult specialized literature on the subject.[4,12,14,23]

4.3.5 *In Vitro* Modification of Plasmid Supercoiling

The most convenient and practical way of changing the degree of supercoiling of a given plasmid population *in vitro* is by resorting to the use of (1) intercalators and (2) topoisomerases. Although the net result is apparently the same, that is, supercoils are removed or added, the fact is that the underlying mechanisms are different in both cases, as described next.

4.3.5.1 *Intercalators*

Intercalators are planar aromatic molecules that, as a result of their geometric and chemical characteristics, are able to position themselves at the center of the double helix, forming DNA intercalator complexes that are stabilized by stacking interactions.[4] The use of DNA intercalators in molecular and cell biology in general, and in plasmid characterization in particular (as described ahead in Chapter 5), is widespread. The introduction of these extraneous molecules within the double helix requires adjacent base pairs to move apart

---

* Since the writhe of a relaxed molecule is 0, the difference in this property is designated as Wr instead of ΔWr.

from each other. This leads not only to the axial stretching of the double helix but also to a decrease in the rotation angle between consecutive base pairs. For example, in the case of the intercalator ethidium bromide (see Chapter 5, Figure 5.1a), the distance between the base pairs that flank the molecule doubles from 0.34 to 0.68 nm, and the angle between them decreases 26° from the standard 34° to approximately 10°.[35] In other words, there is an unwinding of the double helix upon intercalation, that is, the number of base pairs per helical turn, h (the helical pitch of the molecule), continuously increases the more intercalator is added. According to Equation 4.4, this means that the Lk_o gradually decreases with an increasing concentration of intercalator.[4,12] On the other hand, since no breakage of the phosphodiester backbone occurs during intercalation, the linking number, Lk, remains constant. In other words, $-\Delta Lk$ decreases (i.e., the level of supercoiling decreases). At a certain critical concentration of ethidium bromide, the plasmid will become fully relaxed. If more intercalator is added past this threshold value, positive supercoils are gradually introduced in the molecule.[4] Although intercalation is the predominant mechanism by which ethidium bromide binds to DNA, as intercalation sites become saturated, weaker binding to alternate sites in the outside of the double helix takes place.

The effect of intercalation on plasmid supercoiling is qualitatively and graphically illustrated in the plots of Lk_o versus Lk shown in Figure 4.6. In such a plot, any point lying on the diagonal line corresponds to relaxed plasmids ($Lk_o = Lk$), whereas points above and below the line correspond to negatively ($Lk_o > Lk$) and positively ($Lk_o < Lk$) supercoiled plasmids, respectively (Figure 4.6a). Consider now the negatively supercoiled topoisomer of a given plasmid represented by the black circle in Figure 4.6a. The linking number difference, ΔLk, is proportional to the length of either the vertical or horizontal segments that connect the circle to the diagonal (Figure 4.6a). According to the description provided above, the binding of increasing amounts of intercalator to a plasmid will decrease Lk_o without changing Lk. In the plot shown in Figure 4.6b, this corresponds to a downward vertical movement of the black circle marked with "1" toward the diagonal. If sufficient intercalator is added, the plasmid becomes fully relaxed (black circle marked with "2") or even positively supercoiled (black circle marked with "3"). The recovery of supercoiling, which is brought about by a partial or complete removal of the intercalator (e.g., via solvent extraction), will correspond to the upward movement of the circle along the same vertical line toward the original position.

The binding of an intercalator, like any other process that removes negative supercoils for that matter, reduces the unfavorable free energy associated with the original supercoiled plasmid. However, the less supercoiled the plasmid is to start with, the smaller is the amount of energy gained upon intercalation of an equivalent amount. The consequence is that intercalators bind with lower affinity (i.e., less molecules intercalate) the lower the degree of supercoiling of the plasmid.[12] In other words, at the same ethidium bromide concentration,

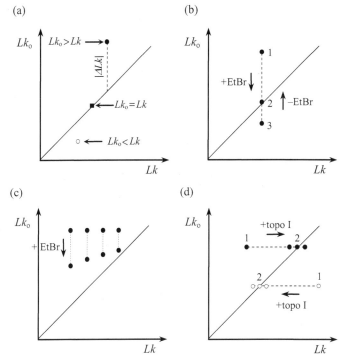

Figure 4.6 In vitro *modification of plasmid supercoiling. (a) In an Lk_o versus Lk plot, points marked above (●) and below (○) the diagonal correspond to negatively or positively supercoiled plasmids, respectively, whereas those that lie on the diagonal (■) correspond to relaxed plasmids. (b) The unwinding of the DNA double helix by intercalation (e.g., of ethidium bromide [EtBr]) decreases the Lk_o of supercoiled plasmids (1 → 2 → 3) without changing Lk; that is, supercoils are removed. Removal of the intercalator restores the original degree of supercoiling (3 → 2 → 1). (c) At the same intercalator concentration, the unwinding of the double helix (i.e., the decrease in Lk_o) is more significant, the more supercoiled is the plasmid. This differential binding is shown by the shorter vertical movement of the more relaxed topoisomers. (d) Topoisomerase I (topo I) relaxation of negatively (●) or positively (○) supercoiled plasmids changes Lk without affecting Lk_o. This is shown by the horizontal movement of the corresponding circles toward the diagonal (1 → 2). The partial or complete relaxation of a plasmid typically produces a Boltzmann–Gaussian distribution of topoisomers (illustrated here by three circles at the positions marked with "2").*

the increase in h (and hence the decrease in Lk_o) is more significant the more supercoiled the plasmid is. This differential binding is qualitatively illustrated in Figure 4.6c by a shorter vertical movement of the circles corresponding to the more relaxed topoisomers of the same plasmid (the ones closer to the diagonal).

Another equivalent way to interpret the topological changes brought about by intercalation is to notice that according to White's equation (Equation 4.13), the corresponding unwinding of the double helix (i.e., a decrease in twist, Tw) must be accompanied by an increase in the plasmid writhe, Wr, in order to maintain Lk constant. In other words, intercalation results in plasmid relaxation, that is, in the loss of supercoils.

4.3.5.2 Topoisomerases

The degree of negative supercoiling in bacterial cells is controlled by specific enzymes called topoisomerases. Enzymes in this category are either able to remove (i.e., increase Lk) or to introduce (i.e., decrease Lk) supercoils in a plasmid. Mechanistically, this requires the breakage and resealing of the phosphodiester backbone. Topoisomerases can be grouped into type I or type II, depending on whether only one or both the strands are broken during the process, respectively.[12] In *E. coli*, the type II ATP-dependent gyrase introduces supercoils, whereas the type I DNA topoisomerase prevents an excess of supercoiling. For a given set of growth conditions, the two enzymes will act synergistically *in vivo* to maintain the supercoiling at a level that is characteristic of those conditions. For instance, an increase in the salt content of the culture media causes a rapid increase in supercoiling, but a nutrient downshift or an extension of growth into the late phase leads to relaxation.[36] Plasmids isolated from cells grown at lower temperatures also exhibit a lower degree of negative supercoiling.[37] Although less common, positively supercoiled plasmids with σ values from +0.006 to +0.017 have been described in a number of hyperthermophilic archaea.[38] The ATP-dependent enzymes which introduce positive supercoils in archaea are known as reverse gyrases.

In vitro, an enzyme like topoisomerase I from wheat germ can catalyze the removal of supercoils either from negatively or positively supercoiled plasmids. Unlike in the case of plasmid relaxation by intercalation, topoisomerase I changes Lk but does not affect Lk_0. Although the net result is also a change in ΔLk, the mechanisms are clearly different. In a plot of Lk_0 versus Lk, topoisomerase-induced relaxation of negatively (black circle marked as "1") or positively (white circle marked as "1") supercoiled plasmids corresponds to a horizontal movement of the corresponding circles toward the diagonal (Figure 4.6d). The partial or complete relaxation of a specific supercoiled topoisomer of a plasmid by a topoisomerase typically produces a population of molecules that follow a Boltzmann–Gaussian distribution around an average Lk value rather than a single topoisomer. This is explained by the existence of thermal fluctuations in the double helix when the strands are rejoined.[34] The materialization of this distribution is illustrated in Figure 4.6d by three circles (black or white) at the positions marked with "2."

4.3.6 Superhelix Dimensions

A plectonemically supercoiled plasmid with superhelix densities, σ, in the −0.07 to −0.05 range, is typically made up of a central interwound core with sequentially distant segments in intimate contact and two or more sharp, hairpin-like ends (the representation in Figure 4.4b is typical). As a first approach, the dimensions of such an irregular shape can be appraised by two

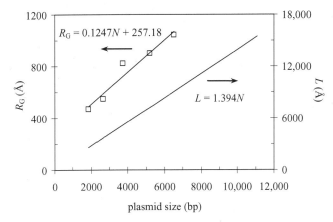

Figure 4.7 *Plasmid dimensions as a function of plasmid size. Experimental data on the radius of gyration (symbols) were taken from the literature: 1868 bp, 468 Å;[79] 2686 bp, 550 Å;[87] 3730 bp, 820 Å;[39] 5200 bp, 900 Å;[14] and 6500 bp, 1040 Å.[94] The line corresponds to a linear fit. The super-helix axis length, L, was estimated by Equation 4.15.*

parameters: the superhelix axis length, L, and the superhelix radius, r. In Figure 4.4b, L corresponds to the sum of the dashed segments that cross the nodes and bisect the area enclosed by the two DNA double strands between adjacent nodes, whereas r is the largest distance between the superhelix axis and the DNA double helix. Using electron microscopy and topological methods, Boles and coworkers have found out that L is independent of the degree of super-coiling and about 41% of the total DNA length* for 3500- and 7000-bp super-coiled plasmids.[30] Since the total length of DNA in a plasmid can be calculated by multiplying the number of base pairs and the average axial rise per base pair (Equation 4.2), L (angstrom) can be estimated by

$$L = 1.394N. \tag{4.15}$$

Given that typical plasmids used in gene therapy and DNA vaccines have a number of base pairs that, in most cases, fall within the 4000–12,000 range, the superhelix axis will thus vary between 5600 and 16,800 Å (Figure 4.7). A comparison of the values of L obtained by the Boles correlation (Equation 4.15) with the diameter of oc plasmid molecules if these were to adopt a per-fectly circular shape, d_{oc} ($=3.4N/\pi$), shows that $L \approx 1.3d_{oc}$.

Boles and coworkers have also determined that the superhelix radius, r, in a plasmid molecule decreases hyperbolically as a function of the superhelix density, σ, and consequently as a function of the number of supercoils, n.[30] The following equation was found to fit the experimental data obtained when analyzing 3500- and 7000-bp plasmids:

---

* Notice that L cannot be larger than 50% of the total DNA length.

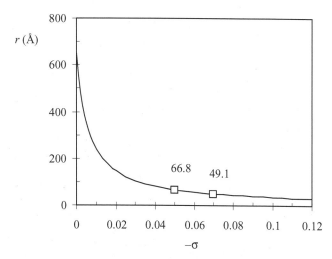

Figure 4.8 *Hyperbolic dependence of the plasmid superhelix radius, r, with the superhelix density, σ, as determined by Boles et al.[30] (Equation 4.11). The symbols and adjacent numbers highlight the radius of the most common topoisomers (−0.07 < σ < −0.05) isolated from prokaryotes.*

$$\frac{1}{r} = 0.00153 - 0.2689\sigma, \tag{4.16}$$

with r in angstrom. The data show that although r decreases sharply as σ decreases down to −0.05, it varies only slightly from 49 to 67 Å within the typical −0.07 to −0.05 range found for plasmids isolated from prokaryotes (Figure 4.8). The fact that the superhelix radius was found to be independent of the plasmid mass is also noteworthy.[30]

4.3.7 Radius of Gyration

The average radius of gyration, R_G, is another parameter that is commonly used to infer the size of plasmids.[14] This quantity is defined as the root mean square average distance of each point in the plasmid from the molecule's center of gravity (see Figure 4.4b). Experimentally, it is derived from a highly averaged set of light scattering data.[39] Figure 4.7 displays experimental R_G values as a function of plasmid size and illustrates that, as a first approach, R_G can be estimated by the linear correlation

$$R_G = 0.1247N + 257.18, \tag{4.17}$$

with R_G in angstrom. The radius of gyration of the corresponding oc and linearized plasmids, R_{Goc} and R_{Gl}, respectively, can be roughly estimated from R_G according to the following relations:[40]

$$R_{Goc} = 1.4R_G \qquad (4.18)$$

$$R_{Gl} \approx 2.0R_G. \qquad (4.19)$$

By introducing the relationship between L and the number of base pairs in a plasmid described above (Equation 4.15), an expression can also be derived to correlate R_G with L:

$$R_G = 0.0895L + 257.18, \qquad (4.20)$$

with R_G in angstrom. Roughly speaking, this last equation shows that the superhelix axis length of a negatively supercoiled plasmid isolated from a prokaryote host is one order of magnitude higher than its radius of gyration.

It is also interesting to compare these plasmid dimensions (L and R_G) with the radius that plasmids were to adopt if they had a globular, protein-like structure. This radius can be estimated using a correlation between the radius of a globular protein, $R_{protein}$, and its molecular weight, MW, such as the one given by Schnabel:

$$R_{protein} = 0.38MW^{0.4}, \qquad (4.21)$$

where $R_{protein}$ is in angstrom.[41] By inserting the molecular weight of typical plasmids in this equation, we readily grasp that "if plasmids were proteins," their dimensions would be much smaller, as schematized in Figure 4.4c.

4.3.8 Area

The adsorption of plasmids onto different types of solid surfaces is often used to facilitate their manipulation and usage. In the context of delivery, for instance, plasmids can be adsorbed onto the surface of gold or polymeric microparticles in order to improve their delivery to the target tissues and cells (see Chapter 6). Additionally, a number of purification strategies like fixed-bed and membrane chromatography rely on the adsorption of plasmid molecules onto the surface of porous and nonporous materials of different types (see Chapter 17). For this reason, it important to have at least a rough idea of the area occupied by a plasmid molecule when it is lying flat on a roughly planar surface. In their landmark study, Boles and coworkers have found that the area enclosed by the DNA supercoils when a plasmid is adsorbed onto a flat surface, A, is related to the superhelix radius and superhelix axis length according to

$$A = \frac{\pi}{2}rL. \qquad (4.22)$$

Combining Equations 4.15 and 4.16, we see that this area is a function of the plasmid size, N, and of the superhelix density, σ:

$$A = \frac{\pi}{2}\left(\frac{1.394N}{0.00153 - 0.2689\sigma}\right) = \frac{0.7\pi N}{0.00153 - 0.2689\sigma}, \qquad (4.23)$$

with A in square angstrom. Using this equation, we estimate that a typical 5000-bp-long plasmid with a superhelix density $\sigma = -0.06$ occupies an area of approximately $62 \times 10^4 \text{Å}^2$.

4.4   ALTERED SECONDARY STRUCTURES

4.4.1   Overview

DNA is a heterogeneous molecule; that is, it has the ability to adopt different conformations.[42,43] Thus, although conformations of the orthodox right-handed B-type, with Watson–Crick base pairing (A•T and G•C), predominate within a plasmid molecule, a whole range of other non-B-DNA configurations of higher energy can be produced locally at sequences characterized by a particular order of bases. Many of these sequences contain some sort of symmetry elements (e.g., direct or inverted repeats) and for the most part are found in noncoding regions.[4] Although at least 10 non-B-DNA structures are known,[43] the most important and studied are probably (1) Z-DNA, (2) stable opened regions, (3) slipped mispaired DNA, (4) cruciforms, and (5) triple helixes (H-DNA). In the first case, Z-DNA, the DNA is fully double stranded, but the geometric parameters of the double helix (e.g., diameter, helical pitch, and helical rise) are distinct from those found in B-DNA (see Section 4.2.1), whereas in the remaining cases, the alternative secondary structures are characterized by a decrease in twist, and hence by a certain degree of single strandedness. In a plasmid, local non-B-DNA structures tend to localize in the apical region of the supercoils.[44]

The presence of specific sequences conducive to non-B-DNA formation in a plasmid does not necessarily mean that the corresponding secondary structures will be present in the molecule. Rather, a number of other factors determine the existence of these alternative secondary structures, namely, the exact nucleotide sequence, the conditions of the surrounding environment, and the presence of supercoiling. Supercoiling, in particular, is especially important because it provides the free energy that is required to generate and maintain the higher-energy, non-B-DNA conformations.[43]

Negatively supercoiled DNA is known to promote the formation and stabilization of non-B-DNA structures. This stabilization can be understood on the basis of the geometric and topological changes involved in the process. A first important notion to be kept in mind is that any B- to non-B-DNA structural transition within a DNA molecule involves some degree of unwinding of the double helix. In a supercoiled plasmid, this negative twist change, ΔTw, will contribute to compensate for the characteristic linking number deficit, ΔLk. This can be appreciated on the basis of the White equation (Equation

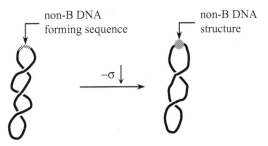

Figure 4.9 *Formation of non-B-DNA structures in negatively supercoiled plasmid DNA. The process is accompanied by the unwounding of superhelical turns, which results in a decrease of the free energy of the supercoiled state and stabilizes the new conformation. Approximately one superhelical turn is relaxed for every 10.5 bp of DNA that forms stably unwound DNA, slipped mispaired DNA, cruciforms, and intermolecular triplexes, whereas two turns are removed for every 10.5 bp of Z-DNA.*[4]

4.13). If the structural transition takes place with no breakage of the backbone, Lk remains constant, and hence $\Delta Lk = 0$. According to Equation 4.13, this means that the sum of ΔTw and Wr is the same before and after the B to non-B transition. For instance, if the formation of a given secondary structure results in the removal of one helical turn of B-DNA (i.e., 10.5 bp), the change in the helical twist, ΔTw, is equal to -1. Since Lk must remain constant, the writhe must also increase by the same amount, that is, $\Delta Wr = 1$. This is equivalent to saying that the structural transition is accompanied by the removal of one supercoil; that is, the molecule becomes partially relaxed (Figure 4.9). This picture may change if other specific sequences (e.g., A-tracts) are also located in the plasmid.[45]

The observation that a number of sequences that are known to induce the formation of non-B-DNA structures (e.g., purine–pyrimidine tracts) are frequently found upstream from eukaryotic genes and in recombination sites, and are overrepresented in eukaryotes, has always constituted an indication that such structures serve important biological functions *in vivo*.[42] This belief has been further consolidated with the discovery of a number of proteins that bind to Z-DNA,[46] cruciforms,[47] and triplexes.[48] The role of some of these non-B-DNA structures in the etiology of human genetic diseases like myotonic disease or Friedreich's ataxia, which involves genetic instabilities such as rearrangements and other types of mutation events, has also been recognized.[43,49] Thus, and in view of the relevance of this issue, the following pages will briefly describe the major features of some of these non-B-DNA structures.

4.4.2   Z-DNA

If a Z-DNA-forming sequence (see Section 4.2.1) is inserted in a plasmid molecule, a B-DNA to Z-DNA structural transition may occur.[4] Since Z conformations are in a higher-energy state when compared with B-DNA, a certain amount of energy is required for the forming sequence to flip from the B- to the Z-form. As we have seen in the previous section, this extra energy which is required to stabilize Z-DNA segments within a plasmid can be obtained by removing torsional stress in the DNA, that is, by removing negative super-coils.[10] In other words, the existence of Z-DNA within a plasmid requires a certain degree of supercoiling. A B- to Z-DNA transition of a region of 10 bp is accompanied by the relaxation of approximately 2 negative supercoils.[4] The coexistence of a Z-DNA region within a B-DNA plasmid molecule requires two junctions to link the right and left-handed helices. Such B-Z junctions are thought to consist of a few (3 to 4) partially unwound base pairs.[4] Thus, although Z-DNA is double-stranded, plasmid molecules with Z-DNA struc-tures may display some sensitivity toward single-stranded nucleases due to the presence of these single-stranded junctions.

A number of studies indicate that there is a strong link between Z-DNA and transcription. The supporting evidence came from the discovery of Z-DNA antibodies which bind to sites of enhanced transcriptional activity, the finding of high concentrations of Z-DNA-favoring sequences near transcription sites and the identification of Z-DNA-binding proteins and respective domains.[10] Although Z-DNA-forming sequences have not been extensively found in *E. coli*, the microbial host used for plasmid production, a number of Z-DNA binding proteins were identified within *E. coli*, most notably recA, a protein involved in genetic recombination.[46] In line with this observation is the fact that the insertion of Z-DNA-forming sequences in plasmids leads to an increase in recombination frequency instability[50-52] in *E. coli*. For example, the construc-tion of several plasmids containing different lengths of monotonous cytosine-phosphate-guanine (CpG) runs was unequivocally associated with a high frequency of deletion events in those regions. Furthermore, the plasmids con-taining those CpG runs were invariably less supercoiled when isolated from *E. coli* than were control plasmids without the sequence.[50] This last observation is consistent with the fact that B to non-B-DNA intramolecular structural transi-tions in plasmids require unwinding of the double helix and are hence accom-panied by the removal of supercoils. The genetic instability of monotonous CpG runs was confirmed in a subsequent study which showed that a number of different deletions occurred in plasmids containing different repetitions of the CpG dinucleotide.[51] Moreover, the interruption of the monotony of the $(CpG)_n$ runs with adenine-phosphate-thymine (ApT) or guanine-phosphate-adenine (GpA) dinucleotides led to a decrease in the rate of deletion within the sequences.[51] One hypothesis put forward to explain these observations cor-relates the instability of the CpG regions with their potential to undergo B- to Z-DNA transitions. According to this model, the formation of the unusual Z-DNA structures within the CpG motifs would trigger an unknown cellular mechanism that originates deletions.[51] Independent of the explanation for the phenomena, the genetic instability of CpG-containing plasmids is especially important in the context of plasmid biopharmaceuticals. This is particularly so in the case of DNA vaccines, since CpG dinucleotides are often introduced in plasmid backbones as a means of stimulating the immune system.[53]

4.4.3 Stable Opened Regions

Regions that are rich in adenine and thymine can potentially form bubbles or stable opened regions. The unwinding of DNA, which characterizes these structures, is more likely to occur at A + T-rich regions due to the weaker stacking contribution of A•T-containing contacts when compared with G•C-containing contacts.[6] These unwound regions are usually associated with replication origins and chromosomal matrix attachment sites.[4,54] Under specific conditions, namely, the absence of Mg^{2+}, A + T-rich regions can be maintained as stably unwound structures in negatively supercoiled plasmid molecules. For every 10.5 bp that is unwound, one supercoil is lost. Such unwound regions can be probed and identified with a single-strand specific nuclease. The addition of Mg^{2+} tends to reverse this situation and promote the reannealing of the strands and the addition of supercoils. Many origins of replication require the presence of nearby A + T-rich regions for the initiation of replication. For instance, the *E. coli* origin of replication, oriC, which is ubiquitous in many plasmid molecules, contains three 13-bp A + T-rich direct repeats, which became stably unwound shortly before the onset of replication. The unwinding of such regions is an important step in the whole process because, in the first instance, it facilitates the access of the helicase protein to the individual strands of DNA. Upon binding to those regions, the helicase further unwinds the double helix, making space for additional proteins to bind (primase, polymerase).[4] If such regions in a plasmid molecule are progressively deleted, the ability to replicate is eventually lost.

4.4.4 Slipped Mispaired DNA

DNA sequences which are repeated in the same strand, that is, direct repeats, can drive the formation of structures known as slipped mispaired DNA or hairpin loops. The opening of these sequences and the subsequent translocation of the pairing between the complementary sequences in the opposing strands can produce two isomeric forms of slipped mispaired DNA (Figure 4.10). In one of the isomers, the target sequences, which are located at the 5′ end of the complementary strands, pair with each other, leaving two protruding loops behind at the 3′ end (Figure 4.10b). In the second isomer, this situation is reversed, with the pairing and loop extrusion of the direct repeats occurring at the 3′ and 5′ ends, respectively (Figure 4.10c). The presence of direct repeats in DNA molecules and the inherent rearrangements are known to drive recombination and mutagenesis events among eukaryotes and prokaryotes.

In the specific case of plasmids that harbor direct repeats, recombination events occur during replication in *E. coli*, which result in the formation of monomeric (M) and heterodimeric forms ([1 + 2] and [1 + 3]). The M form lacks the sequence located between the repeats (i.e., the intervening sequence) and one direct repeat. The [1 + 2] and [1 + 3] forms are head-to-tail dimers,

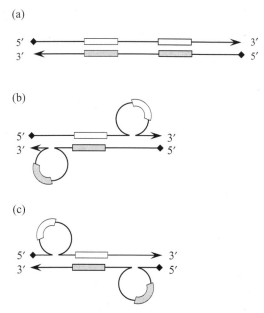

Figure 4.10 *Slipped mispaired DNA. The presence of adjacent or nearby direct repeats in the same DNA strand, shown as white and gray segments in (a), drives the formation of slipped mispaired DNA. Two isomeric forms can be produced following the disruption of hydrogen bonds between the sequences and the subsequent translocation of the pairing between the repeat sequences in the opposing strands. In the isomer shown in (b), single-stranded loops are extruded from the 3′ end, whereas in the isomer shown in (c), the loops are extruded from the 5′ end.*

which combine one native plasmid and one monomeric product, with the [1 + 3] form presenting an additional direct repeat and intervening sequence.[55,56] The frequency of recombination is a function of the length of the direct repeats and of the length of the intervening sequence, which separates them.[57] Additionally, the stress imposed on the growing *E. coli* cells that harbor the plasmid, can profoundly affect the distribution of the recombination products.[58] The fact that this phenomenon occurs both in *recA*+ and *recA*− strains* indicates that in this specific case, the product of this gene is not directly involved in the recombination.[57,59] It is still unclear whether mutation and recombination are driven by the occurrence of slippage during plasmid replication or rather if it is the pre-existing slipped mispaired structures that serve as a substrate for mutagenesis to occur.

These recombination events were observed not only in plasmid molecules that were engineered on purpose to contain direct repeats[59] but also in a commercial plasmid backbone (pCIneo from Promega) and in a DNA vaccine

---

* The disruption of the *recA* gene hampers the expression of a key protein in homologous recombination and should thus decrease the probability of plasmid recombination events.

prototype constructed from this backbone. The recombination frequencies were between 7.8×10^{-7} and 3.1×10^{-5} for DH5α and JM109(DE3) strains, respectively. Furthermore, a quantitative analysis indicated that in a liquid culture of DH5α, 1 out of 13 cells had a molecule of recombined plasmid (in ca. 200–300 molecules of parental plasmid), representing a contamination of about 0.02% in a purified plasmid batch.[58] These results show that caution should be used when constructing a plasmid biopharmaceutical and that attention should be paid both to the transgene sequences being added as well as to the plasmid backbone itself.

Hairpin loop structures may also form within a plasmid provided that certain repeat sequences are present. *E. coli* cells are able to recognize and cleave these hairpin loops *in vivo* via SbcC and SbcD proteins, thus mutating the intervening and flanking regions in the plasmid. This genetic instability can be controlled by modulating the negative supercoil density of the plasmids, as demonstrated by Wojciechowska et al. when working with topoisomerase I ($topA^-$) and gyrase ($gyrB^-$) mutant *E. coli* strains. Specifically, the mutagenesis induced by hairpin removal increased when the mutation favored plasmid supercoiling ($topA^-$) but decreased when the mutation favored plasmid relaxation ($gyrB^-$).[60]

4.4.5 Cruciforms

Adjacent inverted repeats, or palindromic sequences, are widespread among the genomes of pro- and eukaryotes. For instance, they can be found at regions such as promoters, terminators, and replication origins.[47] When present in a DNA segment, these sequences can drive the formation of cruciforms if the appropriate conditions are present. These four-branched structures are formed by the intrastrand base pairing of the inverted repeat-containing segments in each of the complementary strands. In a plasmid, the cruciform presents itself as two hairpin loop harms extruding from the main DNA strands. The presence of unpaired bases at the palindromic center of the sequence, that is, at the tip of the loops, renders the formation of such structures thermodynamically unfavorable.[12] Thus, and like in the case of the non-B-DNA sequences described in the previous sections, the formation of cruciforms within a plasmid requires a certain degree of torsional strain on the DNA, that is, of supercoiling. If such threshold degree of linking difference is present, the structure will form at the expense of the removal of one supercoil for every 10.5 bp involved.[4] The free energy that is lost in the process is proportional to the length of the cruciform. The reversal of cruciforms, on the other hand, requires the introduction of one supercoil and is accompanied by an increase in the free energy.[4] As for the rate of cruciform formation, it depends on the exact base composition and is usually faster with A + T-rich inverted repeats.

Apart from their strong association with supercoiling, cruciforms may also affect the formation of other secondary structures or may directly interact with proteins.[47] Not surprisingly, cruciform structures have been implicated in the regulation of DNA replication and gene expression in various prokaryotic and eukaryotic cells.[44] Upon formation, cruciforms can adopt one of two distinct conformations, which essentially differ from each other by the angle formed between the hairpin arms and the main strands. A more extended conformation is characterized by $90°$ angles, whereas in the more compact, X-type conformation, the angles are acute.[61] The predominance of one or another conformation will depend on the ionic conditions, with the X-type favored at high salt concentrations. The overall topology and the dynamics of a supercoiled plasmid depend on which of the two possible conformations is adopted by the cruciform. For example, atomic force microscopy (AFM) imaging has shown that whereas X-type cruciforms are found mostly at the apical region of supercoils, extended cruciforms have no preference whatsoever. Concomitantly, slithering motions of the supercoiled chains past each other are favored by the extended conformation but are limited by the X-type geometry. The transition between the two forms has been proposed to act as a molecular switch for communication between distant elements in supercoiled molecules.[45]

4.4.6 Triple Helixes

Triple DNA helices can be formed by the binding of a third nucleic acid strand in the major groove of a double helix. The presence of homopurine (or purine-rich)–homopyrimidine (or pyrimidine-rich) sequences at the double helix is a key requisite for triplex formation. If such sequences are present, two types of triplex motifs can form according to the orientation and composition of the third strand. In the case of parallel or pyrimidine (Y·R•Y*) motif triplexes, a homopyrimidine third strand binds to the homopurine strand of the double helix with a parallel orientation.[62] The binding involves the formation of Hoogsteen base pairs (via H-bonds) between thymine (T) and protonated cytosine (C^+) in the third strand, with adenine (A) and guanine (G), respectively (Figure 4.11a). In the case of antiparallel or purine (R·R•Y) motif triplexes, a homopurine third strand binds to the homopurine strand of the duplex with an antiparallel orientation.[62] Here, the binding is brought about by the formation of reverse Hoogsteen base pairs between guanine (G) and adenine (A) in the third strand, with guanine (G) and adenine (A) in the purine strand of the double helix, respectively (Figure 4.11b). The antiparallel motif can also accommodate thymines (T) in the extra strand, which bind with adenine (A) in the duplex. This T·A paring is different from the T·A pairing observed in the parallel motif (Figure 4.11b).

The formation of either parallel or antiparallel motif triplexes can occur within a negatively supercoiled plasmid molecule, provided that the

---

* In Y·R•Y, the symbol • designates a canonic Watson–Crick base pairing between a purine (R) and a pyrimidine (Y) in the double helix, whereas the symbol · designates noncanonical base pairing between a pyrimidine (Y) in the third strand and a purine (R) in the double helix.

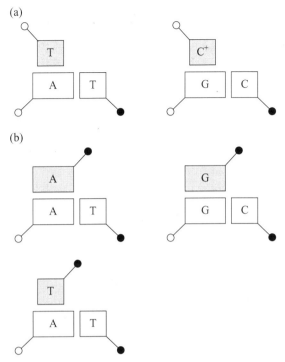

Figure 4.11 *Diagrammatic representations of DNA triplets found in parallel (a) and antiparallel (b) triplex motifs (schemes adapted from Lavery and Zakrzewska[95]). Triplets are formed via (a) Hoogsteen bonds between a third pyrimidine and a purine in a Watson–Crick base pair or (b) reverse Hoogsteen bonds between a third purine and a purine in a Watson–Crick base pair. In the latter case, a T·A•T triplet can also be found, which is different from the T·A•T triplet in the parallel motif. The bases are represented as rectangles (purines) and squares (pyrimidines), whereas the circles represent the strand and the line the glycosidic bond. The parallel or antiparallel orientation of adjacent bases is indicated by circles of the same or different color, respectively. The bases in the third strand are shaded in gray.*

homopurine in one of the strands of the duplex, which is required for triplex formation, is mirror repeated. These palindromes may harbor pyrimidines between the two halves of the repeat. Intramolecular triplexes were discovered in 1985–1986 by Frank-Kamenetskii and colleagues,[63,64] who proposed the two models illustrated in Figure 4.12b,c. According to this model, one half of the mirror repeat must dissociate into separate homopurine and homopyrimidine single strands. Then, two possible isomeric forms of the Y·R•Y type can arise.[64] In the first case, the 5′ end of the homopyrimidine strand must swivel around to bind to the 5′ end of the homopurine tract (H-Y5 conformation, Figure 4.12b). Alternatively, it is the 3′ end of the homopyrimidine that swivels and associates with the 5′ end of the homopurine (H-Y3 conformation, Figure 4.12c). In either case, a parallel triplex motif is formed within the molecule. Although apparently equivalent, structural studies have

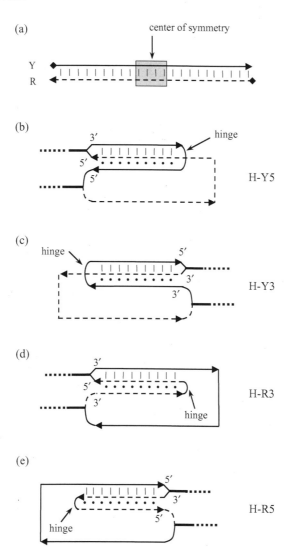

Figure 4.12 *Intramolecular triplex formation. Homopurine–homopyrimidine tracts within a plasmid molecule can originate intramolecular triplexes, provided that there is mirror repeat symmetry (a). The folding back of the homopyrimidine (continuous line) or of the homopurine (dashed line) strand around the center of symmetry of the mirror repeat leads to the formation of two isomers with parallel (b,c) and antiparallel (d,e) triplex motifs, respectively. In the first isomer of the parallel motif (b), the 5′ end of the homopyrimidine strand swivels and binds to the 5′ end of the homopurine (H-Y5 conformation), whereas in the second case (c), it is the 3′ end of the homopyrimidine that swivels and associates with the 5′ end of the homopurine (H-Y3 conformation). In the first isomer of the antiparallel motif (d), the 3′ end of the homopurine strand swivels around and binds to its 5′ end (H-R3 conformation), whereas in the second case (e), it is the 5′ end of the homopurine that associates with its 3′ end (H-R5 conformation).*

indicated that the H-Y3 conformer is usually preferred.[65] Notice that both the portion of the homopurine strand that is left behind and the hinge region that contains the axis of symmetry of the palindrome are single stranded. These two structural features account for the S1 nuclease hypersensitivity of intramolecular triplexes.[64] Although energetically the ideal hinge loop size is four nucleotides, intramolecular triplexes can accommodate more nucleotides in this region.[65] The term H-DNA was used to designate the newly found structures, in part due to the protonation required when the third strand contains cytosines and in part due to the involvement of Hoogsteen base pairing.[4]

Intramolecular antiparallel triplex motifs of the R·R•Y type may also form within plasmids (Figure 4.12d,e), although not as readily as in the case of the parallel Y·R•Y type. Again, and following the dissociation of the palindrome into separate homopurine and homopyrimidine single strands, two isomeric structures can emerge.[4] In the first case, the 3′ end of the homopurine strand swivels around and binds to its 5′ end (H-R3 conformation, Figure 4.12d), whereas in the second case, it is the 5′ end of the homopurine that swivels and associates with its 3′ end (H-R5 conformation, Figure 4.12e).

Two separated homopurine–homopyrimidine tracts that are not mirror repeats and thus cannot form triplexes with each other may nevertheless originate an intramolecular triplex in plasmids, provided that the sequence of the involved nucleotides is the correct one. Such transmolecular triplexes bring distant parts of the plasmid together and give rise to nuclease-sensitive molecules that resemble trefoils, tetrafoils, and dumbbells, which collectively are termed T-loops.[66]

Plasmids that harbor homopurine stretches are known to be more sensitive to the attack of single-stranded nucleases since the intramolecular formation of triplexes results in the appearance of single-stranded regions. Thus, such plasmids are likely to be less stable inside the producer *E. coli* cells. For example, one study has shown that the presence of triplex-forming sequences within a plasmid molecule may lead to a reduction in the relative amount of plasmid in the supercoiled form.[52] This could be associated with the *in vitro* nuclease cleavage of plasmids at the single-stranded regions in the triplex sites. Triplex-containing plasmids may be less stable as well in the nuclease-rich solutions that are encountered during the generation and clarification of cell lysates. The presence of homopurine stretches within a plasmid molecule may also contribute to the formation of plasmid dimers. This propensity has been linked to the putative formation of triplexes under physiological conditions, which would affect the replication process of plasmid DNA.[67] The formation of triple helices between external oligonucleotides and homopurine–homopyrimidine tracts within a plasmid been exploited both for labeling (see Chapter 5, Section 5.2.1) and purification (see Chapter 17, Section 17.2.8) purposes.

4.5 PLASMID DYNAMICS

4.5.1 Configurational Transitions

Supercoiled DNA in solution is not static. Although locally the double-stranded DNA is very stiff as a result of the strong hydrogen bonding and stacking interactions between complementary bases and adjacent base pairs, respectively, plasmid molecules that are larger than the persistence length of double-stranded DNA are highly flexible and dynamic, moving about in space very rapidly. This persistence length, which is a classical measure of the distance over which the direction of the chain is maintained, is about 500 Å (~150 bp) for the case of double-stranded DNA. Thus, and unlike the typical 2- to 10-nm-wide globular protein, which tends to maintain its structure and shape within close boundaries, the micron-sized (>0.1 μm) interwound and super-coiled plasmids freely coil in solution under the influence of Brownian motion. Through a series of bending, twisting, and stretching motions, plasmids reconfigure themselves constantly, with continuous curving of the chain and with branches forming and retracting frequently.[30,32] Such global rearrangements affect geometric properties like the writhe, Wr, the radius of gyration, R_G, and the superhelix length, L, but not a topological property like the linking number, Lk.[68] This means that molecules of a plasmid topoisomer with a specific super-helix density, σ, adopt an enormous variety of energetically accessible, rather irregular, and dynamic conformations in solution. This behavior can be illustrated with molecular images of representative configurations obtained by dynamic simulations of a 1000-bp-long supercoiled DNA molecule in solution (Figure 4.13). The succession of images shown illustrates the transition between an initial three-lobed branched supercoiled DNA form and a final two-lobed interwound structure. The timescales of the motions are in the nanosecond time domain (see original reference for further details).[21]

4.5.2 Site Juxtaposition

Together with supercoiling, the dynamic motions of plasmids contribute to bringing two or more distant sites in a plasmid molecule into proximity (compare Figure 4.14a,b), a mechanism that is thought to be important in processes that regulate replication, recombination, and transcription. For instance, many regulatory proteins involved in such DNA transactions often bind simultaneously to multiple sites on DNA, forming specialized nucleoprotein complexes.[69] Even so, the large-scale distortion of a plasmid DNA molecule required to approximate some sites that are far apart, for example, in the tip of opposing loops, may be energetically unfavorable (Figure 4.14c). In these cases, the sites can be brought into contact through an alternative mechanism known as slithering, in which the base pairs drift in concert along the direction of the central axis until they eventually meet (Figure 4.14d). During this conveyor-belt-like motion of the bases through the supercoil, the global

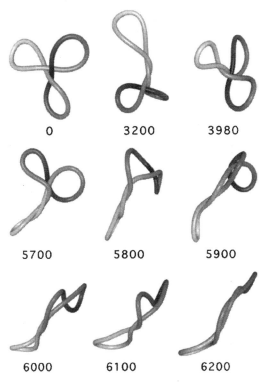

Figure 4.13 Simulation of the dynamic motions of a plasmid molecule. Molecular images of representative configurations obtained by dynamic simulations of a 1000-bp-long supercoiled DNA molecule. The successive images shown illustrate the motions and conversion of an initial three-lobed branched form, and the detailed transition between branched and interwound states, found by simulation. The iteration number (associated with a physical time step of the order of nanoseconds) is shown bellow each image. Reprinted from Biophysical Journal, 73, Liu G, Schlick T, Olson AJ, Olson WK. Configurational transitions in Fourier series-represented DNA supercoils, 1742-1762, Copyright 1997,[21] with permission from Elsevier.

geometry is maintained more or less fixed.[68,70] Molecular dynamics simulations have indicated that the direction of slithering is likely to reverse now and then. Further information gathered from numerical simulations has shown that the local concentration of one particular DNA site near another site, which is separated by at least one persistence length (~50 nm, 150 bp), is around two orders of magnitude greater in supercoiled plasmid DNA than in relaxed DNA. Furthermore, this increase does not appear to depend strongly on the separation between the two sites along the contour.[29] Experimental data also support this, as described in a study on the effect of supercoiling on the stabilization of complexes of the *lac* repressor with DNA molecules containing multiple operator sites. The authors have found that complexes formed by bringing together two operator sites in a supercoiled plasmid, which are approximately 400 bp apart, have a 10-fold longer half-life when compared with their relaxed counterparts.[71]

(a)   (b)

(c)   (d)

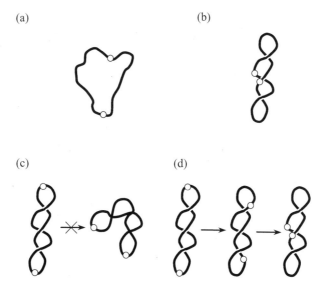

Figure 4.14 *Plasmid dynamics and site juxtaposition. Two distant sites (white circles) in a relaxed plasmid (a) can be brought into close proximity upon supercoiling of the molecule (b). The approximation of two sites that remain far apart after supercoiling, for example, at the loop tips, via the large-scale bending of the plasmid molecule is less likely to occur due to the unfavorable energy change associated (c). In this case, the base pairs can drift in concert along the supercoil through a conveyor-belt-like motion known as slithering, while the global geometry is maintained more or less fixed (d).*

The greater ability of supercoiled plasmids to bring distant sites into proximity and thus to facilitate the binding of regulatory proteins like transcription factors,[72] when compared with relaxed plasmids, provides one explanation for the superior biological activity of the former topoisomers. This biological activity has been measured both in terms of the *in vitro* expression of the transgene[72,73] and of the *in vivo* immunogenicity.[73,74] This recurrent finding is one of the major reasons for the existence of recommendations from regulatory agencies that stress the need for the proportion of the supercoiled isoform in plasmid biopharmaceuticals to be determined and for specifications to be set.[75] Such specifications usually indicate that products should be highly enriched in the supercoiled topoisomer[76] (see Chapter 12, Section 12.3.3).

4.5.3 Effect of Salt

The polyelectrolyte nature of plasmids (and of nucleic acid impurities) renders the structure of these molecules highly susceptible to the presence of ions, as described in Section 4.2.2 and illustrated in Figure 4.2. Thus, and not surprisingly, charge is one of the characteristics that have been explored the most in separation and purification operations (Chapters 14–17). Due to their high charge density, plasmids will readily bind to negatively charged ligands such as those present in anionic matrices like beads and membranes. The addition of salts is the most common way used to modulate such interactions and for this reason, it is important to have an idea of the effect that common cations like Na^+ and Mg^{2+} have on plasmid structure.

As described in Section 4.2.2, an increase in salt (e.g., NaCl) concentration leads to a decrease of the helical repeat of the double helix, h. In the case of a supercoiled plasmid, this will correspond to an increase in the value of Lk_o (Equation 4.4). Since the continuity of the sugar–phosphate backbone is not affected by salt addition, the Lk of the plasmid remains constant. The net result is thus an increase in the linking difference ΔLk; that is, the degree of super-coiling increases.[77] As a consequence of this, distant segments of the double helix that have come into proximity via supercoiling become even closer as the phosphate groups are screened by counterions upon salt addition. This effect of salt on the structure and energetics of supercoiled DNA forms was investigated in detail with computer modeling techniques.[11] These molecular dynamics simulations have shown that the motions of supercoiled DNA are more rigid at high salt, whereas at low salt, the loosely coiled DNA is more dynamic.[11] At high salt, regions where parts of the DNA chain are in intimate contact predominate. At low salt, contacts between sequentially distant segments of the DNA are scarce, with only occasional associations. Under these conditions, parts of the DNA also appear to slither more frequently and rapidly past one another. These simulations indicate that the DNA supercoils change from loose to tight supercoils as the salt concentration approaches the critical 0.1 M value. As an example of this behavior, Figure 4.15 shows the simulated forms of a 1000-bp-long double-stranded, covalently closed DNA molecule at different salt concentrations. It is readily apparent from the molecular configurations obtained that as the salt concentration increases from 5 to

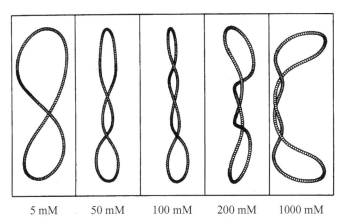

| 5 mM | 50 mM | 100 mM | 200 mM | 1000 mM |

Figure 4.15 *Effect of salt on the structure of supercoiled plasmid. The graphics show simulated forms of a 1000-bp-long double-stranded, covalently closed DNA molecule, at $\Delta Lk = 5$ and different salt concentrations. Reprinted from Biophysical Journal, 67, Schlick T, Li B, Olson WK. The influence of salt on the structure and energetics of supercoiled DNA, 2146-2166, Copyright 1994,[11] with permission from Elsevier.*

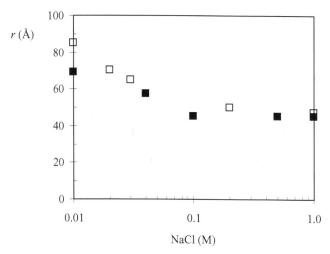

Figure 4.16 *Effect of the salt (NaCl) concentration over the superhelix radius of supercoiled plasmids. Experimental data were taken from Rybenkov et al.[78] (□) and Hammermann et al.[79] (■).*

100 mM, the DNA becomes more compact and tightly interwound, whereas at low salt, the DNA supercoils are much looser.[11] The simulations further show that the extremities of the plasmid molecule bend and the middle segments approach each other as salt is increased to 1000 mM.[11] These theoretical predictions agree rather well with a series of experimental determinations[78,79] which indicate that the superhelix radius of supercoiled plasmids typically varies with the NaCl concentration over the 0- to 100-mM range, flattening off at around 45–50 Å for NaCl > 100 mM (Figure 4.16). Thus, the size of plasmids can also be controlled to some extent by manipulating the concentration and the type of salt in solution. Since the salt concentrations used in plasmid bioprocessing buffers are typically in the 100 mM to 2.0 M range, it is reasonable to assume that $r \approx 50$ Å. When mixed solutions of NaCl and $MgCl_2$ are used, the Na^+ and Mg^{2+} ions will compete for binding DNA. Since magnesium ions have a 100-fold higher affinity for DNA than sodium ions, a more pronounced effect of $MgCl_2$ on the plasmid structures should be expected when compared with NaCl.[77] The experimental determination of sedimentation coefficients of supercoiled plasmids also supports this picture: as NaCl concentration increases, the supercoils become less regular and more compact.[78]

4.5.4 Diffusion Coefficients

The highly dynamic behavior described above determines to some extent how a population of plasmid molecules diffuses from regions of higher concentration to lower concentration, whether these gradients are found in a free solution, within a porous material, or in the extracellular space. Translational plasmid diffusion is particularly important in the context of the design, analysis, and operation of downstream processing operations that involve porous media such as membrane[80,81] and fixed-bed chromatography[82,83] (see Chapter 17). An adequate knowledge of free diffusion may also contribute to a better understanding of the extra- and intracellular trafficking events that are associated with plasmid-mediated gene transfer.[84] This said, it is clear that diffusion coefficients are one of the most important molecular properties of plasmids. However, the enormous variety of irregular shapes and the highly dynamic behavior of plasmids described in the previous section make both the experimental determination and the theoretical prediction of plasmid diffusion coefficients a complicated task. The experimental determination of plasmid diffusion coefficients usually requires the use of sophisticated techniques such as Brownian motion tracking of single molecules[85] or, more often, dynamic light scattering (see Chapter 5, Section 5.4.2).[39,86–88] With these techniques, it is possible to obtain structural and dynamic information of a number of plasmid DNA molecules undergoing conformational and orientational fluctuations. Useful information is then retrieved by adequately treating and averaging this data, usually in terms of statistical mechanics.[14,39] Dynamic light scattering, for instance, can yield estimates of plasmid properties like the molecular weight, MW, average radius of gyration, R_G, and diffusion coefficient, D.[14,39]

The typical diffusion coefficient of a supercoiled plasmid DNA molecule in a dilute solution is of the order of 10^{-8} cm^2/s,[39] while that of a protein with an equivalent mass is one order of magnitude larger.[89,90] This essentially reflects the differences in size and structure between plasmids and proteins. This difference in the magnitude of diffusion coefficients is further stressed in Figure 4.17, which displays a sample of experimental diffusion coefficients of plasmids (determined on the basis of light scattering) and globular proteins, as a function of the molecular weight.[91] A direct consequence of this discrepancy is that popular correlations used to estimate protein diffusion coefficients, like those proposed by Young et al.,[92] Tyn and Gusek,[89] or He and Niemeyer[90] cannot be extended to plasmids per se. This problem has been addressed recently and, as a result, a correlation has been proposed that enables the prediction of the diffusion coefficient of supercoiled plasmid molecules in dilute solutions (<100 μg/mL) with an average error of 6.3%.[91] The number of base pairs of the plasmid, a parameter that is readily available, is used as the single input parameter in the correlation that takes the form

$$D = \frac{AT}{\mu} N^{-2/3}, \tag{4.24}$$

where D (square centimeter per second) is the diffusion coefficient; T (K) is the temperature; μ (pascal second) is the solution; and A is an empirical constant approximately equal to 3.31×10^{-11}. This value of A was estimated by fitting Equation 4.24 to experimental plasmid diffusion coefficients collected from literature on the subject.[91] The 18 data points used correspond to supercoiled

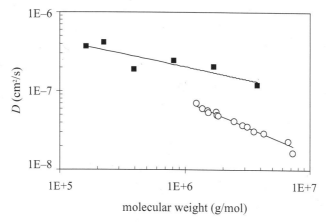

Figure 4.17 *Plasmid diffusion coefficients as a function of plasmid size. Experimental diffusion coefficients of plasmids (○) and proteins (■) are shown, together with predictions for plasmids obtained with the correlation in Equation 4.24 (solid line). Plasmid diffusion coefficients were taken from Prazeres,[91] and protein (γ-globulin, catalase, fibrinogen, R2-myoglobin, satellite tobacco necrosis virus, and pyruvate dehydrogenase) diffusion coefficients were taken from He and Niemeyer.[90]*

plasmids with a number of base pairs ranging from 1800 to 287,100, which were isolated from *E. coli* cells. Experimental determination was typically performed at pH 7–8 and 20°C, with dilute solutions (<100 μg/mL) supplemented with NaCl up to concentrations within 10–150 mM. The temperature, T, and the solution viscosity, μ, were assumed equal to 298 K and 10^{-3} Pa·s, respectively. The correlation can be written as well in the form $D \propto MW^{-2/3}$, since the number of base pairs of the plasmid molecule can be readily converted to molecular weight, MW (Equation 4.1).

4.6 CONCLUSIONS

Plasmids isolated from *E. coli* adopt a topological conformation, which is characterized by the right-handed (i.e., negative) supercoiling of the double helix in space. Molecules in this configuration are long, thin, and sometimes branched. The length of the superhelix axis is typically around 41% of the total length of the DNA, independent of the degree of supercoiling of the molecule. As for the superhelix radius, and although it varies significantly with the supercoiling degree, it assumes values of the order of 50 Å for the average superhelix density of plasmids isolated from *E. coli*. The area circumscribed by the double helix of a plasmid when the molecule lies flat on a plane is a function of both the number of base pairs and of the superhelix density, and usually assumes values of the order of 10^6 Å^2. Supercoiled plasmid molecules are highly dynamic, moving about in space as a consequence of Brownian motion, rotating, bending, branching, and slithering. This enables distant sites in the molecule to come into close proximity. The structure of supercoiled plasmids and, namely, the superhelix radius, is strongly affected by the ionic composition of the surrounding environment. The large mass of plasmids ($>10^6$ Da) translates directly into diffusion coefficients of the order of 10^{-8} cm^{2}s^{-1}. The free energy of supercoiling can drive the formation of higher-energy, non-B-DNA structures like Z-DNA, H-DNA, hairpin loops, or cruciforms within a plasmid molecule, provided that the required base sequence is present. Such local structures are usually characterized by a certain degree of single strandedness, which may render plasmids more prone to nuclease degradation, whereas others are implicated in recombination events. For these reasons, such sequences should, in principle, be eliminated from plasmid biopharmaceuticals.

REFERENCES

1. Marmur J, Rownd R, Falkow S, Baron LS, Schildkraut C, Doty P. The nature of intergeneric episomal infection. *Proceedings of the National Academy of Sciences of the United States of America*. 1961;47:972–979.

2. Campbell A. Episomes. *Advances in Genetics*. 1962;11:101–145.

3. Vinograd J, Lebowitz J, Radloff R, Watson R, Laipis P. The twisted circular form of polyomä viral DNA. *Proceedings of the National Academy of Sciences of the United States of America*. 1965;53:1104–1111.

4. Sinden RR. *DNA structure and function*. San Diego, CA: Academic Press, 1994.

5. Watson JD, Crick FH. Molecular structure of nucleic acids: A structure for deoxyribose nucleic acid. *Nature*. 1953;171:737–738.

6. Yakovchuk P, Protozanova E, Frank-Kamenetskii MD. Base-stacking and base-pairing contributions into thermal stability of the DNA double helix. *Nucleic Acids Research*. 2006;34:564–574.

7. Dickerson RE. DNA structure from A to Z. *Methods in Enzymology*. 1992; 211:67–111.

8. Neidle S. *Oxford handbook of nucleic acid structure*. Oxford: Oxford Science Publications, 1999.

9. Johnston BH. Generation and detection of Z-DNA. *Methods in Enzymology*. 1992;211:127–158.

10. Rich A, Zhang S. Timeline: Z-DNA: The long road to biological function. *Nature Reviews. Genetics*. 2003;4:566–572.

11. Schlick T, Li B, Olson WK. The influence of salt on the structure and energetics of supercoiled DNA. *Biophysical Journal*. 1994;67:2146–2166.

12. Bates AD, Maxwell A. *DNA topology*, 2nd ed. Oxford: Oxford University Press, 2005.

13. Stigter D. Interactions of highly charged colloidal cylinders with applications to double-stranded DNA. *Biopolymers*. 1977;16:1435–1448.

14. Vologodskii AV, Cozzarelli NR. Conformational and thermodynamic properties of supercoiled DNA. *Annual Review of Biophysics and Biomolecular Structure*. 1994;23:609–643.

15. McFail-Isom L, Sines CC, Williams LD. DNA structure: Cations in charge? *Current Opinion in Structural Biology*. 1999;9:298–304.

16. Hud NV, Sklenar V, Feigon J. Localization of ammonium ions in the minor groove of DNA duplexes in solution and the origin of DNA A-tract bending. *Journal of Molecular Biology*. 1999;286:651–660.

17. McFail-Isom L, Shui X, Williams LD. Divalent cations stabilize unstacked conformations of DNA and RNA by interacting with base pi systems. *Biochemistry*. 1998;37:17105–17111.

18. Berman HM, Schneider B. Nucleic acid hydration. In: Neidle S, ed. *Oxford handbook of nucleic acid structure*. Oxford: Oxford Science Publications, 1999: 295–312.

19. Schneider B, Patel K, Berman HM. Hydration of the phosphate group in double-helical DNA. *Biophysical Journal*. 1998;75:2422–2434.

20. Chen YZ, Prohofsky EW. Synergistic effects in the melting of DNA hydration shell: Melting of the minor groove hydration spine in poly(dA).poly(dT) and its effect on base pair stability. *Biophysical Journal*. 1993;64:1385–1393.

21. Liu G, Schlick T, Olson AJ, Olson WK. Configurational transitions in Fourier series-represented DNA supercoils. *Biophysical Journal*. 1997;73:1742–1762.

22. Hickson FT, Roth TF, Helinski DR. Circular DNA forms of a bacterial sex factor. *Proceedings of the National Academy of Sciences of the United States of America*. 1967;58:1731–1738.

23. Cozzarelli NR, Boles TC, White JH. Primer on the topology and geometry of DNA supercoiling. In: Cozzarelli NR, Wang JC, eds. *DNA topology and its biological effects*. New York: Cold Spring Harbor Laboratory Press, 1990:139–184.

24. Glaubiger D, Hearst JE. Effect of superhelical structure on the secondary structure of DNA rings. *Biopolymers*. 1967;5:691–696.

25. Fuller FB. The writhing number of a space curve. *Proceedings of the National Academy of Sciences of the United States of America*. 1971;68:815–819.

26. Crick FH. Linking numbers and nucleosomes. *Proceedings of the National Academy of Sciences of the United States of America*. 1976;73:2639–2643.

27. Wang JC. Interaction between DNA and an *Escherichia coli* protein omega. *Journal of Molecular Biology*. 1971;55:523–533.

28. Pruss GJ, Drlica K. DNA supercoiling and prokaryotic transcription. *Cell*. 1989;56:521–523.

29. Vologodskii AV, Levene SD, Klenin KV, Frank-Kamenetskii M, Cozzarelli NR. Conformational and thermodynamic properties of supercoiled DNA. *Journal of Molecular Biology*. 1992;227:1224–1243.

30. Boles TC, White JH, Cozzarelli NR. Structure of plectonemically supercoiled DNA. *Journal of Molecular Biology*. 1990;213:931–951.

31. Bowater R, Aboul-Ela F, Lilley DM. Two-dimensional gel electrophoresis of circular DNA topoisomers. *Methods in Enzymology*. 1992;212:105–120.

32. Olson WK. DNA higher-order structures. In: Neidle S, ed. *Oxford handbook of nucleic acid structure*. Oxford: Oxford Science Publications, 1999:499–531.

33. Thumm W, Seidl A, Hinz HJ. Energy-structure correlations of plasmid DNA in different topological forms. *Nucleic Acids Research*. 1988;16:11737–11757.

34. Keller W. Determination of the number of superhelical turns in simian virus 40 DNA by gel electrophoresis. *Proceedings of the National Academy of Sciences of the United States of America*. 1975;72:4876–4880.

35. Hayashi M, Harada Y. Direct observation of the reversible unwinding of a single DNA molecule caused by the intercalation of ethidium bromide. *Nucleic Acids Research*. 2007;35:e125.

36. Drlica K. Control of bacterial DNA supercoiling. *Molecular Microbiology*. 1992;6:425–433.

37. Goldstein E, Drlica K. Regulation of bacterial DNA supercoiling: Plasmid linking numbers vary with growth temperature. *Proceedings of the National Academy of Sciences of the United States of America*. 1984;81:4046–4050.

38. Lopez-Garcia P, Forterre P. DNA topology in hyperthermophilic archaea: Reference states and their variation with growth phase, growth temperature, and temperature stresses. *Molecular Microbiology*. 1997;23:1267–1279.

39. Fishman DM, Patterson GD. Light scattering studies of supercoiled and nicked DNA. *Biopolymers*. 1996;38:535–552.

40. Latulippe DR, Zydney AL. Elongational flow model for transmission of supercoiled plasmid DNA during membrane ultrafiltration. *Journal of Membrane Science*. 2009;329:201–208.

41. Schnabel R, Langer P, Breitenbach S. Separation of protein mixtures by Bioran® porous glass membranes. *Journal of Membrane Science*. 1988;36:55–66.

42. Wells RD. Unusual DNA structures. *The Journal of Biological Chemistry*. 1988;263:1095–1098.

43. Wells RD. Non-B DNA conformations, mutagenesis and disease. *Trends in Biochemical Sciences*. 2007;32:271–278.

44. Oussatcheva EA, Pavlicek J, Sankey OF, Sinden RR, Lyubchenko YL, Potaman VN. Influence of global DNA topology on cruciform formation in supercoiled DNA. *Journal of Molecular Biology*. 2004;338:735–743.

45. Shlyakhtenko LS, Hsieh P, Grigoriev M, Potaman VN, Sinden RR, Lyubchenko YL. A cruciform structural transition provides a molecular switch for chromosome structure and dynamics. *Journal of Molecular Biology*. 2000;296:1169–1173.

46. Blaho JA, Wells RD. Left-handed Z-DNA binding by the recA protein of *Escherichia coli*. *The Journal of Biological Chemistry*. 1987;262:6082–6088.

47. Pearson CE, Zorbas H, Price GB, Zannis-Hadjopoulos M. Inverted repeats, stem-loops, and cruciforms: Significance for initiation of DNA replication. *Journal of Cell Biochemistry*. 1996;63:1–22.

48. Musso M, Nelson LD, Van Dyke MW. Characterization of purine-motif triplex DNA-binding proteins in HeLa extracts. *Biochemistry*. 1998;37:3086–3095.

49. Bacolla A, Wells RD. Non-B DNA conformations, genomic rearrangements, and human disease. *The Journal of Biological Chemistry*. 2004;279:47411–47414.

50. Klysik J, Stirdivant SM, Wells RD. Left-handed DNA: Cloning, characterization, and instability of inserts containing different lengths of (dC-dG) in *Escherichia coli*. *The Journal of Biological Chemistry*. 1982;257:10152–10158.

51. Bichara M, Schumacher S, Fuchs RP. Genetic instability within monotonous runs of CpG sequences in *Escherichia coli*. *Genetics*. 1995;140:897–907.

52. Cooke JR, McKie EA, Ward JM, Keshavarz-Moore E. Impact of intrinsic DNA structure on processing of plasmids for gene therapy and DNA vaccines. *Journal of Biotechnology.* 2004;114:239–254.

53. Sato Y, Roman M, Tighe H, et al. Immunostimulatory DNA sequences necessary for effective intradermal gene immunization. *Science.* 1996;273:352–354.

54. Summers DK. *The biology of plasmids.* London: Blackwell Science, 1996.

55. Lovett ST, Drapkin PT, Sutera VA, Gluckman-Peskind TJ. A sister-strand exchange mechanism for recA-independent deletion of repeated DNA sequences in *Escherichia coli. Genetics.* 1993;135:631–642.

56. Feschenko VV, Lovett ST. Slipped misalignment mechanisms of deletion formation: Analysis of deletion endpoints. *Journal of Molecular Biology.* 1998;276:559–569.

57. Oliveira PH, Lemos F, Monteiro GA, Prazeres DMF. Recombination frequency in plasmid DNA containing direct repeats-predictive correlation with repeat and intervening sequence length. *Plasmid.* 2008;60:159–165.

58. Ribeiro SC, Oliveira PH, Prazeres DMF, Monteiro GA. High frequency plasmid recombination mediated by 28 bp direct repeats. *Molecular Biotechnology.* 2008; 40:252–260.

59. Bi X, Liu LF. recA-independent and recA-dependent intramolecular plasmid recombination. Differential homology requirement and distance effect. *Journal of Molecular Biology.* 1994;235:414–423.

60. Wojciechowska M, Napierala M, Larson JE, Wells RD. Non-B DNA conformations formed by long repeating tracts of myotonic dystrophy type 1, myotonic dystrophy type 2, and Friedreich's ataxia genes, not the sequences per se, promote mutagenesis in flanking regions. *The Journal of Biological Chemistry.* 2006;281: 24531–24543.

61. Shlyakhtenko LS, Potaman VN, Sinden RR, Lyubchenko YL. Structure and dynamics of supercoil-stabilized DNA cruciforms. *Journal of Molecular Biology.* 1998; 280:61–72.

62. Wang E, Feigon J. Structures of nucleic acid triplexes. In: Neidle S, ed. *Oxford handbook of nucleic acid structure.* Oxford: Oxford Science Publications, 1999: 355–388.

63. Lyamichev VI, Mirkin SM, Frank-Kamenetskii MD. Structures of homopurine–homopyrimidine tract in superhelical DNA. *Journal of Biomolecular Structure & Dynamics.* 1986;3:667–669.

64. Mirkin SM, Lyamichev VI, Drushlyak KN, Dobrynin VN, Filippov SA, Frank-Kamenetskii MD. DNA H form requires a homopurine–homopyrimidine mirror repeat. *Nature.* 1987;330:495–497.

65. Broitman SL. H-DNA:DNA triplex formation within topologically closed plasmids. *Progress in Biophysics and Molecular Biology.* 1995;63:119–129.

66. Lee JS, Ashley C, Hampel KJ, Bradley R, Scraba DG. A stable interaction between separated pyrimidine.purine tracts in circular DNA. *Journal of Molecular Biology.* 1995;252:283–288.

67. Kato M. Polypyrimidine/polypurine sequence in plasmid DNA enhances formation of dimer molecules in *Escherichia coli.* Dimerization of plasmid DNA in *Escherichia coli. Molecular Biology Reports.* 1993;18:183–187.

68. Sprous D, Tan RK, Harvey SC. Molecular modeling of closed circular DNA thermodynamic ensembles. *Biopolymers.* 1996;39:243–258.

69. Echols H. Multiple DNA-protein interactions governing high-precision DNA transactions. *Science*. 1986;233:1050–1056.

70. Tan RK, Sprous D, Harvey SC. Molecular dynamics simulations of small DNA plasmids: Effects of sequence and supercoiling on intramolecular motions. *Biopolymers*. 1996;39:259–278.

71. Eismann ER, Muller-Hill B. lac repressor forms stable loops *in vitro* with super-coiled wild-type lac DNA containing all three natural lac operators. *Journal of Molecular Biology*. 1990;213:763–775.

72. Weintraub H, Cheng PF, Conrad K. Expression of transfected DNA depends on DNA topology. *Cell*. 1986;46:115–122.

73. Pillai VB, Hellerstein M, Yu T, Amara RR, Robinson HL. Comparative studies on *in vitro* expression and *in vivo* immunogenicity of supercoiled and open circular forms of plasmid DNA vaccines. *Vaccine*. 2008;26:1136–1141.

74. Cupillard L, Juillard V, Latour S, et al. Impact of plasmid supercoiling on the efficacy of a rabies DNA vaccine to protect cats. *Vaccine*. 2005;23:1910–1916.

75. World Health Organization. *Guidelines for assuring the quality and nonclinical safety evaluation of DNA vaccines. Vol Annex 1 (WHO Technical Report Series, No. 941)*. Geneva, 2007.

76. Schleef M, Schorr J. Plasmid DNA for clinical phase I and II studies. In: Walden P, Trefzer U, Sterry W, eds. *Gene therapy of cancer*, Vol. 451. New York: Springer-Verlag, 1998:481–486.

77. Rybenkov VV, Vologodskii AV, Cozzarelli NR. The effect of ionic conditions on DNA helical repeat, effective diameter and free energy of supercoiling. *Nucleic Acids Research*. 1997;25:1412–1418.

78. Rybenkov VV, Vologodskii AV, Cozzarelli NR. The effect of ionic conditions on the conformations of supercoiled DNA. I. Sedimentation analysis. *Journal of Molecular Biology*. 1997;267:299–311.

79. Hammermann M, Brun N, Klenin K, May R, Toth K, Langowski J. Salt-dependent DNA superhelix diameter studied by small angle neutron scattering measurements and Monte Carlo simulations. *Biophysical Journal*. 1998;75:3057–3063.

80. Haber C, Skupsky J, Lee A, Lander R. Membrane chromatography of DNA: Conformation-induced capacity and selectivity. *Biotechnology and Bioengineering*. 2004;88:26–34.

81. Teeters MA, Conrardy SE, Thomas BL, Root TW, Lightfoot EN. Adsorptive membrane chromatography for purification of plasmid DNA. *Journal of Chromatography. A*. 2003;989:165–173.

82. Diogo MM, Queiroz JA, Prazeres DMF. Chromatography of plasmid DNA. *Journal of Chromatography. A*. 2005;1069:3–22.

83. Kepka C, Lemmens R, Vasi J, Nyhammar T, Gustavsson PE. Integrated process for purification of plasmid DNA using aqueous two-phase systems combined with membrane filtration and lid bead chromatography. *Journal of Chromatography. A*. 2004;1057:115–124.

84. Zhou R, Geiger RC, Dean DA. Intracellular trafficking of nucleic acids. *Expert Opinion on Drug Delivery*. 2004;1:127–140.

85. Robertson RM, Laib S, Smith DE. Diffusion of isolated DNA molecules: Dependence on length and topology. *Proceedings of the National Academy of Sciences of the United States of America*. 2006;103:7310–7314.

86. Seils J, Pecora R. Dynamics of a 2311 base pair superhelical DNA in dilute and semidilute solutions. *Macromolecules*. 1995;28:661–673.

87. Chirico G, Baldini G. Rotational diffusion and internal motions of circular DNA. I. Polarized photon correlation spectroscopy. *The Journal of Chemical Physics*. 1996;104:6009–6019.

88. Langowski J, Giesen U. Configurational and dynamic properties of different length superhelical DNAs measured by dynamic light scattering. *Biophysical Chemistry*. 1989;34:9–18.

89. Tyn M, Gusek T. Prediction of diffusion coefficients of proteins. *Biotechnology and Bioengineering*. 1990;35:327–338.

90. He L, Niemeyer B. A novel correlation for protein diffusion coefficients based on molecular weight and radius of gyration. *Biotechnology Progress*. 2003;19: 544–548.

91. Prazeres DMF. Prediction of diffusion coefficients of plasmids. *Biotechnology and Bioengineering*. 2008;99:1040–1044.

92. Young ME, Carroad PA, Bell RL. Estimation of diffusion coefficients of proteins. *Biotechnology and Bioengineering*. 1980;22:947–955.

93. Cohen SN, Miller CA. Multiple molecular species of circular R-factor DNA isolated from *Escherichia coli*. *Nature*. 1969;224:1273–1277.

94. Voordouw G, Kam Z, Borochov N, Eisenberg H. Isolation and physical studies of intact supercoiled, open circular and linear forms of ColE1-plasmid DNA. *Biophysical Chemistry*. 1978;8:171–189.

95. Lavery R, Zakrzewska K. Base and base pair morphologies, helical parameters, and definitions. In: Neidle S, ed. *Oxford handbook of nucleic acid structure*. Oxford: Oxford Science Publications, 1999:39–76.

5

Analytical Characterization

5.1 INTRODUCTION

Over the last 40 years, a vast array of analytical techniques was developed to characterize and probe plasmid DNA molecules and to learn about their interactions with the surrounding environments. As a result, nowadays, it is possible to get hold of powerful analytical techniques to study plasmids that are freely moving in solution, complexed with agents like lipids or polymers, trafficking through the cytoplasm and organelles of live cells, or adsorbed to beads and membranes. These techniques play a key role not only in advancing fundamental research on plasmid biology and structure but also in supporting and sustaining the development of plasmid biopharmaceuticals and processes for their manufacture. Some of the most common and useful techniques like agarose electrophoresis and ultraviolet (UV) absorption are extremely simple, and their use is widespread among research laboratories. Other techniques like atomic force microscopy or circular dichroism, on the other hand, are more sophisticated and require the use of costly equipments. This chapter provides an overview of the range of very different analytical techniques that are used more often today in the context of the development of plasmid biopharmaceuticals.

Plasmid Biopharmaceuticals: Basics, Applications, and Manufacturing, First Edition.
Duarte Miguel F. Prazeres.
© 2011 John Wiley & Sons, Inc. Published 2011 by John Wiley & Sons, Inc.

5.2   CHEMICAL AND ENZYMATIC PROBES

Nucleic acids, in general, can be probed by using a series of chemicals and enzymes that react or interact with different parts of the molecules. These agents can be used not only to probe the DNA structure *in vitro*, but also *in vivo*, within cells. This section briefly describes those compounds and enzymes that have been the most useful for the development of plasmid biopharmaceuticals.

5.2.1   Chemical Probes

A number of chemical compounds react with DNA-forming covalent bonds. Others, on the other hand, can intercalate within consecutive base pairs in the double helix, interact with unpaired bases, or bind to the bases in duplexes through the minor or major grooves, via noncovalent bonds like hydrogen bonding and electrostatic or stacking interactions. The focus of this section is placed on intercalators and oligonucleotide-based probes. Although chemical probes that react with different functional groups in DNA have also contributed to the study of plasmid structure (see, e.g., Sinden[1]), they are seldom used in the context of plasmid biopharmaceuticals and thus will not be described here.

5.2.1.1   Intercalators

Planar aromatic molecules that intercalate within consecutive base pairs and unwind the double helix in the process are among the most important probes of nucleic acid structure. In the case of plasmids, as we have seen in the previous chapter (Section 4.3.5), this intercalation is accompanied by a loss of supercoiling. Intercalators can be used to detect plasmids and other nucleic acids in electrophoresis gels, as sensitive probes in fluorescence *in situ* hybridization assays or for DNA content analysis in flow cytometry studies. Chief among DNA intercalators are those molecules that display a low intrinsic fluorescence when unbound in aqueous solution but become intensely fluorescent when bound to plasmid DNA. This property is especially useful for quantitative purposes, particularly if the fluorescence emission intensity is a linear function of the number of intercalated dye molecules (hence, of the number of plasmid molecules). Ethidium bromide (Figure 5.1a) was one of the first of such compounds to be identified.[2] The weak fluorescence exhibited by free ethidium bromide results from a strong quenching of fluorescence by the surrounding aqueous solvent.[3] When intercalated, on the other hand, ethidium molecules become protected from the aqueous solvent by the hydrophobic environment provided by the stacked bases. This allows the molecule to fluoresce intensely.[3] The importance of ethidium bromide increased significantly after its combined use with agarose gel electrophoresis was first described and proposed.[4] At a concentration of 1 mM, ethidium bromide binds to 57% of base pairs on double-stranded DNA molecules. The resulting DNA–ethidium

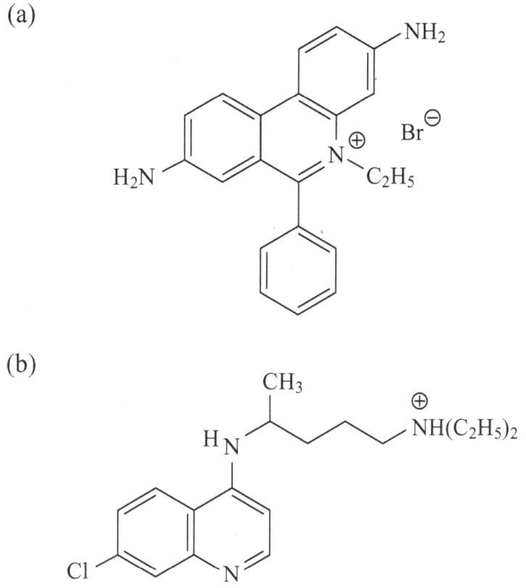

(a)

(b)

Figure 5.1 *Fluorescent dyes used for plasmid DNA quantitation. (a) Ethidium bromide (phenanthridium, 3-amino-8-azido-5-ethyl-6-phenyl, bromide) and (b) chloroquine (N'-(7-chloroquinolin-4-yl)-N,N-diethyl-pentane-1,4-diamine).*

complex is characterized by an association constant of $1.9 \times 10^5\,M^{-1}$ [5] and fluoresces with an orange color when exposed to UV light. Maximum excitation and emission wavelengths are $\lambda_{ex} = 270\,nm$ (for DNA-bound ethidium bromide) and $\lambda_{em} = 605\,nm$, respectively[6] (see also Chapter 12, Table 12.2). Under optimized conditions, the emission of fluorescence from ethidium bromide can increase up to 40-fold after binding to DNA.[6]

The usefulness of ethidium bromide in the context of molecular biology prompted researchers and companies to develop intercalators with improved sensitivity. The unsymmetrical cyanine dye commercially known as PicoGreen (Molecular Probes, Eugene, Oregon), for example, is one of the most sensitive and specific dyes developed so far.[7] The use of PicoGreen to quantitate plasmid DNA in a number of circumstances has been described in detail in the literature.[8–11] The DNA-binding mode of PicoGreen is thought to involve intercalation, as well as surface and groove binding.[7] Characteristics of PicoGreen are excitation and emission wavelengths of $\lambda_{ex} = 480\,nm$ and $\lambda_{em} = 520\,nm$, respectively, a large molar extinction coefficient $(70{,}000\ cm^{-1}M^{-1})$ and a higher than 1000-fold fluorescence enhancement upon binding[7] (see Chapter 12, Table 12.2). Examples of other intercalator dyes that have even superior affinity for DNA are the cyanine fluorochromes YOYO-1 and TOTO-1 (Molecular Probes). Although these molecules yield little fluorescence in solution, they exhibit fluorescence enhancements of the order of 1100- (TOTO) and 3200 (YOYO)-fold, when bound to double-stranded DNA. The extinction coefficients of TOTO $(112{,}000cm^{-1}M^{-1})$ and YOYO $(84{,}000cm^{-1}M^{-1})$ are also superior to that of PicoGreen[12] (see Chapter 12, Table 12.2). The antimalarial drug chloroquine is another intercalator molecule often used in studies of plasmid structure (Figure 5.1b). It is particularly useful as a means to relax plasmids, that is, to remove negative supercoils. Such chloroquine-induced changes in the topology of plasmid molecules are commonly used, together with two-dimensional electrophoresis, to study the formation of local, non-B-DNA secondary structures, as described in Section 5.3.

5.2.1.2   Oligonucleotides

Oligonucleotide molecules complementary to certain base sequences within the target DNA are often used to report the presence of plasmids. Such oligonucleotide probes are designed according to the primary sequence of the plasmid DNA under study and will typically have between 10 and 20 nucleotides. In many cases, a reporter molecule is covalently attached to one of the extremities of the probe oligonucleotide. Although enzymes like horseradish peroxidase or alkaline phosphatase are usual choices, fluorescent molecules are more common reporters since subsequent detection of hybrids is facilitated. When excited with light of a characteristic wavelength, these compounds will emit fluorescence at a particular wavelength. Many fluorescent compounds that span the visible light spectrum and beyond are commercially available nowadays. This spectral flexibility is particularly useful for multicolor applications in which different molecules or subcellular structures within a cell have to be visualized.[13] Fluorescein isothiocyanate (FITC) remains one of the most popular fluorophores for DNA labeling. Fluorescently labeled, sequence-specific oligonucleotide probes are often used to mark plasmid molecules so that they can be tracked down inside cells, particles, or beads. If the plasmid to be detected is located within a live tissue or cell, the hybridization with the oligonucleotide can be promoted *in situ*. Since the canonic Watson–Crick base pairing between A and T and between G and C is usually explored, binding of the probe to a plasmid requires the unwinding of the double helix at the target site, or else the presence of a single-stranded structure at that precise location. Once the hybrids between the probe and the target are formed, fluorescence microscopy is used to image the resulting complexes. This technique is usually designated by fluorescence *in situ* hybridization (FISH).[14] In a recent example of the application of FISH, the relative position of different plasmids in *Escherichia coli* cells was studied using specific oligonucleotides fluorescently labeled with Cy3 ($\lambda_{ex} = 550\,nm$, $\lambda_{em} = 570\,nm$) and Cy5 ($\lambda_{ex} = 649\,nm$, $\lambda_{em} = 670\,nm$) fluorophores.[15]

Sequence-specific oligonucleotide probes can also be used to map protein-binding sites or certain structures within a plasmid molecule. For example, triplex-forming oligonucleotides (see Chapter 4, Section 4.4.6) that bind to double-stranded DNA via the major groove have often been used for this purpose.[16] In some applications, and once the triplex is formed, the extremities of the oligonucleotide probe are ligated to create a circular DNA molecule that thus becomes catenated to the plasmid.[17] This catenation requires the inclusion of extra nucleotides at both ends of the probe, which are selected in such a way as not to bind to the duplex target in the plasmid. The formation of a complex between the oligonucleotide probe and the target plasmid via triple helices (whether catenation is involved or not) results in a local thickening of the DNA. The concomitant increase in the width can then be detected by electron or atomic force microscopy techniques (see Section 5.5). Since the formation of the triple-stranded complex does not require the separation of the strands in the double helix, the superhelicity of the plasmid is not altered.[16] A disadvantage of the technique, on the other hand, is that the presence of homopurine•homopyrimidine sequences at the site of labeling is required to guarantee triplex formation (see Chapter 4, Section 4.4.6). Thus, the targeting sequence must be engineered into the plasmid a priori. Interlocked nanostructures similar to the ones just described can also be created through catenation of a peptide nucleic acid (PNA) oligonucleotide at the designated site in the plasmid. Such PNAs, however, will bind very tightly to complementary sequences in double-stranded plasmid DNA by forming strand invasion complexes.[18] Thus, the unwinding of the double helix that is required for this to happen will lead to the loss of superhelicity of the plasmid molecule under analysis.

5.2.2 Enzymatic Probes

Synthesis, recombination, processing, and degradation of nucleic acids are vital for the survival and proper functioning of living organisms. During the course of natural history, a substantial number of enzymes evolved to play a role in those transactions.[19] Such enzymes act specifically over DNA and RNA molecules, executing tasks like the cleavage and formation of phosphodiester and N-glycosyl bonds, the twisting and untwisting of strands, the methylation of DNA, or the recognition of loops and branched structures. Enzymes that use nucleic acids as substrates can be grouped into categories according to the specific action they perform. For example, topoisomerases are involved in the control of DNA supercoiling; restriction endonucleases recognize specific DNA sequences and cleave the two strands within or nearby that sequence; repair nucleases act over different types of damaged DNA (mismatched pairs, baseless sites, interstrand crosslinks, strand breaks, etc.); and polymerases catalyze the polymerization of deoxyribonucleotides. Many of these enzymes have become indispensible to molecular biology, playing key roles in the *in vitro* manipulation and characterization of DNA molecules.

5.2.2.1 *Restriction and Single-Strand Specific Nucleases*

In the case of plasmids, a series of enzyme-based tests are routinely performed to characterize a specific molecule and probe for features like base sequence, single-stranded regions, and nicks in the phosphodiester backbone. For example, plasmid identity can be inferred by selectively cleaving the molecule into fragments with key restriction enzymes and examining the obtained restriction pattern (see Chapter 12, Section 12.3.1). The number, size, and positioning of the plasmid fragments generated in an agarose gel (see Section 5.3), for instance, should be sufficient in most cases to provide the first clue to the molecule's identity. While restriction enzymes recognize specific base sequences, other specific structural features in a plasmid molecule, like single-stranded or mispaired regions and abasic sites, can be probed using single-strand specific nucleases. For example, the controlled incubation of a plasmid with an enzyme like the S1 nuclease from *Aspergillus oryzae*, followed by an agarose electrophoresis, will reveal the presence of non-B-DNA secondary structures like cruciforms, hairpin loops, or Z-DNA tracts (see Chapter 4, Section 4.4). The precise location of such structures on a plasmid molecule can be further determined by performing sequential digestion with S1 nuclease and with selected restriction enzymes. The determination of the size and number of the resulting fragments should allow the pinpointing of the single-strand locus.[20] Single-stranded segments are also often found in denatured plasmid isoforms. Since these isoforms are usually more sensitive to nucleases that specifically recognize and cleave single strands when compared with "native" supercoiled plasmid DNA, digestion with S1 or other single-stranded nucleases is an expedite way to confirm their presence in a mixture.[21]

Extreme environmental conditions like high temperatures and acidic pH can lead to the cleavage of the glycosidic bond that connects purines to the DNA backbone, leaving an "apurinic" site behind. In a plasmid molecule, this type of damage (i.e., depurination) is not readily visible in an agarose gel since the creation of apurinic sites does not by itself affect the supercoiling degree. In some circumstances, for example, if unit operations that operate at elevated temperatures (e.g., thermal lysis of cells; see Chapter 15, Section 15.3.3) and low pH values are used in the downstream processing, it may be important to probe deeper into the structure of purified plasmids in order to understand if that type of damage was introduced, since this will ultimately translate into a lower biological activity.[22] One way to assess the extent of depurination in a population of plasmid molecules relies on the incubation of samples with endonuclease III or endonuclease VIII.[22] Among other activities, these enzymes specifically recognize abasic sites, cleaving the adjacent phosphate diester bond and thus originating a nick.[23,24] Therefore, supercoiled plasmids with apurinic or apyrimidinic sites are enzymatically transformed into nicked, open circular isoforms. This shift in plasmid topology is easily detected by agarose gel electrophoresis (see Section 5.3). Thus, by measuring the relative proportion of the two isoforms before and after incubation with either endonuclease III or VIII, one can infer about the amount of plasmids that contain abasic sites.[22]

5.2.2.2 *Polymerases*

Information regarding the sequence of plasmid molecules can be obtained by using DNA polymerases in polymerase chain reaction (PCR) assays. These assays are typically designed to amplify a polynucleotide region, which is expected to be present in the plasmid molecule. An example of a sequence that is relevant in the case of plasmid biopharmaceuticals is the transgene or parts of it. A positive PCR test, that is, one that would result in the amplification of the target fragment, would ascertain that cloning was successful or that there were no major instability problems in the transgene region during amplification of the molecule in *E. coli* (see Chapter 12, Section 12.3.1). PCR tests can also be designed to probe for events that alter the plasmid structure like the transposition of *E. coli* insertion sequences (ISs)[25] or the generation of monomeric and heterodimeric plasmid forms via recombination.[26,27] In many cases, these PCR-based tests can be used for quantitative purposes, for example, to determine the proportion of plasmids in a population that underwent a specific recombination event.[27]

PCR tests also play a critical role during preclinical and clinical trials, particularly when the biodistribution, persistence, and integration of a specific plasmid DNA in the tissues and cells of the human/nonhuman recipient are being investigated. The typical experiment involves the collection of different tissues at different times post administration, the isolation of genomic DNA, and then the probing for the presence of the plasmid and derived fragments using a quantitative PCR test.[28] Usually, regions smaller than 100 bp are amplified by resorting to transgene-specific or backbone-specific primers.[29] Sensitivities of the order of 1 plasmid copy/μg of DNA are typically required.[28] Further details can be found in Chapter 7, Section 7.3.2.

5.2.2.3 Topoisomerases

The use of topoisomerases is close to mandatory when performing studies on the topology of plasmids. Such studies often require the preparation of mixtures containing the "complete series" of topoisomers of a particular plasmid (see Section 5.3). This designation refers to the fact that a succession of topoisomers, ranging from the relaxed isoform to the most supercoiled one, and differing by one in their linking number, are present. Such mixtures can be generated by combining the relaxing activity of a topoisomerase (e.g., topoisomerase I from wheat germ) with an intercalating agent like ethidium bromide.[30] The isolated effect of both agents on the supercoiling degree of plasmids has been described in detail in the previous chapter (Section 4.3.5). The combined action of topoisomerases and ethidium bromide in the context of the preparation of sets of topoisomers is now described.

Briefly, the procedure used to prepare a complete series of topoisomers calls for the reaction of the supercoiled plasmid DNA molecules in a sample with an excess of topoisomerase and in the presence of increasing concentrations of ethidium bromide. The process is schematically shown in the Lk_o versus Lk plots in Figure 5.2a. Before proceeding with the rationale behind the method, it should be pointed here again that samples of supercoiled plasmid DNA isolated from *E. coli* consist, in reality, of groups of molecules that differ in their number of superhelical turns around a mean value in a Gaussian-like distribution.[30] For the sake of simplicity of the plot shown, we assume that the sample undergoing treatment contains only three topoisomers

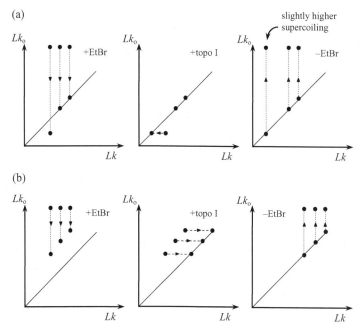

Figure 5.2 *Preparation of mixtures containing the complete series of topoisomers of a particular plasmid by combining the activity of a topoisomerase I with ethidium bromide (EtBr). For the sake of simplicity, the original plasmid sample is assumed to contain only three topoisomers. (a) If EtBr is used in excess, the topoisomers become fully relaxed or slightly positively supercoiled due to intercalation (first panel). Topoisomerase I relaxes the supercoiled specie but does not affect the relaxed ones (central panel). When EtBr is removed by solvent extraction, the topoisomers recover the original Lk_o (right panel). In the case illustrated, the supercoiling degree remains the same for two of the topoisomers but slightly increases for the third one. (b) If EtBr is not used in excess, the topoisomers are only partially relaxed (first panel). Topoisomerase I removes the remaining supercoils, producing fully relaxed molecules (central panel). When EtBr is removed by solvent extraction, the topoisomers recover the original Lk_o, but all species now have a lower degree of supercoiling (right panel).*

(black circles in Figure 5.2a). As we have seen in the previous chapter (see Section 4.3.5), if ethidium bromide is used in excess, the supercoiled plasmids in this distribution become fully relaxed or even positively supercoiled as a consequence of intercalation. In the plot (left-hand panel in Figure 5.2a), this is illustrated by a downward movement of the circles toward the diagonal, because intercalation decreases Lk_o. The higher affinity of ethidium bromide toward the more supercoiled species is reflected by the fact that the final Lk_o is lower the more supercoiled is the topoisomer (as described in Section 4.3.5). Since relaxed plasmid DNA (represented by the circles lying on the diagonal) is a poor substrate for topoisomerase I, those complexes are virtually unaffected by the enzyme.[31] As for the positively supercoiled complexes, topoisomerase I acts upon them, yielding relaxed molecules. In the plot (central panel in Figure 5.2a), this is seen by the horizontal movement of the corresponding

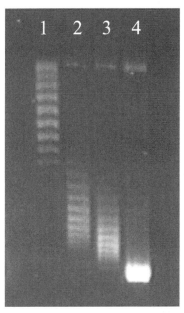

Figure 5.3 *One-dimensional gel electrophoresis of a set of plasmid topoisomers prepared by the combined action of topoisomerase I and ethidium bromide according to the method described by Keller.[30] The concentration of ethidium bromide increases from lanes 1 to 4 (J. Lima and D. M. F. Prazeres, unpublished results).*

specie toward the diagonal, since topoisomerase I operates by decreasing Lk. When the intercalator is subsequently removed, for example, with a phenol:chloroform extraction, the plasmids will reacquire the original, or a slightly increased, degree of supercoiling—in the right-hand panel of Figure 5.2a, the circles move upward until reaching the original level of Lk_o. If after completion of the process the plasmid sample is run on an electrophoresis gel, a single band of unresolved and highly supercoiled species is observed (see lane 4 in Figure 5.3).

If, on the other hand, the ethidium bromide concentration is not high enough, a number of supercoils of the topoisomers in the original distribution will remain to be relaxed. In the Lk_o versus Lk plot shown in the left-hand panel of Figure 5.2b, this is illustrated by the supercoiled species falling short of hitting the diagonal. However, since topoisomerase I is also present, the remaining supercoils can be removed, generating relaxed isoforms. In the figure (central panel), the individual species move horizontally toward the diagonal. By removing the ethidium bromide (right-hand panel, Figure 5.2b), the plasmids will now regain some supercoils, but not as many as they originally had. This will originate mixtures containing a distribution of supercoiled topoisomers with different degrees of supercoiling, as seen in lanes 1–3 on Figure 5.3. The adjacent bands seen in each lane correspond to isomers differing by one in their linking number. By mixing samples prepared with topoisomerase

I and different amounts of ethidium bromide, it is thus possible to obtain a full set of supercoiled topoisomers in a single tube. This procedure is also useful to determine the supercoiling degree of different plasmid preparations. Basically, the smaller the amount of ethidium bromide required to prevent complete relaxation, the lower is the degree of supercoiling.[30]

5.3   ELECTROPHORESIS

First described in 1973,[4] agarose gel electrophoresis with ethidium bromide was readily adopted by researchers and eventually became one of the keystone techniques in molecular biology. The use of agarose gel electrophoresis, especially in the one-dimensional format, is mandatory for all those who work with plasmids. As for the two-dimensional format, it is especially useful for detailed topology studies that require an exact knowledge of the isoform distribution in specific samples.

5.3.1   One-Dimensional Electrophoresis

The establishment of an electric field across a polyelectrolyte solution promotes the separation of charged molecules during migration through the polymeric network of a porous gel matrix. DNA/RNA gel electrophoresis takes advantage of this fact, exploring the dependency of the electrophoretic migration rate of nucleic acids with their molecular size, conformation, and net charge. Although polyacrylamide gels can be used sometimes, agarose is the polymer of choice when it comes to plasmid electrophoresis. The gels are usually casted in a rectangular tray using buffer solutions of melted agarose with concentrations in the 0.6–1.2% (w/v) range. The gels are then placed in an electrophoresis chamber and immersed in a running buffer like tris-acetate-EDTA (40 mM tris base, 20 mM acetic acid, and 1 mM ethylenediamine tetraacetic acid [EDTA], pH 8.0). Once the samples containing the material under analysis are injected in wells located at the cathode side of the chamber, a current (typically 100 V for 30 min with 15 mL of gel) is applied between the anode and cathode using an adequate power supply. Given their polyanionic nature, nucleic acids loaded on the cathode (– charge) side of the gel will migrate in the electric field toward the anode (+ charge). Although a wide variety of migration mechanisms (free-flow, sieving, and reptation) can come into play,[32,33] the different DNA and RNA species are ultimately separated on the basis of size or conformation. The electrophoretic mobility, μ, of a given molecule (i.e., the distance migrated per unit electric field strength and unit time) can be correlated with the concentration of the gel, C_G, and with a retardation coefficient, K_R:

$$\ln \mu = \ln \mu_0 - K_R C_G, \tag{5.1}$$

where μ_0 is the free mobility of the molecule. The migration of linear, double-stranded DNA fragments is proportional to their mass—the smaller the molecule is, the faster it migrates in the gel. In the case of plasmids, however, the picture is not as straightforward since the different topoisomers found in a typical plasmid preparation (i.e., supercoiled, open circular, linear, and denatured) have different geometries and hydrodynamic dimensions. As a result, each will display different frictional properties and will thus be characterized by different retardation coefficients, even if their mass is identical.

Open circular isoforms, whether they are originally relaxed or nicked during purification, typically migrate slower when compared with linear and supercoiled isoforms. The introduction of one negative supercoil in a relaxed, open circular plasmid originates a molecule characterized by a linking difference, ΔLk, equal to -1, which is more compact. Consequently, this specie will migrate slightly faster when compared with the relaxed isoform. The successive introduction of negative supercoils will thus generate a series of supercoiled topoisomers, each with a higher electrophoretic mobility when compared with the previous. However, there are limitations in the ability of agarose gel electrophoresis to resolve supercoiled topoisomers. Thus, for ΔLk values smaller than a given critical value, ΔLk_c, separation becomes impossible, and the more highly supercoiled species will comigrate as a broad band at the lower end of the gel.[34] As for linearized plasmids, they typically migrate between open circular and supercoiled DNA. The typical electrophoresis pattern of a plasmid DNA sample isolated from an *E. coli* culture displays a more intense band of supercoiled isoforms with $\Delta Lk < \Delta Lk_c$, and a less intense band of open circular isoforms (see e.g., Chapter 15, Figure 15.3). The actual proportion of these two species will depend on a number of factors, including the plasmid sequence and the host strain, the growth conditions, and the methods used to isolate and purify the plasmid material.

The positioning of the different nucleic acids after migration is normally visualized with the aid of ethidium bromide, a technique originally developed by Sharp and coworkers in 1973.[4] In one of the options available, the dye is incorporated in the gels and in the running buffer prior to electrophoresis. Alternatively, the gel is immersed in a solution of $0.5\,\mu g/mL$ of ethidium bromide for 30 min or so, after the run is halted. In either case, the planar aromatic ethidium bromide molecules bind to nucleic acids by intercalating between consecutive bases. This bound ethidium bromide can then be detected by exposing the gel to UV light, thus revealing individual "bands" that correspond to different nucleic acid species (e.g., see Figure 5.3). Bands with DNA amounts as small as $0.05\,\mu g$ can be visualized with this technique. Furthermore, lower sensitivities can be obtained using alternative dyes like Sybr®-Gold, Sybr®-Green, or PicoGreen® (Molecular Probes). Although agarose electrophoresis can be used to quantitate the different topoisomers in a plasmid sample by obtaining electropherograms corresponding to each lane in the gel via image analysis, the linear range of quantitation is usually limited.

The use of the fluorescence of resolved bands in an agarose gel to measure the relative amounts of the different plasmid isoforms in an agarose gel is complicated by the fact that the binding constants of intercalated ethidium bromide depend on molecule topology and binding density (see Chapter 4, Section 4.3.5). In the case of nicked circular and linear plasmid forms, for example, the binding constant is equivalent and independent of the number of bound ethidium molecules, that is, of the binding density.[35] In the case of supercoiled plasmids, however, the picture is substantially different. As described in Chapter 4 (Section 4.3.5), ethidium bromide binds with lower affinity, the lower is the degree of supercoiling.[1] Since intercalation is accompanied by relaxation of supercoils, this means that the binding constant of intercalated ethidium bromide decreases the higher is the number of intercalated molecules in the plasmid. As a consequence of this behavior, at low binding densities, the binding constant of ethidium bromide toward supercoiled plasmids is higher when compared with the binding constant toward the corresponding nicked circular and linear isoforms.[35] However, the opposite behavior is observed at higher binding densities. This means that equal amounts of different plasmid isoforms that have been stained with an ethidium bromide solution with a given concentration will not necessarily bind the same amount of dye.[36] Thus, the ratio of the fluorescence emitted by the individual bands is not a direct measure of the mass ratio of the different isoforms.[36]

Although useful to analyze small- to medium-sized plasmids, conventional agarose gel electrophoresis is not able to separate very large plasmid DNA molecules (>20,000 bp). In this latter case, a variation of agarose gel electrophoresis called pulsed-field electrophoresis should be used.[37] The principle of the technique is the periodic change of the direction of the electric field during migration. With this mode of operation, the size of DNA molecules that can be separated in gel electrophoresis is increased by two orders of magnitude.[32]

5.3.2   Two-Dimensional Electrophoresis

Although one-dimensional gels are the most common format used in plasmid analysis, they present limitations when it comes to analyzing the more supercoiled plasmid isoforms (i.e., when $\Delta Lk < \Delta Lk_c$), as described earlier. Alternatively, two-dimensional gels extend the range over which the electrophoretic migration of supercoiled species is a function of the topology, that is, of ΔLk. The technique is especially useful to analyze in detail the topoisomer distribution of plasmid samples and to look for those local structural transitions within a plasmid molecule (e.g., cruciforms, intermolecular triplexes, hairpins) that are a function of supercoiling[34] (see Chapter 4, Section 4.4). Typically, a single plasmid-containing sample is placed on the left top corner of an agarose gel and run under the action of an electric field as usual, without ethidium bromide. If the sample contains a complete set of plasmid topoisomers, that is, a mixture of species with supercoil densities varying from 0 to σ_{max} (see Section 5.2.2.3 on how to prepare such mixtures), this will originate a migration pattern with a succession of bands akin to those observed in lanes 1–3 of the gel in Figure 5.3. The resulting gel is then immersed in a solution of an intercalating dye like chloroquine. Since intercalation unwinds the double helix (i.e., there is a decrease in Lk_o) without breaking the backbone (i.e., Lk remains constant), the ΔLk corresponding to each topoisomer in the distribution increases (see Equation 4.5 in Chapter 4). This means that negative supercoils are removed from the plasmids. For each topoisomer, there will be a point where sufficient chloroquine is intercalated to remove all negative supercoils ($\Delta Lk = 0$). The addition of more dye past this point will originate positively supercoiled isoforms ($\Delta Lk > 0$). Eventually, and if sufficient chloroquine is added, all topoisomers loose their negative supercoiling and a series of positively supercoiled topoisomers is generated. However, those topoisomers that were the most negatively supercoiled before chloroquine intercalation now become the least positively supercoiled.[34] The gel is then rotated 90°, and a second electrophoresis is run with a buffer containing a chloroquine concentration identical to the one used in the previous soaking. But now, the relative order of migration is inverted relatively to the first dimension. This means that in the second dimension, the topoisomer that was originally open circular has the highest mobility, whereas the originally more supercoiled topoisomer has the lowest mobility. Visualization of the gel after completion of the process shows a series of spots aligned as an arc (Figure 5.4). The brightest spot on the top right of the gel corresponds to the originally relaxed plasmid. To the right and below, we find spots that are ascribed to topoisomers that were originally slightly positively supercoiled.[34] As for the spots found when moving to the left, they correspond to the negatively supercoiled topoisomers in the initial mixture. Notice that some resolution of the topoisomers that moved faster in the first dimension is now obtained in the second dimension. If a lower chloroquine concentration is used, not all topoisomers in the original sample become positively supercoiled. The result will be a mixture of

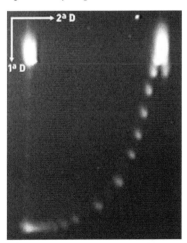

Figure 5.4 *Two-dimensional gel electrophoresis of a set of plasmid DNA topoisomers. Electrophoresis was carried out using a tris–borate buffer (J. Lima and D. M. F. Prazeres, unpublished results).*

plasmid species characterized by different degrees and types (i.e., $\Delta Lk < 0$, $\Delta Lk = 0, \Delta Lk > 0$) of supercoiling. The pattern that emerges in this case is now different from the one shown in Figure 5.4 (see Bowater et al.[34] for more details).

5.3.3 Capillary Electrophoresis

The electrophoretic separation of DNA fragments or plasmid topoisomers can also be carried out within slender, elongated tubes with a very small bore. In this format, the technique receives the name capillary electrophoresis. Capillary electrophoresis is a powerful DNA separation method that combines a high degree of resolution with a fast analysis time.[33] A number of reports can be found in the literature that describe how capillary electrophoresis can be used to quantitate plasmid DNA and its topoisomers.[38–42] Capillaries coated with a layer of poly(vinyl alcohol) and elution with dilute polymer solutions (e.g., 0.1% w/w hydroxypropyl methylcellulose) are typically used.[39,41,43] These elution buffers provide an excellent media for fast electrophoretic separations due to the formation of short-lived complexes between DNA and polymer strands, an effect known as transient entanglement.[44] Furthermore, if intercalating fluorescent dyes such as ethidium bromide,[42] YOYO,[40,43] or YO-PRO[39] are combined with laser-induced fluorescence (LIF), the sensitivity can be improved tremendously and plasmid concentrations as low as 100 ng/mL can be determined.[39,41] Separation of plasmid species in capillary electrophoresis is governed mainly by the topology of the macromolecules and not so much by their size as in one-dimensional slab agarose electrophoresis. This produces what is perhaps one of the most striking features of capillary electrophoresis, that is, an ability to produce baseline resolutions of supercoiled, open circular, and linear plasmid topoisomers.[40] Furthermore, more unusual species like dimeric concatamers can also be separated as well. This is illustrated in Figure 5.5, which shows a typical electropherogram of a plasmid DNA preparation containing different topoisomers and variants of the same plasmid. We see that the different species elute according to their topology, with the more compact supercoiled structures exiting the capillary before linear and open circular structures, independently of whether the plasmids are monomeric or dimeric.[41] This relative order of elution holds when larger plasmids are analyzed.[41] Capillary electrophoresis is especially useful for quality control purposes, for example, to map the topoisomer distribution of bulk plasmids obtained at the end of manufacturing or to monitor the long-term stability of stored plasmid samples.[43] Unfortunately, the superior performance of capillary electrophoresis when compared with one-dimensional gel electrophoresis in terms of resolving power, sensitivity, reproducibility, analysis time, and automation has a high cost associated. Thus, while replacement of conventional gel electrophoresis by capillary electrophoresis in some companies might be economically feasible, it is not likely to happen in most research laboratories in the near future.

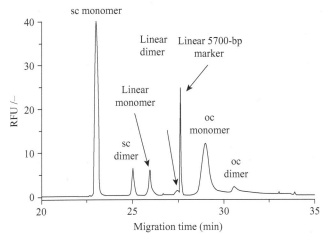

Figure 5.5 *Separation of variants and topoisomers of plasmid pUC19 (2700 bp) by capillary electrophoresis. Reprinted from P/ACE Setter Newsletter, 4, Schmidt T, Friehs K, Schleef M, Voss C, Flaschel E. Assessing the homogeneity of plasmid DNA: An important step toward gene therapy, 1-3, Copyright 2000,[41] with permission from Beckman Coulter.*

5.4 SPECTROSCOPIC TECHNIQUES

Electromagnetic radiation has been explored extensively over the years to probe the structure and the dynamics of biological macromolecules. As a result of these efforts, an array of spectroscopic techniques is currently available that extract information on the basis of the UV, visible, and infrared radiation that is absorbed or scattered when macromolecules in solution are impinged with the corresponding photons. This section reviews those spectroscopic techniques that are most commonly used to characterize plasmid molecules.

5.4.1 Absorbance

Compounds that contain π electrons, and especially those with conjugated double and triple bonds, absorb UV radiation. In the case of nucleic acids, the nitrogenous bases with their characteristic alternating single and double bonds in the purinic and pyrimidinic rings (see Chapter 4, Figure 4.1) are responsible for the UV absorption. Although each of the five bases is characterized by slightly different absorption spectra, the overall spectrum of DNA molecules is characterized by a peak at around 260 nm. RNA and single-stranded DNA will absorb more light when compared with double-stranded DNA molecules like plasmids due to the stacking and partial concealment of the bases inside the double helix of the latter. Accordingly, the denaturation of double-stranded DNA upon heating can be observed by monitoring the increase (~40%) in absorbance at 260 nm associated with strand separation (hyperchromic effect). Additionally, measuring the absorbance at 260 nm is a convenient way to determine the concentration of pure plasmid DNA solutions (see Chapter 12,

Section 12.3.2.1). In chromatography, UV absorption at 260 nm is also the method of choice when it comes to the continuous monitoring of nucleic acid concentration at the outlet of chromatographic columns, membrane stacks, or monoliths (Chapter 17).

5.4.2 Light Scattering

The electric field of light that is shone upon a given molecule induces an oscillating polarization of electrons of that molecule, which then radiates or scatters the incident light. The characteristics of this scattered light (e.g., frequency shifts, intensity, polarization, and angular distribution) strongly depend on characteristics like the size and the shape of the molecule being observed.[45] An adequate analysis of light scattering data can thus yield information on the structure and dynamics of molecules as complex as plasmids.[46] In the typical light scattering setup, light from a laser is polarized before hitting the sample solution. The polarized light that is scattered by the sample is then analyzed and detected, yielding parameters like the scattering angle. Since molecules in solution are constantly translating, rotating, and vibrating, the characteristics of the scattered light continuously change on the same timescale. The recording and analysis of these fluctuations of the scattered light thus provides a convenient way to assess the position, orientation, and movement of molecules.[47] For example, dynamic light scattering data obtained with supercoiled plasmid DNA molecules in solution are consistent with an elongated, interwound structure, which has a high degree of internal motion.[47] The technique is especially useful to determine parameters like the radius of gyration, R_G (see Chapter 4, Figure 4.7), and the translation diffusion coefficient, D (see Chapter 4, Figure 4.17) of plasmid molecules in solution.[46,47] The size of plasmid condensates and aggregates that are formed upon the addition of compacting agents can also be studied with the aid of the technique. For example, dynamic light scattering revealed that the hydrodynamic radius of a 6050-bp plasmid increases from 116 to >1300 nm when formulated with 1 mM $CaCl_2$ and 20% (v/v) t-butanol.[48]

5.4.3 Circular Dichroism

The secondary and tertiary structures of plasmids and the changes they undergo when in solution can be monitored by circular dichroism. Although this spectroscopic technique is not able to provide information at the atomic level of resolution as nuclear magnetic resonance (NMR) and X-ray crystallography are, it is still sensitive enough to describe the overall structural features of biomolecules like proteins and nucleic acids. Furthermore, it is less demanding both in terms of sample and time requirements. Circular dichroism takes advantage of the fact that plane polarized light may be decomposed into left (L) and right (R) circularly polarized components of equal magnitude. The technique essentially measures the differential absorption of these two circularly polarized components after the polarized light is passed through the sample under observation.[49] If the L and R components are equally absorbed, or are not adsorbed at all, by the molecules in solution, the light that is regenerated after passing the solution is unaffected. However, if chiral chromophores are present in the molecules, the L and R components are absorbed differently, originating a circular dichroism signal of elliptically polarized light. If the magnitude of this signal is recorded as a function of the wavelength of the incident light, a circular dichroism spectrum is obtained. The output of a circular dichroism instrument is typically the ellipticity, θ_λ (in degrees), a parameter that is related to the difference in absorbance of the L and R components, ΔA, according to the relation $\theta = 32.98\ \Delta A$.[49] The ellipticity data are usually normalized by taking into account the molar concentration of the whole molecule, or of the repeating monomer in the case of polymers, according to[49]

$$[\theta_\lambda] = 100\frac{\theta d}{m}, \tag{5.2}$$

where $[\theta_\lambda]$ is the molar ellipticity at wavelength λ (degrees); d is the path length of the cell (centimeter); and m is the molar concentration of the solute under observation (molar). The corresponding units of $[\theta_\lambda]$ are hence degree square centimeter per decimole. When comparative studies of circular dichroism of plasmids with different masses are carried out, m should be the concentration of nucleotides in solution. If the same plasmid is under observation, the molar concentration of plasmid can also be used, as long as this is made clear when describing and interpreting the different spectra.

Circular dichroism signals only appear in those wavelength regions where absorption occurs. In the case of nucleic acids, the chromophores of interest are thus the aromatic bases[50] (see Section 5.4.1). Although these have no intrinsic chirality, they acquire chirality and generate circular dichroism signals due to the fact that they are bound to the asymmetric sugars of the backbone. Interactions between the electronic transitions of the bases also originate important circular dichroism signals. As a result of these interactions, the overall circular dichroism spectrum is quite sensitive to changes in the helical parameters of DNA. Consequently, the different alloforms of DNA (A, B, Z, etc.; see Chapter 4, Section 4.2.1) and transitions between them can be readily distinguished by circular dichroism spectra. DNA triplexes have also different circular dichroism characteristics when compared to double-stranded DNA.[50] But perhaps more important in the context of this book is the fact that the local structural changes in the DNA helix (e.g., in the average helical rotation angle) that are brought about by the introduction of supercoils in an open circular plasmid molecule change the optical properties (chirality) of the molecule. In other words, the changes in the circular dichroism spectra of plasmid topoisomers reflect the changes in the average helical rotation of the double helix, which are induced by negative (decrease in helical rotation) or positive (increase in helical rotation) supercoiling.[51] Consequently, differences in the degree of supercoiling can be probed by circular dichroism spectroscopy. Circular dichroism is also particularly useful to measure changes in the optical properties of plasmids that result from alterations in their secondary structure. These alterations, which can be brought about by the addition of denaturing or compacting agents, or by the imposition of denaturing conditions like elevated temperatures, can be conveniently sensed by monitoring the loss or alteration of circular dichroism signals.

The typical spectra of a B-DNA molecule is characterized by a negative ellipticity peak at 250 nm and a positive molar ellipticity peak at approximately 277 nm. These two peaks are separated by a crossover point, which is located at around 260 nm. Although plasmids display a similar spectrum, negatively supercoiled isoforms have an ellipticity in the 277-nm region that is higher when compared with the ellipticity of open circular or linear isoforms.[52] This is illustrated in Figure 5.6a, which compares the circular dichroism spectra of the supercoiled and linear isoforms of the same plasmid. Positively supercoiled plasmids, on the other hand, cause a depression in the 277-nm circular dichroism band relative to nonsupercoiled plasmids. The band at 250 nm, on the other hand, is less affected by supercoiling.[52]

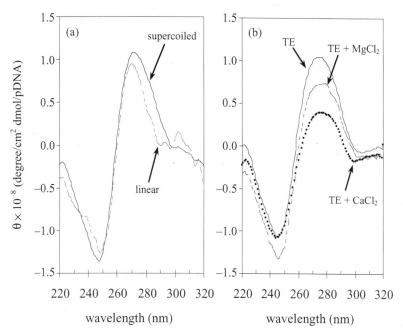

Figure 5.6 *Effect of plasmid topology (a) and cations (b) in the circular dichroism spectra of plasmid DNA. Solutions of the 6050-bp plasmid pVAX1-lacZ (sc:oc ≈ 90:10) were prepared at 60 ng/μL in TE buffer (10 mM tris, 1 mM EDTA, pH 8.0) and supplemented with either 50 mM MgCl₂ or 20 mM CaCl₂ (A. G. Gomes and D. M. F. Prazeres, unpublished results).*

An increase in the salt concentration or temperature of the solution also causes a decrease in the signals around the 270- to 280-nm region together with a shift in the maximum wavelength toward higher values. This effect is exemplified in Figure 5.6b, which compares the circular dichroism spectra of the same supercoiled plasmid molecule in tris-EDTA (TE) buffer (10 mM tris, 1 mM EDTA, pH 8), in TE plus 50 mM $MgCl_2$ and in TE plus 20 mM $CaCl_2$. The changes in the circular dichroism signals are attributable to changes in the average rotation of the double helix, which are brought about by the shielding of backbone phosphates by the added cation.[53] The figure also indicates that different cations will produce different alterations in the plasmid structure— from the spectra shown, it is clear that Ca^{2+} is more effective at changing the rotation of the double helix than Mg^{2+}. This is consistent with the fact that Ca^{2+} compacts DNA more readily and effectively when compared with Mg^{2+}.

Circular dichroism can also be conveniently used to study the ability of many substances (e.g., salts, alcohols, and polymers) to induce the condensation and aggregation of DNA into tertiary structures, which usually have distinctive morphology and optical rotation properties. This phenomenon, whereby plasmid molecules collapse from loose, flexible, and elongated supercoiled plasmid molecules into a condensed and/or aggregated state upon the addition of a specific substance, is called polymer- and salt-induced (ψ) condensation.[54] In a circular dichroism spectra, ψ-type condensation is typically observed as change in the DNA ellipticity near 280 nm either to positive, $\psi(+)$, or negative, $\psi(-)$, values. ψ-Type condensation is explored in the plasmid biopharmaceutical area in a number of different contexts, for example, to produce single-molecule condensates, with the goal of improving delivery[55] (see Chapter 6, Section 6.6.2), to promote the precipitation of plasmid DNA out of a pool of impurities[56] (e.g., see Chapter 16, Section 16.3.2) or to confer protection against mechanical shear during processing[48,57] (e.g., see Chapter 15, Section 15.3.4). The usefulness of circular dichroism in this later situation can be exemplified with a recent study in which the protection against sonication-induced shear provided by mixtures of $CaCl_2$/t-butanol was correlated with a $\psi(-)$ conformational transition.[48] The use of circular dichroism to study interactions between plasmid DNA and molecules like lipids or polymers used to prepare formulations for delivery has also been described in the literature. For example, the complexation of plasmid DNA with a lipopolymer derived from poly(ethyleneimine) was shown by circular dichroism to involve $\psi(-)$ conformational transition.[58]

5.5 MICROSCOPY

A range of modern microscopy techniques can be used to visualize plasmid molecules. These techniques may involve the "illumination" of the specimen with a beam of photons (e.g., fluorescence microscopy and confocal microscopy) or electrons (e.g., electron microscopy). Alternatively, the molecule under observation is "touched" with a highly sensitive probe, a technique known as atomic force microscopy. In any case, the response of the molecule to the perturbation imposed is used to reconstruct an image of the object. This typically involves the usage of computer-assisted image analysis and improved sample preparation methods. A major disadvantage of a number of these microscopy techniques is that they look to plasmids when they are immobilized on a surface and are not free in solution. The observations made are nevertheless biologically relevant since *in vivo*, plasmids will essentially interact with surfaces like membranes.[59] However, a large number of images have to be obtained if one wishes to gather statistically relevant information. Another possible disadvantage of some microscopy techniques relates to the fact that the sample preparation that is required can change the conformation of the plasmid molecules and thus can lead to erroneous conclusions. In spite of their resolving power, most microscopy techniques are extremely sophisticated and expensive, and thus are not readily available to the common researcher.

5.5.1   Electron Microscopy

The structural details of individual macromolecules like plasmids can be visualized using modern electron microscopy techniques. In electron microscopy, the illumination of the specimens with an electron beam generates a shadow image in which the different parts of the object appear with a darkness that depends on their density. Typically, the sample to be imaged is prepared by a process known as negative staining. This involves the immersion of a mesh grid with adsorbed or fixed plasmid in a heavy metal salt solution and subsequent drying. As a result, the plasmid molecules are coated with an electron dense layer that provides the necessary high contrast for visualization in the electron microscope.[60] Two major disadvantages of electron microscopy that can be ascribed to negative staining are low resolution (~20 Å) and the potential distortion of the molecules under observation.[60] Electron microscopy is extensively used to study plasmid DNA. High-quality micrographs obtained with the technique make it possible to measure parameters like the contour length, the number of nodes and branches, or the superhelix radius. The studies published by Boles et al.[61] and Vologodskii et al.[62] constitute good examples of the applicability of the technique. A micrograph of two supercoiled plasmid DNA molecules is shown in Figure 5.7, wherein features like ramification and high twisting are readily observed.[63]

Cryo-electron microscopy is a variation of electron microscopy, which uses a rapid cooling down to −140°C to trap plasmid molecules inside a 50- to 100-nm layer of vitrified water. Typically, a few microliters of a given sample containing the macromolecule of interest are placed on a carbon-coated electron microscopy grid and emerged rapidly in a solution of a coolant like liquid ethane.[64] The fast decrease in temperatures leads to the formation of vitreous (amorphous) ice, a material that has properties similar to those of liquid water.

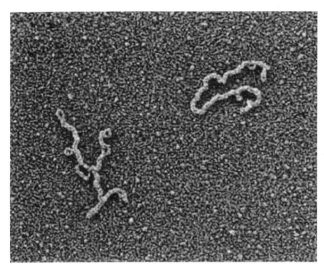

Figure 5.7 *Transmission electron micrographs of supercoiled plasmid DNA isoforms purified by high-performance liquid chromatography (HPLC). Reprinted from Journal of Biotechnology, 121, Weigl D, Molloy MJ, Clayton TM, et al. Characterization of a topologically aberrant plasmid population from pilot-scale production of clinical-grade DNA, 1-12, Copyright 2006,[63] with permission from Elsevier.*

The structure of the molecules is also preserved since no ice crystals are formed.[65] The vitrified specimens are then maintained at subzero temperatures using an adequate holder and observed/photographed with an electron microscope under appropriate magnification.[66] Stereo pairs of micrographs can then be used to yield a three-dimensional reconstruction of the plasmid molecules or macromolecular complex, which is often superior to the ones obtained with conventional electron microscopy. The technique makes it possible to observe macromolecules directly, without the use of metal staining and dehydration, which is characteristic of sample preparation by the negative-staining procedure commonly used with electron microscopy. Furthermore, the low temperature maintained during observation protects the macromolecules against the radiation damage associated with the electron beam.[64] A disadvantage of cryo-electron microscopy relates to the fact that conformational rearrangements can take place during the cooling, even though this process is extremely fast ($\sim 10^{-4}$ s).[66] The technique has been used not only to visualize single plasmid molecules[66] but also to image plasmid–lipid[67] and plasmid–polymer[68] complexes and assemblies prepared for gene therapy and vaccination applications.

5.5.2 Atomic Force Microscopy

Atomic force microscopy relies on the ability of a spatially controlled probe sensor tip carried by a cantilever to detect the atomic scale topography of a given sample.[69] Images of the surfaces are thus obtained by recording the displacement of the cantilever with the aid of a laser as the tip scans the area under observation. This displacement, in turn, is proportional to the force between the tip and the surface. The cantilevers and tips are typically micro-fabricated from materials like silicon (Si), silicon dioxide (SiO_2), or silicon nitride (Si_3N_4).[69,70] In order for a biomolecule to be observed by atomic force microscopy, the specimen must first be positioned on a suitably smooth, strongly adsorbing substrate. In the case of DNA, mica surfaces are modified and prepared by a series of steps designed to create stronger binding sites with the phosphate groups of DNA, to harden the surface, and to render it more hydrophilic. A few microliters of the DNA solution are then deposited over the surface and sufficient time is allowed for adsorption to take place. The surface is then rinsed, dried with nitrogen, and imaged in the atomic force microscope.[69] If adequately sharpened tips are used, the technique can resolve details with sizes of the order of the double helix size.[70]

Atomic force microscopy can be used to directly image wet or dry plasmid DNA molecules adsorbed on modified or unmodified mica surfaces.[69,70] With this technique, the molecular dimensions of plasmid DNA molecules can be measured and the different topoisomers can be clearly identified. Apart from providing information regarding the structure of a particular plasmid, atomic force microscopy is also useful in the context of plasmid manufacturing, to monitor changes in plasmid structure that might occur during processing. For example, in a recent application, atomic force microscopy was used to image alkali-denatured plasmid species (Figure 5.8). A comparison of the images obtained with native supercoiled plasmids and with the corresponding alkali-denatured specie showed that while the former are smooth and have a uniform diameter (Figure 5.8a,c), the latter are characterized by a rougher surface with kinks, an inhomogeneous diameter, and a reduced number of turns and knots (Figure 5.8b,d). The technique also made it possible to measure the contour length of the different plasmid species.[71] Further applications of atomic force microscopy include the localization of protein-binding sites and the mapping/sizing of restriction fragments,[72] the unveiling of the presence of unusual structures like cruciforms[73] and triple helices[74] in plasmid/cosmid molecules, and the study of intercalation-induced changes in the tertiary structure of plasmids.[75] In another application, atomic force microscopy was used to assay the extent of DNA condensation with a number of different agents such as poly-lysine,[59] lipospermine,[76] or poloaxamer.[77] Finally, atomic force microscopy can be operated in such a way that manipulation and even dissection of plasmid molecules becomes possible.[70]

5.5.3   Confocal Fluorescence Microscopy

Laser-scanning confocal microscopes have depth-discriminating properties that enable one to obtain clean and thin optical sections or impressive three-dimensional views of fluorescent specimens. The technique relies on the use of fluorescent molecules, which typically bind to specific molecules or organ-

(a) (b)

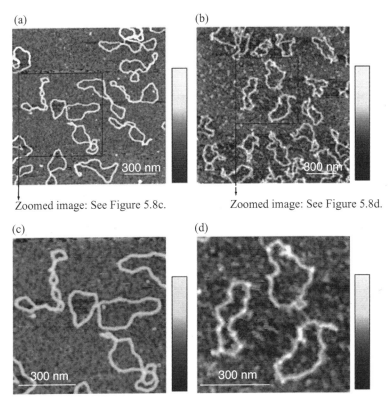

Zoomed image: See Figure 5.8c. Zoomed image: See Figure 5.8d.

(c) (d)

Figure 5.8 *Atomic force images of plasmid pBR322. (a) Images of supercoiled isoforms. (b) Images of alkali-denatured plasmid DNA. (c) Zoomed image of the area highlighted in (a). (d) Zoomed image of the area highlighted in (b). The grayscale represents 5 nm. Reprinted from Biochemical and Biophysical Research Communications, 374, Yu J, Zhang Z, Cao K, Huang X. Visualization of alkali-denatured supercoiled plasmid DNA by atomic force microscopy, 415-418, Copyright 2008,[71] with permission from Elsevier.*

elles in the cells or tissues under observation. After the biological specimen is prepared by combination with the appropriate fluorophores, a laser beam is focused at an appropriate scanning depth and is used to excite the molecules at the corresponding excitation wavelength. The light emitted by the fluorophores then passes through an objective lens and is analyzed by a detector unit. In a conventional microscope, this unit will collect light emitted not only by the in-focus plane but also by the out-of-focus planes. This usually originates a blurred image. Confocal microscopy solves this problem and produces high three-dimensional resolution images with the aid of a confocal pinhole placed before the detection unit. The aperture of this pinhole is such that those signals that come from out-of-focus planes are actively suppressed, while the light from the confocal plane is allowed to reach the detector.[78] The fluorescent image thus obtained is representative of the thin section focused by the laser only. If the laser is focused at different depths by changing the position of the specimen under observation, successive fluorescent images of slices of the object are obtained, which can then be combined into a three-dimensional image of the fluorescent molecule distribution.

Confocal microscopy has been used in a number of cases to visualize the trafficking of naked or encapsulated plasmid molecules through the different compartments of mammalian cells.[13,79] In a recent publication, a strategy is described that calls for the labeling of the plasmid molecule with the fluorescent dye rhodamine and for the staining of endosomes/lysosomes and nucleus with specific dyes.[13] After an *in vitro* transfection of cells with naked or lipid associated plasmid DNA, the subcellular localization of the plasmids can be distinguished by three-dimensional analysis of the living cells with confocal microscopy.[13] With this methodology it is possible to quantitatively analyze the intracellular pharmacokinetics of plasmid DNA. One problem with this approach relates to the fact that conjugation with the fluorescent reporter molecule may alter the plasmid properties, conformation (e.g., supercoiling degree), and intracellular trafficking.[80] For example, the conjugation of plasmid DNA with a fluorescent DNA intercalator molecule like YOYO-1 prior to encapsulation and/or cell transfection will inevitably relax the plasmid molecule (see Chapter 4, Section 4.3.5.1).[81] Hence, confocal microscopy of the transfected cells will observe in reality a modified plasmid molecule, which may thus present a different behavior when compared with the native, nonconjugated plasmid.

Confocal microscopy can also be used to probe the distribution of plasmid molecules within chromatographic beads during the course of adsorption.[82] In this case, the plasmid molecules can be conjugated a priori with the fluorescent dye of choice. After the unbound dye molecules are removed, the plasmid–fluorophore complexes are appropriately diluted with unlabeled plasmid and incubated with the adsorbent beads being analyzed.[83] Alternatively, conjugation can be performed after adsorption of the plasmids to the beads of interest. This latter option might be preferred when fluorophores like intercalators or groove binders are used because these usually tend to alter the plasmid properties and conformation (e.g., supercoiling degree), and hence change the binding behavior of the plasmids.[84] This approach was used to label plasmid DNA molecules previously bound to anion-exchanger beads by using the YOYO-1[84] and TOTO-3[85] fluorophores (Molecular Probes). Both compounds have a high affinity for double-stranded DNA and fluoresce intensely when bound. Whichever labeling strategy is used, the distribution of plasmid molecules inside individual beads can be accurately detected by confocal microscopy imaging. By selecting different incubation times, the intraparticle diffusion and adsorption of plasmid molecules can be adequately monitored. The usefulness of confocal microscopy in the context of plasmid chromatography is perfectly illustrated in the top part of Figure 5.9, which shows confocal laser microscopy images of ordinary chromatographic beads (<200-nm pores) after being exposed to fluorescently labeled plasmid DNA.[83] The depth-discriminating properties of confocal microscopy makes it possible to slice the beads optically into a series of thin sections shown on the top right-hand side of the figure. It

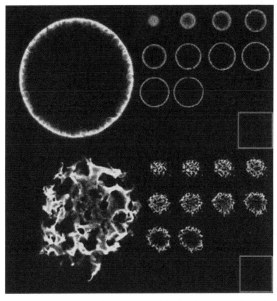

Figure 5.9 *Confocal microscopy of chromatographic (series on top) and microcarrier (series at the bottom) beads, which were incubated with fluorescently labeled plasmid DNA. After the removal of unbound material by washing the beads, different sections of the beads were scanned layer by layer with a confocal laser beam, inducing fluorescence. The result clearly illustrates that, under given conditions, plasmid DNA does not deeply enter into the pores of conventional chromatographic beads, whereas it penetrates the microcarrier beads. Reprinted from Journal of Gene Medicine, 6, Stadler J, Lemmens R, Nyhammar T. Plasmid DNA purification, S54-S66, Copyright 2004,[83] with permission from John Wiley & Sons.*

is clear from these scanned images that plasmid molecules do not enter the core of the beads[84] (further details are given in Chapter 17, Section 17.2.2).

5.6 CHROMATOGRAPHY

In many situations, and especially in the context of plasmid DNA manufacturing, it is important to have relatively rapid techniques capable of quantitating the different components in plasmid-containing samples. Analytical, high-performance chromatography is probably the best technique available for this purpose, and indeed its use is widespread among many laboratories involved in process development. Chromatographic separations explore the differential interactions between solutes in the sample under analysis with a solid matrix. This matrix is typically made of porous or nonporous microscopic beads (10–500 μm), which are packed as a bed in a cylindrical column. For analytic purposes, nonporous beads are preferred since the absence of intrabead solute diffusion directly translates into faster separations. Even when porous beads are used, the large size of plasmids when compared with the average size of pores in most commercial beads prevents access to the inside of the beads any way (see Chapter 17, Section 17.2.2 for further information on this topic). The solutes in the sample are brought into contact with the matrix by continuously flowing a liquid phase through the column. The composition of this so-called mobile phase can be changed in order to modulate the interaction of the different solutes with the matrix. The progressive elution of the different plasmid DNA species is typically monitored at the column outlet by recording the absorbance at 260 nm with an online detector. Although several different types of interactions can be promoted in plasmid chromatography,[86] electrostatic and hydrophobic interactions have been explored the most for analytical purposes, as described next.

5.6.1   Anion-Exchange Chromatography

In the case of anion-exchange chromatography, positively charged ligands are used in the solid matrix specifically to bind to the negatively charged phosphate groups in the DNA backbone.[87–90] An increasing gradient of salt (e.g., NaCl) is then used to displace the different nucleic acid species that elute in order of increasing charge density, a property that is a function of chain length. Molecules with a high charge density such as plasmid DNA isoforms usually bind strongly to most anion-exchange matrices and require NaCl concentrations of the order of 1 M to elute. Figure 5.10a shows a typical anion-exchange HPLC chromatogram of a plasmid standard (pUC18) isolated from *E. coli* cells. The sample is loaded at a high salt concentration and the plasmid topoisomers elute collectively as a single peak during the increasing NaCl gradient. Although no plasmid isoform separation is obtained in this example, in many instances, it is possible to find the correct combination of matrix and elution scheme to resolve open circular from supercoiled topoisomers with anion-exchange columns. The more compact supercoiled isoforms tend to bind stronger (and hence elute later) due to a charge/shape relation that produces a higher charge density relatively to the other isoforms, which are typically less constrained in space.[91–94] When anion-exchange HPLC is used to analyze plasmid-containing *E. coli* extracts, coelution of RNA with plasmid DNA is a recurrent problem. In these situations, a pretreatment of the samples with RNase is usually sufficient to hydrolyze RNA into smaller fragments that, in the subsequent HPLC analysis, will elute at much smaller salt concentration, leaving the plasmid isolated behind (Figure 5.10b).

5.6.2   Hydrophobic Interaction Chromatography (HIC)

Hydrophobic interactions between ligands in a matrix (e.g., phenyl rings) and the hydrophobic bases of DNA have also been explored in the context of analytical chromatography.[95,96] These interactions are typically favored in solutions with high concentrations of salts like ammonium sulfate and are destroyed in low-salt solutions. Thus, in this chromatographic modality, columns are equilibrated at high salt concentration and elution is performed by running negative salt gradients. Since plasmid molecules have the hydrophobic bases

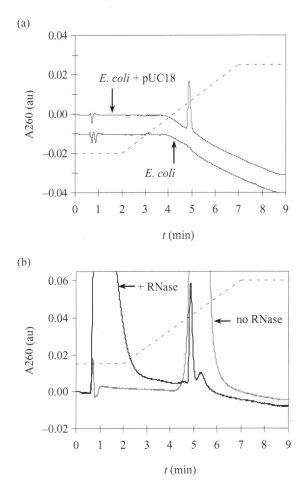

Figure 5.10 *Anion-exchange HPLC analysis of plasmid-containing samples. (a) A plasmid standard (pUC18, 2700 bp) isolated from E. coli cells was loaded at a high salt concentration (0.5 M). The plasmid topoisomers elute collectively as a single peak during the increasing NaCl gradient (up to 2 M). (b) The effect of RNase pretreatment of a plasmid-containing sample in the anion-exchange HPLC chromatogram is shown. A Poros 20 QE strong anion-exchange (4.6 × 100 mm) column from PerSeptive Biosystems (now Applied Biosystems, Foster City, California) was used at 2 mL/min. The salt gradient is shown by the dashed line (D. M. F. Prazeres, unpublished results).*

packed and shielded inside the double helix, interactions with these matrices are typically minimal, especially if compared with single-stranded nucleic acids in which the bases are highly exposed. Thus, plasmids should be expected to bind weakly or not bind at all in HIC columns. The binding mechanisms underlying HIC suggest that plasmid isoforms, which for some reason might differ in the amount of single-stranded material, could be potentially separated. This made it possible, for example, to separate supercoiled and open circular isoforms from denatured plasmids, which typically exhibit large stretches of unpaired, single-stranded DNA.[97] In other cases, and by resorting to highly concentrated salt solutions, the separation of supercoiled from open circular topoisomers is even possible. These separations explore the fact that supercoiled plasmids usually tend to expose bases as a consequence of underwinding of the molecule, a characteristic that is more pronounced at high salt.[97]

5.6.3 Size-Exclusion Chromatography

The ability of size-exclusion chromatography to separate the large plasmid DNA species from the smaller impurities (RNA and proteins), in principle, can be explored for analytical purposes. For example, the relative proportion of plasmid DNA to RNA in different process streams can be conveniently determined by size-exclusion HPLC.[98] This is illustrated in Figure 5.11, which shows results of a size-exclusion analysis of clarified, plasmid-containing alkaline lysates before and after a calcium chloride precipitation step. The group-separation ability of size exclusion is clear from these chromatograms. A more recent publication provides data which shows that such size-exclusion chromatography methods are also able to precisely measure the concentration of plasmid DNA in solutions containing RNA, proteins, and other impurities. Further details are given in the next section.[99] Although size-exclusion chromatography is also able to partially separate topoisomers, its resolving power is not sufficient to enable baseline separation of supercoiled, open circular, and linear plasmid.[100] Thus, it cannot be used to quantitate individual isoforms in a mixture.

5.6.4 Thiophilic Aromatic Chromatography

A method that combines two analytical chromatography steps has been recently described to quantitate plasmid DNA and to determine the relative proportion of supercoiled and open circular isoforms in samples collected throughout a manufacturing process.[99] In the first size-exclusion chromatography step, a short (2.5 cm) column packed with a Sepharose HP resin (GE Healthcare, Uppsala, Sweden) was used to separate total plasmid DNA from RNA, proteins, and other impurities (see Figure 5.12a). The concentration of the ensemble of plasmid species found in the first peak was then determined from calibration curves, which relate absorbance at 260 nm with either peak area or height. The method is fast (2 min) and is claimed to allow determination of plasmid DNA with limits of detection and quantification of 0.28 and 0.83 µg/mL, respectively. The relative proportion of supercoiled and open circular plasmid isoforms in the fraction that is collected from the first size-exclusion chromatography column is then determined by resorting to a thiophilic aromatic chromatography step (see Figure 5.12b). This type of chromatography uses ligands that contain an aromatic ring, as well as a thioether moiety. Under high salt concentration, plasmid isoforms interact with these ligands probably via hydrophobic (π–π) interactions with the aromatic ring and ion pair interactions with the sulfur atom.[101,102] Separation of the two

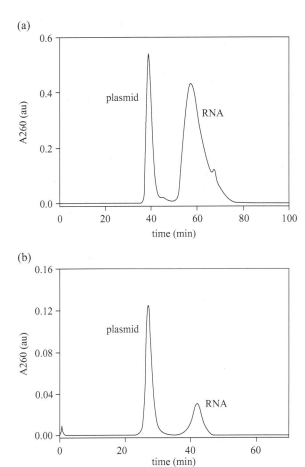

Figure 5.11 *Size-exclusion HPLC analysis of plasmid-containing alkaline lysates before (a) and after (b) 1 M calcium chloride precipitation. A TSKgel G6000 PWXL (7.8 × 300 mm) column from Tosoh-Biosciences (Tokyo, Japan) was used with isocratic elution (0.1 M tris, 300 mM NaCl, 1 mM EDTA, pH 7.5) at 0.5 mL/min. Reprinted from Analytical Biochemistry, 316, Eon-Duval A, MacDuff RH, Fisher CA, Harris MJ, Brook C. Removal of RNA impurities by tangential flow filtration in an RNase-free plasmid DNA purification process, 66-73, Copyright 2003,[98] with permission from Elsevier.*

isoforms becomes possible with this type of chromatography, probably due to the fact that the degree of base exposure to the environment is higher in supercoiled isoforms. A quantitative determination of each isoform is then easily performed on the basis of calibration curves constructed with different amounts of pure standards.

5.6.5 Final Remarks

Overall, HPLC is a fast, reproducible, and robust methodology. Although it is not often used to determine plasmid concentration or topoisomer distribution

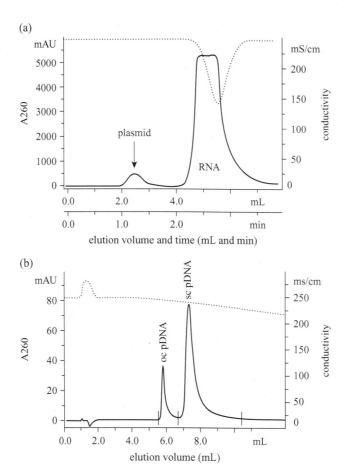

Figure 5.12 *Analysis of plasmid-containing alkaline lysates by tandem size-exclusion and thiophilic interaction chromatography. (a) A size-exclusion column is first used to separate total plasmid DNA (first peak) from RNA, proteins, and other impurities (second peak). (b) The relative proportion of supercoiled and open circular plasmid isoforms in the plasmid-containing fraction is then determined by resorting to a thiophilic aromatic column that uses ligands with an aromatic ring as well as a thioether moiety. Reprinted from Journal of Chromatography B, 877, Bennemo M, Blom H, Emilsson A, Lemmens R. A chromatographic method for determination of supercoiled plasmid DNA concentration in complex solutions, 2530-2536, Copyright 2009,[99] with permission from Elsevier.*

in pure samples obtained in a molecular biology laboratory, for which faster or more usual techniques are used (e.g., A260, gel electrophoresis), it is especially useful throughout manufacturing, both for process monitoring and for quality control (see Chapter 12, Section 12.3.2.3).

5.7 CONCLUSIONS

Analytical techniques are the keystone for all those working with biomolecules, independently of the exact context. The advancement of the area of plasmid biopharmaceuticals, in particular, is critically dependent on the implementation, correct use, and further development of analytical techniques. In the case of plasmids, the handful of well-proven and tested techniques that have stood the test of time (e.g., agarose electrophoresis, UV absorbance, and electron microscopy) have been complemented over the years with a cohort of more sophisticated techniques that make it possibly to probe the molecules in much more detail. Altogether, these methodologies have contributed to facilitate the task of analytically characterizing plasmid molecules, whether they are in solution, adsorbed to beads and particles, or simply trafficking through the cell cytoplasm.

REFERENCES

1. Sinden RR. *DNA structure and function.* San Diego, CA: Academic Press, 1994.

2. LePecq JB, Paoletti C. A fluorescent complex between ethidium bromide and nucleic acids. Physical-chemical characterization. *Journal of Molecular Biology.* 1967;27:87–106.

3. Geall AJ, Blagbrough IS. Rapid and sensitive ethidium bromide fluorescence quenching assay of polyamine conjugate-DNA interactions for the analysis of lipoplex formation in gene therapy. *Journal of Pharmaceutical and Biomedical Analysis.* 2000;22:849–859.

4. Sharp PA, Sugden B, Sambrook J. Detection of two restriction rndonuclease activities in *Haemophilus parainfluenzae* using analytical agarose-ethidium bromide electrophoresis. *Biochemistry.* 1973;12:3055–3063.

5. Hayashi M, Harada Y. Direct observation of the reversible unwinding of a single DNA molecule caused by the intercalation of ethidium bromide. *Nucleic Acids Research.* 2007;35:e125.

6. Bonasera V, Alberti S, Sacchetti A. Protocol for high-sensitivity/long linear-range spectrofluorimetric DNA quantification using ethidium bromide. *Biotechniques.* 2007;43:173–174. 176.

7. Singer VL, Jones LJ, Yue ST, Haugland RP. Characterization of PicoGreen reagent and development of a fluorescence-based solution assay for double-stranded DNA quantitation. *Analytical Biochemistry.* 1997;249:228–238.

8. Ribeiro SC, Monteiro GA, Martinho G, Cabral JMS, Prazeres DMF. Quantitation of plasmid DNA in aqueous two-phase systems by fluorescence analysis. *Biotechnology Letters.* 2000;22:1101–1104.

9. Noites IS, O'Kennedy RD, Levy MS, Abidi N, Keshavarz-Moore E. Rapid quantitation and monitoring of plasmid DNA using an ultrasensitive DNA-binding dye. *Biotechnology and Bioengineering.* 1999;66:195–201.

10. Levy MS, Lotfian P, O'Kennedy R, Lo-Yim MY, Shamlou PA. Quantitation of supercoiled circular content in plasmid DNA solutions using a fluorescence-based method. *Nucleic Acids Research.* 2000;28:E57.

11. Ahn SJ, Costa J, Emanuek JR. PicoGreen quantitation of DNA: Effective evaluation of samples pre- and post-PCR. *Nucleic Acids Research.* 1996;24: 2623–2625.

12. Hirons GT, Fawcett JJ, Crissman HA. TOTO and YOYO: New very bright fluoro-chromes for DNA content analyses by flow cytometry. *Cytometry.* 1994;15: 129–140.

13. Akita H, Ito R, Khalil IA, Futaki S, Harashima H. Quantitative three-dimensional analysis of the intracellular trafficking of plasmid DNA transfected by a nonviral gene delivery system using confocal laser scanning microscopy. *Molecular Therapy.* 2004;9:443–451.

14. Liu F, Shollenberger LM, Conwell CC, Yuan X, Huang L. Mechanism of naked DNA clearance after intravenous injection. *The Journal of Gene Medicine.* 2007;9:613–619.

15. Ho TQ, Zhong Z, Aung S, Pogliano J. Compatible bacterial plasmids are targeted to independent cellular locations in *Escherichia coli. The EMBO Journal.* 2002;21:1864–1872.

16. Escude C, Roulon T, Lyonnais S, Le Cam E. Multiple topological labeling for imaging single plasmids. *Analytical Biochemistry.* 2007;362:55–62.

17. Escude C, Garestier T, Helene C. Padlock oligonucleotides for duplex DNA based on sequence-specific triple helix formation. *Proceedings of the National Academy of Sciences of the United States of America.* 1999;96:10603–10607.

18. Demidov VV, Kuhn H, Lavrentieva-Smolina IV, Frank-Kamenetskii MD. Peptide nucleic acid-assisted topological labeling of duplex dna. *Methods.* 2001;23:123–131.

19. Linn SM, Lloyd RS, Roberts RJ, eds. *Nucleases,* 2nd ed. Cold Spring Harbor Monograph Series. Plainview, NY: Cold Spring Harbor Laboratory Press, 1993.

20. Ribeiro SC, Monteiro GA, Prazeres DMF. The role of polyadenylation signal secondary structures on the resistance of plasmid vectors to nucleases. *The Journal of Gene Medicine.* 2004;6:565–573.

21. Prazeres DMF, Schluep T, Cooney CL. Preparative purification of supercoiled plasmid DNA using anion-exchange chromatography. *Journal of Chromatography. A.* 1998;806:31–45.

22. Carnes AE, Hodgson CP, Luke JM, Vincent JM, Williams JA. Plasmid DNA pro-duction combining antibiotic-free selection, inducible high yield fermentation, and novel autolytic purification. *Biotechnology and Bioengineering.* 2009;104:505–515.

23. Katcher HL, Wallace SS. Characterization of the *Escherichia coli* X-ray endonu-clease, endonuclease III. *Biochemistry.* 1983;22:4071–4081.

24. Saito Y, Uraki F, Nakajima S, et al. Characterization of endonuclease III (nth) and endonuclease VIII (nei) mutants of *Escherichia coli* K-12. *Journal of Bacteriology.* 1997;179:3783–3785.

25. Prather KL, Edmonds MC, Herod JW. Identification and characterization of IS1 transposition in plasmid amplification mutants of *E. coli* clones producing DNA vaccines. *Applied Microbiology and Biotechnology.* 2006;73:815–826.

26. Ribeiro SC, Oliveira PH, Prazeres DMF, Monteiro GA. High frequency plasmid recombination mediated by 28 bp direct repeats. *Molecular Biotechnology.* 2008;40:252–260.

27. Oliveira PH, Prazeres DMF, Monteiro GA. Deletion formation mutations in plasmid expression vectors are unfavored by runaway amplification conditions and differentially selected under kanamycin stress. *Journal of Biotechnology.* 2009;143:231–238.

28. Ledwith BJ, Manam S, Troilo PJ, et al. Plasmid DNA vaccines: Investigation of integration into host cellular DNA following intramuscular injection in mice. *Intervirology.* 2000;43:258–272.

29. Gonin P, Gaillard C. Gene transfer vector biodistribution: Pivotal safety studies in clinical gene therapy development. *Gene Therapy.* 2004;11(Suppl 1):S98–S108.

30. Keller W. Determination of the number of superhelical turns in simian virus 40 DNA by gel electrophoresis. *Proceedings of the National Academy of Sciences of the United States of America.* 1975;72:4876–4880.

31. Camilloni G, Di Martino E, Caserta M, di Mauro E. Eukaryotic DNA topoisomerase I reaction is topology dependent. *Nucleic Acids Research.* 1988;16:7071–7085.

32. Viovy J-L. Electrophoresis of DNA and other polyelectrolytes: Physical mechanisms. *Reviews of Modern Physics.* 2000;72:813–872.

33. Slater GW, Kenward M, McCormick LC, Gauthier MG. The theory of DNA separation by capillary electrophoresis. *Current Opinion in Biotechnology.* 2003; 14:58–64.

34. Bowater R, Aboul-Ela F, Lilley DMJ. Two-dimensional gel electrophoresis of circular DNA topoisomers. *Methods in Enzymology.* 1992;212:105–120.

35. Bauer W, Vinograd J. The interaction of closed circular DNA with intercalative dyes. I. The superhelix density of SV40 DNA in the presence and absence of dye. *Journal of Molecular Biology.* 1968;33:141–171.

36. Shubsda MF, Goodisman J, Dabrowiak JC. Quantitation of ethidium-stained closed circular DNA in agarose gels. *Journal of Biochemistry and Biophysics Methods.* 1997;34:73–79.

37. Maule J. Pulsed-field gel electrophoresis. In: Rapley R, ed. *The nucleic acid protocols handbook.* Totowa, NJ: Humana Press, 2000:81–104.

38. Schleef M, Schmidt T, Flaschel E. Plasmid DNA for pharmaceutical applications. *Developments in Biological Standardization (Basel).* 2000;104:25–31.

39. Schmidt T, Friehs K, Flaschel E. Rapid determination of plasmid copy number. *Journal of Biotechnology.* 1996;49:219–229.

40. Schmidt T, Friehs K, Schleef M, Voss C, Flaschel E. Quantitative analysis of plasmid forms by agarose and capillary gel electrophoresis. *Analytical Biochemistry.* 1999;274:235–240.

41. Schmidt T, Friehs K, Schleef M, Voss C, Flaschel E. Assessing the homogeneity of plasmid DNA: An important step toward gene therapy. *P/ACE Setter Newsletter.* 2000;4:1–3.

42. Nackerdien Z, Morris S, Choquette S, Ramos B, Atha D. Analysis of laser-induced plasmic DNA photolysis by capillary electrophoresis. *Journal of Chromatography. B.* 1996;683:91–96.

43. Schleef M, Baier R, Walther W, Michel ML, Schmeer M. Long-term stability study and topology analysis of plasmid DNA by capillary gel electrophoresis. *BioProcess International.* 2006;September:38–40.

44. Wang S-C, Morris MD. Mechanistic studies of DNA separations by capillary electrophoresis in ultradilute polymer solutions: Effects of polymer rigidity. *Analytical Sciences.* 2001;17:i173–i176.

45. Berne BJ, Pecora R. *Dynamic light scattering: With applications to chemistry, biology, and physics.* Mineola, NY: Courier Dover Publications, 2000.

46. Fishman DM, Patterson GD. Light scattering studies of supercoiled and nicked DNA. *Biopolymers.* 1996;38:535–552.

47. Langowski J, Kremer W, Kapp U. Dynamic light scattering for study of solution conformation and dynamics of superhelical DNA. *Methods in Enzymology.* 1992;211:430–448.

48. Wu ML, Freitas SS, Monteiro GA, Prazeres DM, Santos JA. Stabilization of naked and condensed plasmid DNA against degradation induced by ultrasounds and high-shear vortices. *Biotechnology and Applied Biochemistry.* 2009;53:237–246.

49. Kelly SM, Jess TJ, Price NC. How to study proteins by circular dichroism. *Biochimica et Biophysica Acta.* 2005;1751:119–139.

50. Woody RW. Circular dichroism. *Methods in Enzymology.* 1995;246:34–71.

51. Serban D, Benevides JM, Thomas GJ. DNA secondary structure and Raman markers of supercoiling in *Escherichia coli* plasmid pUC19. *Biochemistry.* 2002;41:847–853.

52. MacDermott AJ, Drake AF. Circular dichroism of positively and negatively super-coiled DNA. *Studia Biophysica.* 1986;115:59–67.

53. Studdert DS, Patroni M, Davis RC. Circular dichroism of DNA: Temperature and salt dependence. *Biopolymers.* 1972;11:761–779.

54. Matzeu M, Onori G, Santucci A. Condensation of DNA by monohydric alcohols. *Colloids and Surfaces B-Biointerfaces.* 1999;13:157–163.

55. Liu G, Li D, Pasumarthy MK, et al. Nanoparticles of compacted DNA transfect postmitotic cells. *The Journal of Biological Chemistry.* 2003;278:32578–32586.

56. Murphy JC, Wibbenmeyer JA, Fox GE, Willson RC. Purification of plasmid DNA using selective precipitation by compaction agents. *Nature Biotechnology.* 1999;17:822–823.

57. Murphy JC, Cano T, Fox GE, Willson RC. Compaction agent protection of nucleic acids during mechanical lysis. *Biotechnology Progress.* 2006;22:519–522.

58. Wang DA, Narang AS, Kotb M, et al. Novel branched poly(ethylenimine)-choles-terol water-soluble lipopolymers for gene delivery. *Biomacromolecules.* 2002; 3:1197–1207.

59. Hansma HG. Surface biology of DNA by atomic force microscopy. *Annual Review of Physical Chemistry.* 2001;52:71–92.

60. Stahlberg H, Walz T. Molecular electron microscopy: State of the art and current challenges. *ACS Chemical Biology.* 2008;3:268–281.

61. Boles TC, White JH, Cozzarelli N-R. Structure of plectonemically supercoiled DNA. *Journal of Molecular Biology.* 1990;213:931–951.

62. Vologodskii AV, Levene SD, Klenin KV, Frank-Kamenetskii M, Cozzarelli NR. Conformational and thermodynamic properties of supercoiled DNA. *Journal of Molecular Biology.* 1992;227:1224–1243.

63. Weigl D, Molloy MJ, Clayton TM, et al. Characterization of a topologically aber-rant plasmid population from pilot-scale production of clinical-grade DNA. *Journal of Biotechnology.* 2006;121:1–12.

64. Saibil HR. Conformational changes studied by cryo-electron microscopy. *Nature Structtural Biology.* 2000;7:711–714.

65. Frank J. Single-particle imaging of macromolecules by cryo-electron microscopy. *Annual Review of Biophysics and Biomolecular Structure.* 2002;31:303–319.

66. Bednar J, Furrer P, Stasiak A, Dubochet J, Egelman EH, Bates AD. The twist, the writhe and overal shape of supercoiled DNA change during counterion-induced transition from a loosely to a tightly interwound superhelix: Possible implications for DNA structure *in vivo*. *Journal of Molecular Biology*. 1994;235:825–847.

67. Tam P, Monck M, Lee D, et al. Stabilized plasmid-lipid particles for systemic gene therapy. *Gene Therapy*. 2000;7:1867–1874.

68. Pitard B, Bello-Roufai M, Lambert O, et al. Negatively charged self-assembling DNA/poloxamine nanospheres for *in vivo* gene transfer. *Nucleic Acids Research*. 2004;32:e159.

69. Bustamante C, Vesenka J, Tang CL, Rees W, Guthold M, Keller R. Circular DNA molecules imaged in air by scanning force microscopy. *Biochemistry*. 1992;31: 22–26.

70. Hansma HG, Vesenka J, Siegerist C, et al. Reproducible imaging and dissection of plasmid DNA under liquid with the atomic force microscope. *Science*. 1992;256:1180–1184.

71. Yu J, Zhang Z, Cao K, Huang X. Visualization of alkali-denatured supercoiled plasmid DNA by atomic force microscopy. *Biochemistry and Biophysics Research Communications*. 2008;374:415–418.

72. Allison DP, Kerper PS, Doktycz MJ, et al. Mapping individual cosmid DNAs by direct AFM imaging. *Genomics*. 1997;41:379–384.

73. Shlyakhtenko LS, Potaman VN, Sinden RR, Lyubchenko YL. Structure and dynamics of supercoil-stabilized DNA cruciforms. *Journal of Molecular Biology*. 1998;280:61–72.

74. Tiner WJ, Potaman VN, Sinden RR, Lyubchenko YL. The structure of intramolecular triplex DNA: Atomic force microscopy study. *Journal of Molecular Biology*. 2001;314:353–357.

75. Pope LH, Davies MC, Laughton CA, Roberts CJ, Tendler SJ, Williams PM. Atomic force microscopy studies of intercalation-induced changes in plasmid DNA tertiary structure. *Journal of Microscopy*. 2000;199:68–78.

76. Dunlap DD, Maggi A, Soria MR, Monaco L. Nanoscopic structure of DNA condensed for gene delivery. *Nucleic Acids Research*. 1997;25:3095–3101.

77. Hartikka J, Geall A, Bozoukova V, et al. Physical characterization and *in vivo* evaluation of poloxamer-based DNA vaccine formulations. *The Journal of Gene Medicine*. 2008;10:770–782.

78. Müller M. *Introduction to confocal fluorescence microscopy*. Bellingham, WA: SPIE Press, 2006.

79. Breuzard G, Tertil M, Goncalves C, et al. Nuclear delivery of NFkappaB-assisted DNA/polymer complexes: Plasmid DNA quantitation by confocal laser scanning microscopy and evidence of nuclear polyplexes by FRET imaging. *Nucleic Acids Research*. 2008;36:e71.

80. Gasiorowski JZ, Dean DA. Postmitotic nuclear retention of episomal plasmids is altered by DNA labeling and detection methods. *Molecular Therapy*. 2005; 12:460–467.

81. Kopatz I, Remy JS, Behr JP. A model for non-viral gene delivery: Through syndecan adhesion molecules and powered by actin. *The Journal of Gene Medicine*. 2004;6:769–776.

82. Hubbuch J, Kula MR. Confocal laser scanning microscopy as an analytical tool in chromatographic research. *Bioprocess and Biosystems Engineering.* 2008;31: 241–259.

83. Stadler J, Lemmens R, Nyhammar T. Plasmid DNA purification. *The Journal of Gene Medicine.* 2004;6:S54–S66.

84. Ljunglöf A, Bergvall P, Bhikhabhai R, Hjörth R. Direct visualisation of plasmid DNA in individual chromatography adsorbent particles by confocal scanning laser microscopy. *Journal of Chromatography. A.* 1999;844:129–135.

85. Tiainen P, Gustavsson P-E, Ljunglöf A, Larsson P-O. Superporous agarose anion exchangers for plasmid isolation. *Journal of Chromatography. A.* 2007;1138: 84–94.

86. Diogo MM, Queiroz JA, Prazeres DMF. Chromatography of plasmid DNA. *Journal of Chromatography. A.* 2005;1069:3–22.

87. Onishi Y, Azuma Y, Kizaki H. An assay method for DNA topoisomerase activity based on separation of relaxed DNA from supercoiled DNA using high-performance liquid chromatography. *Analytical Biochemistry.* 1993;210:63–68.

88. Horn NA, Meek JA, Budahazi G, Marquet M. Cancer gene therapy using plasmid DNA: Purification of DNA for human clinical trials. *Human Gene Therapy.* 1995;6:565–573.

89. Ferreira GNM, Cabral JMS, Prazeres DMF. Monitoring of process streams in the large scale production and purification of plasmid DNA for gene therapy applications. *Pharmacy and Pharmacology Communications.* 1999;5:57–59.

90. Molloy MJ, Hall VS, Bailey SI, Griffin KJ, Faulkner J, Uden M. Effective and robust plasmid topology analysis and the subsequent characterization of the plasmid isoforms thereby observed. *Nucleic Acids Research.* 2004;32:e129.

91. Colpan M, Riesner D. High-performance liquid chromatography of high-molecular-weight nucleic acids on the macroporous ion exchanger, Nucleogen. *Journal of Chromatography.* 1984;296:339–353.

92. Hines R, O'Connor K, Vella G, Warren W. Large-scale purification of plasmid DNA by anion-exchange high-performance liquid chromatography. *Biotechniques.* 1992;12:430–434.

93. Quaak SG, Nuijen B, Haanen JB, Beijnen JH. Development and validation of an anion-exchange LC-UV method for the quantification and purity determination of the DNA plasmid pDERMATT. *Journal of Pharmaceutical and Biomedical Analysis.* 2009;49:282–288.

94. Smith CR, DePrince RB, Dackor J, Weigl D, Griffith J, Persmark M. Separation of topological forms of plasmid DNA by anion-exchange HPLC: Shifts in elution order of linear DNA. *Journal of Chromatography.* 2007;854:121–127.

95. Diogo MM, Queiroz JA, Prazeres DMF. Assessment of purity and quantification of plasmid DNA in process solutions using high-performance hydrophobic interaction chromatography. *Journal of Chromatography. A.* 2003;998:109–117.

96. Iuliano S, Fisher JR, Chen M, Kelly WJ. Rapid analysis of a plasmid by hydrophobic-interaction chromatography with a non-porous resin. *Journal of Chromatography. A.* 2002;972:77–86.

97. Diogo MM, Queiroz JA, Monteiro GA, Prazeres DMF. Separation and analysis of plasmid denatured forms using hydrophobic interaction chromatography. *Analytical Biochemistry.* 2000;275:122–124.

98. Eon-Duval A, MacDuff RH, Fisher CA, Harris MJ, Brook C. Removal of RNA impurities by tangential flow filtration in an RNase-free plasmid DNA purification process. *Analytical Biochemistry.* 2003;316:66–73.

99. Bennemo M, Blom H, Emilsson A, Lemmens R. A chromatographic method for determination of supercoiled plasmid DNA concentration in complex solutions. *Journal of Chromatography. B.* 2009;877:2530–2536.

100. Latulippe DR, Zydney AL. Size exclusion chromatography of plasmid DNA isoforms. *Journal of Chromatography. A.* 2009;1216:6295–6302.

101. Sandberg LM, Bjurling A, Busson P, Vasi J, Lemmens R. Thiophilic interaction chromatography for supercoiled plasmid DNA purification. *Journal of Biotechnology.* 2004;109:193–199.

102. Lemmens R, Olsson U, Nyhammar T, Stadler J. Supercoiled plasmid DNA: Selective purification by thiophilic/aromatic adsorption. *Journal of Chromatography. B.* 2003;784:291–300.

6

Delivery

6.1 INTRODUCTION

The success of plasmid biopharmaceuticals when used to treat the range of diseases described in Chapter 2 depends first on the efficiency of DNA delivery and expression. The word delivery refers to the process by which plasmids and their gene cargo are transported from the exterior into the body of the research subject/patient and all the way through to the nucleus of the target cells. This is a difficult task to accomplish due to the existence of a series of extracellular and intracellular defense barriers and mechanisms that act together to clear the organism from the extraneous DNA molecule. While journeying through capillaries, interstitial spaces, tissues, body fluids, membranes, and the cytoplasm, plasmids may find mononuclear phagocytes, blood components, harsh environmental conditions (e.g., low pH), plasma and cellular endonucleases, cellular membranes, endosomes and lysosomes, and narrow nuclear pore complexes (NPCs) that collectively contribute to reduce the number of molecules arriving at the final destiny, the nucleus.[1] The magnitude of the barriers found within the cytoplasm is illustrated very well by the microinjection experiments performed by Graessman et al., which showed that the level of transgene expression increases more than 30-fold if plasmids (1000–3000 copies) are microinjected directly into the nucleus instead of into the cytoplasm of cultured mammalian cells.[2] Many other experiments have

Plasmid Biopharmaceuticals: Basics, Applications, and Manufacturing, First Edition.
Duarte Miguel F. Prazeres.
© 2011 John Wiley & Sons, Inc. Published 2011 by John Wiley & Sons, Inc.

confirmed this. From the pool of nuclear transgenes, a fraction will eventually undergo transcription and originate a protein product that will hopefully play the molecular role anticipated in the design of the pharmaceutical (see Chapter 2, Section 2.3). However, if the efficiency of these two steps (delivery and expression) is poor to start with, one can hardly expect to obtain a significant therapeutic effect. Unfortunately, it is a well-known fact for those involved in the field that viral vectors are far superior to plasmids (usually >90%) when it comes to delivery and expression of transgenes. Problems with low levels of expression can be tackled by manipulating the structure of plasmids in order to select the promoters, enhancers, or polyadenylation signals best adapted to the target cells and expression needs.[3] Still, and much more than expression, delivery remains the major obstacle for the success of plasmid biopharmaceuticals. The design and development of safe and efficient delivery systems is thus of paramount importance to overcome the lack of performance of plasmid biopharmaceuticals. The first step is to decide how to administer the plasmid biopharmaceutical. The exact route by which plasmids enter the recipient's body will depend in most cases on the nature of the disease under study and of the therapeutic intervention planned (see Chapter 2, Figure 2.4). For example, DNA vaccines for the prevention of infectious diseases are typically administered via muscular or skin tissues;[4] intratumoral administration is used in the treatment of solid tumors,[5] and the airways are usually preferred when addressing diseases that affect the lungs (e.g., cystic fibrosis[6]). The administration route will, to a large extent, constrain the choice of the delivery system used to carry the plasmid from the shelf into the cell nucleus. Likewise, certain delivery systems and devices are specifically designed to serve defined entry routes.

In the first part of this chapter, the most important strategies used to facilitate and mediate the delivery of plasmids to the nucleus of cells in living animals are examined and described. As a first step, the purified target plasmid DNA is first combined and formulated with buffers, stabilizers, and inorganic or organic matrices and molecules (see Chapter 2, Figure 2.2). Depending on the delivery strategy pursued, this formulation may result in (i) a saline solution of plasmid, (ii) gold particles coated with plasmid, (iii) plasmids complexed with cationic lipids or polymers, (iv) nanoparticles of compacted plasmid, or (v) polymeric microparticles with encapsulated or surface-adsorbed plasmid (see Figure 6.1). These formulated plasmids are then introduced in the recipient's body with conventional methods (e.g., needle injection and infusion) or else used in conjunction with a device that is specifically designed to serve the administration route under consideration. While some devices like the gene gun are used essentially to deliver one type of formulation (i.e., plasmid-coated gold particles), others like the conventional needle and syringe or needle-free injectors can be used to administer a plasmid that is formulated in different manners (see Figure 6.1). In the second part of the chapter, an analysis is presented that compares the methodologies used to deliver DNA vaccines developed to provide protection against influenza and to treat mela-

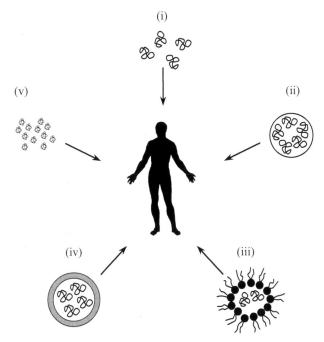

Figure 6.1 *Options for in vivo plasmid delivery. Depending on the delivery strategy pursued, the purified target plasmid DNA is combined and formulated with buffers, stabilizers, and inorganic or organic matrices and molecules. This may result in (i) a saline solution of plasmid, (ii) gold particles coated with plasmid, (iii) plasmids complexed with cationic lipids or polymers, (iv) polymeric microparticles with encapsulated or surface-adsorbed plasmid, or (v) nanoparticles of compacted plasmid. These formulated plasmids are then introduced in the recipient's body with conventional methods (e.g., needle injection and infusion) or else used in conjunction with a device that is specifically designed for the administration under consideration (e.g., gene gun, electroporator, and jet injector).*

noma. The vaccines examined have all undergone or are undergoing trials in humans. This academic exercise is intended to highlight exclusively the differences in the design of each product when it comes to dosage and the delivery methodology used. No considerations are thus made regarding the clinical efficacy of the vaccines themselves.

6.2 NAKED DNA

6.2.1 Introduction

The simplest way of delivering a plasmid biopharmaceutical to the cells of a living recipient is via injection of a saline solution of the plasmid. The proof-of-concept study that supports this methodology was first presented to the scientific community in 1990 by Wolff and coworkers,[7] as described in Chapter

1 (see Section 1.3.3). In the experiments reported in this seminal article, quadriceps muscles of living mice were injected with up to 100 µg of plasmids containing genes coding for the enzymes chloramphenicol acetyltransferase (CAT), luciferase, or β-galactosidase. The breakthrough finding of the study was that such a "naked" plasmid DNA molecule, devoid of any kind of adjuvant, could be taken up by the mice's muscle cells and that the encoded reporter transgenes were expressed within those cells. Histochemical staining of muscles for enzymatic activity revealed that approximately 1.5% of the cells in the entire quadriceps and 10–30% of the cells within the injection area were expressing β-galactosidase 7 days after a single 100 µg shot of plasmid. Additional findings included the observation of a dose–response effect, whereby an increase in the amount of injected plasmid resulted in an equivalent increase in the amount of expressed protein and in a persistence of transgene expression for 2 months that was attributed to the presence of extrachromosomal, nonintegrated plasmid within the transfected cells.[7] The popularity that the naked DNA approach gained as a gene delivery methodology is essentially associated with its inherent simplicity, ease of preparation, and safety.[8] Unfortunately, in most cases, the efficiency of expression of transgenes to the skeletal muscle of large animals (e.g., nonhuman primates) has been shown to be rather poor and variable when compared to alternative delivery methodologies.[8] The fact that thousands of plasmid molecules have to be present at the injection site in order for a single molecule to eventually reach the nucleus and have its transgene expressed[9] underscores the relentless attack to which naked plasmid molecules are subjected *in vivo*.

6.2.2 Mechanisms Underlying Uptake by Muscle Cells

In order to improve the efficiency of naked DNA, an understanding of the mechanisms and route by which plasmids are taken up and expressed by cells in *in vivo* tissues is required. The current thinking regarding this multistep process is described next. Although the focus is on naked plasmid DNA and muscle cells, the description that follows will serve as a benchmark for the analysis of the transfection of other tissues by the alternative delivery methodologies that are described in sections ahead. Following *in vivo* intramuscular needle injection, naked plasmids tend to remain close to the injection site.[10–12] Here, and within the first minutes of administration, the majority of the molecules are rapidly degraded by endogenous nucleases.[13,14] The remaining plasmid is then progressively cleared and degraded from the injection site within a 2- to 6-month period. As a rule, the injection of naked plasmids in muscles does not stimulate the production of anti-DNA or myosin autoantibodies,[15,16] and thus clearance from the injection site is attributable essentially to endonuclease action rather than to an immune response. During their lifetime within the body, plasmids do not disseminate very far from the injection site. Still, plasmid fragments may be sporadically found in organs and tissues (draining lymph nodes, lung, kidney, and liver) due to redistribution via the blood, cells, and lymph to other more distant tissues (see Chapter 7, Section 7.3.2 for more details on the biodistribution and persistence of plasmids after administration). However, and in general, the transfection of distant cells by naked plasmids injected intramuscularly is an unlikely event.[8] The exact mechanism by which plasmid molecules enter muscle cells and travel to the nucleus is not clearly known. The particular structural features of muscle tissue, including its multinucleated cells, sarcoplasmic reticulum, and transverse tubule (T-tubule) system, were initially suggested by Wolff and colleagues to be particularly suited for plasmid uptake and expression.[7] In particular, the deep, perpendicular penetration of T-tubules within muscle fibers and the fact that they are able to transport large amounts of extracellular fluids could constitute a means for plasmids to enter the sarcoplasmic reticulum. Once here, the plasmid would access the cytoplasm of cells during muscle contraction and influx of calcium ions.[7] However, the fact that naked plasmid DNA can also be taken up after injection by tissues other than nonmuscle tissues like the liver,[17] skin,[18] heart,[19] and brain[20] indicates that the T-tubule hypothesis is too restrictive.[13] The mechanical damage imparted to cell membranes by the injection needle, or the induction of small transient membrane pores by the high hydrostatic pressures and velocities generated during injection of the saline solution, were also suggested as mechanisms that could contribute to plasmid uptake.[13] According to this line of reasoning, plasmid molecules would diffuse into the cytoplasm through those cracks and openings. Nevertheless, these mechanisms have been discarded due to a lack of experimental evidence and because they cannot support the fact that plasmid uptake is long-lived.[13]

One of the strongest hypotheses put forward to explain how plasmid molecules overcome the barrier imposed by the cell membrane (see Figure 6.2) suggests the involvement of receptor-mediated endocytosis.[13,21] This hypothesis, which was originally suggested by earlier experimental studies on the *in vivo* uptake of oligonucleotides,[22] has subsequently found support from studies carried out with naked plasmid DNA[13]. According to this model, some plasmid DNA molecules delivered to the extracellular space eventually bind to specific cell receptors, whose exact nature is still unknown. If one assumes that the number of available DNA receptors at the cell surface is limited, this mechanism could explain the slow internalization process that is characteristic of naked plasmid uptake by mammalian cells.[21] The plasmid–receptor complexes at the surface are subsequently engulfed by the cell via the inward folding of the plasma membrane. The plasmid-containing vesicles thus formed are then fused to endosomes, which subsequently fuse with digestive vesicles known as lysosomes. The release of plasmid from those small endosomes and liposomes requires the destabilization of the membranes and the ejection of the internal cargo into the cytoplasm[23]. Endosomes and lysosomes constitute an important barrier, not only because this release is not straightforward but also because internal degradation is likely to occur on account of the acidic

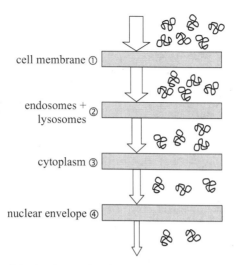

cell membrane ①

endosomes + ② lysosomes

cytoplasm ③

nuclear envelope ④

Figure 6.2 *The intracellular barriers to plasmid-based gene transfer. After passing the physical barrier created by the phospholipidic cell membrane through endocytosis, plasmids have to escape entrapment and degradation in endosomes and lysosomes, resist degradation by cytosolic nucleases, overcome transport limitations imposed by molecular overcrowding in the cytoplasm, and cross the nuclear envelope via translocation through nuclear pore complexes.*

pH and the presence of lysosomal nucleases (see Figure 6.2). After escaping from endosomes and lysosomes, the surviving free plasmid DNA molecules must travel toward the cell nucleus. This is unlikely to occur via free diffusion, since this type of transport is extremely slow on account of the large size and small diffusion coefficient of plasmids (see Chapter 4, Section 4.5.4), and also due to the steric hindrance that is imposed by the highly cross-linked actin cytoskeleton of the cells.[13,14,24] Rather, a mechanism of active transport involving the microtubule network of cells has been proposed to explain the trafficking of plasmid molecules along cytoskeletal elements and toward the nucleus.[24] The interaction between plasmids and microtubules is most likely mediated by cellular proteins like the molecular motor dynein.[24] The fraction of plasmid molecules that eventually reach the rim of the nucleus are faced with an additional barrier—the nuclear envelope—that separates them from their final destiny (see Figure 6.2). If the cells are engaged in division, plasmids can take advantage of the breaking of the nuclear envelope and thus enter the nuclei of descendant cells rather easily before new envelopes are formed.[24] In nondividing cells, however, the NPC, a 125×10^6 Da structure made of more than 100 different proteins, becomes the only gate to access the nucleus.[24,25] The transport of plasmid molecules through the NPC is facilitated if specific DNA targeting sequences (DTSs) like the 72-bp-long SV40 virus enhancer are present in the plasmid backbone.[26,27] The specificity of the SV40 enhancer sequence has been linked to the presence of binding sites for a number of transcription factors (TFs). These factors possess specific amino acid sequences that act as nuclear localization signals (NLSs), enabling and actively directing transport across the nuclear envelope via the NPC. Once in the nucleus, TFs bind to target sites on various promoters and enhancers in the cell DNA.[24,25] The picture that emerges in the case of the import of plasmids that harbor the SV40 enhancer is that TFs will rather bind to the DTS of the enhancer while in the cytoplasm. Thus, the DNA molecule becomes coated with a number of NLSs that signal and facilitate the transportation of the plasmid/TF complex by the protein import machinery across the nucleus envelope.[24,25,27] The few plasmid molecules that have survived the long journey to the nucleus are then ready to undergo transcription.

6.2.3 Needle-Free Intramuscular Injection

The use of needles and syringes to deliver naked plasmids (as any other bio-pharmaceutical for that matter) has some well-known disadvantages, including discomfort to patients, needle phobia, hazardous needle waste, and risk of accidental needlestick injuries with transmission of infectious agents like human immunodeficiency virus (HIV) and hepatitis B virus.[28] One of the best needle-free alternatives available to deliver plasmids and other biopharmaceuticals is to resort to liquid jet injectors. These devices generate fine (~76–360 µm in diameter), high-pressure jets with speeds higher than 100 m/s that puncture through the skin, depositing solutions in the tissue beneath. The Biojector 2000 needle-free jet injection system developed by Bioject Medical Technologies, Inc. (Tualatin, Oregon) is an example of a needle-free device that has been often used to inject naked plasmids intramuscularly and sub-cutaneously[29–31] (see also case studies in Section 6.7). This FDA-cleared injection device relies on a small CO_2 cartridge to force the plasmid solution contained in a disposable needle-free syringe through a tiny orifice. Upon impact, the cylindrical jet that is generated erodes and fractures the skin, creating a hole through which >90% of the fluid is deposited.[28] Following injection, the syringe is disposed off and exchanged for a new one in preparation for the subsequent administration. As for the CO_2 cartridge, it can be used to deliver up to 10–15 injections. Comparative studies with animal models have shown that delivery of DNA vaccines (e.g., HIV[31] and human papillomavirus (HPV)[30]) with a Biojector liquid jet injector elicits cellular and humoral immune responses that are comparable to the ones generated when the vaccines are administered intramuscularly with needle and syringe.[30,31] Since jet injection provides for a standardized, mechanically based delivery, it has been associated with a higher administration consistency when compared with manual needle syringe injection.[30] Delivery by jet injection is sometimes associated with a level of pain that is equivalent to needle injection and with more frequent local site reactions (e.g., swelling).[28]

6.2.4 Hydrodynamic Delivery

As we have seen above, the fact that transfection is essentially restricted to the injection site and that levels of expression are relatively low are characteristics of the intramuscular delivery of naked plasmid DNA, whether needle or needle-free systems are used for administration. These features constitute a drawback, for example, in the case of those pathologies where a systemic delivery of the transgene is sought or when higher levels of expression are required. The early realization of these limitations of naked DNA intramuscular injection prompted the search for alternative, more efficacious means of delivery. One important breakthrough in that quest was the finding that the expression of naked DNA in the muscles in a given limb could be increased substantially by delivering plasmids intravascularly under high hydrostatic pressure.[32] Another important discovery was the realization that the portal, hepatic, and tail vein of mice could also be used to inject naked plasmid DNA and to achieve high expression in hepatocytes.[33,34] This procedure explores the high pressure that is exerted when a large volume (8–10% of the body weight[35]) of a plasmid-containing saline solution is rapidly injected intravenously.[34] Several studies show that when this particular method of delivery is used, plasmids are primarily found in liver cells.[34–36] The mechanisms underlying the liver specificity that is associated with hydrodynamic delivery have been investigated by several authors. The picture that has emerged from these studies is that following the injection of large volumes of solution, a transient heart failure occurs that causes blood and the plasmid solution to back-flow to the liver.[36–39] Here, the increased pressure and shear forces associated with the hydrodynamically injected material originate a series of short-lived morphological liver changes that are ultimately responsible for facilitating plasmid delivery and expression.[37–39] First, an enlargement of venous vessels and an increase in the endothelial discontinuities (also known as fenestrae) in sinusoidal blood vessels are observed[37] (Figure 6.3). As a result, the plasmid solution exits the sinusoidal space, causing an enlarging of the space of Disse that separates the endothelium from hepatocytes.[37,38] Simultaneously, substantial amounts of fluid and associated plasmid molecules are taken up via large endocytic vesicles, which appear very soon (~5 min) after injection[39] (Figure 6.3). Hepatocytes are especially able to cope with this massive rush of fluid since they have a natural ability for microfluidic endocytosis.[37] The incorporated vesicles are thought to be relatively unstable, and thus the release of their plasmid content in the cytoplasm is probably facilitated when compared with the release from the endosomes described in Section 6.2.2.[39] Once in the cytoplasm, those plasmid molecules that remained intact are on their pathway to expression. It has been hypothesized that this trafficking toward the nucleus is facilitated by the significant cytoplasm swelling and partial fragmentation of actin filaments in the cytoskeleton that accompany vesicle uptake.[38] An alternative entry mechanism has also been postulated, which suggests that plasmids could enter hepatocytes directly via convection or diffusion through nonlethal pores formed in the cell

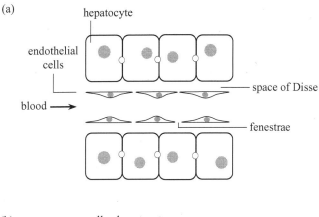

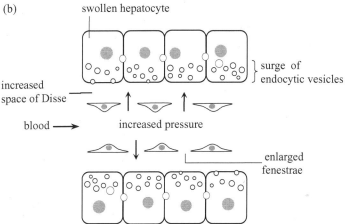

Figure 6.3 *Mechanisms underlying the hydrodynamic delivery of plasmids. Following the injection of large volumes of a plasmid-containing saline solution in the hepatic or portal vein, blood back-flows to the liver, where increased pressure and shear forces originate a series of short-lived changes at the cellular level. The alterations from the normal (a) to the postdelivery (b) status include an enlargement of endothelial fenestrae, the exit of fluid from the sinusoidal space, and a massive intake of plasmid-containing fluidic endocytic vesicles by hepatocytes that are ultimately responsible for facilitating plasmid delivery and expression (adapted from Herrero and Aliño[135]).*

membranes as a result of shear.[39] Thus, hydrodynamic mediated delivery does not seem to require a receptor-mediated mechanism[37] as has been postulated, for example, in the case of intramuscular injection of plasmid DNA (see Section 6.2.2). The effectiveness of the hydrodynamic delivery process when it comes to plasmid-mediated gene transfer to hepatocytes would, in principle, render the technique especially useful to treat those disorders of the liver metabolism that are caused by single gene defects[37] or acute liver failure.[40] However, the fast injection of large volumes of fluid required is an inherently invasive procedure that adds complexity to the technique when it comes to clinical application.[41] Clearly, there are a number of critical aspects of the technique that need to be tested in animal models other than mice (e.g., pigs) before the technique moves into the clinic.[42] Furthermore, the fact that alterations in physiology have been observed in some animal models (e.g., swelling of hepatocytes and consequent increase in the volume of liver, alterations in the levels of liver enzymes, and liver damage[39]) will require a thorough investigation of the safety of the procedure in humans.

6.3   GENE GUN

6.3.1   Introduction

While the low efficiency of gene transfer that is inherent to the simple intramuscular injection of naked DNA was partially overcome by the development of the hydrodynamic delivery technique, the relative complexity of this latter procedure is a complication when it comes to clinical application. In strike contrast, the use of particle bombardment or biolistic is probably one of the most effective and simplest ways devised to deliver plasmids to living cells and tissues. This elegant, device-based delivery technique was originally developed as a means to improve the transfection of plant cells in calluses and leaves,[43] but it soon caught the attention of those working with animal cells.[44] In 1990, the *in vivo* bombardment of liver, muscle, and skin tissues of rat and mice with plasmid-coated microparticles enabled the transient expression of genes (CAT and β-galactosidase) for the first time.[45] The concept behind the delivery of plasmids by a gene gun is straightforward—nonporous metallic microparticles (0.1 to 5 μm) of an adequate material are coated with a layer of plasmid molecules and are then propelled at high speed with an adequate device that allows penetration of target tissues or organs. Although tungsten was initially used, gold microparticles became the benchmark material for medical applications. One of the keys to the success of the gene gun delivery methodology is related to the process used to promote the adsorption of the plasmids to the surface of the microparticles. This is usually accomplished by first mixing a plasmid solution with a suspension of the carrier microparticles and then by promoting the precipitation of the DNA by adding $CaCl_2$ and the polycation spermidine.[43,46] The amount of DNA loaded per milligram of particles is usually kept within 1–5 μg plasmid DNA/mg gold (i.e., 0.1–0.5% w/w) since higher amounts may result in DNA-mediated cross-linking and aggregation of particles. Following centrifugation, ethanol is used to wash and resuspend the microparticles.[46] This suspension may then be loaded in a disposable, sterile cassette or cartridge, which is further subjected to drying to produce a dry powder of plasmid-coated gold particles. The cartridges are then inserted into handheld biolistic systems or "gene guns" specifically designed to propel the particles across specific tissues using pressurized gases such as helium (see Figure 6.4a). When the device is triggered, a helium jet travels across the cartridge, releasing and accelerating the particles. The stream then enters a

(a)

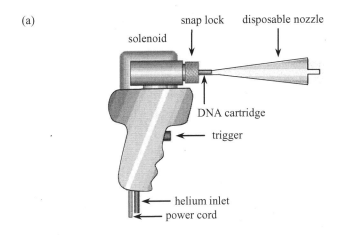

(b)

Figure 6.4 *Gene gun epidermal delivery of plasmid-coated gold microparticles. (a) Handheld gene guns are designed to propel plasmid-coated gold particles preloaded in a cartridge using pressurized gases such as helium. Upon triggering, a helium jet punctures through the cartridge, releasing and accelerating the particles. The gas stream is slowed down while passing through a conical nozzle, whereas the particles maintain the velocity required for skin penetration. (b) Propelled with a gene gun, DNA gold particles (depicted by the black dots) penetrate in the outer layer of the skin, transfecting both resident Langerhans cells and keratinocytes. A cross section of skin punctured by a needle is shown on the left for comparison. (a) Reprinted from Comparative Immunology, Microbiology & Infectious Diseases, 26, Dean HJ, Fuller D, Osorio JE. Powder and particle-mediated approaches for delivery of DNA and protein vaccines into the epidermis, 373-388, Copyright 2003,[4] with permission from Elsevier. (b) Reprinted from Advanced Drug Delivery Reviews, 57, Dean HJ, Haynes J, Schmaljohn C. The role of particle-mediated DNA vaccines in biodefense preparedness, 1315-1342, Copyright 2005,[47] with permission from Elsevier.*

disposable conical nozzle where the gas is slowed down while the particles maintain the velocity required for skin penetration.[4,46]

6.3.2 Underlying Mechanisms

When used specifically to target the top layers of skin, the gene gun/gold microparticle technique is known by the name particle-mediated epidermal delivery (PMED).[47] A distinctive feature of PMED when compared with intramuscular or intradermal needle injection is that plasmids are directly introduced in the cytoplasm of the target cells. Substantial amounts of experimental evidence have shown that the combination of PMED with DNA vaccines is an especially efficient means to obtain strong immune responses. This is first due to the fact that the skin contains antigen-presenting cells (APCs) such as Langerhans cells (LCs), which are able to drive and regulate immune responses against invading antigens.[4] Thus, when impelled at high velocities by gene guns, DNA vaccine-coated microparticles cross past the stratum corneum, puncturing through the membranes and across the cytoplasm and nuclei of LCs and of keratinocytes that reside in the epidermis (Figure 6.4b). The depth of penetration can be fine-tuned by changing the pressure of helium used to shoot the particles. The ability of LCs to process antigens and to migrate out of the delivery site toward the draining lymph node where they present processed antigens both to $CD8^+$ (see Chapter 2, Figure 2.6a) and $CD4^+$ T-helper cells (see Chapter 2, Figure 2.6d) is important to elicit primary cellular responses and immunologic memory.[4,47] On the other hand, the expression of the delivered antigen in the local keratinocytes, its secretion to the extracellular medium, and its subsequent uptake by resident APCs (see Chapter 2, Figure 2.6b) are especially useful to foster the secretion of antibodies.[4,47]

6.3.3 Some Applications

A substantial number of preclinical studies and human clinical trials have been performed to test the validity of the particle-mediated delivery in the context of DNA vaccine immunization against infectious diseases (see reviews by Dean et al.[4,47] and Fuller et al.[48]). The pathogens targeted in nonhuman primate studies include, for example, the Ebola, Japanese encephalitis, rabies, influenza, hepatitis B, dengue, and Hantaan viruses, while human trials have focused on influenza and hepatitis B virus, and on *Plasmodium falciparum*[48]. A key advantage of PMED that emerged within this therapeutic context is that substantially smaller amounts of DNA vaccine (100- to 1000-fold) are required to obtain an immune response (antibody titers and $CD8^+$ T cells) in mice and primates, as compared with intramuscular or intradermal injections.[4,47–49] This means that with PMED, DNA vaccine doses of the order of ~1–10 µg are usually sufficient to induce immune responses in animal models. Direct comparisons also show that when challenging animal models of a given disease, better antibody protection is achieved with PMED.[50,51] These differences are attributable to the fact that plasmids are directly introduced in the cytoplasm of the target cells, whereas with intramuscular or intradermal needle injection, they typically accumulate in the extracellular space.[48] Overall, the experimental demonstration of the superiority of PMED in preclinical and clinical trials has contributed to the established notion that gene gun delivery is probably one of the best ways to overcome the poor immunogenicity of needle-injected DNA vaccines in larger animals and humans.[4,47]

Another important outcome of preclinical and human studies has been the demonstration that delivery of DNA vaccines by PMED technology is safe and well tolerated, with adverse reactions restricted to mild redness, discoloration, flaking, edema, rash, and/or itch that resolve within 1 month after administration.[48] Some disadvantages have been associated with the use of gene gun-propelled gold microparticles as a plasmid delivery technique, which include the cumbersome and time-consuming preparation of the particles, cost, compulsory delivery of DNA in a dry state, burning effects on the bombarded skin, and the skewing of the immune response.[49] In order to bypass these drawbacks, attempts have been made to use low-pressure gene guns to intradermally deliver naked plasmid DNA in solution without using particles. Actually, this procedure is equivalent to the jet injection procedure described in Section 6.2.3. The results of one study show that solutions of DNA vaccines delivered by low-pressure gene guns are able to produce immunologic responses and antitumor effects that are as strong and as potent when compared with the ones generated by the gene gun delivery of gold microparticles.[49] Furthermore, and apart from being more expedite, this delivery also produces fewer side effects.[49]

6.4 ELECTROPORATION

6.4.1 Introduction

Electroporation, or electropermeabilization as it is sometimes called, was one of the first strategies devised to try to improve the low efficiency of gene expression that is associated with the injection of naked plasmid DNA. The technique resorts to the use of electric field pulses to transiently increase the permeability of the target cells, and thus to overcome the membrane barriers that hinder plasmid entrance into cells. Although electroporation was originally developed to improve the uptake of DNA by cells cultured *in vitro*,[52,53] its simplicity and ease of application soon attracted the attention of researchers working on *in vivo* plasmid-mediated gene delivery. In 1991, Titomirov and colleagues described the sub-cutaneous injection of plasmid DNA in newborn mice and then used a special device to deliver two high-voltage pulses with opposite polarities to the corresponding skin area.[54] Later on, the beneficial effect of using electric pulses after the intramuscular delivery of DNA *in vivo* was also demonstrated.[55] These experiments showed for the first time that electroporation was a feasible method to stably transform skin and muscle cells *in vivo*. Subsequent efforts by many researchers contributed to develop the *in vivo* electroporation technology up to a point where it is probably one of the most effective ways to deliver plasmid DNA[56].

6.4.2 Underlying Mechanisms

The exact mechanisms underlying plasmid-based electroporation and expression are still a matter of debate.[57] One view is that the electric fields generated by the high-energy pulses cause ion movement inside the cell and transiently increase the transmembrane potential (up to 0.5–1.0 V and lasting for 10 μs to 10 ms).[58] This results in the opening up of ephemeral (microsecond to second) transbilayer electropores, which are believed to occupy ~0.1% of the surface and have sizes of the order of <10 nm[58], or in the creation of structural defects in the membrane sides of the cell that face the electrodes.[57] At the same time, an electrophoretic effect is created, which actively drives the negatively charged plasmids toward the anode side, fostering its interaction with the membrane and passage across pores and into the cell cytoplasm.[57,58] This model, however, is not consensual. For example, some authors have suggested that the transit of plasmids across the perturbed membranes occurs by passive diffusion rather than by electrophoresis.[59] Other possible mechanisms are the formation of charged plasmid vesicles or stable DNA/membrane complexes,[60] and their subsequent endocytosis, or the aggregation of ion pumps and their concomitant opening to give way for plasmid entrance. The delivery of plasmids by electroporation is affected by a number of electrical parameters that include, for example, the number, length (few micrograms to milliseconds), voltage (50–1500 V), and waveform (exponential decay or square wave) of the pulses.[58]

6.4.3 Preclinical and Clinical Development

Overall, a substantial amount of preclinical and clinical data has been accumulated so far which shows that electroporation constitutes an effective means of increasing the transfer of plasmid biopharmaceuticals *in vivo* to tissues like the skin and muscle. Furthermore, this increase in plasmid uptake is accompanied by high levels of expression of transgenes and clinical improvements.[61] An interesting and useful feature of electroporation, particularly in the context of DNA vaccines, is that the technique by itself (i.e., independent of the DNA) is able to mobilize cells of the immune system and to foster the release of cytokines.[59] The clinical usefulness of electroporation is strongly dependent on the availability of devices capable of a safe and consistent delivery of DNA. A number of companies have accepted this challenge and, as a result, a few devices have been developed, which are being evaluated in clinical trials.[56] For example, Ichor Medical Systems (San Diego, California) designed a handheld integrated device (TriGrid™) that combines an injection needle for intramuscular administration with a system that delivers the required electric pulses[56,62] (Figure 6.5b,c). A critical component of the TriGrid electroporation device is a single-use cartridge that contains four penetrating electrodes surrounding a central injection needle, which is connected to an off-the-shelf syringe (Figure

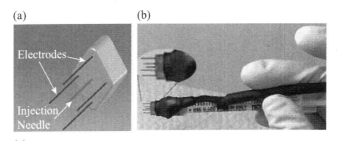

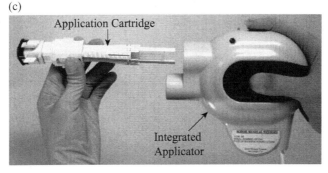

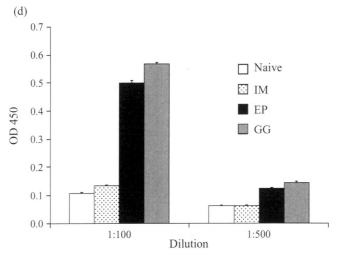

Figure 6.5 In vivo *electroporation (EP)-mediated delivery of plasmid DNA with the intramuscular TriGrid delivery system (Ichor Medical Systems). (a) The diamond-like arrangement of the four penetrating electrodes and the central needle is designed to maximize the propagation of electric fields to fluid-filled regions. This array is central to integrated systems designed for use in rodents (b) and in larger animals and humans (c). The devices integrate a pulse generator with a cartridge that encloses the electrode array and accommodates an off-the-shelf syringe. (d) Evaluation of the efficiency of EP, gene gun (GG), and intramuscular injection (IM) in the delivery of a DNA vaccine against human papillomavirus. The figure shows the serum levels of E7-specific antibodies elicited in C57BL/6 mice (four per group) vaccinated with 2μg in alternating hind legs on days 0, 3, and 6. E7-specific antibodies were measured by enzyme-linked immunosorbent assay (ELISA) 2 weeks after the last immunization at a mean absorbance of 450 nm. (a-c) Reprinted from Vaccine, 24, Luxembourg A, Hannaman D, Ellefsen B, Nakamura G, Bernard R. Enhancement of immune responses to an HBV DNA vaccine by electroporation, 4490-4493, Copyright 2006,[62] with permission from Elsevier. (d) Reprinted from Vaccine, 27, Best SR, Peng S, Juang CM, et al. Administration of HPV DNA vaccine via electroporation elicits the strongest CD8+ T cell immune responses compared to intramuscular injection and intradermal gene gun delivery, 5450-5459, Copyright 2009,[65] with permission from Elsevier.*

6.5a). The electrodes are connected to an electric pulse generator that generates the electric signals at the same time that the plasmid solution is injected from the syringe. The relative positioning of the electrodes and of the needle is designed so as to maximize the propagation of electric fields to the muscle regions, which are characteristically filled with fluid upon injection. The administration relies on a correct alignment of the electrodes with the direction of the muscle fibers. Other electroporation devices developed to meet the requirements of a clinical delivery of plasmid DNA include the Elgen™ intramuscular delivery device from Inovio Biomedical Systems (San Diego, California), the Cellectra™ DNA delivery device from VGX Pharmaceuticals (Blue Bell, Pennsylvania), and the Easy Vax™ device from Cyto Pulse Sciences Inc. (Glen Burnie, Maryland).[56]

Numerous preclinical trials and a significant number of clinical trials have been conducted or are under way to demonstrate the effectiveness and safety of electroporation for the delivery of plasmids. The diseases addressed in the clinic include, for example, cancer (melanoma, head and neck, pancreatic, and breast), HIV, HPV, and hepatitis. Collectively, the results obtained so far have indicated that with a few administrations and decreased doses, the delivery of plasmids by electroporation increases cellular and humoral responses while prolonging the beneficial effects of the intervention.[61] Still, and in spite of its effectiveness, a number of negative features have been associated with electroporation, namely, muscle stimulation, patient discomfort, and tissue damage.[58] While these trials have focused on the therapeutic applications of electroporation, the use of the technique in the context of DNA vaccine immunization is being actively pursued at the preclinical level.[63–66]

Comparative studies are crucial when trying to evaluate the merits of the different delivery methodologies. In one of such studies, the benefits associated with electroporation-mediated intramuscular delivery and gene gun epidermal delivery of a DNA vaccine for HPV have been compared side by side and evaluated against the conventional intramuscular injection.[65] In this study, uniform $2\,\mu g$ doses of a plasmid encoding the E7 antigen of HPV subtype 16 were administered to mice. While gene gun vaccination resulted in higher levels of circulating E7-specific antibody responses as compared to the other two methods, the ability to generate antigen-specific cytotoxic $CD8^+$ T-cell responses was highest in mice vaccinated by electroporation (Figure 6.5d). Together, the cytotoxic $CD8^+$ T cells and E7-specific antibodies elicited by both electroporation and gene gun delivery of the DNA vaccine contributed to the generation of potent antitumor responses in mice inoculated with an E7-expressing tumor cell line.[65]

6.5 CATIONIC LIPIDS AND POLYMERS

6.5.1 Introduction

The formulation of plasmids with specific molecules like cationic lipids and soluble polymers is one of the most widely used ways to improve the transfection ability of plasmid biopharmaceuticals. In generic terms, the methodology explores the electrostatic interaction between the polyanionic plasmids with a cationic counterpart (e.g., a lipid or a polymer). One of the important characteristics of this association is that it usually results in the collapse and condensation of the plasmid molecules. Thus, each molecule will "shrink," acquiring dimensions that are substantially smaller than the usual size of the individual plasmids in solution. This change in shape and size is one of the reasons behind the improvement in the uptake of plasmid by target cells that is often reported. The complexes formed by cationic lipids (lipopexes) and polymers (polyplexes) may harbor several molecules of compacted plasmids. One of the rationales behind the use of lipoplexes and polyplexes is that the coating of the negatively charged plasmids with cationic "envelopes" will protect plasmids against the attack of external agents that are likely to be found extra- and intracellularly (e.g., plasma, lysosomal and cytosolic nucleases, and proteins). Furthermore, the positively charged coating facilitates fusion of the complexes with the negatively charged cell membranes (e.g., on account of the presence of sulfated proteoglycans[67]) and thus fosters plasmid internalization by endocytosis.

6.5.2 Lipoplexes

The use of lipoplexes in *in vivo* gene delivery dates back to the work of Nicolau and coworkers, as described in Chapter 1 (Section 1.3.2). These researchers proved that liposomes made up of phospholipids and cholesterol were able to encapsulate a plasmid harboring the preproinsulin gene, and that these lipolexes could effectively mediate the uptake and expression of the transgene upon intravenous injection in rats.[68] Soon after, Felgner et al. described the effectiveness of lipoplexes formed with a tailored lipid, *N*-[1-(2,3-dioleyloxy) propyl]-*N*, *N*, *N*-trimethylammonium chloride (DOTMA) and dioleoylphosphatidylethanolamine (DOPE),* in the transfection of cells *in vitro*.[69] Since then, the use of the so-called lipofection methodology for the plasmid-based, *in vivo* delivery of transgenes has been the subject of countless publications. Furthermore, the variety of formulations and procedures used to prepare these lipoplexes has increased enormously, leading to a disparity of results and interpretations. A brief description of the basics of lipoplex preparation and usage is given next.

Above a certain critical concentration, lipids in aqueous solutions have a tendency to self-aggregate into multilamellar, microscopic vesicular structures with a double bilayer called liposomes. Lipid molecules in this bilayer are organized back-to-back in such a way that their polar hydrophilic heads face outward, while the hydrophobic tails are shielded from the aqueous solution. The extrusion of these multilamellar structures through porous membranes

---

* These liposomes are commercially available under the trade name Lipofectin™.

may generate either a small (~30–100 nm) or large unilamellar vesicle (~150–250 nm).[70] When mixed with liposomes that are preformed from cationic lipids, plasmids become confined to a large extent to an aqueous compartment that is encapsulated by a lipidic shell, originating a heterogeneous population of more complex microstructures. If the adequate ratio of lipid to DNA is used, positively charged complexes that are able to adsorb to the negatively charged (due to the presence of glycoproteins and glycolipids) surface of cells are formed.[70] This is thought to facilitate both the passing of the cell membrane barrier, either through endocytosis[71] or membrane fusion, and the internalization process when compared, for example, with naked plasmid DNA[72]. Experimental evidence has shown that once internalized, the endocytosed complexes may coalesce into larger structures that accumulate close to the cell nucleus.[71] The lipid/DNA complexes within these aggregates often display a highly ordered structure.[71] Then, the lipoplexes must somehow disrupt endosomal membranes (e.g., via fusion) in order to access the cytoplasm. During the release process, plasmids may remain associated with lipolexes or may dissociate from them. In this latter case, traces of lipids may remain bound to the plasmids, thus providing some compaction and degree of protection.[72] However, when reaching the fringes of the nucleus, plasmids should be freed from any coating, since lipids have been known to inhibit transcription.[71] While lipoplex formation may occur spontaneously, extrusion is usually used to facilitate the process of lipoplex preparation. Examples of popular cationic lipids used to form liposomes for plasmid delivery include the two-chained and monovalent DOTMA, 1,2-dioleoyl-3-trimethylammonium propane (DOTAP), and N-(2-hydroxyethyl)-N,N-dimethyl-2,3-bis(tetradecyloxy)-1-propanaminium bromide (DMRIE) (see Figure 6.6a). Structurally, such cationic lipids possess three characteristic features: a hydrophobic anchor, a linker, and a polar group. While the possibilities are numerous within such a general structure, three-carbon skeletons derived from glycerol are often used to link double-chain hydrocarbon hydrophobic anchors (e.g., oleyl chains) to tertiary or quaternary ammonium (e.g., trimethyl ammonium in DOTMA and DOTAP) polar groups[73] (see Figure 6.6a). These cationic lipids are usually associated with helper colipids such as DOPE and cholesterol since these combinations produce liposomes that display an improved ability to mediate cell transfection.[72] More specifically, the introduction of colipids is thought to originate liposomes with more flexible bilayers, a characteristic that is likely to facilitate fusion with cell membranes, endocytosis, destabilization of endosome membranes, and disassembling of lipoplexes. The exact geometry of lipoplexes is dependent on a range of factors such as the lipid and colipid structure, the ratio of lipid to DNA, the ratio of lipid to colipid, and the process used to prepare them[74]. Structures and morphologies like (1) multilamellar aggregates that originate from the merging of the large and small unilamellar cationic liposomes described above with plasmids, (2) lipid-coated nucleic acids, (3) liposomes coated with DNA, and (4) two-dimensional hexagonal lattices have all been described.[70,72] An illustrative example of a possible structure is given in Figure 6.6b, which shows a cryo-electron microscopy photo-

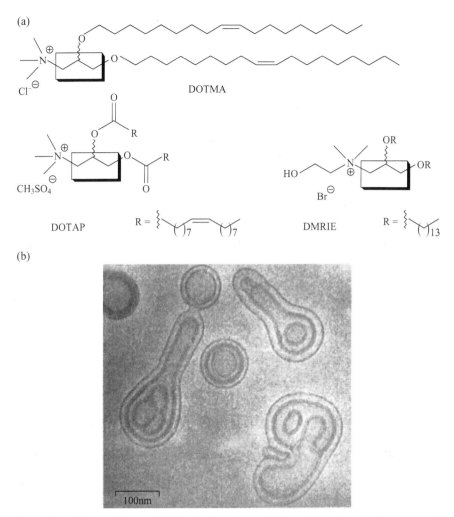

Figure 6.6 *Delivery of plasmid DNA with lipoplexes. (a) Examples of glycerol-based cationic lipids used to complex plasmid DNA. The rectangular box highlights the three carbon glycerol linkers. (b) Cryo-electron microscopy photographs of lipoplexes prepared by complexing plasmid DNA with DOTAP:cholesterol liposomes. (a) Reprinted from Medicinal Research Reviews, 27, Karmali PP, Chaudhuri A. Cationic liposomes as non-viral carriers of gene medicines: resolved issues, open questions, and future promises, 696-722, Copyright 2007,[70] with permission from John Wiley & Sons. (b) Reprinted by permission from Macmillan Publishers Ltd.: Nature Biotechnology, 15, Templeton NS, Lasic DD, Frederik PM, Strey HH, Roberts DD, Pavlakis GN. Improved DNA: liposome complexes for increased systemic delivery and gene expression, 647-652, Copyright 1997.[74]*

graph of lipoplexes obtained by complexing plasmid DNA with DOTAP: cholesterol liposomes.[74] In this case, plasmid DNA was found to condense in the interior of invaginated liposomes between two lipid bilayers, producing lipoplexes with sizes of the order of 200–450 nm[74]. Given the diversity of morphologies, sizes, and charged densities of complexes that can be obtained when mixing a certain liposome composition with a specific amount of plasmid DNA, it is not surprising to find that the biological activity of lipolexes is quite sensitive to the preparation methods used. The stability of lipolexes *in vivo* (e.g., in the presence of serum) is also an important issue.[73] Nevertheless, several studies have demonstrated that lipoplexes can be used to deliver plasmid DNA to a range of different tissues *in vivo*, by local administration or intravenous injection. The strategy has also moved to the clinic, and as of today, more than 100 trials* have been conducted or are under way, which rely on lipofection to deliver genes.[75–77] A good example of these efforts to incorporate cationic and neutral lipids in clinical candidates is Allovectin-7®, a cancer DNA vaccine designed by Vical Inc. (San Diego, California) to treat melanoma, which is currently in phase 3[78] (see Section 6.7). The same company has also developed a new cationic and neutral lipid formulation termed Vaxfectin, which is especially suitable to deliver DNA vaccines and to increase antigen-specific antibodies.[79]

6.5.3 Poliplexes

Poliplexes made by combining plasmids with soluble cationic polymers like polyethyleneimine (PEI),[80–82] polylysine,[81,82] polypropylamine dendrimers, chitosan, and cationic dextran; nonionic polymers like polyethylene glycol (PEG); and nonionic block copolymers like poloxamers,[83–87] to name but a few, have also been prepared and tested as a means to improve transfection efficiency *in vivo*. The rationale behind the preparation of these microstructures is much in line with the one that is pursued when preparing lipoplexes: A coating (cationic or not) is used to foster plasmid condensation into small particles, to provide protection from external agents (e.g., nucleases), to mediate interaction with negatively charged cell surfaces, and to facilitate the passing of the cell membrane via endocytosis.[88] Since the literature on the topic is abundant, in the following lines, only a short description of two polymers used to complex plasmids and to facilitate delivery and expression is provided.

PEI is a water-soluble, nitrogen-rich synthetic polymer that is prepared by polymerizing ethanolamine (CH_2CH_2NH-).[67] The high density of positive charges found in PEI molecules, which results from the protonation of its amine groups, is responsible for the ability of the polymer to condense the anionic plasmid DNA. The properties and characteristics of plasmid/PEI polyplexes, and hence their transfection efficiency, depend on a range of factors, which include the plasmid-to-PEI ratio, the molecular weight and structure (linear and branched) of PEI, the concentration of plasmid and PEI, and so on. The superficial charge of the polyplex is of course important, since the interaction with the negatively charged membranes occurs via ionic interac-

---

* Clinical trial data were extracted from *The Journal of Gene Medicine* Gene Therapy Clinical Trials Worldwide Web site at http://www.wiley.co.uk/genmed/clinical (accessed May 23, 2010).

tions. Furthermore, the size of the polyplexes, which may vary anywhere from the few nanometers typical of isolated complexes to the several microm-eters characteristic of larger aggregates, is especially important in terms of transfection activity. Specifically, sizes smaller than 100 nm seem to facili-tate internalization by endocytosis and thus are usually associated with improved transfection.[67] An important property of PEI, which derives from the presence of numerous amine groups in its structure, is its ability to act as a proton sponge.[67] Essentially, this means that after endocytosis, the amine groups in the PEI coating of the polyplexes are able to uptake protons from the acidic interior of endosomes. It has been postulated that this buffering effect is coupled to an inflow of chloride ions, which in turn produces an osmotic swelling that ultimately ruptures endosomes and facilitates polyplex release into the cytoplasm[67]. This picture, however, has been challenged by some authors.[89] The mechanisms that enable the polyplexes to access the cell nucleus are not clearly known, but some experimental evidence suggests that PEI is able to target plasmids to the nucleus, moving alongside its interior in the form of ordered structures.[90] While polyplex disassembly is in principle required to ensure expression of the transgene, the hypothesis that the transcription machinery of the cell could transiently separate plasmids from PEI has also been put forward.[67] Numerous studies with animal models have been published in the literature describing the usefulness of PEI poly-plexes as a plasmid delivery agent.[80–82,91] PEI/plasmid complexes have also been tested in the clinic. For example, reports of phase 1 and phase 2 clinical trials that assess the safety and preliminary efficacy of intravesical infusions of a PEI-complexed plasmid coding for diphtheria toxin A chain into patients with bladder cancer can be found at the clinical trials database of the United States.[92,93]

Poloxamers constitute a good example of nonionic block copolymers that have been used to facilitate plasmid delivery. The fact that they have been already been used in a number of biomedical applications (e.g., drug delivery, medical imaging, and management of vascular diseases and disorders) is the first important advantage of these polymers.[83,94] The molecules feature a central polyoxypropylene (POP) molecule flanked on both sides by two hydrophilic chains of polyoxyethylene (POE), yielding structures of the $(POE)_a(POP)_b(POE)_a$ type.[94] Plasmid molecules are thought to complex with poloxamers through the formation of weak interactions (e.g., hydrogen bridges) with the central POE[83]. Several studies have shown that formulation with poloxamers increases the efficiency of the intramuscular expression of plasmids. The technique has been tested both at the preclinical[83–85] and clinical level.[86,87] Poloxamers have hemorrheological, antithrombotic, and neutrophil-inhibitory properties, are able to enhance immunologic responses (e.g., by increasing antibody formation), and can activate the human complement system. Although this variety of biological activities may be interesting from a clinical point of view, they may also be responsible for unwanted toxic effects, which must be properly addressed during trials.[94]

6.6 MICRO- AND NANOPARTICLES

6.6.1 Introduction

The polyplexes described in the previous section are usually prepared by mixing given amounts of plasmid DNA with solubilized polymers. However, polymers and plasmids can also be combined in such a way as to produce plasmid-loaded, solid microparticles of a defined size (0.5–10.0 μm) instead of submicron complexes. The methodology was first described in 1997 by Jones and coworkers[95] and has since gained an enormous popularity among researchers involved with plasmid biopharmaceuticals. A key advantage of polymeric, plasmid-loaded microparticles is that they provide the means for a more prolonged release of plasmids instead of the bolus-type delivery that is characteristic of polyplexes.[96] Poly(DL-lactide-co-glycolide) (PLG) and poly(DL-lactic acid) (PLA) are two of the most popular polymers used in this context, mostly due to their biocompatible and biodegradable nature, and due to the fact that they have been safely used in other biomedical applications. After *in vivo* administration, for example, via sub-cutaneous or intramuscular needle injection, such microparticles can be phagocytosed by professional APCs (macrophages and dendritic cells) and then transported to the lymph nodes where the plasmid can be gradually released.[97] The particle dimensions are important since sizes lower than 5–10 μm appear to improve particle uptake.[98] On account of their biodegradability, the polymeric microparticles that are taken up should undergo bulk hydrolysis within the cell cytoplasm or endosomes, generating lactic acid and glycolic acid, and thus progressively releasing the entrapped plasmids from within their cores.[99]

Polymeric plasmid-loaded microparticles can be obtained essentially by two distinct strategies. In the first case, microparticles can be designed and produced so as to encapsulate plasmid molecules within their inner core.[95,100–102] While PLG and PLA have been the polymers of choice to prepare the particles, alternatives like chitosan[96,103] have also been tested. The particles are usually prepared by double emulsification, a process whereby specified amounts of polymers, plasmid, and other reagents (e.g., organic solvents) are first brought together and homogenized. Next, evaporation of the organic solvent is promoted until solid microspheres are finally obtained. The stability of the plasmid during this process is crucial since the shear forces, temperatures, and organic chemicals involved may lead to plasmid degradation and hence loss of biological activity.[97,101] Additionally, the entrapment of plasmids may be too strong to provide for a release of sufficient amounts of plasmid within an acceptable time frame. As an alternative to encapsulation, the microparticles can be prepared in advance and then mixed with the target plasmids. With this strategy, both the problem of plasmid degradation during preparation and of very slow plasmid release from the particles are circumvented.[97] The goal here is to promote the adsorption of plasmids to the outer surface of the particles, in a similar way to what is done with gold particles (see Section 6.3). The best way to achieve this surface loading of DNA is to produce particles that have a cationic surface.[99,104–106] The preparation of particles of PLG and PLA functionalized with the cationic surfactant cetyltrimethylammonium bromide (CTAB), constitute a good example of this strategy.[99,106] By controlling the particle composition and polymerization conditions, it is possible to prepare particles with sizes of the order of 1 μm and with varying properties (e.g., zeta potential and plasmid loading and release). The plasmid loading in these particles is typically of the order of 1% (w/w), whether entrapment or surface adsorption is being explored.[97,99,101,106]

Numerous reports have described the use of microparticles for plasmid delivery *in vivo*, focusing on aspects like the preparation of the particles[96,100–103] and their usefulness in the context of diseases like tuberculosis,[107] hepatitis C,[105] and B[106], AIDS,[108] and cancer.[104,109] Researchers have found that microparticle formulations with surface-adsorbed or encapsulated plasmids are usually characterized by a low toxicity and are often able to mediate an increased gene expression and augment the immunogenicity of DNA vaccines.[104–106] For example, cationic PLG microparticles loaded with a plasmid DNA vaccine encoding HIV antigenes were shown to be substantially more potent than the corresponding naked DNA vaccines.[110] This increased immunogenicity has been associated with an increase in the half-life of the plasmid *in vivo*, which is associated with the prolonged release of plasmid from the microparticles.[106] As examples of clinical application, plasmid-loaded polymeric microparticles were used in phase 1 trials to evaluate the safety and immunogenicity of DNA vaccines to treat anal dysplasia[109] or to prevent HIV infection.[108]

6.6.2 Compacted Nanoparticles

The microparticles and lipid/polymer complexes described in the previous sections have sizes in the 200-nm to 5-μm range and typically contain several molecules of plasmid DNA, which maybe more or less compacted. This means that in order for the plasmid molecules to pass through the nuclear envelope of nonmitotic cells, some kind of disaggregation or dismantling process must take place beforehand in the cytoplasm. This will generate individual molecules that are small enough to pass through the NPC, a structure with an approximate inner diameter of 25 nm. One way to overcome the need for dismantling before nuclear entry, which is inherent to encapsulated and coated microparticles and complexes, is to compact plasmid molecules into individual nanoparticles with sizes lower than 100 nm. For example, one process has been described whereby a 30-mer lysine peptide with an N-terminal cysteine is conjugated via a maleimide linkage to 10 kDa polyethylene glycol ($CK_{30}P10k$) and is then used to condense individual plasmid DNA molecules into nanoparticles with neutral charge density.[6,111–113] The shape of the $CK_{30}P10k$-plasmid

(a)

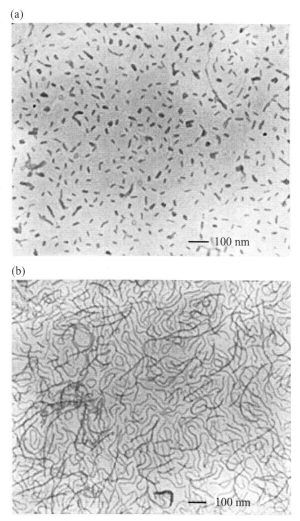

100 nm

(b)

100 nm

Figure 6.7 *Plasmid DNA nanoparticles. Nanoparticles were prepared by mixing a 5300-bp plasmid with a 30-mer lysine peptide with an N-terminal cysteine that is conjugated via a maleimide linkage to 10 kDa polyethylene glycol ($CK_{30}P10k$). By changing the amine counterions of $CK_{30}P10k$ from trifluoroacetate to acetate, ellipsoidal (a) or rodlike (b) nanoparticles can be produced. Reprinted by permission from Macmillan Publishers Ltd.: Gene Therapy, 13, Fink TL, Klepcyk PJ, Oette SM, et al. Plasmid size up to 20 kbp does not limit effective* in vivo *lung gene transfer using compacted DNA nanoparticles, 1048-1051, Copyright 2006.[113]*

nanoparticles can be adjusted from ellipsoidal to rodlike by changing the counterions of the lysine polymers used in the formulation from trifluoroac-etate to acetate[112] (see Figure 6.7). Such particles are stable and can be stored at 4°C in a saline buffer solution for at least 23 months.[113]

The *in vitro* transfection of cultured nonmitotic cells with these compacted DNA nanoparticles shows that transgene expression is significantly enhanced when compared to naked DNA. In a specific experiment, when the $CK_{30}P10k$-plasmid nanoparticles were combined with liposomes and were used to transfect growth-arrested cells, transgene expression increased up to 6900-fold when compared with a situation wherein naked plasmids were combined with liposomes.[111] This superiority of the nanoparticles was not so evident when log-phase cells were transfected.[111] Experiments in which nanoparticles of different sizes are microinjected in the cell cytoplasm further indicate that expression is maximized as long as size is kept bellow 24–25 nm. This observation is consistent with a mechanism whereby the nanoparticles access the cell nucleus by traveling through the 25-nm-wide NPC[111]. Other features of the plasmid nanoparticles that might explain their superior transfection ability when compared with naked DNA are an increased resistance to nuclease action and a faster diffusion.[112] This later situation can be illustrated by comparing the diffusion coefficient of a naked 5000-bp supercoiled plasmid ($\sim 3.3 \times 10^{-8}$ cm^2/s)* and of a spheroid nanoparticle of the same plasmid ($\sim 14 \times 10^{-8}$ cm^2/s)† in water. In this particular situation, the diffusion of the nanoparticle is fourfold faster than that of a noncompacted supercoiled plasmid. The ellipsoidal and rodlike plasmid nanoparticles described are also effective when it comes to transfecting murine[112,113,115,116] and human[6] cells *in vivo*. Preclinical animal studies demonstrated that the DNA nanoparticles could be delivered to the lung of mice, through inhalation,[112,113] and to the retina, through subretinal needle injection.[115,116] In the latter case, for example, rodlike nanoparticles were taken up by the target retina cells of a mouse model of retinitis pigmentosa; the transgene was expressed and a significant rescue of the disease phenotype was observed.[6] The clinical safety and effectiveness of the condensed nanoparticles as vehicles for the transfer of the cystic fibrosis transmembrane regulator (CFTR) gene were also studied in a phase 1 double-blind, placebo-controlled dose escalation study.[6] An 8234-bp plasmid was condensed with the aid of the $CK_{30}P10k$ peptide–PEG biconjugate into 100- to 300-nm-long rods with diameters of around 12–15 nm. The monitoring of the 12 cystic fibrosis subjects enrolled in the trial showed that single administrations of up to 8 mg of the plasmid DNA nanoparticles to the nasal mucosa did not cause any adverse event. Furthermore, the DNA nanoparticles were able to transfect nasal epithelial cells and express the CFTR gene. The results of this study and the characteristics of the nanoparticles suggest that direct delivery to the lung of CF subjects could be achieved via inhalation of mists of DNA nanoparticles.[6] Overall, the data accumulated so far suggest that single-plasmid nanoparticles constitute a highly effective means of transfering genes *in vivo*.

---

* Calculated by Equation 4.4 in Chapter 4.
† The diameter of a compacted plasmid spheroid is estimated at 33 nm by Equation 4.21, and the corresponding diffusion coefficient is estimated on the basis of the He and Niemeyer correlation for globular macromolecules[114].

6.7 COMPARATIVE ANALYSIS OF DELIVERY MODES

6.7.1 Background

The active principle at the core of a plasmid biopharmaceutical is genetic information. Depending on the particular case, this information can code for a therapeutic protein, a vaccinating antigen or a silencing RNA molecule (see Chapter 2). In any case, it is presently very clear that, depending on the intended clinical goal, the exact nature/composition of the formulated plasmid biopharmaceutical product and the way it will be used can vary widely. The different strategies and options that have been experimented and tested imply that a wide range of products is possible, from the simplest naked DNA vaccine in saline, which is delivered by intramuscular injection, to the more sophisticated multi-plasmid products, which are formulated with specially designed adjuvants and facilitators and are administered with specific devices (see Figure 6.1). One important variable is the dose (i.e., mass) of plasmid per single administration. An overview of the literature shows that single doses can vary from a few tenths of a microgram, for instance, in the case of a hepatitis B vaccine,[117] up to 8 mg as in the case of a DNA vaccine for Ebola.[118] A single administration of 42 mg has also been reported in a case where a plasmid coding for the cystic fibrosis conductance regulator is administered by inhalation.[119] But perhaps more important and relevant from a safety point of view than the amount of extraneous DNA material that is administered each time is the cumulative amount introduced in a patient's body during the course of a whole treatment. Whereas in the case of DNA vaccines against infectious diseases less than a handful of inoculations might suffice to generate a protective immune response, the treatment of diseases like single genetic disorders, cancer, and others could require a lifelong chronic administration. For example, subjects with intermittent claudication secondary to peripheral arterial disease (PAD) enrolled in a phase 2 clinical trial received a cumulative dose of up to 84 mg following multiple injections of a plasmid during the course of the experiment.[86,87]

Although the amount of plasmid used per patient depends strongly on the nature of the target disease, the way the final product is formulated and delivered may significantly impact the dosage adopted. The evidence abounds to support the idea that an adequate selection and development of adjuvants and delivery methods can significantly improve the performance (i.e., the biological activity) of plasmid biopharmaceuticals. This means that if a suitable delivery methodology is adopted, less mass of plasmid material is required to achieve the same efficacy. This dose sparing effect may be important, for example, in the context of a crisis situation like pandemic influenza, wherein speed of response is critical and manufacturing capacity may be limited (see Chapter 9, Section 9.2). The expectation is thus that the most successful plasmid biopharmaceuticals will comprise not only the target gene(s) cloned in a suitable plasmid vector and a few stabilizers/excipients, but also a number of components acting as delivery/adjuvant aids. Although a large number of such delivery/adjuvant platforms are currently being developed by research centers and firms, the passing of the years will, in all likelihood, see the emergence and survival of a few "dominant designs," as is typically the case in many industries[120] (see Chapter 19, Section 19.2). These dominant designs will be the ones that companies involved in plasmid biopharmaceuticals must adhere to and adopt if they hope to conquer significant fractions of the market. In this section, a brief analysis is presented, which compares some of the methodologies used to deliver DNA vaccines developed to provide protection against influenza and to treat melanoma. These vaccines have all underwent or are undergoing clinical trials in humans. This academic exercise is intended to highlight the differences in the design/formulation of each plasmid product when it comes to dosage and delivery methodology used. No considerations whatsoever are made here regarding the clinical efficacy of the vaccines themselves, even though this is of course one of the most critical performance parameters for any biopharmaceutical.

6.7.2 Case Study Vaccines

The context in which a prophylactic DNA vaccine is likely to be used is, in principle, very different from the one involving a therapeutic DNA vaccine. In the first case, the vaccine is administered to healthy individuals as a preventive measure against an infectious disease, whereas in the second case, a therapeutic action is taken to treat a particular medical condition that affects patients. Accordingly, a limited number of administrations are to be expected in the case of prophylactic DNA vaccines. The uses of therapeutic DNA vaccines, on the other hand, and especially for the conditions against which they are currently being developed (e.g., cancer), are likely to require chronic administration. For the sake of the comparison being made in this section, DNA vaccines against influenza and melanoma were selected in order to examine whether the differences in the circumstances in which prophylactic and therapeutic vaccines are used are somehow reflected upon the intrinsic nature of the products themselves. Given that the potency or biological activity of plasmid pharmaceuticals is highly dependent on the delivery mode used, three different platforms were selected: gene gun, needle-free liquid jet injection, and cationic lipids. The major characteristics of the vaccines examined are briefly described next.

6.7.2.1 Pandemic and Seasonal Influenza

The unparalleled poultry mortality that has been recorded in Asia in the recent years has increased the fear that a world influenza pandemic, caused by a highly pathogenic and transmissible avian flu virus, may be lurking around the corner[121] (see Chapter 9, Section 9.2). This inevitability of a global flu pandemic, as it has been classified by the World Health Organization (WHO)[121], has prompted a number of research institutions and firms to develop scientific and technological platforms that could support the swift development of a vaccine in response to an outbreak.[122] DNA vaccines and a number of players are at the forefront of this race, as described next. PowderMed, the Oxford-based company acquired by Pfizer in 2006 (Pfizer, *2006 Annual Review*), is currently leveraging on its proprietary PMED platform to develop a prophylactic influenza DNA vaccine. As we have seen in Section 6.3, PMED relies on the use of pressurized helium to propel micron-sized gold particles coated with plasmid DNA through the epidermal layer of the skin. The ability of this gene gun technology to elicit both humoral and cellular responses translates into a product portfolio, which also includes early-stage vaccine candidates against herpes simplex virus and chronic hepatitis B[123]. The PowderMed flu vaccine, which successfully underwent phase 1 clinical trials, contains the hemagglutinin H3 gene from the A/Panama/2007/99 strain cloned into a pPJV1671 plasmid.[124] This plasmid construct is coated on 1- to 3-μm gold particles, at a mass ratio of 1 μg of DNA/500 μg of gold, and the microparticles are dried onto the inner surface of a 0.5-in. length fluoropolymer tubing. This cartridge is then attached to a handheld device (PowderJect XR-1), which propels the DNA/gold powder into the epidermis via pressurized helium[123]. The clinical study showed that a single 4 μg plasmid dose (i.e., 2000 μg of gold) was sufficient to elicit serum hemagglutinin inhibition antibody responses (eightfold increase) with only mild to moderate reactions[124] (see Table 6.1). This is probably one of the smallest amounts of plasmid DNA being tested in a human DNA vaccine. The vaccine is expected to enter phase 2 studies soon.

The flu vaccine sponsored by the U.S. National Institute of Allergy and Infectious Diseases (NIAID), which is currently undergoing a safety and immunogenicity phase 1 study,[125] provides an interesting counterpart to the PowderMed flu vaccine. The vaccine contains a plasmid that encodes hemagglutinin 5 (H5), an influenza protein similar to the one encoded in the PowderMed vaccine. Vaccine vials contain this plasmid in phosphate buffered saline (PBS) at a concentration of 4 mg/mL. The clinical study is intended to examine the effect of three intramuscular injections of 1000 or 4000 μg doses, given about 4 weeks apart (see Table 6.1). The Biojector 2000 needle-free jet injection system described in Section 6.2.3 is used to administer 1 mL of the vaccine in the deltoid muscle of the upper arm. PBS is used as the diluent to prepare 1000 μg doses (at 1 mg/mL) from the original vaccine vials.

6.7.2.2 Melanoma

Melanoma has one of the most rapidly increasing incidence rates of any cancer worldwide. Although in its early stage melanoma is curable by surgical excision, patients with metastatic melanoma have median survival rates in the 6- to 9-month range.[126] The search for immune-potentiating vaccines against melanoma has attracted the attention of several researchers.[127] A variety of components, which range from allogeneic or autologous tumor cells to proteins, peptides, glycolipids, and monoclonal antibodies, have been formulated and tested as vaccines.[127] The potential of DNA vaccines in the treatment of mela-

TABLE 6.1. Characteristics of Selected Human Plasmid Biopharmaceuticals

		Flu			Melanoma		PAD	Cystic Fibrosis
Sponsor		PowderMed[124]	NIAID[125]	Vical Inc.[78]	MSKCC/NCI[130]		Valentis[86,87]	Imperial College[119]
Clinical phase		1	1	3	Pilot study		2	1
Delivery		Gene gun	Jet injection	Lipoplex	Gene gun	Jet injection	Polyplex	Lipoplex
Delivery agent		Gold	None	Lipids	Gold	None	Poloxamer 188	Lipids
Number of doses/treatment		1	3	6	16	16	42	1
[pDNA] (mg/mL)		–	4	1	–	2	1	2.1
Mass/dose	pDNA (µg)	1	1000	1000	2	1000	2000	1
	Adjuvant (µg)	2000	0	1000	1000	0	100,000	229,000
	Water (mg)	0	1000	1000	0	500	2000	20,000
	Total (mg)	2	1001	1002	1	501	2102	20,271
Mass/treatment	pDNA (µg)	4	3000	6000	32	16,000	84,000	42,000
	Adjuvant (µg)	2000	0	6000	16,000	0	4.2×10^6	229,000
	Water (mg)	0	3000	6000	0	8000	84,000	20,000
	Total (mg)	2	3003	6012	16	8016	88,284	20,271

The data highlight the differences in the design/formulation of each product when it comes to dosage and delivery methodology used (see text for more details).

noma has also been the focus of attention for almost 15 years. Some of these efforts have culminated in the approval and marketing of a veterinary DNA vaccine for canine malignant melanoma, as described in Chapter 10 (Section 10.4). The efforts to come up with a human counterpart are ongoing.

For example, Allovectin-7 is a cancer DNA vaccine designed by Vical Inc. to induce a proinflammatory response and express allogenic major histocompatibility complex (MHC) class I antigen upon intratumoral injection. This vaccine contains a bicistronic plasmid (VCL-1005) with genes that code for the human leukocyte antigen HLA-B7 and the β2-microglobulin. These two genes encode an allogeneic form of the MHC class I antigen.[76,128] The high uptake of the DNA by the tumor cells is facilitated by the complexation of the plasmid with a mixture (1:1 molar ratio) of the cationic lipids DMRIE and DOPE. A series of phase 1, 1/2, 2, and 3 trials have been carried out or are under way using Allovectin-7 to treat a variety of malignancies.[75,76] Overall, results have been promising, and no significant toxicity or serious adverse events have been reported. For instance, a high-dose phase 2 study completed in 2004 has indicated that intratumoral injection of Allovectin-7 is a safe and active treatment for stage III/IV metastatic melanoma patients with cutaneous, sub-cutaneous, or nodal lesions.[129] A phase 3 clinical trial is currently recruiting patients with recurrent metastatic melanoma to evaluate the safety and efficacy of treatment with 2000 μg intralesional Allovectin-7 compared to standard chemotherapy.[78] This total dose contains 1 mL of water and approximately 1000 μg pDNA and 1000 μg cationic lipids (B. Paxton, Vical Inc., pers. comm.). In this trial, each treatment cycle consists of weekly injections of Allovectin-7 alone for 6 weeks[78] (see Table 6.1).

Another melanoma DNA vaccine pilot study in humans is currently under way, which is jointly sponsored by the Memorial Sloan–Kettering Cancer Center (MSKCC) and the National Cancer Institute (NCI).[130] The plasmid in the vaccine encodes gp100, a glycoprotein that is one of the most prevalent antigens recognized on melanomas (see Chapter 10, Section 10.4). The goal of the study is to compare two different methods of immunization with plasmid DNA, namely, PowderMed's PMED and Bioject's needle-free intramuscular jet injection. In the first case, and as in the PowderMed flu trial described above, the plasmid construct is coated on 1- to 3-μm gold particles, at a mass ratio of 2 μg of DNA/1000 μg of gold. These particles are then adequately formulated into a cartridge and administered to the first group of patients using the ND10 device, a commercial version of the XR-1 design. The vaccination schedule comprehends 2 actuations every 2 weeks for 4 months, making a total of 16 actuations. Since each actuation delivers 2 μg of plasmid DNA coated onto 1000 μg of gold, each patient will receive 32 μg DNA and 16,000 μg gold[131] (see Table 6.1). A second group of patients is being vaccinated with 1000 μg of the gp100 plasmid via intramuscular administration using the Biojector 2000 needle-free delivery system. The plasmid concentration in vaccine vials is equal to 2 mg/mL. The vaccination schedule consists of 2 injections/day, administered every 2 weeks for 4 months. This makes up 16 injections and a total of 16,000 µg of plasmid (see Table 6.1). The proponents of the study have hypothesized that delivery of plasmid DNA as a gold particle conjugate into the skin will augment the immune response compared to standard delivery by intramuscular injection.[131]

6.7.2.3 Others

Although influenza and melanoma DNA vaccines constitute the focus of the comparative study presented here, data concerning two additional plasmid-based gene therapy products are also examined given some of their associated peculiarities. The first case deals with a phase 2 trial designed to investigate the safety and efficacy of a plasmid-mediated approach to induce angiogenesis/arteriogenesis with the angiomatrix protein Del-1 in subjects with intermittent claudication secondary to PAD.[86,87] The plasmid was formulated at 1 mg/mL with the nonionic polymer poloxamer 188* at a concentration of 5% (w/v)[85] and was injected intramuscularly. Although the delivery of the formulated plasmid was well tolerated and safe, no differences in outcome measures were obtained when comparing patients in the study (plasmid + poloxamer 188) and control (poloxamer 188) groups.[87] Despite this failure to demonstrate efficacy, what makes this trial an interesting case study is the fact that the massive amounts of plasmid material that have been administered in the form of 42 intramuscular injections (2 mL, 2000 µg plasmid and 100 mg of poloxamer 188 per injection) during the course of the study are probably among the highest ever used in humans[86,87] (see Table 6.1).

The second case in appreciation refers to a clinical trial designed to investigate the performance of a plasmid coding for the cystic fibrosis transmembrane conductance regulator (CFTR). A mutation in this gene is responsible for cystic fibrosis, a condition that affects organs of cystic fibrosis patients like the lungs and the intestinal tract. This inherited monogenic disease has been one of the favorite targets for gene therapy, albeit one of the most elusive. Although successful gene transfer and partial correction have been demonstrated in many of these studies,[6,119] the question that remains unaddressed is whether this level of efficiency is sufficient to improve clinical parameters. In the particular case selected for analysis here, the plasmid encoding CFTR is complexed with a mixture of lipids: GL-67 (Genzyme Lipid-67), DOPE, and 1,2-dimyristoyl-sn-glycero-3-phosphoethanolamine-N-(polyethylene glycol 5000 (DMPE–PEG$_{5000}$). GL-67 is a cationic lipid amphiphile made up of a spermine head group linked to a cholesterol anchor in a "T-shape" configuration.[132] The molar ratio of each lipidic component in the mixture is 1.0:2.0:0.05. The active complex was administered by nebulization, first into the lungs (42.2 mg plasmid + 229 mg lipid in 20 mL) and then into the nose (11.8 mg plasmid + 229 mg lipid in 4.5 mL) of patients.[119] The single administration of

---

* The structure of poloxamer 188 is $(POE)_{52}(POP)_{30}(POE)_{52}$ (see Section 6.5.3) and its average molecular weight is 8400[94].

42.2 mg of plasmid into the lungs, which is one of the highest reported in humans, makes this an interesting case study (see Table 6.1).

6.7.3   Comparison of Product Profiles

Some of the characteristics of the five plasmid biopharmaceuticals described above are listed in Table 6.1. The mass of plasmid, delivery agent, and water (when applicable) per single dose is given, together with the cumulative mass associated with the full treatment/intervention described in the corresponding clinical experiment. The very different nature of the delivery modes used (gene gun discharge of plasmid-coated gold particles, jet injection or nebulization of naked plasmids, and needle injection of lipoplexes or polyplexes) translates into products that have very different compositions. This is highlighted in Figure 6.8, which compares the relative masses of active principle (i.e., plasmid DNA) and delivery agent in the different products. Water and other hypothetical components contained in the formulation (e.g., stabilizers) are not accounted for in this analysis. Whereas the delivery agent accounts for more than 99% (w/w) and 98% (w/w) of the product in the case of the gold particle and poloxamer 188 based delivery, respectively, the vaccines delivered by the Bioject needle-free jet injection system are simply formulated in PBS buffer, and require no specific delivery agent whatsoever. The lipofection methodology used in Allovectin-7, which forms the basis of Vical's delivery system, lies between these two extremes, resulting in a product that is composed of roughly 50% (w/w) of plasmid and 50% (w/w) of delivery agent. The lipid mixture used to formulate the plasmid in the case of the cystic fibrosis accounts for 85% (w/w) of the product (Figure 6.8).

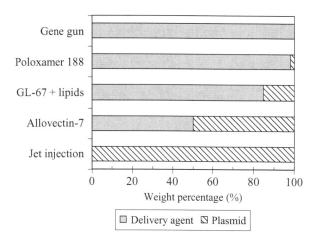

Figure 6.8 *Effect of the delivery mode on plasmid product profile. The relative masses of plasmid DNA and delivery agent in the different plasmid products presented in Table 6.1 are shown for comparison.*

The total mass of plasmid DNA plus delivery agent (gold, lipids) per dose is not very different in the melanoma and influenza cases reported, ranging from ~1 mg to ~2 mg. The cystic fibrosis and PAD trials were exceptional in this regard, with single doses delivering 42 mg of plasmid and 229 mg of lipids in the first case, and 2 mg of plasmid and 100 mg of poloxamer 188 in the second case (see Table 6.1). However, the picture is radically different when one compares the plasmid DNA mass used in each dose of the different products. The major observation which can be drawn from the corresponding data in Table 6.1 is that the amount of plasmid used per dose does not correlate with the prophylactic or therapeutic nature of the DNA vaccine, but is rather highly dependent on the delivery platform used. The gene gun technology can often achieve stronger immune responses with lower amounts of DNA when compared with other inoculation routes.[4] The data in Table 6.1 confirms this superiority, making it clear that the gene gun platform supports the use of plasmid amounts (2–4 μg) per dose which are around three orders of magnitude lower when compared with the typical plasmid masses (1–2 mg) present in single doses of vaccines delivered by jet injection or via lipoplexes and polyplexes. The reasons for this superiority of the gene gun approach are associated with the fact that, unlike intramuscular injection, the gene gun directly propels the DNA vaccine to both nonprofessional and professional APCs of the viable epidermis (see Section 6.3). Moreover, a fraction of the DNA coated particles are delivered directly to the nucleus of the target cell, whereas other particles are deposited in the cytoplasm[4].

It is also instructive to look to the cumulative amount of plasmid DNA that is introduced in a patient's body during the course of a whole treatment/ intervention. These data, which are shown on the lower part of Table 6.1, is also plotted in Figure 6.9 as a function of the total cumulative mass of plasmid plus delivery agent administered. The corresponding number of administrations ranges from 1 in the case of the PowderMed flu vaccine to 42 in the case of the PAD plasmid. These two cases are also at the extremes of the spectra of overall plasmid DNA mass used, with 4 μg for the flu vaccine and 84 mg for arterial disease. The data in Figure 6.9 are delimited by two boundaries. The upper boundary corresponds to the needle-free jet injection delivery system, which requires no delivery agent other than water (i.e., the plasmid is naked), whereas the lower boundary corresponds to the gene gun delivery systems in which gold particles account for 99.8% of the product. The products, which rely on the use of complexing agents like lipids and polymers, lie within these boundaries, as previously seen in Figure 6.8 (notice that logarithmic scales are used in both axes in Figure 6.9). The distinction between the delivery technologies is confirmed here—smaller amounts of plasmid for a full intervention are administered with the gene gun technology when compared with the other options under analysis.

The profile of plasmid products delivered with alternative technologies other than PMED, needle-free liquid jet injection, and lipoplexes/polyplexes might find its own place in the space confined between the two boundaries

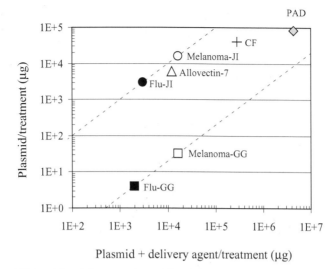

Figure 6.9 *Effect of the delivery mode on plasmid dosage. The cumulative amount of the different plasmid products presented in Table 6.1 that is introduced in a patient's body during the course of a whole treatment/intervention is shown as a function of the cumulative amount of plasmid plus delivery agent. CF, cystic fibrosis; GG, gene gun; JI, jet injection; PAD, peripheral arterial disease.*

shown in Figure 6.9. For instance, electrically mediated delivery methods like electroporation, which most commonly require no adjuvant but have the potential to deliver plasmids directly to the cytoplasm of cells, are likely to give rise to products and treatments that use smaller amounts of plasmids.[1,56] Given that electroporation can (1) increase DNA vaccine potency by 100-fold or more, improving the magnitude and consistency of responses, as well as their functionality and breadth,[56] and (2) significantly increase the magnitude of gene expression by 400-fold and more[133,134] compared to conventional injection of naked plasmid DNA, we may expect such products to lie on the top boundary but closer to the left-hand region of the figure. Another method that is gaining popularity relies on the use of polymeric microparticles (1–5 μm) such as those made up of PLG to enhance delivery of plasmid DNA after intramuscular injection[97] (see Section 6.6.1). The PLG-based delivery is more effective if the microparticle surface is modified to display a positive surface charge for plasmid DNA adsorption. For example, the phase 1 trial of PLG-loaded HIV DNA vaccines alluded to in Section 6.6.1 is currently looking at the safety of triple administrations of 0.25, 0.5, and 1.0 mg of plasmid.[108] Since the plasmid to microparticle loadings typically used are of the order of 1% (w/w),[97] this places products based on this delivery system close to the bottom boundary of Figure 6.9 but closer to the right-hand side of the graphic.

If one compares the data within the same delivery platform, it is also evident that larger amounts of plasmid material are required per intervention in the case of therapeutic DNA vaccines. Furthermore, it should be stressed that repeated treatments and chronic administration are likely to be required in the case of the melanoma DNA vaccines, given the potential difficulties in inducing a long-lasting immune response against tumors. This means that in a real setting, we should expect the open symbols in Figure 6.9 to move upward, toward the right-hand corner of the chart. The same reasoning applies to cystic fibrosis and PADs.

6.8 CONCLUSIONS

The number of cells *in vivo* that express plasmid-borne transgenes, as well as the amount of the transgene product itself, is strongly dependent on the delivery method used. For this reason, much of the future success of plasmid biopharmaceuticals rests on the correct choice of the delivery system. A correct understanding of the mechanisms underlying the transfer and intracellular trafficking of plasmids to the cell nucleus, as well as of the associated barriers, is crucial for the development of a successful delivery system. On top of this understanding, the selection of the best delivery methodology should take into account a series of factors that are interconnected, namely, the nature of the disease being targeted, the function of the plasmid-borne genes, the entry route, the impact on patient safety, and the administration regimen being planned. The costs associated with a given delivery methodology may also constrain the choice in some cases. Today, there is a whole ensemble of delivery options available, from the simplest needle injection of naked or complexed plasmids to the more sophisticated device-based delivery methods like electroporation or the gene gun. Apart from the impact on the transfection efficiency, some delivery options also provide an adjuvant effect, for example, by activating the immune system. While gene gun and electroporation-based delivery are probably the most effective means of achieving an efficient delivery of DNA vaccines, other options may be more appropriate in the context of other plasmid product types. In spite of the progress made so far, and without any doubt, advancements and innovative ideas in the delivery area are essential to move plasmid biopharmaceuticals forward.

REFERENCES

1. Nishikawa M, Huang L. Nonviral vectors in the new millennium: Delivery barriers in gene transfer. *Human Gene Therapy.* 2001;12:861–870.
2. Graessman M, Menne J, Liebler M, Graeber I, Graessmann A. Helper activity for gene expression, a novel function of the SV40 enhancer. *Nucleic Acids Research.* 1989;17:6603–6612.
3. Gill DR, Pringle IA, Hyde SC. Progress and prospects: The design and production of plasmid vectors. *Gene Therapy.* 2009;16:165–171.

4. Dean HJ, Fuller D, Osorio JE. Powder and particle-mediated approaches for delivery of DNA and protein vaccines into the epidermis. *Comparative Immunology, Microbiology & Infectious Diseases.* 2003;26:373–388.

5. Mahvi DM, Henry MB, Albertini MR, et al. Intratumoral injection of IL-12 plasmid DNA—Results of a phase I/IB clinical trial. *Cancer Gene Therapy.* 2007; 14:717–723.

6. Konstan MW, Davis PB, Wagener JS, et al. Compacted DNA nanoparticles administered to the nasal mucosa of cystic fibrosis subjects are safe and demonstrate partial to complete cystic fibrosis transmembrane regulator reconstitution. *Human Gene Therapy.* 2004;15:1255–1269.

7. Wolff JA, Malone RW, Williams P, et al. Direct gene transfer into mouse muscle *in vivo. Science.* 1990;247:1465–1468.

8. Wolff JA, Budker V. The mechanism of naked DNA uptake and expression. *Advances in Genetics.* 2005;54:3–20.

9. Little SR, Langer R. Nonviral delivery of cancer genetic vaccines. *Advances in Biochemical Engineering and Biotechnology.* 2005;99:93–118.

10. Sheets RL, Stein J, Manetz TS, et al. Biodistribution of DNA plasmid vaccines against HIV-1, Ebola, severe acute respiratory syndrome, or West Nile virus is similar, without integration, despite differing plasmid backbones or gene inserts. *Toxicological Sciences.* 2006;91:610–619.

11. Pilling AM, Harman RM, Jones SA, McCormack NA, Lavender D, Haworth R. The assessment of local tolerance, acute toxicity, and DNA biodistribution following particle-mediated delivery of a DNA vaccine to minipigs. *Toxicologic Pathology.* 2002;30:298–305.

12. Manam S, Ledwith BJ, Barnum AB, et al. Plasmid DNA vaccines: Tissue distribution and effects of DNA sequence, adjuvants and delivery method on integration into host DNA. *Intervirology.* 2000;43:273–281.

13. Satkauskas S, Bureau MF, Mahfoudi A, Mir LM. Slow accumulation of plasmid in muscle cells: Supporting evidence for a mechanism of DNA uptake by receptor-mediated endocytosis. *Molecular Therapy.* 2001;4:317–323.

14. Levy MY, Barron LG, Meyer KB, Szoka FC, Jr. Characterization of plasmid DNA transfer into mouse skeletal muscle: Evaluation of uptake mechanism, expression and secretion of gene products into blood. *Gene Therapy.* 1996;3:201–211.

15. Nabel EG, Gordon D, Yang ZY, et al. Gene transfer *in vivo* with DNA-liposome complexes: Lack of autoimmunity and gonadal localization. *Human Gene Therapy.* 1992;3:649–656.

16. Choi SM, Lee DS, Son MK, et al. Safety evaluation of GX-12. A new DNA vaccine for HIV infection in rodents. *Drug and Chemical Toxicology.* 2003;26:271–284.

17. Hickman MA, Malone RW, Lehmann-Bruinsma K, et al. Gene expression following direct injection of DNA into liver. *Human Gene Therapy.* 1994;5:1477–1483.

18. Choate KA, Khavari PA. Direct cutaneous gene delivery in a human genetic skin disease. *Human Gene Therapy.* 1997;8:1659–1665.

19. Ardehali A, Fyfe A, Laks H, Drinkwater DC, Qiao J-H, Lusis AJ. Direct gene transfer into donor hearts at the time of harvest. *The Journal of Thoracic and Cardiovascular Surgery.* 1995;109:716–720.

20. Schwartz B, Benoist C, Abdallah B, et al. Gene transfer by naked DNA into adult mouse brain. *Gene Therapy.* 1996;3:405–411.

21. Budker V, Budker T, Zhang G, Subbotin VM, Loomis A, Wolff JA. Hypothesis: Naked plasmid DNA is taken up by cells *in vivo* by a receptor-mediated process. *The Journal of Gene Medicine.* 2000;2:76–88.

22. Yabukov LA, Deeva EA, Zarytova VF, et al. Mechanism of oligonucleotide uptake by cells: Involvement of specific receptors. *Proceedings of the National Academy of Sciences of the United States of America.* 1989;86:6454–6458.

23. Lechardeur D, Lukacs GL. Intracellular barriers to non-viral gene transfer. *Current Gene Therapy.* 2002;2:183–194.

24. Vaughan EE, DeGiulio JV, Dean DA. Intracellular trafficking of plasmids for gene therapy: Mechanisms of cytoplasmic movement and nuclear import. *Current Gene Therapy.* 2006;6:671–681.

25. Dean DA, Strong DD, Zimmer WE. Nuclear entry of nonviral vectors. *Gene Therapy.* 2005;12:881–890.

26. Dean DA. Import of plasmid DNA into the nucleus is sequence specific. *Experimental Cell Research.* 1997;230:293–302.

27. Dean DA, Dean BS, Muller S, Smith LC. Sequence requirements for plasmid nuclear import. *Experimental Cell Research.* 1999;253:713–722.

28. Mitragotri S. Current status and future prospects of needle-free liquid jet injectors. *Nature Reviews in Drug Discovery.* 2006;5:543–548.

29. Raviprakash K, Ewing D, Simmons M, et al. Needle-free Biojector injection of a dengue virus type 1 DNA vaccine with human immunostimulatory sequences and the GM-CSF gene increases immunogenicity and protection from virus challenge in Aotus monkeys. *Virology.* 2003;315:345–352.

30. Trimble C, Lin CT, Hung CF, et al. Comparison of the CD8+ T cell responses and antitumor effects generated by DNA vaccine administered through gene gun, biojector, and syringe. *Vaccine.* 2003;21:4036–4042.

31. Rao SS, Gomez P, Mascola JR, et al. Comparative evaluation of three different intramuscular delivery methods for DNA immunization in a nonhuman primate animal model. *Vaccine.* 2006;24:367–373.

32. Budker V, Zhang G, Danko I, Williams P, Wolff JA. The efficient expression of intravascularly delivered DNA in rat muscle. *Gene Therapy.* 1998;5:272–276.

33. Budker V, Zhang G, Knechtle S, Wolff JA. Naked DNA delivered intraportally expresses in hepatocytes. *Gene Therapy.* 1996;3:593–598.

34. Liu F, Song YK, Liu D. Hydrodynamics-based transfection in animals by systemic administration of plasmid DNA. *Gene Therapy.* 1999;6:1258–1266.

35. Dagnaes-Hansen F, Holst HU, Sondergaard M, et al. Physiological effects of human growth hormone produced after hydrodynamic gene transfer of a plasmid vector containing the human ubiquitin promotor. *Journal of Molecular Medicine.* 2002;80:665–670.

36. Miao CH, Thompson AR, Loeb K, Ye X. Long-term and therapeutic-level hepatic gene expression of human factor IX after naked plasmid transfer *in vivo. Molecular Therapy.* 2001;3:947–957.

37. Crespo A, Peydro A, Dasi F, et al. Hydrodynamic liver gene transfer mechanism involves transient sinusoidal blood stasis and massive hepatocyte endocytic vesicles. *Gene Therapy.* 2005;12:927–935.

38. Sebestyen MG, Budker VG, Budker T, et al. Mechanism of plasmid delivery by hydrodynamic tail vein injection. I. Hepatocyte uptake of various molecules. *The Journal of Gene Medicine.* 2006;8:852–873.

39. Budker VG, Subbotin VM, Budker T, Sebestyen MG, Zhang G, Wolff JA. Mechanism of plasmid delivery by hydrodynamic tail vein injection. II. Morphological studies. *Journal of Gene Medicine.* 2006;8:874–888.

40. Zhu CL, Li YW, Gao RT. Gene therapy for acute liver failure. *Current Gene Therapy.* 2010;10:156–166.

41. Sawyer GJ, Rela M, Davenport M, Whitehorne M, Zhang X, Fabre JW. Hydrodynamic gene delivery to the liver: Theoretical and practical issues for clinical application. *Current Gene Therapy.* 2009;9:128–135.

42. Sawyer GJ, Zhang X, Fabre JW. Technical requirements for effective regional hydrodynamic gene delivery to the left lateral lobe of the rat liver. *Gene Therapy.* 2010;17:560–564.

43. Klein TM, Wolf ED, Wu R, Sanford JC. High-velocity microprojectiles for delivering nucleic acids into living cells. *Nature.* 1987;327:70–73.

44. Zelenin AV, Titomirov AV, Kolesnikov VA. Genetic transformation of mouse cultured cells with the help of high-velocity mechanical DNA injection. *FEBS Letters.* 1989;244:65–67.

45. Yang NS, Burkholder J, Roberts B, Martinell B, McCabe D. *In vivo* and *in vitro* gene transfer to mammalian somatic cells by particle bombardment. *Proceedings of the National Academy of Sciences of the United States of America.* 1990;87: 9568–9572.

46. Bio-Rad Laboratories. *Helios gene gun system: Instruction manual.* Hercules, CA: Bio-Rad Laboratories, 2000.

47. Dean HJ, Haynes J, Schmaljohn C. The role of particle-mediated DNA vaccines in biodefense preparedness. *Advanced Drug Delivery Reviews.* 2005;57:1315–1342.

48. Fuller DH, Loudon P, Schmaljohn C. Preclinical and clinical progress of particle-mediated DNA vaccines for infectious diseases. *Methods.* 2006;40:86–97.

49. Chen CA, Chang MC, Sun WZ, et al. Noncarrier naked antigen-specific DNA vaccine generates potent antigen-specific immunologic responses and antitumor effects. *Gene Therapy.* 2009;16:776–787.

50. Fynan EF, Webster RG, Fuller DH, Haynes JR, Santoro JC, Robinson HL. DNA vaccines: Protective immunizations by parenteral, mucosal, and gene-gun inoculations. *Proceedings of the National Academy of Sciences of the United States of America.* 1993;90:11478–11482.

51. Leitner WW, Seguin MC, Ballou WR, et al. Immune responses induced by intramuscular or gene gun injection of protective deoxyribonucleic acid vaccines that express the circumsporozoite protein from *Plasmodium berghei* malaria parasites. *Journal of Immunology.* 1997;159:6112–6119.

52. Wong TK, Neumann E. Electric field mediated gene transfer. *Biochemical and Biophysical Research Communications.* 1982;107:584–587.

53. Neumann E, Schaefer-Ridder M, Wang Y, Hofschneider PH. Gene transfer into mouse lyoma cells by electroporation in high electric fields. *The EMBO Journal.* 1982;1:841–845.

54. Titomirov AV, Sukharev S, Kistanova E. *In vivo* electroporation and stable transformation of skin cells of newborn mice by plasmid DNA. *Biochimica et Biophysica Acta.* 1991;1088:131–134.

55. Aihara H, Miyazaki J. Gene transfer into muscle by electroporation *in vivo. Nature Biotechnology.* 1998;16:867–870.

56. Luxembourg A, Evans CF, Hannaman D. Electroporation-based DNA immunisation: Translation to the clinic. *Expert Opinion on Biological Therapy.* 2007;7: 1647–1664.

57. Escoffre JM, Portet T, Wasungu L, Teissie J, Dean D, Rols MP. What is (still not) known of the mechanism by which electroporation mediates gene transfer and expression in cells and tissues. *Molecular Biotechnology.* 2009;41:286–295.

58. Denet AR, Vanbever R, Preat V. Skin electroporation for transdermal and topical delivery. *Advanced Drug Delivery Reviews.* 2004;56:659–674.

59. Chiarella P, Massi E, De Robertis M, et al. Electroporation of skeletal muscle induces danger signal release and antigen-presenting cell recruitment independently of DNA vaccine administration. *Expert Opinion on Biological Therapy.* 2008;8:1645–1657.

60. Faurie C, Rebersek M, Golzio M, et al. Electro-mediated gene transfer and expression are controlled by the lifetime of DNA/membrane complex formation. *The Journal of Gene Medicine.* 2010;12:117–125.

61. Bodles-Brakhop AM, Heller R, Draghia-Akli R. Electroporation for the delivery of DNA-based vaccines and immunotherapeutics: Current clinical developments. *Molecular Therapy.* 2009;17:585–592.

62. Luxembourg A, Hannaman D, Ellefsen B, Nakamura G, Bernard R. Enhancement of immune responses to an HBV DNA vaccine by electroporation. *Vaccine.* 2006;24:4490–4493.

63. Hooper JW, Golden JW, Ferro AM, King AD. Smallpox DNA vaccine delivered by novel skin electroporation device protects mice against intranasal poxvirus challenge. *Vaccine.* 2007;25:1814–1823.

64. Zhang X, Divangahi M, Ngai P, et al. Intramuscular immunization with a monogenic plasmid DNA tuberculosis vaccine: Enhanced immunogenicity by electroporation and co-expression of GM-CSF transgene. *Vaccine.* 2007;25:1342–1352.

65. Best SR, Peng S, Juang CM, et al. Administration of HPV DNA vaccine via electroporation elicits the strongest CD8+ T cell immune responses compared to intramuscular injection and intradermal gene gun delivery. *Vaccine.* 2009;27: 5450–5459.

66. Livingston BD, Little SF, Luxembourg A, Ellefsen B, Hannaman D. Comparative performance of a licensed anthrax vaccine versus electroporation based delivery of a PA encoding DNA vaccine in rhesus macaques. *Vaccine.* 2010;28:1056–1061.

67. Guillem VM, Aliño SF. Transfection pathways of nonspecific and targeted PEI-polyplexes. *Gene Therapy and Molecular Biology.* 2004;8:369–384.

68. Nicolau C, Le Pape A, Soriano P, Fargette F, Juhel MF. *In vivo* expression of rat insulin after intravenous administration of the liposome-entrapped gene for rat insulin I. *Proceedings of the National Academy of Sciences of the United States of America.* 1983;80:1068–1072.

69. Felgner PL, Gadek TR, Holm M, et al. Lipofection: A highly efficient, lipid-mediated DNA-transfection procedure. *Proceedings of the National Academy of Sciences of the United States of America.* 1987;84:7413–7417.

70. Karmali PP, Chaudhuri A. Cationic liposomes as non-viral carriers of gene medicines: Resolved issues, open questions, and future promises. *Medicinal Research Reviews.* 2007;27:696–722.

71. Zabner J, Fasbender AJ, Moninger T, Poellinger KA, Welsh MJ. Cellular and molecular barriers to gene transfer by a cationic lipid. *The Journal of Biological Chemistry.* 1995;270:18997–19007.

72. Pedroso de Lima MC, Simoes S, Pires P, Faneca H, Duzgunes N. Cationic lipid-DNA complexes in gene delivery: From biophysics to biological applications. *Advanced Drug Delivery Reviews.* 2001;47:277–294.

73. Chesnoy S, Huang L. Structure and function of lipid-DNA complexes for gene delivery. *Annual Reviews in Biophysics and Biomolecular Structure.* 2000;29: 27–47.

74. Templeton NS, Lasic DD, Frederik PM, Strey HH, Roberts DD, Pavlakis GN. Improved DNA: Liposome complexes for increased systemic delivery and gene expression. *Nature Biotechnology.* 1997;15:647–652.

75. Gonzalez R, Hutchins L, Nemunaitis J, Atkins M, Schwarzenberger PO. Phase 2 trial of Allovectin-7 in advanced metastatic melanoma. *Melanoma Research.* 2006;16:521–526.

76. Galanis E. Technology evaluation: Allovectin-7, Vical. *Current Opinion in Molecular Therapy.* 2002;4:80–87.

77. Matsumoto K, Kubo H, Murata H, et al. A pilot study of human interferon beta gene therapy for patients with advanced melanoma by *in vivo* transduction using cationic liposomes. *Japanese Journal of Clinical Oncology.* 2008;38: 849–856.

78. Vical Inc. A phase 3 pivotal trial comparing Allovectin-7® alone vs chemotherapy alone in patients with stage 3 or stage 4 melanoma. Available at: http://www.clinicaltrials.gov/ct2/show/NCT00395070. Accessed May 12, 2010.

79. Hartikka J, Bozoukova V, Ferrari M, et al. Vaxfectin enhances the humoral immune response to plasmid DNA-encoded antigens. *Vaccine.* 2001;19:1911–1923.

80. Zhang C, Yadava P, Hughes J. Polyethylenimine strategies for plasmid delivery to brain-derived cells. *Methods.* 2004;33:144–150.

81. Ziady AG, Davis PB, Konstan MW. Non-viral gene transfer therapy for cystic fibrosis. *Expert Opinion in Biological Therapy.* 2003;3:449–458.

82. Farrell LL, Pepin J, Kucharski C, Lin X, Xu Z, Uludag H. A comparison of the effectiveness of cationic polymers poly-L-lysine (PLL) and polyethylenimine (PEI) for non-viral delivery of plasmid DNA to bone marrow stromal cells (BMSC). *European Journal of Pharmaceuticals and Biopharmaceuticals.* 2007;65: 388–397.

83. Lemieux P, Guerin N, Paradis G, et al. A combination of poloxamers increases gene expression of plasmid DNA in skeletal muscle. *Gene Therapy.* 2000;7: 986–991.

84. Hartikka J, Sukhu L, Buchner C, et al. Electroporation-facilitated delivery of plasmid DNA in skeletal muscle: Plasmid dependence of muscle damage and effect of poloxamer 188. *Molecular Therapy.* 2001;4:407–415.

85. Zhong J, Eliceiri B, Stupack D, et al. Neovascularization of ischemic tissues by gene delivery of the extracellular matrix protein Del-1. *Journal of Clinical Investigation.* 2003;112:30–41.

86. Rajagopalan S, Olin JW, Young S, et al. Design of the Del-1 for therapeutic angiogenesis trial (DELTA-1), a phase II multicenter, double-blind, placebo-controlled trial of VLTS-589 in subjects with intermittent claudication secondary to peripheral arterial disease. *Human Gene Therapy.* 2004;15:619–624.

87. Grossman PM, Mendelsohn F, Henry TD, et al. Results from a phase II multicenter, double-blind placebo-controlled study of Del-1 (VLTS-589) for intermittent claudication in subjects with peripheral arterial disease. *American Heart Journal.* 2007;153:874–880.

88. Gao X, Kim KS, Liu D. Nonviral gene delivery: What we know and what is next. *The AAPS Journal.* 2007;9:E92–104.

89. Godbey WT, Barry MA, Saggau P, Wu KK, Mikos AG. Poly(ethylenimine)-mediated transfection: A new paradigm for gene delivery. *Journal of Biomedical Materials Research.* 2000;51:321–328.

90. Godbey WT, Wu KK, Mikos AG. Tracking the intracellular path of poly(ethylenimine)/DNA complexes for gene delivery. *Proceedings of the National Academy of Sciences of the United States of America.* 1999;96: 5177–5181.

91. Shi L, Tang GP, Gao SJ, et al. Repeated intrathecal administration of plasmid DNA complexed with polyethylene glycol-grafted polyethylenimine led to prolonged transgene expression in the spinal cord. *Gene Therapy.* 2003;10: 1179–1188.

92. Hebrew University of Jerusalem. Safety and proof of concept study of intravesical DTA-H19 in patients with superficial bladder cancer. Available at: http://clinicaltrials.gov/ct2/show/NCT00393809. Accessed May 23, 2010.

93. BioCancell Therapeutics Ltd. Phase 2b, trial of intravesical DTA-H19/PEI in patients with intermediate-risk superficial bladder cancer. Available at: http://clinicaltrials.gov/ct2/show/NCT00595088. Accessed May 23, 2010.

94. Moghimi SM, Hunter AC. Poloxamers and poloxamines in nanoparticle engineering and experimental medicine. *Trends in Biotechnology.* 2000;18:412–420.

95. Jones DH, Corris S, McDonald S, Clegg JC, Farrar GH. Poly(DL-lactide-co-glycolide)-encapsulated plasmid DNA elicits systemic and mucosal antibody responses to encoded protein after oral administration. *Vaccine.* 1997;15: 814–817.

96. Aral C, Akbuga J. Preparation and *in vitro* transfection efficiency of chitosan microspheres containing plasmid DNA:poly(L-lysine) complexes. *Journal of Pharmacy and Pharmaceutical Sciences.* 2003;6:321–326.

97. Singh M, Briones M, Ott G, O'Hagan D. Cationic microparticles: A potent delivery system for DNA vaccines. *Proceedings of the National Academy of Sciences of the United States of America.* 2000;97:811–816.

98. Rafati H, Coombes AG, Adler J, Holland J, Davis SS. Protein-loaded poly(DL-lactide-co-glycolide) microparticles for oral administration: Formulation, structural and release characteristics. *Journal of Controlled Release.* 1997;43: 89–102.

99. Basarkar A, Devineni D, Palaniappan R, Singh J. Preparation, characterization, cytotoxicity and transfection efficiency of poly(DL-lactide-co-glycolide) and poly(DL-lactic acid) cationic nanoparticles for controlled delivery of plasmid DNA. *International Journal of Pharmaceutics.* 2007;343:247–254.

100. Mok H, Park TG. Direct plasmid DNA encapsulation within PLGA nanospheres by single oil-in-water emulsion method. *European Journal of Pharmaceuticals and Biopharmaceuticals.* 2008;68:105–111.

101. Hao T, McKeever U, Hedley ML. Biological potency of microsphere encapsulated plasmid DNA. *Journal of Controlled Release.* 2000;69:249–259.

102. Tse MT, Blatchford C, Oya Alpar H. Evaluation of different buffers on plasmid DNA encapsulation into PLGA microparticles. *Internationl Journal of Pharmaceutics.* 2009;370:33–40.

103. Bozkir A, Saka OM. Chitosan nanoparticles for plasmid DNA delivery: Effect of chitosan molecular structure on formulation and release characteristics. *Drug Delivery.* 2004;11:107–112.

104. Luo Y, O'Hagan D, Zhou H, et al. Plasmid DNA encoding human carcinoembryonic antigen (CEA) adsorbed onto cationic microparticles induces protective immunity against colon cancer in CEA-transgenic mice. *Vaccine.* 2003;21: 1938–1947.

105. O'Hagan DT, Singh M, Dong C, et al. Cationic microparticles are a potent delivery system for a HCV DNA vaccine. *Vaccine.* 2004;23:672–680.

106. He X, Jiang L, Wang F, et al. Augmented humoral and cellular immune responses to hepatitis B DNA vaccine adsorbed onto cationic microparticles. *Journal of Controlled Release.* 2005;107:357–372.

107. Mollenkopf HJ, Dietrich G, Fensterle J, et al. Enhanced protective efficacy of a tuberculosis DNA vaccine by adsorption onto cationic PLG microparticles. *Vaccine.* 2004;22:2690–2695.

108. United States National Institute of Allergy and Infectious Diseases. Safety of and immune response to a combination HIV vaccine regimen in HIV uninfected adults. Available at: http://clinicaltrials.gov/ct2/show/NCT00073216. Accessed May 23, 2010.

109. Klencke B, Matijevic M, Urban RG, et al. Encapsulated plasmid DNA treatment for human papillomavirus 16-associated anal dysplasia: A Phase I study of ZYC101. *Clinical. Cancer Research.* 2002;8:1028–1037.

110. O'Hagan D, Singh M, Ugozzoli M, et al. Induction of potent immune responses by cationic microparticles with adsorbed human immunodeficiency virus DNA vaccines. *Journal of Virology.* 2001;75:9037–9043.

111. Liu G, Li D, Pasumarthy MK, et al. Nanoparticles of compacted DNA transfect postmitotic cells. *The Journal of Biological Chemistry.* 2003;278 :32578–32586.

112. Fink TL, Klepcyk PJ, Oette SM, et al. Plasmid size up to 20 kbp does not limit effective *in vivo* lung gene transfer using compacted DNA nanoparticles. *Gene Therapy.* 2006;13:1048–1051.

113. Ziady AG, Gedeon CR, Miller T, et al. Transfection of airway epithelium by stable PEGylated poly-L-lysine DNA nanoparticles *in vivo. Molecular Therapy.* 2003;8:936–947.

114. He L, Niemeyer B. A novel correlation for protein diffusion coefficients based on molecular weight and radius of gyration. *Biotechnology Progress.* 2003;19: 544–548.

115. Farjo R, Skaggs J, Quiambao AB, Cooper MJ, Naash MI. Efficient non-viral ocular gene transfer with compacted DNA nanoparticles. *PLoS One.* 2006;1:e38.

116. Cai X, Nash Z, Conley SM, Fliesler SJ, Cooper MJ, Naash MI. A partial structural and functional rescue of a retinitis pigmentosa model with compacted DNA nanoparticles. *PLoS One.* 2009;4:e5290.

117. Tacket CO, Roy MJ, Widera G, Swain WF, Broome S, Edelman R. Phase 1 safety and immune response studies of a DNA vaccine encoding hepatitis B surface antigen delivered by a gene delivery device. *Vaccine.* 1999;17:2826–2829.

118. Martin JE, Sullivan NJ, Enama ME, et al. A DNA vaccine for Ebola virus is safe and immunogenic in a phase I clinical trial. *Clinical and Vaccine Immunology.* 2006;13:1267–1277.

119. Alton EW, Stern M, Farley R, et al. Cationic lipid-mediated CFTR gene transfer to the lungs and nose of patients with cystic fibrosis: A double-blind placebo-controlled trial. *Lancet.* 1999;353:947–954.

120. Utterback J. *Mastering the dynamics of innovation.* Boston: Harvard Business School Press, 1996.

121. World Health Organization. *Avian influenza: Assessing the pandemic threat.* Geneva: World Health Organization, 2005.

122. Subbarao K, Murphy BR, Fauci AS. Development of effective vaccines against pandemic influenza. *Immunity.* 2006;24:5–9.

123. Roberts LK, Barr LJ, Fuller DH, McMahon CW, Leese PT, Jones S. Clinical safety and efficacy of a powdered hepatitis B nucleic acid vaccine delivered to the epidermis by a commercial prototype device. *Vaccine.* 2005;23:4867–4878.

124. Drape RJ, Macklin MD, Barr LJ, Jones S, Haynes JR, Dean HJ. Epidermal DNA vaccine for influenza is immunogenic in humans. *Vaccine.* 2006;24: 4475–4481.

125. United States National Institute of Allergy and Infectious Diseases. Safety study of avian flu vaccine. Available at: http://www.clinicaltrials.gov/ct2/show/ NCT00408109. Accessed May 12, 2010.

126. Becker JC, Kirkwood JM, Agarwala SS, Dummer R, Schrama D, Hauschild A. Molecularly targeted therapy for melanoma: Current reality and future options. *Cancer.* 2006;107:2317–2327.

127. Chapman PB. Melanoma vaccines. *Seminars in Oncology.* 2007;34:516–523.

128. Stopeck AT, Jones A, Hersh EM, et al. Phase II study of direct intralesional gene transfer of Allovectin-7, an HLA-B7/beta2-microglobulin DNA-liposome complex, in patients with metastatic melanoma. *Clinical Cancer Research.* 2001;7: 2285–2291.

129. Richards JM, Bedikian A, Gonzalez R, et al. High-dose Allovectin-7 in patients with advanced metastatic melanoma: Final phase 2 data and design of phase 3 registration trial. *Journal of Clinical Oncology.* 2005;23:7543.

130. Memorial Sloan–Kettering Cancer Center. Vaccine therapy in treating patients with stage IIB, stage IIC, stage III, or stage IV melanoma. Available at: http:// www.clinicaltrials.gov/ct2/show/NCT00398073. Accessed May 12, 2010.

131. Wolchok J, Chapman PB, Houghton AN, et al. *Injection of AJCC Stage IIB, IIC, III and IV melanoma patients with mouse gp100 DNA—A pilot study to compare intramuscular jet injection with particle mediated delivery. MSKCC therapeutic/ diagnostic protocol: IRB#: 06-113A(2).* New York: Memorial Sloan–Kettering Cancer Center, 2007.

132. Lee ER, Marshall J, Siegel CS, et al. Detailed analysis of structures and formulations of cationic lipids for efficient gene transfer to the lung. *Human Gene Therapy.* 1996;7:1701–1717.

133. Pringle IA, McLachlan G, Collie DD, et al. Electroporation enhances reporter gene expression following delivery of naked plasmid DNA to the lung. *The Journal of Gene Medicine.* 2007;9:369–380.

134. Jaini R, Hannaman D, Johnson JM, et al. Gene-based intramuscular interferon-beta therapy for experimental autoimmune encephalomyelitis. *Molecular Therapy.* 2006;14:416–422.

135. Herrero MJ, Aliño SF. Naked DNA liver delivery by hydrodynamic injection. *Gene Therapy Review. Technology Overview #2.* Available at: http://www.genetherapyreview.com/gene-therapy-education/technology-overview/137-hydrodynamic-liver-injection.html. Accessed May 19, 2010.

Part II

Applications

7

Ethical and Safety Issues

7.1 INTRODUCTION

Concerns about the ethics and safety of innovative medical interventions and technologies are recurrent in the field of biomedical research.[1] These two topics are of significant importance to stakeholders involved with new medical interventions—clinical researchers, biotechnology companies, disease advocates, regulatory bodies, institutional review boards (IRBs), media, and desperately ill research subjects—no matter which specific area or type of treatment is being dealt with. Although significant progress can be made nowadays on the basis of well-planned and conducted laboratory experiments and clinical observations, the approval of new treatments or medicines inevitably involves experimenting with humans (see Chapter 3, Section 3.2.2). Consequently, and in order to guarantee maximum protection of the human research subjects who voluntarily participate in the different clinical trial phases, the majority of the activities undertaken within the context of such experiments are strongly regulated and controlled. Part of this regulation effort is directed toward the elaboration, establishment, and enforcement of a number of ethical principles and safety guidelines. A number of texts are important in this framework, namely, (1) the *Declaration of Helsinki*,* an

* World Medical Association. *Declaration of Helsinki: Ethical Principles for Medical Research Involving Human Subjects*, 6th ed. adopted on the 52nd WMA General Assembly, Edinburgh, Scotland, October 2000.

Plasmid Biopharmaceuticals: Basics, Applications, and Manufacturing, First Edition.
Duarte Miguel F. Prazeres.
© 2011 John Wiley & Sons, Inc. Published 2011 by John Wiley & Sons, Inc.

ethical code that contains general standards for human experimentation and provides guidance to physicians and other participants in medical research involving human subjects, and (2) good clinical practice documents, which set international ethical and scientific standards for research trials involving human subjects.[2,3] Agencies and organizations like the National Institutes of Health (NIH) and the Food and Drug Administration (FDA) in the United States, the European Medicines Agency (EMA) in Europe, or the World Health Organization (WHO) also provide guidance in ethical questions and safety issues associated with specific types of medical interventions (e.g., gene and cell therapy and xenogeneic transplantation), through documents of the "Points to Consider" or "Guidance to Industry" type. The subject matter covered in many of the documents mentioned is typically found at the ethical and scientific interface, and includes issues like research design, informed consent, risk–benefit analysis, privacy, and accuracy in reporting research results.

Although ethical and safety questions are transversal to biomedical research, perhaps in no other context are they more readily evoked and discussed as in the field that is generically and popularly termed "gene therapy."[4-7] This is clearly demonstrated by the fact that the ethics and safety of gene therapy have been under close scrutiny and attention ever since the days when the first experiments in humans were carried out (e.g., see the papers by Friedmann[8] and Walters[6]). Furthermore, every time milestone and polemic events like the Martin Cline thalassemia experiments[9] or the Jesse Gelsinger case[10] emerge (see Chapter 1, Sections 1.1.2 and 1.1.4), the discussion on the ethics and safety of gene transfer is spurred and the topics are revisited with increased acumen. As a result, a number of guidance documents have been produced over the years by governmental (e.g., FDA and EMA) and nongovernmental (e.g., WHO) organizations to address the specificities of what can be broadly classified as "human gene transfer research."[11-14] These documents are regularly updated as the years go by in order to reflect the evolution in thinking and the increased knowledge on the subject. Apart from perusing through the quality issues associated with gene transfer medicinal products (see Chapter 11), be them recombinant viruses or plasmids, some of these documents also provide important recommendations on how to evaluate the clinical efficacy and safety of those products.

In the particular case of the usage of nonviral plasmid vectors, some of the ethical and safety worries are probably not as prevalent as in the case of recombinant viral vectors. One of the reasons for this is related to the current belief that plasmid vectors are safer. Actually, a number of scientific and clinical studies have demonstrated that plasmid DNA is, in general, well tolerated and safe.[15-18] Some of the concerns that were associated with the use of plasmid vectors as biopharmaceuticals in the earlier years have thus not materialized, at least in the preclinical and clinical development context. Another reason for the favorable appreciation surrounding plasmid biopharmaceuticals is related to the fact that they are, in the vast majority of cases, designed to promote transient expression of the encoded protein in the target human tissues. Furthermore, in those cases where the disease is life threatening, no alternative therapy is available, and the benefits clearly outweigh the risks, the stakeholders are more likely to accept a relaxation of the safety and ethical boundaries. Those plasmid-based gene therapy approaches that aim at treating diseases like cancer fall within this category. In the case of prophylactic DNA vaccines, which are designed to be used in healthy people and often in children, on the other hand, the risk/benefit ratio is clearly different.[14] In this case, harmful events are virtually unacceptable even if they are rare, since the large number of individuals typically subjected to immunization warrants that a significant number of them might become affected.[19] This means that a more strict approach will have to be taken when pondering the safety and ethical issues associated with DNA vaccination of large segments of a given population.

A widespread usage of plasmid biopharmaceuticals also raises concerns regarding the safety of people other than the recipients of the product themselves. For example, risks of accidental exposure or of an inadvertent self-administration of plasmids are inherent to the activities of the health professionals involved in the treatment.[20] The importance of this issue has prompted professional associations to raise awareness of their members, as illustrated by a recent guidance on the pharmacy handling of gene medicines issued by the European Association of Hospital Pharmacists.[21] Apart from establishing the procedures to be carried out in the case of an accidental exposure to a gene medicine, the document also provides practical recommendations on issues like storage, preparation, transportation, dispensing, administration, waste disposal, and decontamination of spill.[21] Furthermore, and since recipients of plasmid biopharmaceuticals are expected in most cases to lead a normal life in the midst of society and not be confined to a well-controlled hospital environment, there is always the probability that shedding of the genetic material from the treated individual may originate horizontal transfer to other individuals and even other species. Although in the future these safety concerns may not materialize or may even be considered irrelevant, the pioneering nature of gene therapy makes close scrutiny inevitable.

In the first part of this chapter, the major ethical issues associated with the administration of exogenous DNA sequences into humans, whether for curative or preventive purposes, are addressed. The intention is not to present an exhaustive and detailed discussion on the topic, but rather to produce an overview of those ethical aspects that have been identified as the most critical in recent years. A more in-depth treatment of the subject can be found in the specialized literature.[1,4–8,22] In the second section of the chapter, specific issues related to the clinical safety of plasmid biopharmaceuticals are examined. A special focus is directed to those particular aspects that recurrently capture the attention of the scientific and medical community, that is, integration, autoimmunity, and tolerance. Finally, the last section deals with ethical and safety issues that are raised in the specific case of plasmid biopharmaceuticals developed for veterinary applications. This is a topic that deserves special consideration particularly in those cases where products are to be used in food-producing species, given that in such situations, the probability of human exposure to the extraneous genetic material is increased.

7.2 ETHICAL ISSUES

7.2.1 Introduction

The risk, complexity, and uncertainty associated with human gene transfer are very high, and the reasons for this are several. Perhaps most importantly, and even though almost 30 years have passed since the first human experiments took place (see Chapter 1, Sections 1.1.2 and 1.1.3), there is still a significant scarcity of scientific understanding of the mechanisms (e.g., genetic recombination and gene regulation) that underlie many gene transfer strategies and approaches. This lack of knowledge adds to the persistent feeling that the outcome of gene therapy may be irreversible and heritable (i.e., vertical transmission), independently on whether this has been accidental or designed on purpose, as would be the case if germline cells had been targeted. The potential for horizontal transmission of genes and its vectors from an individual to other persons or into the environment is another concern.[11]

Gene therapy's potential for promoting oncogenesis, particularly when recombinant viruses are used as gene delivery vectors, is one of the roots of the uneasiness associated with the technique. This risk is a real one, as already shown in a number of cases where patients have developed leukemia as a result of insertional mutagenesis events.[23] But perhaps in no other instance has the high risk associated with gene therapy been so evident as in the case of Jesse Gelsinger, the young man suffering from ornithine transcarbamylase deficiency, who died as a result of a fulminant systemic inflammatory response syndrome developed in reaction to an adenovirus vector[10] (see Chapter 1, Section 1.1.4). The complexity and uncertainty surrounding the delivery of genes to humans are also particularly well illustrated by the outcome of the Merck-sponsored, phase 2 efficacy trial of an adenovirus serotype 5 (Ad5) vector-based HIV-1 vaccine.[24] In the course of this experiment, and unexpectedly, researchers found that the candidate vaccine not only was ineffective at lowering plasma viremia postinfection but also increased the susceptibility of subjects who had pre-existing antibodies against Ad5 to HIV-1 infection. This increased infection risk has been linked to a vaccine-induced immune activation and expansion of Ad5-specific memory CD4 T cells. Since CD4 T cells are the main target of HIV, the cell population expanded upon vaccination is thought to have encouraged HIV infection uptake.[25]

The realization of the risk, complexity, and uncertainty of current human gene transfer constitutes an important starting point for the discussion of its ethics. This task can be facilitated by broadly separating the types of interven-

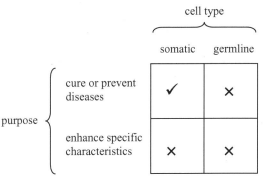

Figure 7.1 *The ethics of human gene transfer. The ethical discussion can be facilitated by broadly separating the types of intervention according to their ultimate goal (disease treatment or prevention vs. enhancement) and to the cells that are targeted and affected (somatic vs. germline) (based and adapted from Walters[5]).*

tion according to their ultimate goal and to the cells that are targeted and affected, as proposed by Walters[5] (Figure 7.1). In the first case, the relevant distinction to be made is between a gene transfer procedure that is designed to cure or prevent a disease and a gene transfer procedure that aims to enhance specific characteristics of individuals. The ethical challenges in this case are discussed in Section 7.2.2. The second distinction separates target cells into two groups, somatic (i.e., nonreproductive) and germline (i.e., reproductive) cells. This distinction is crucial because it raises the question of whether the result of a gene transfer intervention should be or should not be passed to future generations. This is examined in Section 7.2.3.

7.2.2 Disease Management versus Enhancement

Genes are usually transferred into humans with the purpose of tackling and managing specific diseases or disorders, whether via treatment, prevention, or monitoring. Although several ethical aspects like informed consent, privacy and confidentiality, patient selection, and so on, deserve due consideration (see Section 7.2.4) and should always be discussed on a case-by-case basis, it is usually consensual that somatic cell gene transfer should be pursued if the potential benefits to recipients are likely to outweigh its risks. This view has been expressed in a survey of 1299 American scientists involved in human genetics research, who were pooled for their opinions regarding the ethical issues of gene transfer. In that study, 96% of the responders declared to be in favor of the use of gene transfer techniques that target somatic cell therapy, as long as the goal is to cure a life-threatening genetic disease both in adults and in children.[7] Somatic cell gene transfer is thus viewed by many as "a natural and logical extension of current techniques for treating disease."[7] As such, its development and application is close to a moral imperative.

Apart from managing disease, however, gene transfer approaches and technologies have also been equated as a means to improve or enhance human traits beyond normal levels.[26] Physical performance (e.g., muscle mass and endurance), mental capacity (e.g., memory and alertness), behavioral aspects (e.g., societal competences), and appearance (e.g., weight, height, and hair), in principle, could all be ameliorated by gene transfer. As a matter of fact, there are already a number of results from animal studies which clearly show that the transfer of genes to somatic cells of an individual has the potential to enhance and improve his/her specific traits. Examples of genes that could be used in this context include those that code for (1) erythropoietin (EPO), a key regulator of erythrocyte production, to enhance endurance; (2) vascular endothelial growth factor (VEGF), a protein that promotes the formation of new blood vessels, to improve the supply of oxygen and nutrients to the muscles, heart, and other tissues in athletes; (3) insulin-like growth factor, a regulator of muscle growth, to increase muscle strength; (4) estrogen and glucocorticoid receptors, to enhance spatial memory; and (5) leptin and growth hormone, to control weight and height, respectively.[26]

The ethics of such gene transfer-based enhancement strategies should be discussed in a broader societal context and by first realizing that a variety of more conventional methods (e.g., plastic surgery, hair transplantation, and Botox) are already accepted as means to enhance a number of human traits. Furthermore, although approaches like the use of steroids, beta-blockers, and other drugs/biologics (e.g., EPO) for social, aesthetic, or athletic reasons are promptly rejected on the basis of an unfavorable risk/benefit ratio, we know that their use is recurrent despite the inherent legal penalties. In the case of sports, the unfairness of competing under the action of doping substances, which boost the performance of healthy athletes, is an ethical issue that further adds to the safety problem[27]. In view of these antecedents, and provided that sufficient time passes for the science to evolve and the technology to mature, gene therapy may well be just another tool to be used in the context of enhancement. This perspective is so real that the World Anti-Doping Agency (WADA, Montreal, Canada) has created a specific panel to deal with the issue and declared "gene doping" illegal in sports by stating that "The non-therapeutic use of cells, genes, genetic elements, or of the modulation of gene expression, having the capacity to enhance athletic performance, is prohibited."[28] Some people also defend that given the high risks and the current uncertainties associated, to use gene transfer for doping would be "scientifically stupid," on top of being ethically unacceptable.[27]

In the survey mentioned above, a clear majority of the scientists inquired (67%) considered it unacceptable to use gene transfer for enhancement purposes, while 25% think it could be acceptable to some degree if the goal is to render humans "healthier," not "better."[7] However, some researchers have pointed out that in some cases, it may be difficult to distinguish between therapy and enhancement. For instance, how much should an individual weigh in excess to be eligible for a weight control treatment using a gene transfer procedure developed to treat morbid obesity? At what weight will we draw the line and who will be responsible for taking the decision?

7.2.3 Somatic versus Germline Gene Therapy

In theory, genes could be introduced into human sperm and egg cells (fertilized or not), for example, by using microinjection techniques, with the goal of passing on the gene-associated changes to the offspring of the cell donors. This has already been accomplished successfully in animal models.[29] A number of reasons can be put forward to justify the targeting of germline cells (Table 7.1). The major justification is found in the context of patients who suffer from single-gene, hereditary defects. Clearly, a somatic cell gene transfer approach, even if successful, will not eliminate the hereditary nature of those diseases. On the other hand, by targeting germline cells, gene therapy would enable those successfully treated individuals to reproduce without the risk of transmitting malfunctioning genes to their descendants, which would thus be spared from the disease.[5,6] On these grounds, germline gene transfer is considered ethically acceptable by many researchers.[7] Another very strong argument in favor of germline therapy is one of social effectiveness—if and when technically feasible, such a single intervention would cure an entire family line, reducing the incidence and burden of the disease in a population. The cost-effectiveness of such an intervention would also be unbeatable when compared with a somatic cell gene therapy approach or with conventional

TABLE 7.1. Major Arguments in Favor and against Germline Gene Therapy

Reasons to Perform Germline Gene Therapy
To spare descendants from transmission of disease-related genes
To spare descendants from undergoing somatic cell gene transfer
Accord with health professional's role
More efficient and economical than treating successive generations
To replace abortion and selective discard alternatives
To protect those afflicted
Moral imperative (fits with duty to remove harm)
Back science's freedom to explore treatment and preventive alternatives

Reasons to Prohibit Germline Gene Therapy
Unanticipated, inheritable negative effects
Pressures to use techniques for enhancement
Possible malevolent uses
Excessive cost for most couples to use
Reduction in diversity of human genome
Unnecessary methods, alternatives available
Interference with evolution/natural selection
Violates a child's right to a genome not tampered with
Contrary to religious beliefs

Source: Based on Rabino.[7]

treatments like protein replacement. An interesting and thought-provoking argument is the one which contends that successful germline gene transfer interventions would avoid the need to perform selective discard alternatives like abortion, which are viewed as unethical by many. Other not so strong arguments have also been put forward to justify germline modification (see Table 7.1).

Interestingly, the argument that the treatment of a single individual can impact its descendants can also be used to support the major objection against germline therapy. The line of argument here is that any unanticipated mistakes will be inevitably passed on to future generations (Table 7.1). At the current stage of research, these risks are too high to be acceptable, and thus germline therapy is banned from most countries. The perspective that gene transfer techniques could be used already at a preconception stage with the goal of enhancing specific features of an individual and its descendants (see Section 7.2.2) is even more disturbing from an ethical and moral point of view.

Other concerns raised suggest that germline gene transfer may lead to (1) an imprudent acceleration of human evolution, (2) a widespread genetic homogenization that could affect the long-term survival of the species, and (3) the implementation of eugenic practices.[26] Others argue that such strategies would shift limited resources away from more pressing problems and would essentially favor those of a higher socioeconomic status, increasing social disparities. Finally, strong arguments have also been put forward claiming that the manipulation of germline cells would essentially change what makes us humans.[4–7]

7.2.4 Further Ethical Issues

The large majority of human gene transfer interventions currently under study aim to manage disease by targeting somatic cells. As we have seen in the previous sections, this is the type of intervention that is more acceptable from an ethical point of view. Even so, a number of ethical issues that are transversal to biomedical research should be considered in order to guarantee maximum protection of the human volunteers engaged in the corresponding clinical trials. These ethical issues can be divided for simplicity into technical and nontechnical, as proposed and discussed by Walters.[6]

7.2.4.1 Technical Issues
The technical questions have to do essentially with the assessment and balancing of the potential risks and benefits of gene transfer. This should start well before the preclinical and clinical development stages (see Chapter 3) by examining whether the specific gene therapy approach under consideration is acceptable. This implies that a series of ethical and scientific criteria must be satisfied (Figure 7.2). First, an appraisal of the target disease should be made, which includes an examination of its severity. Given the complexity, risk, and degree of uncertainty currently associated with gene therapy, only those

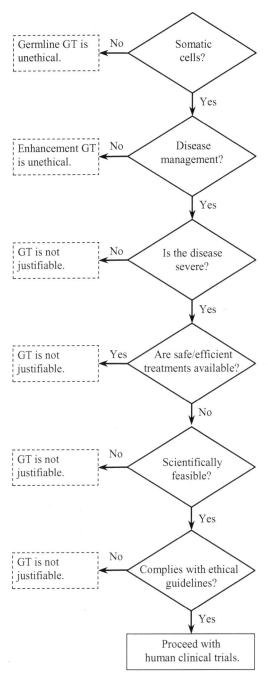

Figure 7.2 *Justifications for human gene therapy (GT) clinical trials. The treelike graph of decisions and their possible consequences shown in this figure provides an overview of the most relevant issues that need to be considered when deciding whether GT is justifiable or not.*

diseases that have a high degree of mortality and morbidity associated should be considered.[6] To put it simply, people will be willing to tolerate a higher degree of risk in the medical treatment of the more serious conditions.[8] This typically includes most types of cancer, some single-gene hereditary disorders, and cardiovascular and neurologic diseases. In the context of prophylactic DNA vaccines, on the other hand, infectious diseases like AIDS, multiresistant tuberculosis, pandemic flu, or Ebola are typical candidates. Although the seriousness of a disease should be relatively easy to assess, at least in most cases,* it may, however, be a bit difficult to pinpoint which specific diseases have the greatest cure potential and should thus be the primary target for gene therapy research. Some may argue that inherited rare single-gene genetic diseases are potentially easier to cure and thus should be the major focus for human gene transfer experimentation. Others, on the other hand could favor those diseases that involve complex genetic interactions on the grounds that research on such diseases is likely to generate more valuable information on the underlying mechanisms.[7]

Once the severity of the disease has been judged, the safety and efficacy of available treatments, if any exist, have to be examined (Figure 7.2). The criterion here is that only if patients find themselves left with no reasonable treatment options should a gene therapy approach be considered.[5] This is probably the current situation for most of the diseases listed above. If the final conclusion is that gene transfer should be considered as an option to treat or prevent a specific disease, researchers must then investigate the scientific and technical feasibility of doing so. Important questions here are the following: (1) How much is known about the specific disease? (2) Do we have good candidate gene(s) and vector(s)? (3) Are the techniques under consideration mature enough and adequately understood to justify application in humans? (4) Do we have adequate animal models in which the probable safety and effectiveness of the intervention can be investigated? Most of these questions can be addressed by performing research experiments and are thus amenable to verification by laboratory data.[5]

7.2.4.2 *Nontechnical Issues*

If the overall result of the previous assessment supports the decision to embark on human experimentation, the ensuing clinical trials will have to be designed in accordance with existing codes of ethics like the *Declaration of Helsinki* and good clinical practice documents, which set international ethical and scientific standards for research trials involving human subjects.[2,3] This is especially important in the context of a conceptually new intervention like gene transfer, which has a number of risks and uncertainties associated.[30] For this

---

* For example, in the case of the H1N1 influenza pandemic that emerged in 2009, it became apparent in early 2010 that the severity of the disease was overrated at the onset of the crisis by health officials and authorities.

reason, supplementary guidance is provided in documents like the *Points to Consider in the Design and Submission of Human Somatic-Cell Gene Therapy Protocols*.[11]

A trial protocol describing the design and performance of the clinical experiment and with information on ethical aspects must be carefully and clearly prepared by the sponsor of the research and submitted for consideration, comment, guidance, and approval to an independent IRB or ethics committee. The document prepared by Nabel and coworkers, which describes a trial involving immunotherapy for cancer by direct gene transfer, is a good example of such a clinical protocol.[31] The first important issue has to do with the selection of the research subjects who will participate in the trial. Objective eligibility and ineligibility criteria should be in place beforehand, in order to ensure a fair and equitable selection of subjects among a pool of potential candidates. Many of these criteria have to do with the past medical history and the current health status of the research subjects, whereas others, like the ability to provide informed consent (see below), are more generic.[31]

One of the underlying principles of medical research states that "each potential subject must be adequately informed of the aims, methods, sources of funding, any possible conflicts of interest, institutional affiliations of the researcher, the anticipated benefits and potential risks of the study and the discomfort it may entail" (from the *Declaration of Helsinki*). Such information is usually contained in an informed consent document, which is associated with the clinical protocol. In this document, the research subjects are made aware of the experimental nature of the intervention and are informed that the objective of the trial they are about to enter is to obtain scientific information and not to provide a cure.[6] Furthermore, they must understand that, depending on the trial design, there is a chance that they may be randomly allocated to a placebo control group. Sometimes, subjects may also be informed that in the event of their death, a request for autopsy is likely to be placed with a next-of-kin in order to obtain as much information as possible about the gene transfer procedure used.[31] Other pertinent information like the policy regarding research-related injuries or the requirement for long-term follow-up may also be included. After making sure that the research subjects have clearly understood the information conveyed to them, the sponsors should secure his/her freely given informed consent, usually by requesting their signature. Procedures for seeking the permission of parents or guardians should also be considered in those cases where children are enrolled.[11]

The preservation of the psychological integrity of research subjects is another important aspect. Concomitantly, every possible measure should be taken to guarantee the privacy and the confidentiality of the subject's information, for example, by withholding the identification of those involved when reporting results of the trial in meetings or journals. This may be difficult to achieve in some instances due to the public and media interest that usually surrounds gene transfer. Additional provisions contained in clinical protocols deal with the accuracy of reporting and publishing results.

7.3 SAFETY

7.3.1 Introduction

Like any other biologic that is administered to humans, plasmid biopharmaceuticals hold in them the potential to cause deleterious effects in the recipients. A number of these effects may be directly related to the poor quality of the finished product, as a result of problems in the manufacturing process. Possible quality defects introduced in a plasmid product would be, for example, a level of lipopolysaccharides (see Chapter 12, Section 12.3.4.5, and Chapter 14, Section 14.2) that exceeds the accepted threshold level or a lack of sterility. As will be seen further in Chapter 11, the best way for a plasmid DNA manufacturer to minimize the risk of facing these problems is to comply with the established manufacturing practices and to accept the vigilance and control exerted by regulatory agencies. Although the manufacturing-related safety problems just alluded to are important, in this chapter, we will focus our attention to a number of safety issues that are directly related to the inherent properties of plasmid biopharmaceuticals. Some of these issues may be related with the manifestation of generic and unspecific effects like local reactions at the site of injection administration, fever, and other systemic reactions. Thus, a standard procedure during preclinical and clinical development is to study local reactogenicity by performing clinical observations of the administration site and a histological analysis of tissue samples from biopsies.[13] But apart from these local reactions, a number of very specific safety issues are usually associated with the clinical use of plasmid molecules. Chief among these are (1) the potential for integration of the plasmid molecule or derived fragments into the host genomic DNA, (2) the induction of anti-DNA antibodies and autoimmune reactions, and (3) the induction of immune tolerance (especially important in the case of DNA vaccines).[15] These issues should be conveniently addressed during the preclinical development stage (see Chapter 3, Section 3.2.1) by performing pharmacological and toxicological studies with adequate animal models, and according to the recommendations of regulatory bodies detailed in the specific guidance documents.[12–14,32] The selection of the test species used in these studies is especially important, since the better the animal model can mimic the pharmacological response in humans, the more reliable will be the conclusions of the study.[12] In general terms, the goal of such studies is to determine the toxicity (i.e., the ability to harm recipients) of the particular plasmid product under study and to establish whether it might cause any damage to clinical volunteers in the subsequent human clinical trials. Specific objectives include the definition of safe starting doses and escalation regimens and the identification of organs at risk and parameters to monitor toxicity. In the specific case of plasmids, the nature of the evaluation studies will depend on the clinical use (e.g., prophylactic vs. therapeutic DNA vaccine), the target populations, and the intended duration of the treatment (e.g., single vs. multiple administrations).

7.3.2 Integration

7.3.2.1 The Risks

Plasmid biopharmaceuticals are usually designed to promote the extrachromosomal, transient expression of the transgenes. These episomal plasmids are eventually cleared from the cells and tissues as a result of degradation within the cytosol and nucleus. Although the integration of the exogenous DNA material into the host genomic DNA is clearly not sought for, there is always the probability that this might occur. For example, earlier projections estimated that the probability of an insertion event following DNA vaccination was one in one million.[33] Theoretically, such an integration of DNA could activate oncogenes, inactivate tumor suppressor genes, or mutate other important genes, resulting in unforeseeable adverse events.[15] The inadvertent modification of germline cells via integration could also lead to the vertical transmission of the mutated sequences. In this case, and even if there might be no further safety consequences to the recipients, the ethical concerns raised are highly relevant, as was discussed in Section 7.2.3 (see also Section 7.4 on veterinary applications). The biological significance of an event like the integration of foreign DNA into genomic DNA has been dramatically demonstrated in the case of the recombinant viral vectors used to treat X-linked severe combined immunodeficiency (SCID-X1). As was described briefly in Chapter 1 (Section 1.1.4), a number of recipients of the treatment developed a leukemia-like clonal lymphocyte proliferation as a direct consequence of the integration of the retrovirus vector in a number of sites.[34,35] Whether similar consequences could result following the integration of plasmids *in vivo* is still an open question.

The insertion of plasmid DNA sequences into the host cell genome can occur by one of three possible mechanisms: (1) random integration of the plasmid or derived fragments into the genome (e.g., via nonhomologous end-joining mechanisms[36]), (2) homologous recombination between homologous sequences present in the plasmid and in the genome, or (3) direct integrating mechanisms such has those characteristic of retroviruses.[14] Random integration is the most likely to occur since the type of sequences that drive homologous recombination and direct integration (insertion sequences, retroviral-like long terminal repeats, and sequences homologous to the packaging sequences of retroviruses) is usually removed during the construction of plasmid biopharmaceuticals (see Chapter 11, Section 11.5.1), as recommended by regulatory documents.[14,37] Surprisingly, random integration occurs at rates that are three to four orders of magnitude higher when compared with targeted integration directed by homologous sequences (frequency $< 10^{-6}$).[36] Apart from the nature of the sequences present in the plasmid, factors that affect the uptake of plasmid and the type of cells exposed, like the delivery method, adjuvants, and route used, can also impact the frequency of integration.[38] Finally, the protein encoded in the plasmid may also possibly affect integration, as has been demonstrated in the case of proteins E6 and E7 from the human papillomavirus.[39] Finally, one should keep in mind that not all integration events will necessarily translate into the disruption of tumor suppressor genes or activation of oncogenes, and might hence be inocuous.[37] Nevertheless, the realization of studies like the ones described below is critical to provide experimental evidence of the unlikelihood of integration events.

7.3.2.2 *Biodistribution and Persistence*

Biodistribution and persistence studies are particularly important in the context of plasmid integration, since these events and their impact may be more or less significant depending on the type of cells exposed to the plasmid. For example, higher risks and impact are foreseen in the case of actively dividing cells (e.g., neonatal tissues in children) and gonadal cells.[38] The distribution of plasmids will depend on the type of formulation and delivery method used (see Chapter 6). Biodistribution studies are precisely designed to assess the presence of plasmid DNA in various fluids, tissues, and organs (e.g., blood, draining lymph nodes, liver, lungs, kidneys, gonads, muscle at the site of administration, and subcutis at the injection site) both at early (e.g., 1–7 days) and late (e.g., 2–3 months) time points after administration (Figure 7.3).[13,14,40] The collected samples are then probed for the presence of the plasmid and derived fragments, or of the transgene product. Although reporter genes (e.g., luciferase and green fluorescent protein) are often used in the context of animal studies to enable the precise localization of transgene expression, techniques that look for the presence of remaining plasmid fragments like Southern blotting, fluorescence *in situ* hybridization, and polymerase chain reaction (PCR) assays are more common (see Chapter 5, Section 5.2).[40] In the case of quantitative real-time PCR assays, the recommendations of the FDA are that this method should be sensitive enough to quantify less than 100 copies of plasmid/µg of host DNA. If the amount of plasmid DNA at the test sites and tissues is lower than this figure, "nonpersistence" can be claimed. Such studies are very important because their outcome helps in determining whether integration studies are further required or not. For instance, in the case of DNA vaccines, the current recommendation of the FDA, which has been issued on the basis of published studies, is that "integration studies are warranted only when plasmid persists in any tissue of any animal at levels exceeding 30,000 copies/µg of host DNA by study termination."[13]

A number of studies that investigate the possibility for *in vivo* integration of plasmids using animal models have been described in the literature.[38,41–43] As described above, a previous assessment of plasmid biodistribution should be performed to identify the tissues and cells that are at higher risk. In the typical experiment, and following the administration of the plasmid material, the distribution and persistence of plasmid is assessed by collecting tissue samples from the animal at certain time points post administration. Then, DNA material in these tissues is isolated and assayed to probe for plasmid sequences using a PCR method[42] (Figure 7.3). In order to obtain sensitivities of the order of 10–100 copies/µg of gDNA, regions smaller than 100 bp should

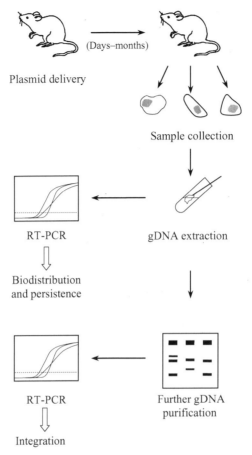

Figure 7.3 *Plasmid biodistribution, persistence, and integration studies. In the typical experiment, and following the administration of the plasmid to a relevant animal model, tissue samples (e.g., kidney, liver, spleen, lung, and lymphatic nodes) are collected at certain time points post administration. Genomic DNA material is then isolated from these tissues and probed for plasmid sequences (e.g., by real-time polymerase chain reaction (RT-PCR)). Since the detection of plasmids associated with gDNA is not sufficient to conclude that integration took place, the gDNA can be further purified (e.g., by gel electrophoresis) to eliminate nonintegrated plasmid isoforms. In principle, the detection of plasmid sequences in these highly purified samples represents integrated DNA, even though persistent contamination by free plasmid cannot be discarded.*

be amplified using either transgene-specific or backbone-specific primers.[40] The sensitivity of such assays is of the order of 1 plasmid copy/µg of DNA—in mice, this is roughly equivalent to 1 plasmid copy per 150,000 diploid cells.[42] Given that the method will detect plasmid sequences independently of whether they are integrated or not, high-molecular-weight genomic DNA (HMW gDNA) in the tissues can be further purified by size fractionation/gel electrophoresis assays in order to remove free plasmid topoisomers (supercoiled, open circular, linear concatamers). In these experiments, the typical size of the isolated gDNA fragments is within the 50- to 200-kb range. During this crucial procedure, special precautions have to be taken to prevent shearing and any type of contamination that might cause interference in the following PCR analysis[42] (Figure 7.3).

The many plasmid biodistribution studies performed so far have collectively shown that the majority of the plasmid molecules that are administered intramuscularly (e.g., by needle injection, needless jet, or particle-mediated delivery) tend to remain in the muscle and subcutis (extracellularly or inside the transfected cells) close to the injection site.[16,18,38,44,45] Furthermore, the majority of the plasmid molecules are rapidly degraded by endogenous nuclease within the first minutes of administration. The remaining plasmid is then progressively cleared and degraded from the injection site within a 2- to 6-month period.[16,18,45] An illustrative example of this trend can be given on the basis of the experiments performed by Ledwith and coworkers, who dosed mice twice and 3 weeks apart with intramuscular injections of 100 μg of plasmid in the quadriceps ($\sim10^{13}$ molecules).[42] Their results showed that the level of plasmid in muscle at 6–9 and 26 weeks post administration decreased from around 1000–4000 to about 200–800 copies/μg of gDNA[42]. Similar amounts of extrachromosomal plasmid in mice muscle tissue after intramuscular injection have been reported in other studies.[46]

Although plasmids are essentially confined to the administration region, a certain fraction may be redistributed by the blood, cells, and lymph to other more distant tissues. Thus, plasmid fragments can be sporadically found in organs and tissues (draining lymph nodes, lung, kidney, and liver) that are located more or less apart from the administration site. Still, levels of intramuscularly injected plasmids at distal sites hardly exceed the 1–16 copies/μg of gDNA (e.g., see the study by Manam et al.[38]). A recent study with a larger animal model, the pig, also confirms that plasmids injected intramuscularly (1) remain transiently present in the muscle for at least 4 weeks and (2) can be detected in distal organs (spleen, liver, kidney, lung, ovaries, and lymph nodes) for shorter periods.[47] While some experiments have shown that the biodistribution and persistence pattern is independent of the specific transgene and promoter used, as illustrated by a study that examined the biodistribution of DNA vaccine candidates against HIV-1, severe acute respiratory syndrome virus, West Nile virus, and Ebola virus,[16] in other cases, however, different plasmids have been shown to persist and distribute differently.[47] Although not yet explained, this phenomenon is probably ascribable to the physical properties of the plasmid molecules involved (size, secondary structures, and topoisomer distribution).[47]

As was described above, the fact that plasmid copies are found at different tissues and organs after administration says nothing about whether integration did take place or not. In order to assess this, any free plasmid DNA must be removed from the gDNA fragments, typically by a gel electrophoresis method, before running quantitative PCR. In the studies by Ledwith et al.[42] and Manam et al.[38] described above, this typically reduced the detectable plasmid levels to less than 1 copy/µg of gDNA. In principle, these residual amounts could represent integrated plasmid, even though persistent contamination by free plasmid cannot be discarded. Since 1 µg of gDNA is roughly equivalent to 150,000 diploid cells, this would represent 6.7×10^{-6} integrations per cell, or 8.9×10^{-11} integrations per gene (assuming 75,000 genes per mouse genome).[46] This rate is at least 2.5×10^4 lower than the spontaneous rate of gene-inactivating mutations (2.2×10^{-6}),* and thus the risk of mutation due to integration is clearly negligible. Another preclinical safety study conducted in mice found out that levels of a malaria DNA vaccine associated with gDNA could reach 30 copies/µg 1–2 months after intramuscular injection of 100 µg of the vaccine.[46] But even if residual levels of plasmid associated with gDNA in different tissues and organs of the order of 1000 copies/µg were detected, the rate of spontaneous mutation would still be slightly higher. Of course, it is obvious that the amount of plasmid administered is an important variable to consider—in principle, the risk of integration will be higher the higher is the dose used. However, studies conducted with higher plasmid doses $(4 \times 400 \mu g/$ mice) revealed no traces of plasmid associated with muscle gDNA 45 days post administration.[48] Overall, the studies published so far have essentially reached the same conclusion; that is, the integration of plasmid in muscle following injection is a low-probability event.

Although the experiments described above indicate that risk of mutation due to integration is low, it cannot be dismissed or neglected. Furthermore, as more efficient vectors and delivery techniques are developed, plasmids will persist longer within the interior of cells, increasing the probability of integration. This situation has been confirmed in a number of experimental studies. For instance, Wang and coworkers have found out that the number of plasmid copies in tissues increased from 780×10^3, 12×10^3, and 2.9×10^3 to 5100×10^3, 410×10^3, and 60×10^3 copies/µg of gDNA after 1, 6, and 16 weeks of administration, respectively, when the delivery method used changed from intramuscular injection to electroporation.[43] In the study, gel purification was further used to separate free plasmid in the samples from HMW gDNA isolated from the quadriceps of mice. After several rounds of purification, 17 copies of plasmid DNA were found associated per microgram of genomic DNA in the case of intramuscular injection. However, electroporation increased this figure to 980 copies/µg DNA, a clear indication of an increase in the level of integration.[43] The authors were also able to identify four independent and random integration events, which nevertheless involved the participation of short homologous segments in the vector and insertion site.[43] Experiments like this show that the possibility that plasmid DNA integrates into host genomic DNA should be investigated as part of the evaluation of the safety of a new plasmid biopharmaceutical.

---

* Calculated assuming that an average gene has 10^6 base pairs (bp)[41] and that the average mammalian genome mutation rate is 2.2×10^{-9}/bp/year.[48]

The plasmid biodistribution pattern can be radically different when a systemic administration method like intravenous injection is used. Here, a plasmid solution is typically injected directly into the blood stream. Typically, the plasmid concentration in the blood will peak a short while after administration and then decline progressively down to undetectable levels. Still, there is sufficient time for the circulatory system to promote the rapid distribution of molecules to the different organs of the body.[49–52]

The impact of systemic delivery in plasmid biodistribution and persistence when compared with local administration can be illustrated in the case of hydrodynamic delivery, a particular method of intravenous injection (see Chapter 6). The procedure explores the high pressure that is exerted when a large volume of a plasmid-containing solution is rapidly injected intravenously.[50] Several studies show that when using this particular method, plasmids are primarily found in liver cells.[50,53,54] This liver specificity is probably related to a phenomenon of backflow to liver vessels.[53,54] In one of the longest-term mice studies performed so far, a 2 mL solution containing 50 µg of a plasmid coding for human factor IX was injected via the tail vein over 6–8 s.[53] The results showed that although the amount of plasmid in liver cells peaked 1 day post administration, traces of it could still be found after 240 days.[53] Interestingly, when the intravenous injection was performed at a slower rate (hence lower pressure), the plasmid also distributed to other tissues (e.g., lungs, spleen, and heart) and not exclusively to the liver.[53] Further analysis revealed that the plasmid persisted in liver cells at an extraordinary amount of approximately 2.3 copies per diploid genome. When expressed as number of plasmid copies per microgram of gDNA (3,450,000/µg gDNA), this figure corresponds to at least a three orders of magnitude increase when compared with the maximum values found after local administration.

Since at such a high level of persistence the need for integration studies is clearly warranted, total liver DNA isolated 240 days post administration was subjected to further rounds of purification to separate any extrachromosomal plasmid. Subsequent Southern analysis revealed that most plasmid in liver cells is episomal. The decrease in transgene expression after partial hepatectomy provided another convincing argument against genomic integration.[53] Another important finding of this study was that therapeutic levels of the encoded transgene could be sustained in plasma for more than 1.5 years after hydrodynamic delivery. The results in this study show that plasmids can persist in a functional state as episomes for prolonged periods of time. As a general conclusion, the likelihood of finding plasmid in tissues like the lung, kidney, spleen, and liver after intravenous injection increases when compared with local regional administration.

7.3.3   Autoimmunity and Adverse Immune Reactions

7.3.3.1   Anti-DNA and Antimyosin Autoantibodies

Autoimmunity is characterized by an uncontrolled attack of the immune system of an organism on its own cells or biomolecules, due to a failure in recognizing those components as self. The number of diseases presenting an autoimmune etiology is large (~80), and includes psoriasis, rheumatoid arthritis, systemic lupus erythematosus, and multiple sclerosis.[55] The possibility that the administration of plasmids and the *in vivo* expression of the encoded transgenes could somehow disturb the network of cellular and biochemical pathways that enable the immune system to differentiate self from nonself has been put forward as one of the possible risks of plasmid biopharmaceuticals right from the beginning.[56] One of the specific safety concerns that have been recurrently associated with the clinical use of plasmids is the possibility that their administration to healthy individuals could induce the production of anti-DNA antibodies and thereby contribute to the development of some kind of systemic or organ-specific autoimmune diseases.[56–58] This issue could be even more critical if the individuals undergoing the treatment already suffer from some kind of autoimmune disease. The concern is rooted on the fact that autoimmune diseases such as systemic lupus erythematosus are characterized by abnormally elevated levels (100- to 1000-fold) of specific, high-affinity anti-DNA antibodies in the serum[37]. These antibodies can form immune complexes with the DNA (e.g., released from apoptotic cells), which circulate throughout the body, damaging various tissues and blood vessels in critical areas of the body. A typical example is the lodging of these anti-DNA antibodies/DNA complexes in the kidney, with the consequent development of glomerulonephritis.[56] For this reason, anti-DNA antibodies are considered one of the markers and pathogenesis triggers of renal systemic lupus erythematosus.[58] Thus, one of the key safety tests made to the recipients of plasmid DNA is to look for the presence of anti-DNA autoantibodies and to look for an associated autoimmune response. The expression of specific transgene products may also negatively impact the immune system of the recipient. In the case of DNA vaccines that are administered intramuscularly, for example, and although an immunogenic response against the transgene product is of course the desired outcome, the expression of the encoded antigen could convert a normal non-antigen-presenting cell (i.e., the muscle cell) into an antigen-presenting cell.[12] This would trigger an attack from antigen-specific T cells and the induction of antimyosin antibodies, which would ultimately result in an inflammation of the muscles (myositis).[57]

A number of experiments have been designed and carried out with animal models to investigate the capacity of plasmid DNA to generate and promote the development of autoimmunity and other deleterious immunologic responses.[49,56,57,59] For example, in one of the earlier studies, increases in the population of IgG anti-DNA autoantibodies producing B cells and in the titers of serum anti-DNA autoantibodies were detected after the repeated intramuscular administration of plasmid DNA in normal and lupus-prone mice.[56] However, no evidence of glomerulonephritis or immune complex deposition was found following histological examination of kidney tissue from normal mice. Furthermore, immunization with DNA had no impact in the age of onset and severity of the disease in lupus-prone mice when compared with control mice that were treated with saline.[56] The development of myositis following immunization with plasmid DNA was also discarded, since antimyosin antibodies, a characteristic marker of muscle inflammation, were also not detected.[56] These results have been confirmed by other studies in mice—the injection of a naked DNA vaccine did not stimulate the production of anti-DNA or myosin autoantibodies nor induced the development of myositis or glomerulonephritis.[59]

There is also some evidence that plasmid-encoded proteins that interact directly or indirectly with nucleic acids may stimulate the secretion of anti-DNA antibodies in recipients.[58] The results of one study in which the viral nucleic acid binding and adapter proteins HIV-1 reverse transcriptase (RT), nef, and human hepatitis C virus core were tested showed that a primary immune response first developed toward the encoded proteins. Then, a secondary antibody response against DNA was detected in two-thirds of the subjects who had received either the genes or their products. However, this response was transient and no evidence for the enhancement of pre-existing autoimmunity was obtained.[58]

And finally, gene products that are designed into plasmids to modulate the immune system (e.g., cytokines) may lead to overstimulation, triggering a series of immunopathological reactions, including immunosuppression, chronic inflammation, and autoimmunity.[12,14]

7.3.3.2 Cytosine–phosphate–guanine (CpG)-Induced Inflammation and Suppression of Transgene Expression

The ability of the mammalian innate immune system to recognize foreign DNA and to mount a response against it is especially vigorous when unmethylated CpG motifs are present.[60] Although extremely rare in vertebrate DNA, CpGs are often found in viral and bacterial DNA. Since the majority of the DNA backbones used in the context of plasmid biopharmaceuticals contain many sequences of bacterial and viral origin, it is thus not surprising to find out that a typical plasmid could contain more than 200–300 CpGs.[60] When administered alone or alongside a plasmid, such motifs interact with the host toll-like receptor 9 (TLR-9), activating B cells and plasmacytoid dendritic cells, promoting the proliferation of T cells, macrophages, monocytes, and natural killer cells.[60] These, in turn, trigger the production of chemokines, cytokines, and antibodies such as IgM, and inflammatory responses.[56,57] These events can be advantageously explored when the generation of an adaptive response to a given antigen is being sought. For example, in view of these immunostimulatory properties, unmethylated CpG motifs are many times purposely designed into DNA vaccines or simply coadministered as an adjuvant to step up and improve specific antibody responses[60,61] (see Chapter 2, Section 2.5.2).

In spite of their usefulness as immunostimulators, there is also a downside to the presence of CpG motifs in plasmid biopharmaceuticals, since the underlying inflammatory response may be acute enough to cause severe adverse effects. As a matter of fact, there is abundant evidence showing that CpG sequences are a major driver of acute inflammatory responses (e.g., see the review by Yew and Cheng[60]). Furthermore, the seriousness of the responses mounted due to the presence of CpGs is more pronounced when methods that are more efficient at delivering plasmids to the cell cytoplasm (e.g., cationic lipids) are used.[60] This toxicity can be substantially reduced if such CpG motifs are reduced or eliminated from the vector. This is not an easy task since the number of such motifs in a typical plasmid may exceed 200–300. Typically, one would start by exploring the fact that most amino acids are coded by more than one codon to eliminate CpGs from coding regions (e.g., from the transgene). Next, CpGs from other regions could be eliminated or replaced, as long as this does not strongly impact their regulatory functions. A couple of experiments have confirmed that the toxicity of these CpG-reduced plasmids is, in fact, reduced when compared to the original vector.[60,62] For example, one study showed that the systemic delivery of lipid complexes of a vector that had been depleted in 80% of its CpG content produced less inflammation, reduced levels of inflammatory cytokines, and decreased liver toxicity.[62]

Apart from their toxic effects, CpGs in a plasmid have also been associated with the suppression of the expression of the transgene.[63] This is thought to occur through a tandem mechanism that involves the methylation of the CpGs in the plasmids that have reached the nucleus by DNA methyltransferases, and then the recruitment of methyl-CpG binding proteins that contribute to repress transcription of the transgene.[63] In line with this observation, the depletion of CpG from a plasmid vector can substantially improve the duration of the expression of the encoded transgene. This beneficial effect is illustrated in Figure 7.4, which shows the time course evolution of the circulating levels of human-galactosidase A (HGA) in mice following the hydrodynamic delivery of plasmid constructs encoding the reporter protein.[63] In this experiment, a CpG-reduced plasmid was constructed by removing 388 CpG dinucleotides out of 484 from different regions (cytomegalovirus (CMV) promoter, kanamaycin resistance gene, transgene) of the original plasmid. It is clear from the plot that the CpG-reduced plasmid generated a higher and more sustained level of the transgene product when compared with the corresponding unmodified plasmid. Thus, apart from reducing vector toxicity, CpG elimination brings with it an increase in potency as an added benefit.[63]

7.3.3.3 Conclusions

Further preclinical animal studies on the topic essentially reached the same conclusions—although in some cases transient increases in IgG anti-DNA autoantibodies have been detected following the administration of plasmid DNA, the levels detected are substantially lower when compared with the ones characteristic of lupus and therefore can be considered not significant. Furthermore, no clinical evidence of autoimmune disease has been detected so far as a consequence of plasmid administration. Clinical experiments with human volunteers, to date, have also failed to demonstrate the existence of a correlation between the administration of plasmid DNA and the secretion of anti-DNA antibodies or the onset of autoimmune disease.[49] In view of the available preclinical and clinical data, which suggest that plasmid DNA

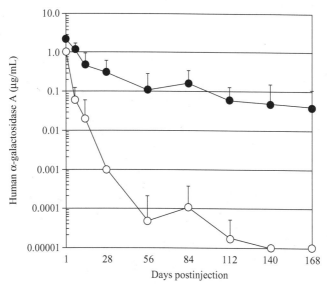

Figure 7.4 Effect of the depletion of CpG dinucleotides on plasmid potency. BALB/c mice were injected intravenously by hydrodynamic delivery with CpG-reduced (96 dinucleotides, black circles) and CpG-replete (484 dinucleotides, white circles) plasmids encoding the human-galactosidase A (HGA) reporter protein. The plot shows the circulating levels of HGA in sera after plasmid administration. Reprinted by permission from Macmillan Publishers Ltd.: Molecular Therapy, 10, Hodges BL, Taylor KM, Joseph MF, Bourgeois SA, Scheule RK. Long-term transgene expression from plasmid DNA gene therapy vectors is negatively affected by CpG dinucleotides, 269-278, Copyright 2004.[63]

administration is unlikely to trigger autoimmune responses, the FDA's current thinking on the matter is clear: "we no longer recommend that preclinical studies be performed to specifically assess whether vaccination causes autoimmune disease, but recommend that the general welfare of animals in preclinical immunogenicity and toxicity studies continue to be carefully monitored."[13] Still, preclinical testing with adequate animal models is encouraged in those cases where the plasmids harbor immunomodulatory genes (e.g., cytokine) to determine whether modulation of immunity can cause inflammation, immune suppression, autoimmunity, and immunopathological reactions.[13]

7.3.4   Immune Tolerance

One of the critical safety issues associated with the use of DNA vaccines is their potential to induce immune tolerance in response to the persistent expression of antigens.[57,64] Tolerance will arise if the immune system fails to recognize the antigenic protein encoded by the DNA vaccine and expressed endogenously as foreign.[65] In other words, the immune system ignores the antigen that is being expressed. Concerns regarding immune tolerance are especially important in the case of vaccines developed for use in children and newborns, since the immaturity of their immune systems may render them more susceptible.[57] However, and in spite of these worries, in the vast majority of cases, the immunization of newborn mice or nonhuman primates with DNA vaccines coding for a vast array of antigens has resulted in the induction of a variety of immune responses (humoral, CTL, Th), rather than unresponsiveness.[64]

Still, the potential for DNA vaccines to induce tolerance rather than immunity has been demonstrated in a couple of animal studies. For instance, a study with a DNA vaccine encoding the circumsporozoite protein of malaria showed that immune tolerance but not immunity was induced upon vaccination of newborn mice.[65,66] This tolerance persisted for more than 1 year and was found to correlate with the poor immunogenicity of the encoded antigen, since plasmids encoding other malaria antigens were not tolerogenic. This seems to indicate that the specific nature of the antigen is an important determinant of tolerance. Additionally, mice older than 1 week developed immunity instead of tolerance, confirming the higher susceptibility of newborns.[65] Interestingly, tolerance could not be induced in newborns when the exogenous circumsporozoite protein was administered. This indicates that the mode of antigen presentation is also an important determinant of tolerance susceptibility.[66]

Even if in the majority of cases DNA vaccines administered to newborns are immunogenic rather than tolerogenic, it is nevertheless prudent to focus a special attention to immune tolerance issues during the preclinical and clinical development of DNA vaccines, which are intended for the prophylaxis of childhood diseases.[67] This calls for the design and execution of specific immunization tests in animal models possessing immune systems with a maturity equivalent to those of the human recipients.[65] Finally, the problem of immunologic tolerance is also important in the context of cancer DNA vaccines, which target "self" antigens that are expressed by tumor cells. The effectiveness of such vaccines can be greatly compromised if the immune system develops tolerance and ignores the target antigen. A number of strategies may be pursued to break or avoid tolerance, including the use of xenogeneic antigens described in Chapter 10 (Section 10.4) and the use of DNA vaccines encoding alphaviral replicons.[68]

7.4 VETERINARY PLASMID PRODUCTS

The veterinary use of plasmid biopharmaceuticals also raises a number of concerns regarding the risks posed to the environment, to the treated specie, and to humans. Special attention is usually given when the animals are bred specifically to produce meat, fish, milk, or eggs for human nutrition. In these cases, biosafety studies that focus on the persistence, biodistribution, and integration of plasmid DNA in livestock animals are critical to enable a correct assessment of the potential risks posed to human health and are mandatory to obtain regulatory approval and license to market.[69] The generic discussion of these safety issues, which is presented in this section, is complemented and further illustrated in Chapter 10 (Section 10.3) by examining the specific case of the DNA vaccine that was approved in Canada in 2005 to protect farm-raised salmon against infectious hematopoietic necrosis.

7.4.1 Environmental Risks

The risks posed to the environment when administering plasmid biopharma-ceuticals to animals are usually at the forefront of the concerns of regulatory agencies.[70] This issue deserves due consideration not only because in many cases those risks are still poorly understood but also because of the potential it has to stir strong objections from environmentalist groups, lobbies, and political forces. The most important environmental risk associated with the veterinary use of plasmid DNA is the potential for the horizontal transfer of the administered DNA (intact or fragmented) from the recipient animals to other nontargeted species and microorganisms (e.g., *Escherichia coli*).[71] In the likelihood of this event, genes harbored in the plasmid like antibiotic resis-tance markers or transgenes coding for antigens of the disease-causing micro-organisms (in the case of DNA vaccines) could be expressed outside the target organism with unknown consequences. In principle, this risk is likely to be low since we can foresee that most plasmid biopharmaceuticals will be used in animals like pigs, cattle, poultry, sheep, horses, companion animals, and captive wild species, which are bred and/or kept in more or less confined environments (see Chapter 8, Section 8.4); that is, there will be some degree of control over the whereabouts of the treated individuals. Still, we may expect that in the future, some plasmid products might be administered to wild species, which are then released into their natural environment. This has already happened in the case of the DNA immunization of the California condor against West Nile virus infection, as described in the case study presented in Chapter 10 (Section 10.2). But even if the animals in question are confined, there is always the possibility that in some circumstances, a number of individuals might escape and breed with wild animals.[71,72] For example, in the case of the farming of Atlantic salmon, millions of fish escape every year from the marine and estuarine mesh cages where they grow (see Chapter 10, Section 10.3). Thus, it is clear that some degree of release of plasmid material into the environment will inevitably occur once the administration of plasmid biopharmaceuticals to animals becomes a routine. This could be especially problematic if the DNA accidentally integrates in the chromosomes of germline cells and thus acquires the ability to pass on to future generations. A genetically modified organism (GMO) would thus be created that could perpetuate itself out in the open through breeding. The consumption of the evaded individuals by other organ-isms is another way to promote the horizontal dissemination of the DNA. Although in these cases most DNA should be readily degraded in the gastro-intestinal tract through the action of gastric acid, pancreatic/bile secretions, and nucleases,[73] some experiments have shown that a fraction of the ingested DNA may persist long enough to render the uptake by intestinal bacteria possible.[74] Still, the amounts of viable DNA material involved in such a sporadic transfer from an individual treated with plasmid DNA to a predator are probably small enough to warrant that risks of integration and transmission are negligible. Finally, the release of the plasmid into the environment could also occur by gradual expulsion (i.e., shedding) from the body of the target animal (e.g., via feces) or by accidental spilling. Environmental contamination from additives, inactivating agents, and adjuvants, which might be included in the formulation of the plasmid product, is also a possibility, even though this issue is clearly not as relevant.

7.4.2 The Safety of Target Animals and Humans

Apart from the risks posed to the environment, a number of the safety concerns raised by the veterinary applications of plasmid biopharmaceuticals are usually examined in regard to the target animal species, which is being subjected to plasmid administration, and to humans. In the first case, laboratory and field tests should be designed to look for adverse reactions (e.g., inflammation and skin darkening), behavioral changes (e.g., lethargy and abnormal return to feed), and unusual weight loss or mortality rates among the treated animals. Furthermore, and as in the case of human products, the risks for integration of the injected plasmids into the host genome and for germline transmission should be evaluated in accordance to regulatory recommendations.[69] If such tests demonstrate that the plasmid biopharmaceutical is in anyway unsafe and deleterious to the animal's health, it is clear that it should not be licensed. As of now, however, and similarly to what has been observed in humans, no severe adverse effects have been reported in connection with the veterinary use of plasmids.

Although animals are obviously the target for veterinary products, there are circumstances in which humans can come into intimate contact with the plasmid material. For example, the persons responsible for the administration of the biopharmaceutical can accidentally self-administer the product. These risks can, however, be minimized by an adequate training of the operators. As an illustration of this later claim, no self-injection events were reported following the administration of 6.1 million doses of a fish DNA vaccine during prelicensing field trials.[70] The risk of self-administration is of course limited to the small number of operators involved with the manipulation of plasmid biopharmaceuticals. The administration of plasmid biopharmaceuticals in animals intended to enter the human food chain also deserves careful consideration. This calls for the implementation of a number of tests to confirm safety to consumers.

7.5 CONCLUSIONS

The ethical and safety implications associated with the medical use of genes are several. In order for plasmid biopharmaceuticals to gain acceptance from society, these implications should be faced and dealt with without reserves. For example, we have seen in this chapter that the possibility that a plasmid or parts of it might integrate into the genome of the host recipient, whether it is nonhuman or human, raises important safety issues. The consequences associated with the specific case of integration into germline cells are also highly relevant, since this opens up the door for vertical transmission of the genetic material to subsequent generations. However, integration into the host genome also raises an important societal question, which has to do with the genetic status of the animal in question—should it be, or not be, considered a GMO? In the case of nonhuman animals, the attribution of a GMO label will make a huge difference when it comes to public perception and consumer acceptance, especially in countries where GMOs are banned. Many people will simply reject the consumption of products derived from food animals that are considered GMOs. This issue has already been raised in the case of the farmed Atlantic salmons, which are immunized with a DNA vaccine against infectious hematopoietic necrosis. This is discussed in more detail in Chapter 10 (Section 10.3). Other people may also move away from any plasmid biopharmaceutical that might render their companion animals into GMOs. The inquiry received by the Environmental Risk Management Authority (ERMA) in New Zealand from someone who was seeking to know if a dog vaccinated with the canine melanoma DNA vaccine (manufactured by Merial, Athens, Georgia) would make that animal a GMO[75] is a good illustration of the type of uneasiness that is likely to be raised once the use of plasmid biopharmaceuticals becomes widespread. More information on this case can also be found in Chapter 10 (Section 10.4). In the case of humans, the issue is far more complicated. Nevertheless, the question should not be eluded—should a human being be considered a GMO if it becomes demonstrated that pieces of extraneous DNA used as a medicine (whether originating from plasmids or viral vectors) have integrated into their genome? And are there risks that such people might be discriminated by others?

REFERENCES

1. McKneally MF, Daar AS. Introducing new technologies: Protecting subjects of surgical innovation and research. *World Journal of Surgery*. 2003;27:930–934; discussion 934–935.

2. European Medicines Agency. ICH Topic E6R1. Note for guidance on good clinical practice (CPMP/ICH/135/95). London, July 2002.

3. Fromell GJ. Good clinical practice standards: What they are and some tools to support them. *Human Gene Therapy*. 2008;19:431–440.

4. Kimmelman J. The ethics of human gene transfer. *Nature Reviews in Genetics*. 2008;9:239–244.

5. Walters L. Ethical issues in human gene therapy. *Journal of Clinical Ethics*. 1991;2:267–274; discussion 274–268.

6. Walters L. The ethics of human gene therapy. *Nature*. 1986;320:225–227.

7. Rabino I. Gene therapy: Ethical issues. *Theoretical Medicine*. 2003;24:31–58.

8. Friedmann T, Roblin R. Gene therapy for human genetic disease? *Science*. 1972;175:949–955.

9. Wade N. UCLA gene therapy racked by friendly fire. *Science*. 1980;210:509–511.

10. Raper SE, Chirmule N, Lee FS, et al. Fatal systemic inflammatory response syndrome in a ornithine transcarbamylase deficient patient following adenoviral gene transfer. *Molecular Genetics and Metabolism*. 2003;80:148–158.

11. United States National Institutes of Health—Human Gene Therapy Subcommittee. *Points to consider in the design and submission of human somatic-cell gene therapy protocols*. Bethesda, MD: NIH, 1986.

12. European Medicines Evaluation Agency. ICH Topic Q6b. Note for guidance on quality, pre-clinical and clinical aspects of gene transfer medicinal products (CPMP/BWP/3088/99). London, April 24, 2001.

13. United States Food and Drug Administration. *Guidance for industry: Considerations for plasmid DNA vaccines for preventive infectious disease indications*. Rockville, MD: FDA, 2007.

14. World Health Organization. Guidelines for assuring the quality and nonclinical safety evaluation of DNA vaccines. Vol. Annex 1 (WHO Technical Report Series, No. 941). Geneva, 2007.

15. Schalk JAC, Mooi FR, Berbers GAM, van Aerts LAGJM, Ovelgönne H, Kimman TG. Preclinical and clinical safety studies on DNA vaccines. *Human Vaccines*. 2006;2:45–53.

16. Sheets RL, Stein J, Manetz TS, et al. Biodistribution of DNA plasmid vaccines against HIV-1, Ebola, severe acute respiratory syndrome, or West Nile virus is similar, without integration, despite differing plasmid backbones or gene inserts. *Toxicological Sciences*. 2006;91:610–619.

17. Sheets RL, Stein J, Manetz TS, et al. Toxicological safety evaluation of DNA plasmid vaccines against HIV-1, Ebola, severe acute respiratory syndrome, or West Nile virus is similar despite differing plasmid backbones or gene-inserts. *Toxicological Sciences*. 2006;91:620–630.

18. Pilling AM, Harman RM, Jones SA, McCormack NA, Lavender D, Haworth R. The assessment of local tolerance, acute toxicity, and DNA biodistribution following particle-mediated delivery of a DNA vaccine to minipigs. *Toxicologic Pathology*. 2002;30:298–305.

19. Global Advisory Committee on Vaccine Safety (GACVS). Global safety of vaccines: Strengthening systems for monitoring, management and the role of GACVS. *Expert Reviews in Vaccines*. 2009;8:705–716.

20. Watson M, Stoner N. Safe handling of gene medicines. *European Journal of Hospital Pharmacy Practice*. 2007;13:24–26.

21. Vulto AG, Stoner N, Balásová H, et al. European Association of Hospital Pharmacists (EAHP) Guidance on the pharmacy handling of gene medicines. *European Journal of Hospital Pharmacy Practice*. 2007;13:2939.

22. Anderson G. Ethical preparedness and performance of gene therapy study co-ordinators. *Nursing Ethics*. 2008;15:208–221.

23. Edelstein ML, Abedi MR, Wixon J. Gene therapy clinical trials worldwide to 2007-an update. *The Journal of Gene Medicine*. 2007;9:833–842.

24. Moore JP, Klasse PJ, Dolan MJ, Ahuja SK. AIDS/HIV: A step into darkness or light? *Science*. 2008;320:753–755.

25. Benlahrech A, Harris J, Meiser A, et al. Adenovirus vector vaccination induces expansion of memory CD4 T cells with a mucosal homing phenotype that are readily susceptible to HIV-1. *Proceedings of the National Academy of Sciences of the United States of America*. 2009;106:19940–19945.

26. Kiuru M, Crystal RG. Progress and prospects: Gene therapy for performance and appearance enhancement. *Gene Therapy*. 2008;15:329–337.

27. Filipp F. Is science killing sports? Gene therapy and its possible abuse in doping. *EMBO Reports*. 2007;8:433–434.

28. World Anti-Doping Agency. The 2007 prohibited list. World anti-doping code. Montreal, September 16, 2006.

29. Cavard C, Grimber G, Dubois N, et al. Correction of mouse ornithine transcarbamylase deficiency by gene transfer into the germ line. *Nucleic Acids Research*. 1988;16:2099–2110.

30. Cohen-Haguenauer O. Gene therapy: Regulatory issues and international approaches to regulation. *Current Opinion in Biotechnology*. 1997;8:361–369.

31. Nabel GJ, Chang AE, Nabel EG, et al. Immunotherapy for cancer by direct gene transfer into tumors. *Human Gene Therapy*. 1994;5:57–77.

32. United States Food and Drug Administration. *Guidance for industry: Guidance for human somatic cell therapy and gene therapy*. Rockville, MD: FDA, 1998.

33. Kurth R. Risk potential of the chromosomal insertion of foreign DNA. *Annals of the New York Academy of Sciences*. 1995;772:140–151.

34. Hacein-Bey-Abina S, Von Kalle C, Schmidt M, et al. LMO2-associated clonal T cell proliferation in two patients after gene therapy for SCID-X1. *Science*. 2003;302: 415–419.

35. Cavazzana-Calvo M. Gene therapy for SCID-X1. *Human Gene Therapy*. 2007;18:944.

36. Iiizumi S, Kurosawa A, So S, et al. Impact of non-homologous end-joining deficiency on random and targeted DNA integration: Implications for gene targeting. *Nucleic Acids Research*. 2008;36:6333–6342.

37. Cichutek K. DNA vaccines: Development, standardization and regulation. *Intervirology*. 2000;43:331–338.

38. Manam S, Ledwith BJ, Barnum AB, et al. Plasmid DNA vaccines: Tissue distribution and effects of DNA sequence, adjuvants and delivery method on integration into host DNA. *Intervirology*. 2000;43:273–281.

39. Kessis TD, Connolly DC, Hedrick L, Cho KR. Expression of HPV16 E6 or E7 increases integration of foreign DNA. *Oncogene*. 1996;13:427–431.

40. Gonin P, Gaillard C. Gene transfer vector biodistribution: Pivotal safety studies in clinical gene therapy development. *Gene Therapy*. 2004;11(Suppl 1):S98–S108.

41. Nichols WW, Ledwith BJ, Manam SV, Troilo PJ. Potential DNA vaccine integration into host cell genome. *Annals of the New York Academy of Sciences*. 1995;772: 30–39.

42. Ledwith BJ, Manam S, Troilo PJ, et al. Plasmid DNA vaccines: Investigation of integration into host cellular DNA following intramuscular injection in mice. *Intervirology*. 2000;43:258–272.

43. Wang Z, Troilo PJ, Wang X, et al. Detection of integration of plasmid DNA into host genomic DNA following intramuscular injection and electroporation. *Gene Therapy.* 2004;11:711–721.

44. Bureau MF, Naimi S, Torero Ibad R, et al. Intramuscular plasmid DNA electro-transfer: Biodistribution and degradation. *Biochimica et Biophysica Acta.* 2004; 1676:138–148.

45. Vilalta A, Mahajan RK, Hartikka J, et al. I. Poloxamer-formulated plasmid DNA-based human cytomegalovirus vaccine: Evaluation of plasmid DNA biodistribution/persistence and integration. *Human Gene Therapy.* 2005;16:1143–1150.

46. Martin T, Parker SE, Hedstrom R, et al. Plasmid DNA malaria vaccine: The potential for genomic integration after intramuscular injection. *Human Gene Therapy.* 1999;10:759–768.

47. Gravier R, Dory D, Laurentie M, Bougeard S, Cariolet R, Jestin A. *In vivo* tissue distribution and kinetics of a pseudorabies virus plasmid DNA vaccine after intramuscular injection in swine. *Vaccine.* 2007;25:6930–6938.

48. Kang KK, Choi SM, Choi JH, et al. Safety evaluation of GX-12, a new HIV therapeutic vaccine: Investigation of integration into the host genome and expression in the reproductive organs. *Intervirology.* 2003;46:270–276.

49. Nabel EG, Gordon D, Yang ZY, et al. Gene transfer *in vivo* with DNA-liposome complexes: Lack of autoimmunity and gonadal localization. *Human Gene Therapy.* 1992;3:649–656.

50. Liu F, Song Y, Liu D. Hydrodynamics-based transfection in animals by systemic administration of plasmid DNA. *Gene Therapy.* 1999;6:1258–1266.

51. Parker SE, Borellini F, Wenk ML, et al. Plasmid DNA malaria vaccine: Tissue distribution and safety studies in mice and rabbits. *Human Gene Therapy.* 1999;10: 741–758.

52. Koshkina NV, Agoulnik IY, Melton SL, Densmore CL, Knight V. Biodistribution and pharmacokinetics of aerosol and intravenously administered DNA-polyethyleneimine complexes: Optimization of pulmonary delivery and retention. *Molecular Therapy.* 2003;8:249–254.

53. Miao CH, Thompson AR, Loeb K, Ye X. Long-term and therapeutic-level hepatic gene expression of human factor IX after naked plasmid transfer *in vivo. Molecular Therapy.* 2001;3:947–957.

54. Dagnaes-Hansen F, Holst HU, Sondergaard M, et al. Physiological effects of human growth hormone produced after hydrodynamic gene transfer of a plasmid vector containing the human ubiquitin promotor. *Journal of Molecular Medicine.* 2002;80:665–670.

55. Bluestone JA. A balanced attack. *The Scientist.* 2007;21:32–44.

56. Mor G, Singla M, Steinberg AD, Hoffman SL, Okuda K, Klinman DM. Do DNA vaccines induce autoimmune disease? *Human Gene Therapy.* 1997;8:293–300.

57. Mor G, Eliza M. Plasmid DNA vaccines. Immunology, tolerance, and autoimmunity. *Molecular Biotechnology.* 2001;19:245–250.

58. Isaguliants MG, Iakimtchouk K, Petrakova NV, et al. Gene immunization may induce secondary antibodies reacting with DNA. *Vaccine.* 2004;22:1576–1585.

59. Choi SM, Lee DS, Son MK, et al. Safety evaluation of GX-12. A new DNA vaccine for HIV infection in rodents. *Drug and Chemical Toxicology.* 2003;26:271–284.

60. Yew NS, Cheng SH. Reducing the immunostimulatory activity of CpG-containing plasmid DNA vectors for non-viral gene therapy. *Expert Opinion in Drug Delivery.* 2004;1:115–125.

61. Zhao H, Hemmi H, Akira S, Cheng SH, Scheule RK, Yew NS. Contribution of toll-like receptor 9 signaling to the acute inflammatory response to nonviral vectors. *Molecular Therapy.* 2004;9:241–248.

62. Yew NS, Zhao H, Przybylska M, et al. CpG-depleted plasmid DNA vectors with enhanced safety and long-term gene expression *in vivo. Molecular Therapy.* 2002;5:731–738.

63. Hodges BL, Taylor KM, Joseph MF, Bourgeois SA, Scheule RK. Long-term transgene expression from plasmid DNA gene therapy vectors is negatively affected by CpG dinucleotides. *Molecular Therapy.* 2004;10:269–278.

64. Bot A, Bona C. Genetic immunization of neonates. *Microbes and Infection.* 2002;4:511–520.

65. Ichino M, Mor G, Conover J, et al. Factors associated with the development of neonatal tolerance after the administration of a plasmid DNA vaccine. *Journal of Immunology.* 1999;162:3814–3818.

66. Mor G, Yamshchikov G, Sedegah M, et al. Induction of neonatal tolerance by plasmid DNA vaccination of mice. *Journal of Clinical Investigation.* 1996;98: 2700–2705.

67. Smith HA, Klinman DM. The regulation of DNA vaccines. *Current Opinion in Biotechnology.* 2001;12:299–303.

68. Leitner WW, Hwang LN, deVeer MJ, et al. Alphavirus-based DNA vaccine breaks immunological tolerance by activating innate antiviral pathways. *Nature Medicine.* 2003;9:33–39.

69. Salonius K, Simard N, Harland R, Ulmer JB. The road to licensure of a DNA vaccine. *Current Opinion in Investigational Drugs.* 2007;8:635–641.

70. Canadian Food Inspection Agency, Veterinary Biologics Section, Animal Health and Production Division. *Environmental assessment for licensing infectious haematopoietic necrosis virus vaccine, DNA vaccine in Canada.* Ottawa: CFIA, 2005.

71. Gillund F, Dalmo R, Tonheim TC, Seternes T, Myhr AI. DNA vaccination in aquaculture—Expert judgments of impacts on environment and fish health. *Aquaculture.* 2008;284:25–34.

72. Gillund F, Kjolberg KA, von Krauss MK, Myhr AI. Do uncertainty analyses reveal uncertainties? Using the introduction of DNA vaccines to aquaculture as a case. *Science of the Total Environment.* 2008;407:185–196.

73. Maturin L Sr., Curtiss R, 3rd. Degradation of DNA by nucleases in intestinal tract of rats. *Science.* 1977;196:216–218.

74. Wilcks A, van Hoek AH, Joosten RG, Jacobsen BB, Aarts HJ. Persistence of DNA studied in different *ex vivo* and *in vivo* rat models simulating the human gut situation. *Food Chemistry and Toxicology.* 2004;42:493–502.

75. New Zealand Environmental Risk Management Authority. To determine whether a dog vaccinated with the canine melanoma vaccine is a new organism (Application Number: S2608008, ERMA New Zealand Evaluation and Review Report). Wellington, 2008.

8

Human and Veterinary Markets

8.1 INTRODUCTION

One of the ultimate goals of science and engineering is to translate scientific advances into products for the benefit of society as a whole. In the case of gene therapy, and of plasmid biopharmaceuticals in particular, this goal remains elusive in spite of the significant efforts and resources that have been devoted both by academia and industry to the advancement of the field. Nevertheless, a first hint of what is yet to come has been given by the handful of plasmid biopharmaceuticals for veterinary applications, which have received regulatory approval in the last 5 years (see Chapter 1, Section 1.3.6 and Chapter 10, Sections 10.3 and 10.4). The expectation is that in the coming years, products for human use will start to emerge gradually from the pipeline of the different companies that have decided to invest in plasmid biopharmaceuticals. But the fact is that the commercialization of the first plasmids for human use will open up a market whose overall size and value is still unknown. Even if the scientific and technological challenges of developing a successful plasmid DNA product (i.e., one that is able to effectively and safely fulfill the intended therapeutic or prophylactic goal) are met, at this stage, it is hard to predict the impact of plasmid biopharmaceuticals on health care and to forecast which products will be blessed with market success. Will therapeutic DNA vaccines for the oncology market perform better than DNA vaccines aimed at preventing infectious

Plasmid Biopharmaceuticals: Basics, Applications, and Manufacturing, First Edition.
Duarte Miguel F. Prazeres.
© 2011 John Wiley & Sons, Inc. Published 2011 by John Wiley & Sons, Inc.

diseases? What about dual vaccination strategies, which combine the priming of the immune system with a DNA vaccine administration, with a subsequent boost of protein or viral elements? Also, can we expect products that target single-gene disorders to succeed, given that the transient nature of gene expression, which is inherent to the majority of plasmid vectors, is likely to call for chronic administration in these cases?

A number of factors other than safety and efficacy will dictate which products will succeed in the market place, that is, which products will generate the highest revenues. For once, the exact nature of the condition being addressed is important. A plasmid product is likely to be adopted more easily by customers if it targets a life-threatening disease to which there is no alternative treatment (see Chapter 7, Section 7.2). Since in many cases the decision to use a specific therapeutic is left at the discretion of physicians and patients, adequate advertising and marketing campaigns should be in place to educate and inform these two groups. Their attitude toward the new form of therapy/vaccination is no doubt one of the keys to success. The role of governments, official bodies, and insurance companies is also crucial, given the power that they have to decide whether a given therapeutic will be subsidized and reimbursed or not. In the end, it will all depend on the social value of the treatment, that is, on the cost savings and gains in quality of life that can be harnessed with the new product.[1] Revenues will also correlate directly with the number of patients treated per year. This could be low, for instance, in the case of single-gene diseases, or extremely high, as in the case of a vaccine against a high-impact disease like malaria or HIV/AIDS. The number of treatments per patient per year is also important. This will depend on the nature of the disease being targeted and of the intervention planned. For instance, vaccination against an infectious disease usually requires a single shot plus one or two boosts at most. The treatment of chronic diseases, on the other hand, might not be so effective, requiring regular administration of the biopharmaceutical.[1] Price, of course, will play a key role as well as the marketing strategy adopted by the firms. Some of the safety issues that have been raised (see Chapter 7, Section 7.3) may also adversely affect the perception that the different stakeholders have toward DNA biopharmaceuticals, and hence may influence the sales of the product. Together with the existence of alternative, more conventional therapies, this may preclude stakeholders from adopting such innovative biopharmaceuticals at an early stage, even if they can be made available at a lower price.

The best way to have an idea of the overall value of the plasmid biopharmaceutical market in the years to come is to focus on those target applications that have received the most attention from researchers in academia and industry, since these are the most likely to hit the market first. In this chapter, and following the first section where the societal context that will be faced by plasmid biopharmaceuticals in the next decade is given, the potential value of human and veterinary markets is addressed. The human applications of plasmid biopharmaceuticals are divided into two major groups, communicable and noncommunicable diseases, whereas veterinary applications are essentially segmented into companion and farm animals. The chapter concludes with a section where a sample of key plasmid biopharmaceutical companies and their products is briefly described.

8.2   A CHANGING WORLD

8.2.1   Population, Life Expectancy, and Wealth

The world has changed dramatically over the course of the last 30 years. For once, people are healthier, wealthier, and live longer today, even though this progress has not reached all countries and segments of the population alike.[2] Although the increase in the world population has been under control, with the annual growth rate decreasing from a yearly average of 1.6% in the 1986–1996 period to 1.3% in the 1996–2006 period, more than 6500 million inhabit the planet today. In 2006, the average age of an earth inhabitant was 28 years, and around 45% of the population was either under 15 (28%) or over 60 (15%).[3] The breakdown of numbers according to the different world regions shows that the average age is significantly lower in Africa, in the Eastern Mediterranean region, and in Southeast Asia when compared with Europe, the Americas, and the West Pacific region, where the eldest constitute a significant fraction of the population (Figure 8.1). And today, more than 50% of the world's population lives in cities and urban areas, as compared to 38%

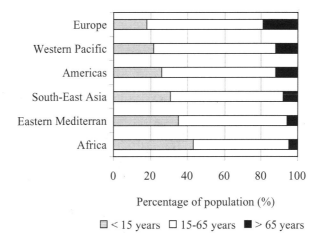

Figure 8.1   *Age distribution of the human population in different regions of the world in 2006. The number of people and their average age in each of the regions are as follows: Africa: 774 million, 18 years; Eastern Mediterranean region: 540 million, 22 years; Southeast Asia: 1721 million, 25 years; Europe: 887 million, 37 years; Americas: 895 million, 30 years; and West Pacific, 1763 million, 33 years. The average age of the 6500 million inhabitants was 28 years* (data from World Health Statistics 2008. Part 2: Global Health Indicators[3]).

only 30 years ago.[2] This geographic shift carries with it new challenges, especially in terms of health, since the quality of life in urban and suburban areas, particularly in those that are overpopulated, is many times very poor when compared with the one in rural areas.

The overall health of the world population can be gauged by noting that from the end of the 1970s until today, life expectancy at birth increased more than 20% to 74 years or more. This extraordinary improvement can be attributed to the increase in world wealth. Estimates of the gross national income per capita indicate that from 1990 to 2006, the figure almost doubled to 10,223 PPP int. US$.* The additional financial resources enabled populations to access better nutrition, education, and health technologies. These assets are a key determinant of health status and have thus contributed to improve longevity. However, there are strong inequalities between life expectancy in the different regions of the globe, which can be as low as 35 years and as high as 85 years. This fact should not be surprising given the strong correlation between health and wealth, and the skewed distribution of wealth in the world.[2]

8.2.2 Climate Change, Ecosystem Deterioration, and Globalization

The changes in ecosystems and climate have also been dramatic at a planetary scale. The devastation of tropical forests and other ecological niches, the destruction of many wild life habitats, and global warming have contributed to the spreading of disease-causing agents, which were once confined to specific territories. The outbreak of West Nile virus in North America, which is described in Chapter 10 (see Section 10.2), is paradigmatic of this situation. Furthermore, there are strong arguments indicating that by disturbing and invading more and more ecological niches, humans have inadvertently contributed to the emergence of zoonoses (see Section 8.4.1), which would have otherwise remained latent in the corresponding animal reservoirs. The interference with the African rainforest, for instance, has been implicated with the emergence of Ebola and HIV[4].

Globalization is now firmly entrenched, linking populations, economies, and societies. The exchange of people and goods across borders and different world regions increased beyond any expectation over recent years. For example, as a consequence of the ease and affordability of air travel, over 1 billion people are transported annually between different regions of the world.[5] The fact that 50 million of these passengers travel to the developing world, where many infectious diseases are endemic, has contributed to the perception that commercial aircrafts play a pivotal role in the spread of pathogens and their

---

* PPP int. US$—purchasing power parity at international dollar rate. An international dollar is a hypothetical currency that is used as a means of translating and comparing costs from one country to the other using a common reference point, the U.S. dollar. Costs in local currency units are converted to international dollars using purchasing power parity (ppp) exchange rates (http://www.who.int/cost/ppp/en).

vectors, and in the dissemination of emerging infections or pandemics.[5] A good example of this danger was seen in the case of the severe acute respiratory syndrome (SARS) epidemic, which emerged in Asia in the first years of the twenty-first century, and was carried almost overnight to Canada by infected people in planes. The role played by air travel in bringing pathogens from areas of outbreaks to distant regions of the globe is also perfectly illustrated by the recent case of the H1N1 influenza A pandemic. The disease was originally detected in Mexico and in the United States in late April 2009, but within 2 months, close to 71,000 laboratory-confirmed cases had been recorded in more than 100 countries,* the majority of which were associated with traveling from the affected zones. Although air travel is the key concern for health authorities, other means of transportation (ships, trains, and trucks) used to move goods and people can also contribute to the spread of airborne, foodborne, and vectorborne zoonotic and nonzoonotic infectious diseases.

8.2.3 The Global Burden of Disease

The comparative importance of diseases and injuries in causing premature death, loss of health, and disability in different populations has been examined in detail in the Global Burden of Disease study prepared by the WHO on the basis of data from the year 2004.[6] The study clusters the leading causes of death and burden of diseases into three major cause groups: (1) Group 1: communicable, maternal, perinatal, and nutritional conditions; (2) Group 2: noncommunicable diseases; and (3) Group 3: injuries. The conditions in Group 1, which include infectious and parasitic diseases, occur essentially in the poorer countries of the developing world. The majority of diseases in Group 2 are chronic conditions like cancer, diabetes, chronic respiratory diseases, and cardiovascular disease, which are often associated with old age and lifestyle (e.g., smoking, alcohol consumption, diet, and lack of exercise).[6] As for the causes in Group 3, they include mostly injuries sustained as a consequence of road traffic accidents and wars. The breakdown of the estimated 58.8 million deaths in 2004 according to this classification shows that the nature of the health problems that affect humanity has changed alongside the transformations described in Sections 8.2.1 and 8.2.2. Specifically, recent years have witnessed an epidemiological transition in which the pattern of mortality has shifted from Group 1 causes (30.6%) to Group 2 causes (59.6%) (Figure 8.2).[6] The fact that Group 2 diseases are on the rise is partially a consequence of the aging of the population, ill-managed urbanization, and increased income. The most frequent causes of death in 2004 are listed in Table 8.1. Together, ischemic heart disease and cerebrovascular disease, the leading causes of heart attacks and stroke, respectively, were responsible for approximately 22% of the deaths registered in 2004. Lower respiratory infections (including pneumonia), chronic obstructive

---

* Data from the World Health Organization (WHO), influenza A (H1N1) update 55 of June 29, 2009 (http://www.who.int/csr/don/2009_06_29/en/index.html, accessed on May 9, 2010).

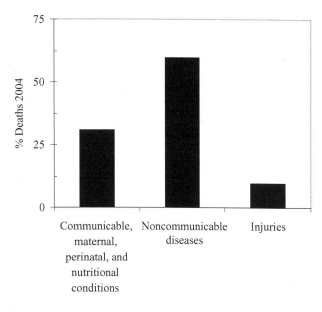

Cause of death

Figure 8.2 *Distribution of world deaths in 2004 according to cause of death (data from the WHO Global Burden of Disease study[6]).*

TABLE 8.1. The Top 10 Leading Causes of Death in 2004

Disease or Injury	Deaths (millions)	Percentage (%)
Ischemic heart disease	7.2	12.2
Cerebrovascular disease	5.7	9.7
Lower respiratory infections	4.2	7.1
Chronic obstructive pulmonary disease	3.0	5.1
Diarrheal diseases	2.2	3.7
HIV/AIDS	2.0	3.5
Tuberculosis	1.5	2.5
Trachea, bronchus, and lung cancers	1.3	2.3
Road traffic accidents	1.3	2.2
Prematurity and low birth weight	1.2	2.0

Source: Data from the Global Burden of Disease study.[6]

pulmonary disease, and diarrheal diseases accounted for 16%, while AIDS and tuberculosis were the sixth and seventh most common causes of death.[6] The ranking of death is different when the numbers are broken down according to the level of income of nations. As expected, in low-income countries, the dominant causes are due to Group 1 conditions (infectious and parasitic diseases like malaria and perinatal conditions), while in high-income countries, 90% of the leading causes of death are noncommunicable conditions (including four

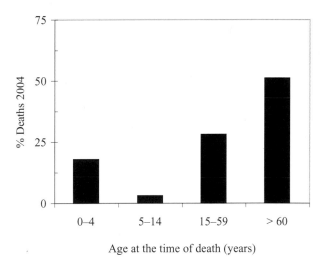

Figure 8.3 *Distribution of world deaths in 2004 according to age at time of death (data from the WHO Global Burden of Disease study[6]).*

types of cancer).[6] Further examination of the data highlights the fact that more than half of all deaths involved people 60 years and older. Nevertheless, around one-fifth of the deaths still occurred among children under the age of 5 (Figure 8.3).

The trends observed in 2004 are expected to continue in the coming years. Current projections estimate that by 2030, the number of deaths associated with the major communicable diseases (including HIV/AIDS, tuberculosis, and malaria) will decline significantly, while the four leading causes of death are predicted to be ischemic heart disease, cerebrovascular disease (stroke), chronic obstructive pulmonary disease, and lower respiratory infections (mainly pneumonia).[6] In other words, death and disease will become more prevalent in older ages, essentially due to noncommunicable conditions, whereas decades ago, it was the youngest who were mostly at risk of dying, essentially due to infections and perinatal and maternal causes.

8.3 HUMAN MARKETS

The scientific knowledge produced since the inception of the new technologies described in this book shows very clearly that plasmid biopharmaceuticals are potentially useful in the context of both communicable and noncommunicable human diseases. The plethora of specific diseases addressed by researchers in the plasmid biopharmaceuticals field is a first indication that the potential market for these products, if successful, is likely to be very large. The following sections provide some estimates of the size of the communicable and noncommunicable disease markets. From these numbers, one can provisionally infer the market share that could eventually be occupied by plasmid biopharmaceuticals.

8.3.1 Communicable Diseases

8.3.1.1 Infectious Diseases and Vaccination
In spite of the significant progress made in recent decades, infectious diseases continue to constitute a burden to world health. According to the WHO, infectious diseases are responsible for two-thirds of all childhood deaths and for half of the premature deaths. Unfortunately, the successful management and control of diseases like poliomyelitis and measles, which once devastated entire populations, has been counteracted by the emergence of new epidemics like AIDS, or by the re-emergence of more virulent forms of diseases like tuberculosis, once thought to be under control. In this context, evidence abounds to support the idea that the best strategy to manage communicable diseases within communities at risk relies on a combination of adequate prevention of transmission and widespread immunization coverage.

Many vaccines were developed and introduced in the wake of Edward Jenner's pioneering work on smallpox immunization in 1790[7] (Figure 8.4). These efforts, led by renowned scientists like Louis Pasteur,[8] Robert Koch,[9] or Jonas Salk,[10] have reduced the mortality of several infectious diseases and have contributed to the increase in life expectancy referred to in the previous section. The eradication of smallpox from the face of the planet constitutes the best example of the power of vaccines. Although this viral disease killed 2 million people every year until the late 1969, the last case of natural infection was detected in 1977 as a result of a global and systematic immunization

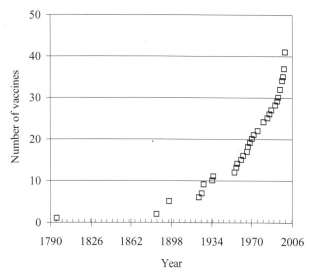

Figure 8.4 *Rate of introduction of commonly used vaccines (based on data from Andre[12]).*

effort.[11,12] No other medical procedure has been able to match the impact of vaccination in such a way. Indeed, vaccines are probably the greatest success of modern medicine. Other major successes of vaccination are, for instance, the eradication of neonatal tetanus in two-thirds of developing countries, or the lowering of the global incidence of poliomyelitis by 99% in 2005[13] from over 300,000 cases/year in the 1980s.[14] Apart from curtailing the impact of disease on individuals, the improvements in health brought about by vaccination also contribute significantly to the wealth of nations by impinging on aspects like education, productivity, or income.[14]

Vaccines are also one of the most cost-effective technologies available to humankind when it comes to dealing with infectious diseases and reducing the associated morbidity and mortality. It has been estimated that every year of healthy life gained via immunization costs less than US$50 and that the average cost per death avoided is under US$1000.[13] These figures are at least two orders of magnitude lower when compared with the costs of treating a noninfectious disease like hypertension. The only human intervention that can parallel with vaccines in terms of the lives and millions of dollars saved is the supplying of potable water.[15] The value of vaccination has been examined in detail in a recent paper, which reviews both cost-effectiveness analysis and cost–benefit analysis, and in recent research showing the relationship between health and wealth.[14] Among other findings, the authors conclude that

> immunization does appear to be an important tool for improving survival and strengthening economies. By boosting cognitive abilities, it improves children's prospects of success when reaching working age. And it does so in an extremely cost-beneficial way. Immunization provides a large return on a small investment— higher than most other health interventions, and at least as high as non-health development interventions such as education.[14]

Currently, more than 25 infectious diseases can be prevented by vaccination.[12] Indicative and preliminary numbers cited by the WHO and the United Nations Children's Fund (UNICEF) in 2005 estimate that 1–2 million child deaths were prevented by immunization in 2000 and forecast that this figure will increase up to 4–5 million child deaths averted per year in 2015. This would mean that in the 2006–2015 decades, a sustainable immunization program could prevent more than 38 million premature deaths.[13] In spite of this, a significant part of the developing world remains vulnerable to a number of infectious diseases (e.g., measles) simply due to lack of coverage. As a result of this, around 3 million people die every year from diseases that can be prevented by vaccines. On top of this, major infections (e.g., malaria and HIV/AIDS), new threats (e.g., pandemic influenza), re-emerging diseases (e.g., tuberculosis), and a number of tropical (e.g., African trypanosomiasis, leishmaniasis, and dengue) diseases continue to threaten public health, thus pushing scientists toward the development and introduction of new vaccination strategies and technologies.[16] Tropical infectious diseases, for example, affect more than 1 billion people around the world, of which the poor and marginalized in under-developed nations make up the larger fraction.[17] For this reason, such diseases have been systematically neglected by pharmaceutical companies who are unwilling to invest large sums in the development of vaccines for those diseases, given the meager returns anticipated. This picture, however, is beginning to change, thanks to the emergence of a series of public–private partnerships and alliances between charities, large pharmaceutical companies, and small biotech firms, which are joining efforts in order to translate basic research findings into effective and affordable vaccines.[17] The world's vulnerability in the face of infectious disease has been underscored dramatically with the emergence of the 2009 influenza A/H1N1 pandemic.[18] The worldwide mobilization, which took place as soon as the speed and extent of distribution of the disease became apparent, has no parallel in history. Not surprisingly, vaccines were immediately identified as one of the key measures required to minimize the progress, morbidity, and mortality of the disease. This prompted a race to produce effective and safe vaccines, which led to the first lots being ready for distribution 5–6 months after the disease had been recognized. By the end of the year, millions of people had already been immunized all over the world.

8.3.1.2 The Vaccine Market

The revenues generated by vaccines worldwide in 2005 were close to US$10,000 million (Figure 8.5). Although this represents but a small fraction of 2.0% of the total revenues of the pharmaceutical industry (greater than US$300,000 million[19]), the global vaccine market is expected to grow at a compound annual growth rate (CAGR) of 10.5%, reaching US$20,000 million in 2012[20] (Figure 8.5). The side-by-side comparison of drugs used to treat noncommunicable diseases and vaccines shows that the sales of the latter are rather limited.

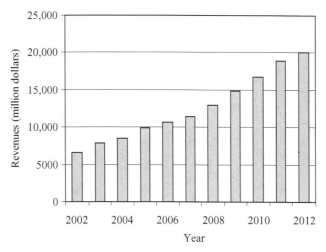

Figure 8.5 *Revenue forecasts for the world vaccine markets, 2002–2012 (data from Frost & Sullivan[20]).*

Paradoxically, the poor market performance of vaccines is directly related to their high efficacy since in most cases, a few doses are sufficient to provide long-lasting immunity to a child or an individual. Thus, markets for prophylactic vaccines are rather small, even if the potential number of users and societal impact is very large.

Geographic segmentation shows that in 2005, North America, Europe, and the rest of the world accounted for 47.5, 32.0, and 20.5% of the vaccine market, respectively.[20] This distribution will be maintained through the next years since each of the market segments is expected to grow at approximately the same rate. The revenues and growth of developed markets like the North American and European markets are directly associated with the launching of innovative products, the development of new technologies, and the improvement of coverage. As for emerging (e.g., India, China, and Brazil) and underdeveloped markets (e.g., African countries), the key drivers for growth are the increased efforts led by governmental and aid agencies to insure public vaccination and extended coverage. The developing world vaccine market is estimated at just 10–15% of the world total market.[14] For example, it is interesting to note that UNICEF accounted for 40% of the global vaccine doses used in 2004, even though this corresponded only to 5% (US$440 million) of the market value.[21] Clearly, profitability in this geographic segment is less attractive when compared with the North American and the European markets.

Almost two-thirds of the global vaccine sales correspond to childhood vaccines that prevent infectious diseases like measles, tetanus, or diphtheria.[20] Although such essential vaccines (i.e., "vaccines of public health importance that should be accessible to all people at risk"[19]) have dominated the scene so far, the market is increasingly moving toward adult diseases and adapting itself to the new circumstances of the twenty-first century. For instance, specific travel vaccines are needed as a result of the ever-increasing mobility of the world population. Furthermore, resurgent outbreaks (e.g., yellow fever) and threatening global pandemics (e.g., influenza and SARS) have increased the importance of the so-called emergency response vaccines. Global bioterrorism threats have also contributed to boost the research and development spending in vaccines against diseases like anthrax or smallpox.[19,22]

The number of licensed manufacturers producing vaccines has decreased dramatically from 26 in 1967 to only 12 in 2002.[15] The small size of the industry results from an ensemble of factors, which include low profit margins, liability issues, and costs of the good manufacturing practice (GMP) compliant processes, which are nowadays mandatory to manufacture vaccines.[22] Furthermore, of the eight pediatric vaccines that are currently recommended, five have a single supplier.[15] This dependency on single or few manufacturers creates a high-risk situation, since the failure of one company can dramatically affect the worldwide supply of a given vaccine. The global vaccine market is dominated by five major manufacturers, GlaxoSmithKline (22.5%), Sanofi Pasteur Inc. (21.2%), Wyeth (14.8%), Merck & Co., Inc. (10.5%), and Chiron Corporation (6.5%), which together collect approximately 85% of the revenues.[20] The preponderance of these giants leaves little room for other players. Nevertheless, and after a long period of relative stagnation, the attractiveness of the vaccine market has increased significantly. Today, the double-digit growth in sales makes the vaccine market highly appellative when compared with other areas of the healthcare sector.[22] Once a sector that was characterized by a small number of players, government-fixed prices, a restricted number of technologies, and a mature collection of low-margin products that sell for less than US$1–US$3 per dose, vaccines are now attracting more and more investment and witnessing a surge of technological innovation. The increased research and development efforts devoted to the development of new vaccines have already paid off, as illustrated by the cases of Wyeth's heptavalent pneumoccocal conjugate vaccine (Prevenar®) and Merck's human papillomavirus (Gardasil®) and rotavirus (Rotateq®) vaccines. Prevenar, which sells around US$232 per four-dose series, became one of the first vaccine blockbusters, with sales close to US$1.5 million in 2005. One of the major reasons why companies have managed to improve pricing is related to the innovative character of these products. There are currently a number of niche opportunities for companies willing to bet on and adopt new technologies that could originate new vaccines or replace currently approved products and conventional production processes (e.g., egg-based manufacturing).

The share of the world vaccine market that could be captured by DNA vaccines is an unknown at this stage, especially because the technology has still to prove its worth in the case of humans. Furthermore, since the purchasing of vaccines is many times intimately linked to public health policy recommendations, precise predictions are difficult to make.[22] Assuming for the sake of argument that this share could be around 1%, this would represent revenues of the order of US$200 million by 2012 (see Figure 8.5).

8.3.1.3 Implementation of DNA Vaccines

The overall picture described above makes it clear that the potential market for DNA vaccines for infectious diseases is huge. The major targets selected by DNA vaccine researchers have been the most obvious, and include major killers like malaria, HIV/AIDS[23], hepatitis C,[24] and tuberculosis,[25] but also threats like pandemic influenza[26] or anthrax.[27] DNA vaccines are also under development to protect against other lower-impact infectious diseases like Ebola,[28] dengue,[29] Japanese encephalitis,[30] and West Nile virus.[31] However, before the potentialities of DNA vaccines are harnessed, a series of technological and nontechnological barriers have to be surmounted. First, the safety and efficacy of DNA vaccines for the prevention of specific diseases must be scientifically and unambiguously proven. Also, manufacturing technologies should be in place so that the vaccines can be mass-produced at a reasonable cost. If these challenges are met, the potential for application of DNA vaccines is huge, not only in developed countries but also, most importantly, in developing countries.[16] In fact, there are a number of features associated with DNA vaccines that make them especially adequate for the poorer and less developed areas of the world (see Chapter 19, Section 19.3). For once, the relative simplicity of the technology makes it accessible to scientists and researchers in nations with less developed research and development systems. The higher thermal stability of DNA when compared to proteins is another characteristic, which will hopefully facilitate the handling, transportation, and delivery of vaccines to patients. In this case, the expectation is that the requirements for a network of freezers and refrigerators, that is, for a cold chain, are not as stringent as compared to conventional vaccines. This could be highly relevant in tropical and subtropical areas where high temperatures, malfunctioning equipment, and a lack of a proper energy supply often hamper the distribution of vaccines. The fact that different DNA vaccines can, in principle, be manufactured by the same generic process is another feature that will hopefully contribute to facilitate the dissemination of the technology.

The implementation of DNA vaccines in the field will call for a joint effort of pharmaceutical companies, governments, and international organizations like the WHO and UNICEF. Given the discrepancy among world nations in terms of population and wealth, tiered pricing will be practiced as is common with other vaccines. This means that organizations like the UNICEF and the WHO will be responsible for purchasing DNA vaccines to be distributed to the poorest countries. Although most scientific evidence shows that DNA vaccines are safe, public perception and ethic arguments may constitute a barrier to market success. Many will find it difficult to accept the worldwide dissemination of genetic material across healthy and young populations, which will be inherent to a DNA vaccination program against a disease like malaria or HIV/AIDS. Furthermore, the fact that this massive use of an unproven technology will likely take place largely in developing countries may lead some to question whether the recipient populations are not being in reality used as subjects in a large-scale clinical trial.

8.3.2 Noncommunicable Diseases

8.3.2.1 *Target Diseases*

The human population is aging. This trend is expected to continue in future years, especially affecting rich countries, which form the so-called developed world (Figure 8.1). These changing demographics, together with the improvements obtained in the health of the elderly since the early 1980s, have been accompanied by an increase in a constellation of age-related diseases and disabilities, of which cancer and cardiovascular diseases are the most important. Gene therapy is well positioned to play a role in the treatment and management of diseases, which can be grouped into three major clinical domains: cancer, cardiovascular, and monogenic diseases.[32] A number of facts support the focus on these diseases: (1) They have been favorite targets for gene therapy research, accounting for 83.9% of all gene therapy clinical trials reported between 1989 and 2007;[33] (2) the associated fatality rates are high; (3) the risk-to-benefit ratio is highly favorable, given that many of the

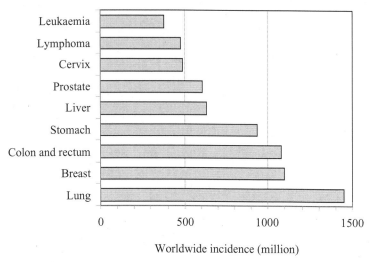

Figure 8.6 *Worldwide incidence of major cancers in 2004 (data from the WHO Global Burden of Disease study[6]).*

diseases are terminal; and (4) the medical need has been unmet to a large extent.

Cancer   The impact of cancer in modern societies is extremely high. In 2004, 11.4 million people were diagnosed with cancer[6] (Figure 8.6). The breakdown of numbers shows that more cancers occur in high-income countries than in low- and middle-income countries. In 2004, Europe (27%), the Americas (20%), and the West Pacific region (20%) accounted for 74% of the total incidence, whereas the contributions of Africa (6%), the Eastern Mediterranean region (4%), and Southeast Asia (15%) were more modest.[6] The correlation between cancer incidence and age is also striking—cancer is definitely a disease of elders. Given the expected increases in the age of the world population, it is thus not surprising to find that the number of cancer-related deaths is projected to increase from ~8 million in 2004 to approximately ~12 million in 2030.[6] In the United States, cancer has already replaced heart disease as the leading cause of death,[34] whereas in most developed nations, it ranks in second place. Apart from the physical and psychological burden that cancer imposes on patients and their families, the economical load on healthcare systems is also significant. Costs are especially high in the case of breakthrough biopharmaceuticals like monoclonal antibodies, which typically cost 300–500% more than conventional drugs. Also, the marginal gains in survival rate and life expectancy obtained with some of these innovative treatments, although highly desirable, translate into more prolonged treatments, and thus more costs.[34] Cancer is one of the clinical domains in which gene therapy is most likely to have the largest impact.[35] Several facts attest to this, namely, the more than 1000 clinical trials with recombinant viruses and plasmids targeting oncological diseases,* the large body of scientific literature devoted to the subject, and the number of distinct therapeutic strategies devised to kill tumor cells on the basis of genes (see Chapter 2, Section 2.4.2.2). In comparison with other technologies, and together with early detection, therapeutic cancer vaccines appear to provide the best potential value when measured as marginal costs per year of life gained.[34]

Cardiovascular Diseases Cardiovascular diseases are one of the plagues of modern-day societies. Millions die every year from stroke or heart disease, and the predictions are that these will constitute one of the major causes of death in years to come (see Section 8.2.3). The economic impact of cardiovascular diseases is huge, not only due to the costs associated with health care but also due to losses in productivity incurred as a result of the poor physical condition of many of the afflicted individuals. Although most strategies devised to minimize the effect of cardiovascular diseases in the socioeconomic development of communities and nations, like the promotion of lifestyle changes or the creation of healthy environments, are preventive and nontherapeutic in nature, the medical control of cardiovascular diseases will remain crucial for all those already afflicted. The world market for cardiovascular disease therapies is certainly huge, as a result of the large numbers of people affected. This provides a substantial ground for the development of gene therapy approaches, and as a result, this group of diseases accounted for 9% of the gene therapy trials registered between 1989 and 2007 in the clinical trial database of *The Journal of Gene Medicine*.[33]

A number of cardiovascular diseases have been addressed by gene therapy, including hypertension, thrombosis, vascular bypass graft occlusion, restenosis, coronary arterial disease (CAD) and peripheral arterial disease (PAD).[36] The applicability of plasmid biopharmaceuticals to the treatment of critical limb ischemia, a specific manifestation of PAD, is described in detail in Chapter 9 (Section 9.3). Other cardiovascular diseases that have been addressed by gene therapy include atherosclerosis, thrombosis, and hypertension. Although significant progress has been made in recent years, major obstacles for the successful treatment of cardiovascular disease by gene therapy include the identification of the best candidate gene and delivery option.

Single-Gene Disorders Congenital disorders are characterized by deficiencies at the single-gene level, which either originate defective proteins or hamper their synthesis altogether. As a result, afflicted individuals display a series of symptoms whose severity may vary widely. Although in many cases it is possible to manage the disease, normalizing both life expectancy and quality of life, for example, by resorting to protein replacement therapies or appropriate dietary regimens, other disorders are severe and life threatening.

* Data from *The Journal of Gene Medicine* Gene Therapy Clinical Trials Worldwide Web site at http://www.wiley.co.uk/genmed/clinical (accessed May 9, 2010).

While some single-gene disorders are extremely rare, others affect considerable numbers of individuals. Additionally, the incidence of such diseases can vary widely across populations, racial groups, and genders. Gene therapy has long promised to cure and treat such disorders. Among others, favorite targets for gene therapy are (1) hemophilia,[37] (2) cystic fibrosis,[38] (3) severe combined immunodeficiencies (SCIDs),[39] (4) lysosomal storage disorders,[40] and (5) Duchenne muscular dystrophy[41] (see also Chapter 2, Section 2.4.1). Although the number of people affected by monogenic diseases is not as high as in the case of cancer and cardiovascular disease, gene therapy is still expected to have an impact on the treatment. Around 20 different monogenic diseases have been studied at the clinical trial level, with cystic fibrosis and immunodeficiencies accounting for one-third and one-fifth of the total number of registered trials during 1989–2007.[33]

8.3.2.2 The Gene Therapy Market

According to a market report published by Frost & Sullivan in 2005, the global gene therapy market was expected to grow at a CAGR of 68.3%, with revenues increasing from US$150 million in 2005, up to US$5744 million in 2011[42] (Figure 8.7). The large number of people afflicted by cancer and cardiovascular diseases and the fact that many of them live in the wealthier regions of the globe renders the prospective market for the corresponding products and interventions highly appellative. Furthermore, all projections indicate that the number of deaths attributed to these diseases will increase in all countries, whichever the level of income. Thus, it is not surprising to find that the predictions indicate that gene therapy products for cancer and cardiovascular diseases will lead the way and dominate the market, generating revenues of US$3159 and US$1149 million, respectively, in 2011 (Figure 8.7). By that time,

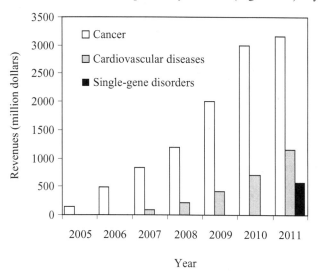

Figure 8.7 *Revenue forecasts for the world gene therapy markets, 2005–2011 (data from Frost & Sullivan[42]).*

and although more modest, the single-gene disorder segment will still amount to US\$574 million[42] (Figure 8.7). Plasmid biopharmaceuticals will hopefully capture a fraction of the gene therapy market. One way of appraising this fraction is to look into the distribution of gene therapy clinical trials in terms of delivery vector used. Recent data show that strategies that rely on the use of naked plasmid DNA alone accounted for 18% of all clinical trials that had been performed or were ongoing worldwide between 1989 and 2007[33] (see Chapter 2, Figure 2.3). Although this percentage refers to all diseases, we may assume for the sake of argument that plasmid biopharmaceuticals will account for 18% of revenues as well. Using the data for cancer, cardiovascular diseases, and single-gene disorders quoted above,[42] this would translate into sales of the order of US\$1000 million by 2011. However, these estimates are probably overoptimistic in view of the fact that no plasmid biopharmaceutical for human use as yet received regulatory approval and marketing authorization. Furthermore, it should be stressed that the estimates for the gene therapy market mentioned above were made in 2005. More recent data indicate that the projections made then may have overestimated the size of the market by one order of magnitude.

8.4 VETERINARY MARKETS

8.4.1 Animal Disease

Animal diseases constitute a significant burden to society. First, many animal species are reservoirs of pathogenic agents that are transmissible to humans, causing a range of diseases that are collectively referred to as zoonoses. Such diseases constitute a risk to individuals who live or work with animals (e.g., veterinarians, farmers, and pet owners). The risks are especially heightened in immunocompromised individuals like HIV patients or transplant recipients.[43] The breeding, manipulation, and handling of exotic and unusual pets should be especially controlled since such species can potentially introduce previously unknown pathogens in specific areas or continents.[43] Zoonosis outbreaks also constitute a threat to entire communities and populations.[43] The black death, the plague that hit medieval Europe as a pandemic wave, is a classical example of an uncontrolled zoonosis of deadly proportions. The disease is caused by the bacterium *Yersinia pestis*, which lives in wild rodents and is transmitted to humans by fleas.[44] Many of the infectious diseases that have emerged in the last 50 years are also zoonoses. These include, for example, the pulmonary syndrome caused by the hantavirus, which is carried by the deer mouse,[4,45] the H5N1 "bird flu" and the H1N1 influenza A of 2009 whose primary reservoirs are believed to be wild aquatic birds[4] (see Chapter 9, Section 9.2 for more details), or the mosquito-borne Chikungunya disease, which is caused by an alphavirus that lurks in primates.[46]

A large array of pathogens, including bacteria (e.g., *Salmonella* and *Brucella*), viruses (e.g., influenza and rabies), and parasites (e.g., *Leishmania* and

TABLE 8.2. A Sample of Veterinary Diseases Affecting Companion and Food Animal

Disease/Specie	Agent	Disease/Specie	Agent
Bovine		Poultry	
Foot-and-mouth	Virus	Colibacillosis	Bacteria
Rinderpest	Virus	Chlamydiosis	Bacteria
West Nile	Virus	Newcastle disease	Virus
Brucellosis	Bacteria	Avian influenza	Virus
Hearthwater	Bacteria	Coccidiosis	Protozoa
Babesiosis	Protozoa	Fish	
Ovine		Furuncolosis	Bacteria
Blue tongue	Virus	Vibriosis	Bacteria
Toxoplasmosis	Protozoa	Hematopoietic necrosis*	Virus
Anthrax	Bacteria	Pancreatic necrosis	Virus
Porcine		Cats	
Swine fever	Virus	Leukemia	Virus
Porcine circovirus	Virus	Rabies	Virus
Aujesky's disease	Virus	Dogs	
Equine		Rabies	Virus
Bronchopneumonia	Bacteria	Canine distemper	Virus
West Nile*	Virus	Leishmaniasis	Protozoa
Influenza	Virus	Babesiosis	Protozoa

*A DNA vaccine has been approved that provides immunization against the disease.

Trypanossoma) can infect animals, causing respiratory, enteric, systemic, and reproductive diseases, among others. Table 8.2 shows some of the major veterinary diseases that affect a number of highly valued animal species, as well as the causative pathogen. Some of the diseases listed in the table have been associated with high economic impact outbreaks in specific regions (e.g., foot-and-mouth disease, blue tongue, and avian influenza), whereas others have made headlines because of their potential danger to humans (e.g., H5N1 avian influenza) and proven pandemic impact (e.g., the H1N1 "swine" influenza A of 2009). The economic viability of developing a given veterinary product depends on the incidence and number of individuals affected by the specific disease in question, as well as on the economic burden associated with it. Some veterinary diseases will never be sufficiently attractive from an economic point of view to justify the development of a new product. Still, the market opportunities for manufacturers of veterinary products abound. Two major categories can be distinguished within this market: companion and food animals.

8.4.1.1 Food Animals

The threats posed by zoonoses to human health are particularly important in our modern days as a result of the global transformations we have witnessed in human lifestyle. Especially important are the changes in livestock production, from a more traditional approach (which still subsists in many developing countries) based on free-roaming animals, to a more intensive industrial production based on the raising of animals with a similar genotype in confined spaces.[47] Furthermore, the establishment of worldwide agrofood networks has contributed to an increase in the trade and mobility of animals and animal products among human populations.[47] The control and surveillance of the health and disease status of many of wild and domestic animal reservoirs is thus crucial to prevent zoonoses from hitting human populations. Although the transmission of zoonoses is usually airborne (e.g., influenza), waterborne (e.g., salmonellosis and toxoplasmosis), or vectorborne, via bites (e.g., malaria and rabies), animal diseases can also affect humans via the food chain. Foodborne transmission is especially important in a context where human nutrition is becoming more and more dependent on animal-derived products like meat, fish, milk, or eggs. Thus, the control of the health of producer animals is essential to guarantee a supply of uncontaminated, animal-derived food, and minimize health risks to consumers. Safety measures should also be extended beyond the animal level, throughout the entire production, processing, and storage chain to prevent contamination with pathogens like *Salmonella* or *Lysteria*.

Apart from their obvious impact on human health, animal diseases have also a direct impact in the economies of countries. For example, the commercial success of the production of food animals depends heavily on the ability of producers to maintain healthy animals. Infectious diseases (whether they are zoonoses or not) are especially important in this context, constituting a recurrent threat to poultry and livestock. Some outbreaks can devastate entire populations of animals, whereas in other cases, the infection of a few individuals often makes it mandatory to isolate and kill the other individuals in the herd or flock and in the neighboring farms. For instance, close to 2 million animals were slaughtered within 2 months of the outbreak of the foot-and-mouth disease epidemic that hit Great Britain in 2001.[48] More recently, and since 2004, hundreds of millions of chickens have been killed by sanitary authorities in Southeast Asian countries in an attempt to control the spreading of the highly pathogenic H5N1 avian influenza virus (see Chapter 9, Section 9.2). In any case, the costs associated with disease in food animals are huge.

The control of highly infectious diseases in densely populated farms or animal houses depends on the implementation of effective surveillance measures and on the rapid destruction of the infected herds or flocks.[48] Another option relies on the widespread, prophylactic vaccination of healthy animals. When available and if adequately used, vaccines contribute both to improve the productivity of the food animal industry and to decrease or eliminate the health risks to the consumer. Furthermore, vaccinated, healthy animals are likely to require less veterinary pharmaceuticals and hormones. This will indirectly impact human health since fewer residues of those medicines will pervade through the human food chain.[49]

8.4.1.2 *Companion Animals*

The value that many pet owners in the developed world countries put on the life of their companion animals makes this segment of the veterinary market highly appellative to the major industrial players of the area. For example, in 2006, nearly half of the pet owners in the United States considered their pets to be family members.[50] With this mindset, the fact that people are willing to pay large amounts of money to extend or improve the life of pets, even if it is just for a few months or years, is not surprising at all. In 2006, the average veterinary expenditure per U.S. household for all pets was US$366, totalling an approximate US$19,000 million annually. This nearly doubled the US$11,000 million expenditure recorded in 1996.[50] The European market for companion animal health products is expected to be of this same order of magnitude as well. Thus, and roughly speaking, the annual market for companion animal products is probably of the order of a few tenths (15–20) of billion dollars every year.[51]

8.4.2 The Veterinary Vaccine Market

Veterinary health is an extremely large and fast-growing market. A handful of species dominate the scene, namely, cats and dogs in the companion animal segment, and pigs, cattle, poultry, sheep, and horses in the livestock segment. With the advent and rapid growth of fish and marine product production by aquaculture technologies, aquatic species are also becoming more and more important in this context[52] (see the case study on the Atlantic salmon described in Chapter 10, Section 10.3). For companion animal products, the market can be broadly segmented into the following categories: anti-infectants, biologics, dietetics, ectoparasiticides, endoparasiticides, and pharmacologicals.[51] A similar product categorization can be made for the food animal segment. Biologics, and specifically the vaccine subcategory, constitute the most important sector. For example, the expenditures associated with vaccines against diseases of dogs (e.g., canine parvovirus, canine distemper, canine parainfluenza, canine leptospirosis, and canine hepatitis) or cats (e.g., feline leukemia, panleucopenia virus, rhinotracheitis, and calicivirus) are likely to account for 20–25% of the yearly market and sales in the companion animal segment.[51] Vaccines for companion animals are typically sold at a higher price per dose than vaccines for food animals, which tend to be cheaper.[53] However, the quantities of livestock vaccines produced every year are much larger.[53] Roughly speaking, pet vaccines represent one-third of the veterinary vaccine market, which is clearly dominated by livestock vaccines. In 2004, the worldwide sales of veterinary vaccines amounted to US$3.2 billion, representing approximately one-fifth of the global revenues generated by animal health products.[54] Recent estimates project that the market will grow at a CAGR of more than 6%, reaching US$5.1 billion by 2012. Although Europe and North America lead the market with a combined share of 60%, the increase in revenues is expected to be highest in the Asia Pacific region.[55]

The market is dominated by a handful of major players, including Intervet/Schering-Plough Animal Health and Fort Dodge Animal Health, a division of Wyeth. This latter company has led the way in the DNA vaccine field, gaining approval from the United States Department of Agriculture (USDA) in July 2005 to market a West Nile virus vaccine for horses. This vaccine was launched in December 2008 under the trade name West Nile-Innovator® DNA and is sold exclusively to veterinarians.[56] The vaccine contains plasmid DNA material combined with MetaStim, a proprietary lipid/surfactant adjuvant that stimulates both antibody and cell-mediated immune responses. The recommended dosage is a first 2 mL intramuscular dose followed by a second 2 mL boost 2–4 weeks after. Yearly revaccination with one 2 mL shot is further advised. According to Fort Dodge Animal Health, the vaccine (1) is 99% reaction free, as shown when administered intramuscularly to a cohort of 645 horses of various breeds and ages; (2) confers a 12-month duration of immunity; and (3) is effective, as demonstrated in challenge studies evaluated on the basis of viremia.[56]

A third category within the veterinary market should probably be referred here, one that includes wildlife. This niche of the market would include specific DNA vaccines developed and deployed in response to zoonotic diseases or to specific infectious threats to endangered species. The protection of the Californian condor population against the West Nile virus is the benchmark case in this context (see Chapter 10, Section 10.2). In overall terms, however, the value of this market segment is probably close to irrelevant.

Successful plasmid products could eventually capture a fraction of the US$3 billion to US$6 billion a year veterinary vaccine market. Already a significant number of DNA vaccine prototypes are being developed against a range of animal diseases. The interested reader should consult specialized reviews for a more comprehensive information on veterinary DNA vaccines.[57-59] Major successes in this context are the West Nile virus vaccine developed for horses and condors, and the infectious hematopoietic necrosis virus vaccines developed for salmons (see Chapter 10, Section 10.3). In the last case, for example, around 10 million doses of vaccine are sold every year in Canada at a cost of US$0.4 per dose. This amounts to an annual volume of sales of the order of US$4 million.*

8.4.3 Concluding Remarks

Although the market for veterinary plasmid biopharmaceuticals is not likely to match its human counterpart in terms of value by orders of magnitude, its importance and relevance are nonetheless significant. First, the vast amount of knowledge accumulated in the research and development of plasmids for a multitude of veterinary diseases and animal hosts constitutes an important resource for scientists who address human applications. Furthermore, the codevelopment of plasmid therapeutics in humans and closely related animal species, particularly in the case of those diseases that jump from animals to humans (e.g., SARS and avian influenza), is an approach that is expected to speed up the development of human products. This bridging of medical and veterinary medi-

* Kira Salonious, AquaHealth R&D, private communication.

cine can also contribute to speed up progress in the therapy of human/animal noninfectious diseases, as described in Chapter 10 (Section 10.4) for the case of DNA vaccines against dog/human melanoma. Another important feature of the animal health market is related to the fact that regulatory requirements and ethical barriers to the development of plasmid biopharmaceuticals are much more relaxed when compared with the human health markets. Among other things, this translates into a development process that is faster and less costly. Thus, and not surprisingly, plasmid biopharmaceuticals for veterinary applications are leading the way in terms of market approval (see Chapter 1, Section 1.3.6). Although this gap between approved/marketed plasmids designed for veterinary and human applications is likely to persist in the near future, it is clear that the growth of human and animal markets will be intertwined.

8.5 KEY COMPANIES AND THEIR PRODUCTS

A number of new companies were created in the past 20 years with the specific goal of harnessing the potential of plasmid-based therapeutics and vaccines (Figure 8.8). The prospect of establishing new markets with plasmid biopharmaceuticals has also lured traditional, well-established pharmaceutical com-

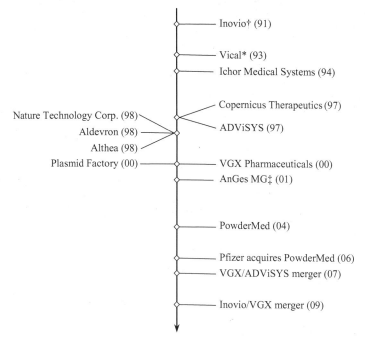

Figure 8.8 *A sample of companies active in different areas of plasmid biopharmaceutical development (product development, contract manufacturing, delivery, etc.). *Originally founded 10 years earlier, 1993 was the date for the initial public offering. †A drug and gene delivery division is added to Inovio, a Biotech company founded in 1983. ‡Founded earlier in 1999, the Japanese-based company MedGene changed its corporate name to AnGes MG in 2001.*

panies into the new business opportunity. By acting alone or in alliance, these players have pushed the development of new products, both for human and veterinary markets. Although these different players all work in the plasmid biopharmaceutical arena, different firms have adopted different strategies and business models to build value.

A number of emerging companies were created on the basis of research and development findings originating from universities and research institutes. Such start-ups typically have access (e.g., via licensing from universities) to proprietary technologies or competences that are enabling for a given part of the plasmid biopharmaceutical development process. Some companies may spend their first years investing in research and development on their platform technology in order to build and expand their intellectual property portfolio and expertise. In these cases, revenues are typically produced on the basis of licensing deals, consulting, and contract research. In the plasmid biopharmaceutical area, one can find such companies, which have specialized in aspects like plasmid delivery (e.g., Ichor Medical Systems, San Diego, California), vector development (e.g., Nature Technology Corporation, Lincoln, Nebraska), process development (e.g., Nature Technology Corporation), or manufacturing of plasmid material for clinical trials (e.g., Aldevron, Fargo, North Dakota; Althea, San Diego, California; Plasmid Factory, Bielefeld, Germany). A number of companies (e.g., Geneart, Regensburg, Germany; Eurogentec, Seraing, Belgium) also offer GMP plasmid manufacturing as a part of a broader range of services in other areas.

However, if the technology is powerful enough, it can form the scientific foundation upon which the firm can discover and develop their proprietary plasmid biopharmaceuticals. Vical (San Diego, California), PowderMed (Oxford, United Kingdom), Inovio Biomedical Corporation (San Diego, California), VGX Pharmaceuticals (Blue Bell, Pennsylvania), and Copernicus Therapeutics (Cleveland, Ohio) constitute typical examples of platform companies that managed to transform themselves into plasmid biopharmaceutical companies. Vical was originally founded in 1987 to research and develop the proprietary lipid chemistry for DNA transfection described by Felgner et al.,[60] whereas PowderMed was founded in May 2004 to develop the proprietary Particle Mediated Epidermal Delivery (PMED™) technology. A proprietary, electroporation-based technology used to deliver and enhance the potency of DNA vaccines was also at the inception of Inovio Biomedical Corporation (previously Genetronics Biomedical Corporation). As for VGX Pharmaceuticals, it was originally created in 2000 to explore a technology developed at the University of Pennsylvania that uses viral proteins as a basis for developing drugs.[61] A technology that provides effective delivery and expression of nucleic acids, including plasmids, is also one of the key assets of Copernicus Therapeutics. The company has licensed, developed, and optimized a process to compact single molecules of DNA into minimally sized nanoparticles. This ability to produce such small plasmid particles has pushed the company into the development of specific products to treat cystic fibrosis and a series of diseases that cause blindness.

Although these companies were created on the basis of relatively focused and narrow technology expertise, they have reshaped themselves in such a way that they are currently pushing the development of plasmid biopharmaceutical past preclinical experimentation and into clinical trials. This transformation and growth has called for the vertical integration of extensive and complementary capabilities, either via licensing agreements with academic research institutions or through the acquisition of other players. For example, by acquiring the Texas-based firm ADViSYS, Inc. (The Woodlands, Texas), VGX gained access not only to its proprietary electroporation technology (cellectra™) electroporator but also to its manufacturing operations and animal health business. This move was crucial for the successful approval of the veterinary plasmid product LifeTide™ SW5, which is marketed by VGX Animal Health, Inc. (The Woodlands, Texas), the company subsidiary dedicated to veterinary medicine.[62] Furthermore, the Cellectra™ electroporation technology is central to all other plasmid biopharmaceuticals being developed by the company. By way of this transformation from a technology-based company into a product company, Vical, VGX, Inovio, and PowderMed currently have strong product candidates for the treatment of infectious diseases (e.g., HIV, influenza, and hepatitis), as well as cancer and inflammatory diseases at the different stages of the development pipeline (research and development, preclinical, and clinical) (Table 8.2). However, given the high risks and large investment required to bring a pharmaceutical into the market, these companies typically form some sort of alliance or strike licensing deals with larger, capital-intensive firms at a certain time along the road. This brings capital in, minimizes entrance barriers due to the dominance of the established players, and gives the smaller company access to the distribution and marketing channels of the larger firm. Thus, it is not surprising to find that most products in clinical trials are being codeveloped by a small/medium company and a larger pharmaceutical company (Table 8.3). The involvement of Vical in (1) Merial's canine melanoma vaccine, (2) Aqua Health's (Prince Edwards, Canada) infectious hematopoietic necrosis virus salmon vaccine, and (3) AnGes's (Osaka, Japan) therapeutic plasmid for PAD is a paradigmatic example of this strategy. For the big incumbent firms, on the other hand, partnering with young companies that have innovative products or solutions is an excellent way to extend their own core competences by tapping into the research and development strengths of the newcomers. Sometimes, it may be difficult for companies to keep independency, especially if they meet success along the product development track. PowderMed, for example, was acquired by Pfizer in 2006. Merging with a similarly sized company in the area is another option. For example, in a characteristic move, VGX Pharmaceuticals recently (June 2009) merged with Inovio Biomedical Corporation to form a leading company in vaccine discovery, development, and delivery.

The sample of candidate plasmid biopharmaceuticals that are currently undergoing preclinical and clinical trials (Table 8.3), together with the fact that major pharmaceutical companies are investing in their development, is one indicator that market success may be lurking around the corner for some of

TABLE 8.3. A Sample of Plasmid Biopharmaceutical Companies and Their Lead Products

Target/Indication	Status	Primary Developer
Company: Vical (San Diego, California)*		
Allovectin-7®, metastatic melanoma	Phase 3	Vical
Cytomegalovirus (CMV)	Phase 2	Vical
Influenza	Phase 1	Vical
Congenital CMV	Preclinical	Vical
Collategene™, PAD, and Buerger's disease	NDA filed in Japan, phase 2 over in the United States	AnGes
Ischemic heart disease	Phase 1	AnGes
PAD	Phase 3	Sanofi-Aventis
Apex-IHN® (salmon)	Marketed in Canada	Aqua Health
Melanoma (dogs)	Conditional approval in the US	Merial
Cancer (ovary, breast, colorectal, and lung)	Phase 1	Merck
HIV	Phase 2	NIH
Company: VGX Pharmaceuticals (Blue Bell, Pennsylvania)†		
LifeTide SW5 (pigs)	Marketed in Australia	VGX Animal Health
HIV (preventive)	Phase 1	HIV vaccine trial network
HIV (therapeutic)	Phase 1	NIAID
Pandemic/seasonal influenza	Preclinical	VGX
Avian influenza	IND	VGX
Cervical cancer	Phase 1	VGX
Cancer cachexia	IND	VGX
Company: Inovio Biomedical Corporation (San Diego, California)‡		
Malignant melanoma	Phase 1	Moffit Cancer Center
Metastatic melanoma	Phase 1	Vical
Prostate cancer	Phase 1	University of Southampton
Cancer (ovary, breast, colorectal, and lung)	Phase 1	Merck
Hepatitis C	Phase 1	Tripep
CMV	IND	Vical
HIV	Preclinical	NCI
Melanoma	Preclinical	VGX
Other companies		
Leishmaniasis	Preclinical	Mologen AG
West Nile virus (horses)	Marketed in the United States	Fort Dodge Animal Health

*http://www.vical.com/.

†http://www.vgxp.com.

‡http://www.inovio.com/.

HIV, human immunodeficiency virus; IND, investigational new drug; NCI, National Cancer Institute; NDA, new drug application; NIH, National Institutes of Health; NIAID, National Institute of Allergy and Infectious Diseases; PAD, peripheral arterial disease.

the products. The plasmid biopharmaceutical Collategene, which encodes the hepatocyte growth factor (HGF) and is being codeveloped by AnGes and Vical to treat PAD, might be one of such products (see Chapter 9, Section 9.3). The plasmid has proved its safety and efficacy in a phase 3 trial conducted in Japan, and consequently, AnGes has submitted a new drug application (NDA) to competent authorities.[63] The same product is undergoing phase 2 trials in the United States. Another plasmid biopharmaceutical that is closer to getting regulatory approval is Vical's melanoma cancer vaccine, Allovectin-7. The product has successfully completed the first two phases of clinical development and is currently undergoing phase 3 studies. Like Allovectin-7, a significant number of the prototype plasmid products under development that are listed in Table 8.2 fall within the category of therapeutic cancer vaccines.

8.6   CONCLUSIONS

The market opportunities for those plasmid biopharmaceuticals that can be judged efficient and safe are huge, both in the context of management of communicable (infectious) and noncommunicable (chronic) human diseases. The impact of plasmid biopharmaceuticals in veterinary health (and indirectly in human health) may also be significant. However, it is difficult to estimate how the plasmid biopharmaceutical market will evolve in the coming years. What is clear is that there are a substantial number of opportunities, both in the veterinary and human healthcare arenas. Veterinary products like DNA vaccines are likely to enter the market more easily, whereas human products for therapy or prevention will continue to face many of the obstacles (lack of efficacy, regulation, and ethics) that have precluded their success up to now. The highest revenues will likely come from the human market, and especially from those plasmid biopharmaceuticals designed for the management of chronic diseases like cancer or cardiovascular disease. The highest impact on society and humankind as a whole, however, will occur if a DNA vaccine against a major disease like AIDS or malaria finds its way through the scientific, technological, and regulatory maze that is still ahead. Although data are scarce at this time, the plasmid biopharmaceutical market is likely to reach hundreds of million dollars during the coming decade.

REFERENCES

1. Danzon P, Towse MA. The economics of gene therapy and of pharmacogenetics. *Value in Health*. 2002;5:5–13.
2. World Health Organization. *The world health report 2008: Primary healthcare now more than ever*. Geneva: World Health Organization, 2008.
3. World Health Organization. *World health statistics 2008. Part 2: Global health indicators*. Geneva: World Health Organization, 2008.

4. Ryan F. *Virus X: Understanding the real threat of the new pandemic plagues*. London: HarperCollins, 1998.

5. Mangili A, Gendreau MA. Transmission of infectious diseases during commercial air travel. *Lancet*. 2005;365:989–996.

6. World Health Organization. *The global burden of disease: 2004 update*. Geneva: World Health Organization, 2008.

7. Mullin D. Prometheus in Gloucestershire: Edward Jenner, 1749–1823. *Journal of Allergy and Clinical Immunology*. 2003;112:810–814.

8. Bordenave G. Louis Pasteur (1822–1895). *Microbes and Infection*. 2003;5: 553–560.

9. Gradmann C. Robert Koch and the white death: From tuberculosis to tuberculin. *Microbes and Infection*. 2006;8:294–301.

10. Pearce JM. Salk and Sabin: Poliomyelitis immunisation. *Journal of Neurology, Neurosurgery, and Psychiatry*. 2004;75:1552.

11. Liu MA. Overview of DNA vaccines. *Annals of the New York Academy of Sciences*. 1995;772:15–20.

12. Andre FE. Vaccinology: Past achievements, present roadblocks and future promises. *Vaccine*. 2003;21:593–595.

13. World Health Organization and United Nations Children's Fund. GIVS: Global immunization vision and strategy 2006–2015. Geneva and New York, October 2005.

14. Bloom DE, Canning D, Weston M. The value of vaccination. *World Economics*. 2005;6:15–39.

15. Danzon PM, Pereira NS, Tejwani SS. Vaccine supply: A cross-national perspective. *Health Affairs (Millwood)*. 2005;24:706–717.

16. Robinson HL, Ginsberg HS, Davis HL, Johnston SA, Liu MA. *The scientific future of DNA for immunization*. Washington, DC: American Society of Microbiology, 1997.

17. Butler D. Lost in translation. *Nature*. 2007;449:158–159.

18. Neumann G, Noda T, Kawaoka Y. Emergence and pandemic potential of swine-origin H1N1 influenza virus. *Nature*. 2009;459:931–939.

19. Milstien J, Lambert S. Emergency response vaccines—A challenge for the public sector and the vaccine industry. *Vaccine*. 2002;21:146–154.

20. Frost & Sullivan. Global vaccines markets (report no. F499-52). Palo Alto, CA, 2006.

21. Dorland Healthcare Information. *The medical & healthcare marketplace guide*, 19th ed. Philadelphia: Dorland Healthcare Information, 2004.

22. Sheridan C. The business of making vaccines. *Nature Biotechnology*. 2005;23: 1359–1366.

23. Giri M, Ugen KE, Weiner DB. DNA vaccines against human immunodeficiency virus type 1 in the past decade. *Clinical Microbiology Reviews*. 2004;17:370–389.

24. Duenas-Carrera S. DNA vaccination against hepatitis C. *Current Opinion in Molecular Therapy*. 2004;6:146–150.

25. Haile M, Kallenius G. Recent developments in tuberculosis vaccines. *Current Opinion in Infectious Disease*. 2005;18:211–215.

26. Drape RJ, Macklin MD, Barr LJ, Jones S, Haynes JR, Dean HJ. Epidermal DNA vaccine for influenza is immunogenic in humans. *Vaccine*. 2006;24:4475–4481.

27. Luxembourg A, Hannaman D, Nolan E, et al. Potentiation of an anthrax DNA vaccine with electroporation. *Vaccine*. 2008;26:5216–5222.

28. Sullivan NJ, Sanchez A, Rollin PE, Yang ZY, Nabel GJ. Development of a preventive vaccine for Ebola virus infection in primates. *Nature*. 2000;408:605–609.

29. Imoto J, Konishi E. Dengue tetravalent DNA vaccine increases its immunogenicity in mice when mixed with a dengue type 2 subunit vaccine or an inactivated Japanese encephalitis vaccine. *Vaccine*. 2007;25:1076–1084.

30. Zhai YZ, Li XM, Zhou Y, Ma L, Feng GH. Intramuscular immunization with a plasmid DNA vaccine encoding prM-E protein from Japanese encephalitis virus: Enhanced immunogenicity by co-administration of GM-CSF gene and genetic fusions of prM-E protein and GM-CSF. *Intervirology*. 2009;52:152–163.

31. Martin JE, Pierson TC, Hubka S, et al. A West Nile virus DNA vaccine induces neutralizing antibody in healthy adults during a phase 1 clinical trial. *Journal of Infectious Diseases*. 2007;196:1732–1740.

32. Goldman DP, Shang B, Bhattacharya J, et al. Consequences of health trends and medical innovation for the future elderly. *Health Affairs (Millwood)*. 2005;24(Suppl 2):W5R5–W517.

33. Edelstein ML, Abedi MR, Wixon J. Gene therapy clinical trials worldwide to 2007—An update. *The Journal of Gene Medicine*. 2007;9:833–842.

34. Ramsey S. What do we want from our investment in cancer research? *Health Affairs (Millwood)*. 2005;24(Suppl 2):W5R101–W5R104.

35. Shekelle PG, Ortiz E, Newberry SJ, et al. Identifying potential health care innovations for the future elderly. *Health Affairs (Millwood)*. 2005;24(Suppl. 2):W5R67–W5R76.

36. Dishart KL, Work LM, Denby L, Baker AH. Gene therapy for cardiovascular disease. *Journal of Biomedicine and Biotechnology*. 2003;2003:138–148.

37. Hoeben RC, Schagen FHE, Van der Eb MM, Fallaux FJ, Van der Eb AJ, Hormondt HV. Gene therapy for haemophilia. In: Meager A, ed. *Gene therapy technologies, applications and regulations*. Chichester: John Wiley & Sons, 1999:195–206.

38. Caplen N. Cystic fibrosis: Gene therapy approaches. In: Meager A, ed. *Gene therapy technologies, applications and regulations*. Chichester: John Wiley & Sons, 1999:207–226.

39. Thrasher AJ, Gaspar HB, Kinnon Ć. Gene therapy for severe combined immunodeficiency. In: Meager A, ed. *Gene therapy technologies, applications and regulations*. Chichester: John Wiley & Sons, 1999:179–193.

40. Lashford LS, Fairbairn LJ, Wraith JE. Lysosomal storage disorders. In: Meager A, ed. *Gene therapy technologies, applications and regulations*. Chichester: John Wiley & Sons, 1999:267–290.

41. Murphy S, Dickson G. Gene therapy approaches to Duchenne muscular dystrophy. In: Meager A, ed. *Gene therapy technologies, applications and regulations*. Chichester: John Wiley & Sons Ltd, 1999:243–266.

42. Frost & Sullivan. World gene therapy market (report no. F300-52). Palo Alto, CA, 2005.

43. Kahn LH. Confronting zoonoses, linking human and veterinary medicine. *Emerging Infectious Diseases*. 2006;12:556–561.

44. Kiple K. *Plague, pox and pestilence*. London: Weidenfeld & Nicolson, 1997.

45. Hughes JM, Peters CJ, Cohen ML, Mahy BW. Hantavirus pulmonary syndrome: An emerging infectious disease. *Science*. 1993;262:850–851.

46. Enserink M. Infectious diseases. Chikungunya: No longer a third world disease. *Science*. 2007;318:1860–1861.

47. Otte J, Roland-Holst D, Pfeiffer D, et al. *Industrial livestock production and global health risks*. Baltimore, MD: John Hopkins University Bloomberg School of Public Health, 2007.

48. Ferguson NM, Donnelly CA, Anderson RM. The foot-and-mouth epidemic in Great Britain: Pattern of spread and impact of interventions. *Science*. 2001;292: 1155–1160.

49. Meeusen EN, Walker J, Peters A, Pastoret PP, Jungersen G. Current status of veterinary vaccines. *Clinical Microbiology Reviews*. 2007;20:489–510, table of contents.

50. American Veterinary Medical Association. *U.S. pet ownership & demographics sourcebook*. Schaumburg, IL: AVMA, 2007.

51. Frost & Sullivan. *European companion animal product markets: Competitive benchmarking*, Vol. 1. Palo Alto, CA: Frost & Sullivan, 1996.

52. Lorenzen N, LaPatra SE. DNA vaccines for aquacultured fish. *Revue Scientifique et Technique*. 2005;24:201–213.

53. Heldens JG, Patel JR, Chanter N, et al. Veterinary vaccine development from an industrial perspective. *Veterinary Journal*. 2008;178:7–20.

54. Wesley T. *Animal pharm reports: Veterinary vaccines*. London: T&F Informa, 2005.

55. Research and Markets. *Veterinary vaccines*. Dublin: Research and Markets, 2008.

56. Anonymous. *West Nile-Innovator DNA—The first USDA approved DNA vaccine*. Fort Dodge, IA: Fort Dodge Animal Health, 2008.

57. Dhama K, Mahendran M, Gupta PK, Rai A. DNA vaccines and their applications in veterinary practice: Current perspectives. *Veterinary Research Communications*. 2008;32:341–356.

58. Beard CW, Mason PW. Out on the farm with DNA vaccines. *Nature Biotechnology*. 1998;16:1325–1328.

59. Krishnan BR. Current status of DNA vaccines in veterinary medicine. *Advanced Drug Delivery Reviews*. 2000;43:3–11.

60. Felgner PL, Gadek TR, Holm M, et al. Lipofection: A highly efficient, lipid-mediated DNA-transfection procedure. *Proceedings of the National Academy of Sciences of the United States of America*. 1987;84:7413–7417.

61. Key P. Penn: Tech-transfer hotbed. *Philadelphia Business Journal*. September 13, 2002.

62. Person R, Bodles-Brakhop AM, Pope MA, Brown PA, Khan AS, Draghia-Akli R. Growth hormone-releasing hormone plasmid treatment by electroporation decreases offspring mortality over three pregnancies. *Molecular Therapy*. 2008;16: 1891–1897.

63. Kim S, Peng Z, Kaneda Y. Current status of gene therapy in Asia. *Molecular Therapy*. 2008;16:237–243.

9

Human Case Studies: Pandemic Influenza and Critical Limb Ischemia

9.1 INTRODUCTION

Plasmid biopharmaceuticals have a number of specific attributes that may render them especially adequate to manage certain diseases. Given the wide variety of illnesses that are potentially addressable by plasmid biopharmaceuticals (see Chapter 2), the characteristics of a plasmid that might be advantageous in a specific case are not necessarily the ones that will favor the development of a product in another situation. For example, the context in which a prophylactic DNA vaccine is likely to be used is, in principle, very different from the one where a therapeutic DNA vaccine could be beneficial. In the first situation, the vaccine is administered to healthy individuals as a preventive measure against an infectious disease, whereas in the second case, a therapeutic action is taken to treat a particular medical condition that affects patients. Accordingly, a limited number of administrations are to be expected in the case of prophylactic DNA vaccines. The uses of other plasmid biopharmaceuticals, on the other hand, and especially for the conditions against which they are currently being developed (e.g., cancer and cardiovascular disease) are likely to require chronic administration.

In this chapter, we will examine two case studies that underscore some of the competitive advantages of plasmid biopharmaceuticals when compared to

Plasmid Biopharmaceuticals: Basics, Applications, and Manufacturing, First Edition.
Duarte Miguel F. Prazeres.
© 2011 John Wiley & Sons, Inc. Published 2011 by John Wiley & Sons, Inc.

the existing therapeutic/prophylactic alternatives. The two cases are representative of the major categories of diseases described in Chapters 2 and 8: communicable and noncommunicable diseases. In the first part of the chapter, we examine the potential of the highly pathogenic avian influenza virus H5N1 to mutate into a pandemic (i.e., a geographically widespread epidemic) influenza strain and to spread havoc among the world population. The inevitability of such a global flu pandemic, as it was classified by the World Health Organization (WHO) in 2005,[1] has prompted a number of research institutions and firms to develop scientific and technological platforms to support the swift development, deployment, and mass production of a cost-effective vaccine. The relevancy of this issue increased dramatically with the very recent emergence, in April 2009, of a H1N1 virus of swine origin. This new virus spread so rapidly among humans that it prompted the WHO to declare the first flu pandemic in 40 years.[2] A number of arguments will be presented in this chapter that support DNA vaccines as one of the best choices to protect millions of individuals during the critical early months of a future pandemic outbreak.[3] The drawbacks of DNA vaccines in the same context are also presented alongside.

The second case study deals with critical limb ischemia (CLI), a cardiovascular disease that affects numerous people worldwide and remains difficult to treat. Gene transfer has been studied both at preclinical and clinical levels as an alternative to conventional approaches used in the treatment of CLI. The lead taken by plasmids when compared to recombinant viruses as gene transfer vectors is directly linked to their safety profile and to the transient nature of the treatment required. The rationale behind the plasmid-based management of CLI will be presented, together with the progress made so far in the development of specific products.

9.2   PANDEMIC INFLUENZA

9.2.1   Influenza

Influenza, or flu as it is more popularly known, is a viral disease usually transmitted from human to human via droplets released by coughing, sneezing, or breathing. The disease is recurrent on a yearly basis, affecting some 500 million people (approximately 10% of the world's population) and usually peaking somewhere during the colder months.[4] The most common symptoms of flu are runny nose, sore throat, fever, chills, and aching muscles and joints. The incubation period is from 1 to 2 days, and patients typically regain their normal health status after a week or so.[5] The characteristic explosive nature of influenza, which is related to its short incubation period and contagiousness, produces epidemics that sweep over entire populations very rapidly. The death rate associated with seasonal influenza is less than 0.1%, with most victims being either very young or very old.[2] The disease is particularly dangerous when complicated by coinfection with bacterial pneumonia.[5]

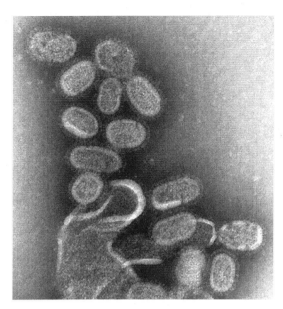

Figure 9.1   *Negative stained transmission electron micrograph (TEM) of recreated 1918 influ-enza virions (courtesy of Dr. Terrence Tumpey, Centers for Disease Control and Prevention, Atlanta, Georgia).*

The exact geographic origin of influenza is unknown, but it is more or less consensual that the disease emerged somewhere in Europe, Africa, or Asia.[5] Historical records have described the occurrence of several epidemics and pandemics of flu at irregular intervals over the centuries. The 1918–1919 pandemic was unprecedented because it killed an estimated 40–50 million people worldwide[1,2] (Figure 9.1). The global attack rate (i.e., the percentage of the population who fell ill) of that pandemic was also high, with one-fifth of the world's human population becoming infected in less than 1 year.[6] Another distinctive characteristic of the 1918 flu was the fact that, unlike what normally occurs with seasonal flu, most of its victims were between 20 and 40 years old.[5] The 1918 pandemic became known as the "Spanish flu," not because Spain was the epicenter of the outbreak, but rather because in a time when the world was engulfed by the First World War, the neutral Spain was one of the few countries that did not censor reports on the invasion of the country by the disease.[1,6] The high-profile Spanish news coverage thus associated the name of the country with the disease.

Influenza viruses are enveloped viruses containing negative-sense seg-mented RNA genomes that belong to the Orthomyxoviridae family. Three genera are known to cause the disease: A, B, and C. Influenza B and C are essentially human viruses that cause mild respiratory illness (C) or eventually, a more severe respiratory disease (B). Influenza A, on the other hand, is clearly the most problematic member in the family in terms of disease acuteness and pandemic potential. This is due to the fact that influenza A is able to evolve much more rapidly when compared with influenza B and C[1]. A wide variety of mammals (pigs, horses, sea mammals, etc.) and birds (both domestic and wild) are also susceptible to infection by influenza A[7]. Extensive genetic evidence suggests that the influenza A viruses that infect mammals, including humans, have their origin in aquatic birds (ducks, gulls, and geese). Although influenza A is found across a multitude of organisms, some species are not susceptible to influenza viruses that infect other species. For example, transmission of influenza from pigs to humans is a known fact, whereas human infection with avian influenza viruses is a rare event, limited to a few virus subtypes.[8] These transmission patterns are consistent with laboratorial observations, which show that influenza A viruses from aquatic birds replicate poorly in human cells and vice versa, and that both expand very well in pig cells.[6]

The ability of influenza A viruses to change and their versatility in terms of the range of species infected are intimately linked to their molecular structure. The genome of the typical influenza A virus contains eight single-stranded negative-sense RNA segments that encode 11 known polypeptides. Two glycoproteins that spike out of the virus surface are especially important due to their ability to elicit protective immune responses in infected recipients: hemagglutinin (HA) and neuraminidase (NA). From a functional point of view, HA is responsible for virus binding to cellular receptors and entry into cells via endocytosis, whereas NA facilitates and controls the release of newly formed viruses from infected cells by cleaving sialic acids from HA and NA.[1,2] The two proteins constitute the major antigenic targets for the immune system of the afflicted host when it responds to an infection. This antigenicity of the two proteins forms the basis of the classification of individual virus strains of influenza A into subtypes. According to this classification, a given strain is identified by the letters H and N followed by the number of the subtype. The Spanish flu of 1918–1919, for example, was caused by an avian-like H1N1 influenza A virus.[2] Sixteen HA subtypes (H1–H16) and nine NA subtypes (N1–N9) are currently recognized.[2]

Influenza viruses are continually evolving, either through major changes (antigenic shift) or through slight alterations (antigenic drift) in their viral structure.[6] An antigenic shift occurs when a virus with a new HA, with or without an accompanying new NA, emerges. The surfacing of new HA and NA subtypes constitutes a strong indication that a pandemic may be lurking around the corner. Nevertheless, the dissemination of a new subtype will depend on whether the virus is able to pass from human to human and whether the population lacks immunity against the new viral strain.[3,7] Antigenic shifts are thought to originate when human and avian viruses coincide in one animal host, usually the pig, or less commonly in humans. At this time, the viruses reshuffle and a new strain appears.

Slight alterations are also continually taking place in and around the antibody recognition sites of the HA and NA antigens, through pinpoint changes in some amino acids. This process is known as antigenic drift and allows the modified virus to escape neutralization by antibodies generated during a previous episode of the infection. Thanks to this selective pressure, which is imposed by the immune system of the infected host, the population of newly modified viruses will eventually take over the pre-existing ones. This genetic instability is responsible for the short-lived immunity, which is elicited during each episode of the disease. Hence, influenza outbreaks are recurrent and, as a consequence, vaccines have to be produced specifically for every flu season and are used to reimmunize risk groups every year.

9.2.2 The H5N1 Influenza Pandemic Fear

The unparalleled poultry mortality recorded in Asia in the recent years ignited the fear that a world influenza pandemic, caused by a highly pathogenic and transmissible avian flu virus, could hit the globe.[1] Far from being irrational, this fear was and is real and supports itself on the basis of historic evidence, which shows that influenza pandemics arise, on average, three to four times each century. In the twentieth century, for example, the Spanish flu occurred in 1918–1919, the "Asian" flu in 1957–1958 and the "Hong Kong" flu in 1968–1969. The current concerns of a pandemic influenza started more precisely in 1997, with the emergence of a highly pathogenic form of an avian strain of the influenza A virus in Hong Kong poultry farms and live markets. The mortality of chicken infected with this strain was close to 100%. Avian influenza viruses do not usually infect humans, but on that year, 18 cases were recorded, 6 of which were fatal. The serologic analysis of viral material isolated from a patient revealed that the virus belonged to the H5N1 subtype.[9] This highly pathogenic virus subtype had first been identified in Scottish chicken in 1959. From then on, and until the 1997 outbreaks, the activity of H5N1 among birds was almost inexistent. In order to control the epidemic in poultry, and in view of the potential danger posed to humans, the Hong Kong authorities took swift action, destroying close to 1.5 million birds. The virus then became dormant for some years, but subsequently re-emerged in 2003–2004, hitting different Southeast Asian countries (Thailand, Vietnam, China, Indonesia, etc.) in the following years.[3,7] The 2004 outbreaks of H5N1 influenza in poultry were historically unprecedented. Within 3 months, more than 120 million birds died as a result of direct infection or destruction by health authorities. At the time, the number of human cases also constituted a record of human infection with an avian influenza virus—46 cases were registered, of which 32 were fatal.[10] Such a high mortality among the infected is one of the most striking features of H5N1 infection in humans.[1] From 2004 on, outbreaks of avian influenza (H5N1) in poultry have never ceased to occur. Although Asian countries remained the epicenter of viral activity, the infection moved progressively toward the west into countries from Europe, the Middle East, and Africa in a series of waves[8] (Figure 9.2). The virus has also been detected in a number of wild bird species across different countries. The trade of contaminated poultry and poultry products and the circulation of people and equipment have been pinpointed as the most likely cause for transmission. Additionally, migratory birds may have also contributed to the spreading of the virus over extended

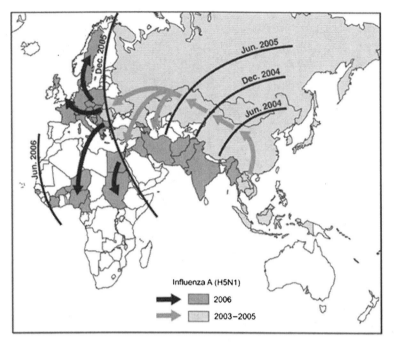

Figure 9.2 *Geographic distributions of cases of avian influenza A (H5N1) in wild birds and poultry, December 2003–May 2006. The solid lines (isochrones) show the approximate position of the panzootic wave front at 6-month intervals, whereas arrows indicate the inferred corridors of virus diffusion. Reprinted from Annals of the Association of American Geographers, 98, Smallman-Raynor M, Cliff AD. The geographical spread of avian influenza A (H5N1): panzootic transmission (December 2003-May 2006), pandemic potential, and implications, 553-582, Copyright 2008,[8] Association of American Geographers, reprinted by permission of Taylor & Francis Ltd., (http:// www.tandf.co.uk/journals) on behalf of the Association of American Geographers.*

distances.[8] As a direct or indirect result of the disease, hundreds of millions of poultry heads were lost in only 4 years, causing declines in stocks as high as 20% in severely affected countries like Thailand and Vietnam[8]. The implications for the international poultry market (valued at more than US$10 billion per year) and trade were also significant. The overall economic costs incurred since 2004 have been estimated to be higher than $10 billion. Furthermore, a restructuring of the international trade flows of poultry products took place, shifting the leading producers from Asia to countries like Brazil.[11]

The yearly outbreaks of avian influenza recorded since 2004 were always accompanied by episodes of human infection, which affected mostly children and young adults, and usually occurred in family clusters and in the winter/ spring months.[8] A total number of 494 cases were recorded in more than 15 countries from January 2004 to May 6, 2010 (Figure 9.3). Of these, 290 cases resulted in the death of the patients, setting the fatality rate of human cases of avian influenza A (H5N1) at 59%.[10] This high fatality rate is a strong indication that natural immunity against H5N1 is largely lacking in human popula-

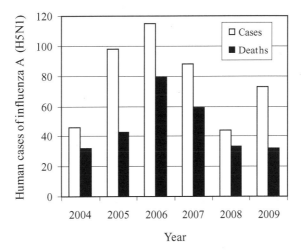

Figure 9.3 *Cumulative number of laboratory-confirmed human cases of avian influenza A (H5N1) reported to the World Health Organization as of May 6, 2010.[10] The total number of cases includes number of deaths and dates refer to the onset of illness.*

tions. Clinically, the disease is characterized by the typical influenza symptoms, breathing difficulties and the development of pneumonia. In most cases, death occurs 9–10 days after the onset of the disease, primarily due to progressive respiratory failure.[8] The available epidemiological evidence indicates that humans typically become infected with H5N1 via direct or close contact with sick or dead poultry.[12] For the time being, there is no data supporting the sustained human-to-human transmission of H5N1 virus, even though rare cases have been described in some family clusters. However, if the H5N1 virus adapts itself sufficiently to spread from human to human, a pandemic is almost inevitable. Since absence of immunity in the general population is almost warranted, the virus will likely spread over the world in months or even weeks due to the intensity of transcontinental air travel and commerce.[13]

The worldwide mortality associated with an influenza pandemic will depend on the lethality of the virus.[14] According to the WHO, if a mild pandemic like the 1968 one emerges, the number of deaths could be anywhere between 2.0 and 7.4 million. However, projections that assume the global spreading of a highly virulent virus like the one responsible for the 1918 Spanish flu estimate that deaths could reach a staggering 70 million.[14] Still, influenza is not a particularly deadly infectious disease, with mortality rates typically falling in the 0.1–2.0% range. Even the mortality rate of the 1918–1919 flu, one of the deadliest ever recorded, has been estimated at a meager 2.5%.[2] This shies away in comparison with case fatality rates of viral infectious diseases like the Zairian Ebola, which killed 90% of those infected in 1976.[15] Rather, what makes pandemic influenza a high-impact and extremely dangerous disease is its highly contagious nature, which translates into a high attack rate; that is, millions become easily infected over a short period of time. A similar situation occurs every year with seasonal influenza—millions are infected by the virus, and for this reason, thousands die, even though the fatality rate is low.

9.2.3 Pandemic Preparedness

As is usual with pandemics, the economic impact would also be tremendous, not only due to death, illness, worker absenteeism, hospitalization, and efforts to avoid and control infection but also as a consequence of the disruption of commerce, services, travel, and other aspects of life in society. According to World Bank estimates, the direct and indirect costs of a severe influenza pandemic would amount to $1.25–$2.00 trillion, which is equivalent to 3–5% of the global domestic product.[16] These figures underscore dramatically the need for countries and international organizations to prepare and plan for an eventual outbreak. The close monitoring and control of the avian H5N1 virus in the source animals can prevent the occurrence of an influenza pandemic, and for this reason, the setup of an adequate surveillance system is key to any pandemic preparedness plan.[13] At a global level, the Global Influenza Surveillance Network of the WHO*, which recommends twice annually the content of the influenza vaccine for the subsequent influenza season, serves also as a global alert mechanism for the emergence of influenza viruses with pandemic potential. However, if surveillance actions are not effective enough to prevent the disease from spreading, the best strategy to manage the pandemic is to take active and aggressive prophylactic measures to protect populations at risk from infection and to reduce morbidity and mortality. Although a number of public health measures such as social distancing will certainly play an important role, the use of drugs and vaccines will be inevitable. This has actually been confirmed by the course of events that took place in response to the H1N1 influenza A of 2009.

Antiviral drugs have been highlighted as one of the most important medical interventions under pandemic conditions, especially during the first waves of infection when vaccines are not yet available.[1] This expectation is based on the fact that some antivirals have proven effective in the treatment and prevention of seasonal influenza. When used for therapeutic purposes, antivirals must be administered shortly after the symptoms of infection become apparent. An aggressive mass administration of antivirals within communities where cases of pandemic influenza might start to accumulate could also contribute to reduce the opportunities for the virus to improve its transmissibility. Thus, if adequate antiviral drugs are stockpiled in prepandemic periods, sufficient amounts could be ready to use in the first weeks of the disease while the pandemic strain is being identified and vaccines are being produced. The expectation is that for each day gained by the use of antivirals, a couple of million extra doses of vaccines can be manufactured. However, a number of uncertain-

* http://www.who.int/csr/disease/influenza/surveillance/en/, accessed on January 18, 2009.

ties are associated with the use of antivirals. For once, the new virus subtype might be resistant to available drugs. Additionally, since antiviral protection is usually short-lived when the drug is taken for a short period, prophylatic administration should be regular while the disease is spreading.[13] Also, the therapeutic impact of antivirals will be highly dependent on the ability to identify cases of the disease and to administer the drug rapidly, a task that might be difficult to accomplish in a situation where the disease is spreading very fast. The NA inhibitors oseltamivir and zanamivir are probably the most effective antivirals available, even though they are more expensive when compared with older drugs.[1]

Some suggestions have also been made that statins, a set of drugs with anti-inflammatory and antioxidative properties commonly used to prevent cardiovascular disease, could reduce mortality from pandemic influenza among patients.[17] One of the great advantages of statins is the fact that many of them are produced and distributed worldwide as generics to treat millions of people. Therefore, if the epidemiological signals of protection obtained in preliminary studies are confirmed, statins could be promptly made available globally at a considerable lower cost compared with antivirals. However, the value of statins to influenza patients needs to be fully assessed with more epidemiological, animal, and clinical studies.[17]

Despite the role that antiviral drugs (and eventually, statins) might play during the earlier stages of the pandemic, vaccines are clearly the best option to prevent the spread of the disease. A key advantage, when compared with antivirals, is that vaccines will probably be more effective in the longer run, while simultaneously providing long-term immunity.[13] The major problem with the vaccination approach has to do with the fact that an effective and true pandemic vaccine can only be prepared once the pandemic strain is identified and isolated. Although "mock-up" vaccines providing protection against the circulating H5N1 subtypes can be developed, produced, and stored in advance, their effectiveness is unpredictable since there is no guarantee that the reassortant pandemic virus will be antigenically equivalent.[1,7] Clearly, the best option will be to develop a vaccine for the specific pandemic strain once it emerges.

9.2.4 Influenza Vaccine Platforms

One of the key decisions to be made in preparation for a pandemic scenario will be to decide which types of vaccines to deploy and which manufacturing technology to use. The importance of this assessment has to do with the fact that (1) the effectiveness of the vaccine will depend on the type of vaccine made and that (2) the manufacturing technology used will dictate the amount of vaccine doses that can be made in the short time available. The influenza vaccines available in the market or under development can be broadly divided into six types, according to the nature of the "active principle" they contain: (1) inactivated vaccines (whole virion or split), (2) live attenuated vaccines,

TABLE 9.1. Vaccine Technologies under Consideration for Pandemic Influenza

Platform	Vaccine Type
Embryonated eggs	Inactivated whole virion, inactivated split virus, inactivated antigens, live attenuated
Mammalian cells	Inactivated whole virion, inactivated split virus, inactivated antigens, live attenuated, viral vector based
Insect cells	Virus-like particles (VLPs), recombinant antigen
Yeast	Recombinant antigen
Bacteria	Recombinant antigen, plasmid DNA

Source: Adapted from Thomas et al.[22]

(3) virus-like particle (VLP) vaccines, (4) recombinant antigen vaccines, (5) DNA vaccines, and (6) viral vector-based vaccines. The first two types of influenza vaccines are clinically used on a regular basis, whereas the others are undergoing preclinical and clinical development.[18] A number of platforms are available to produce the different types of influenza vaccines, all of which might be considered in a pandemic scenario (Table 9.1).

If an influenza pandemic emerges, the first and most obvious option would be to explore the experience and installed manufacturing capacity of established pharmaceutical companies like Chiron, GlaxoSmithKline, and Sanofi Pasteur that are used to produce the regular seasonal flu vaccine every year. The WHO international surveillance system alluded to in the previous section plays a key role in the process by identifying which of the new strains of the circulating influenza virus should be included in the vaccine for the coming year. On the basis of these recommendations, candidate high-growth seed strains of attenuated influenza viruses are prepared by genetic reassortment, a process that combines viral segments that code for the HA and NA antigens of the circulating strains with segments from different vaccine strains.[4,18] The recombinant virus may be further attenuated by mutating specific amino acids in key proteins.[18] Vaccine manufacturers then have approximately 6 months to produce and distribute the vaccines. This production cycle is repeated twice a year, once in the Northern hemisphere and once in the Southern hemisphere.[19] The seasonal influenza vaccines are typically produced in bulk by growing the selected and modified seed strain in the allantoic cavity of embryonated chicken eggs. Following harvest of the injected eggs, different methodologies can be used to prepare different types of vaccines (e.g., inactivated whole or split virus and inactivated surface antigens). For example, the virus can be inactivated by formalin or β-propriolactone and can be purified by ultracentrifugation.[19] Next, antigen fractions are prepared by splitting the viral particles with ether or detergent, and an equivalent 15 μg of HA antigen is formulated into a monovalent vaccine.[20] One egg typically produces material sufficient for three of such doses. Alternatively, trivalent vaccines can be produced by combining 15 μg of HA antigen from three strains. The current capacity for the manufacturing of such egg-based vaccines is approximately 1 billion doses of monovalent vaccine or slightly higher than 300 million doses of trivalent vaccine.[20] The whole process of producing egg-based influenza vaccines, including the management of the egg supply organization, has to be carefully planned in advanced so that the market demand is met at the proper time.[4] Even so, problems with lack of manufacturing consistency and poor yields are a common concern.[21]

Although egg-based vaccines have a proven 60-year-long track record, a number of problems may limit their use in the context of a pandemic influenza emergency: (1) The candidate vaccine has to grow well in eggs; (2) a steady supply of healthy eggs must be available; (3) the biological safety containment of the viral strains has to be guaranteed; and (4) mass production capabilities have to be in place. These caveats, together with a number of effectiveness and tolerability limitations of egg-based vaccines, have supported investments in alternative vaccine and manufacturing technologies. As a result, inactivated or live attenuated vaccines can be produced nowadays by replicating the modified viral strains in cell lines derived from mammalian species that are grown in large-scale bioreactors. The procedures used to purify and inactivate the live viruses produced in the cells are roughly identical to the ones used in the egg platform. This type of manufacturing is more amenable to scale-up and is more controlled and expedite compared with egg-based production. A number of different mammalian cell platforms (e.g., Vero, PER.C6, and Madin–Darby canine kidney [MDCK]) are under development by well-established companies to take full advantage of these characteristics.[20,22] The current expectation among many of the stakeholders is that egg-grown vaccines will eventually loose their current share of the market to this type of cell-based vaccine.

The egg and cell technologies described above produce whole-virus vaccines, which are then inactivated or attenuated, and are used as such or further purified into antigenic fractions. This means that many viral components are present alongside the antigenic HA and NA proteins. An alternative to this approach would be to design vaccines containing only the key HA and NA antigens. Such antigens can be produced by recombinant DNA technology in a number of different hosts, which range from microbes (yeast and *Escherichia coli*[23]) to plant,[24] insect,[25] and mammalian cells.[26] An important advantage of this approach has to do with the fact that the recombinant antigens can be designed solely on the basis of the genetic sequence of the viral strain. Thus, since no handling of live virus is required unlike in the cases of egg-based and of most mammalian cell-based vaccines, there are no infection risks to operators in the manufacturing facility and to the people being vaccinated. The downside of this approach, however, has to do with the fact that the potency of the resulting vaccines is many times inferior when compared with the potency of traditional vaccines. An important reason for the superior immunogenicity of whole-virus attenuated vaccines is related to the fact that many of the nonantigenic virus components in these vaccines act as immunostimulators.[20] As a result, powerful adjuvants and complex delivery systems have to be included in vaccines made up of purified recombinant antigens in order to guarantee the immunogenicity of the final product. In the case of the traditional, inactivated, or live attenuated vaccines, the use of adjuvants may also contribute to decrease the amount of antigen required per dose of the vaccine. This so-called dose-sparing effect may be particularly important in the event of a pandemic, since substantially lower amounts of antigenic material would have to be produced.[18] Another way to improve the immunogenicity of influenza vaccines is to resort to expression systems that promote the assembling of particles from individual key components of the flu virus. For example, the U.S.-based company Novavax (Rockville, Maryland) uses insect cells and recombinant baculovirus to express the proteins of the outer shell (e.g., HA and NA) and core (e.g., M1) of the virus.[25] These proteins self-assemble into RNA-free VLPs, which have been claimed to trigger robust immune responses.[25]

Recombinant viruses (e.g., adenovirus and poxvirus) can also be used as vectors to transport the influenza antigenic genes to the host cells of the vaccinated individual.[18] The rationale behind this approach is to take advantage of the *in vivo* expression of the encoded antigens in order to stimulate strong humoral and cellular responses. In the case of an adenovirus encoding the HA protein from H5N1 virus, for example, this has resulted in the cross-protection of mice models against a lethal viral challenge.[27] The manufacturing of such viral vector-based influenza vaccines relies on the cultivation of appropriate mammalian cells (e.g., MDCK[27]).

Finally, DNA vaccines encoding influenza genes complete the palette of options available. Several studies have confirmed that immune responses can be elicited in several animal models using this approach (e.g., see Chen et al.[28]). Human clinical studies have also shown that DNA vaccines elicit serum HA inhibition antibody responses with only mild to moderate reactions.[29]

9.2.5   Advantages of Influenza DNA Vaccines

Developing, manufacturing, and administering a vaccine will not be an easy task given the specific characteristics of flu and the explosive and global nature of a pandemic. Apart from the safety and efficacy requirements that must be met by a pandemic vaccine, as like in the case of any other vaccine, a number of key challenges have to be addressed: (1) speed, (2) scalability, (3) biocontainment, and (4) cost.[22] A judicious assessment of the ability of a given technology to accommodate these design criteria will determine, to a large extent, whether it will be selected or discarded.

9.2.5.1   Speed

Pandemic influenza typically occurs in two or more waves of infection separated several months apart.[1] Each wave may last about 2–3 months, and generally, second and later waves are more severe in terms of mortality when compared with first waves. Thus, and although a pandemic influenza could take 18 months to run its full course, the majority of casualties and infirmity are likely to occur within the first 6 months of the outbreak (Figure 9.4). Assuming

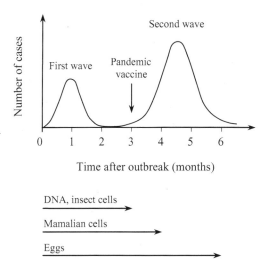

Figure 9.4 *Matching vaccine deployment and manufacturing strategy with the typical pandemic influenza epidemic curve. The average manufacturing time for the different influenza vaccine platforms available is indicated. An effective pandemic influenza vaccine should be available 3 months after the outbreak in order to maximize the number of immunized people before the second wave of infection peaks. During the first 3 months, the impact of the disease should be mitigated by taking public health measures (e.g., social confinement) and by promoting the use of antivirals and mock-up vaccines stockpiled in advance.*

that a future influenza pandemic will display a similar pattern, an effective vaccination strategy will call for the production of millions of doses of an effective vaccine within the first 6 months of an outbreak, preferably before the infection and associated mortality reaches its peak (Figure 9.4). If this calendar is not met, the impact of vaccination in the control and mitigation of the disease will be lost to a large extent.

Therefore, once the new strain is identified and isolated, the antigens have to be incorporated swiftly into a vaccine. This means that human, material, and technological resources must be available at a global scale to develop, mass produce, and equitably distribute the vaccine in a very short period (6 months). One of the major catches with egg and mammalian cell-based technologies is that they are unlikely to provide such a fast and momentous response due to the slow nature of the underlying manufacturing processes. The production cycle of egg-based vaccines, for example, typically lasts 6 months.[19] Although faster, the production of inactivated, live attenuated, and viral vector-based vaccines by mammalian cell culture is nevertheless a slow and complex process, which can take around 4 months.[30] Thus, meeting the required demand in the short time window available might be complicated.

With microbial or insect cell platforms, on the other hand, vaccines can be produced at a much faster pace (Figure 9.4). For example, the manufacturing of a vaccine based on VPLs by insect cells is expected to require from 10 to 9 weeks.[25] This includes the time needed to prepare recombinant baculovirus seed stocks and to formulate, fill, and package the final product.[25] A similar time frame of under 3 months, starting from strain identification to initiation of vaccination, has been suggested for the deployment of an influenza DNA vaccine delivered by particle bombardment.[21] Shorter manufacturing times of around 1 month have even been put forward by some authors.[31] Furthermore, when balancing DNA vaccines with *E. coli*-based recombinant antigens, it is clear that the downstream processing used to purify the former is less demanding than the one used to purify the later. Major reasons for this are the higher stability of plasmids when compared with proteins and the eventual need for refolding recombinant antigens produced in *E. coli*. Thus, the combination of cultivation of *E. coli* cells for plasmid amplification with a fast-track downstream processing renders DNA vaccines unbeatable when it comes to speed of manufacturing.

9.2.5.2 Scalability
Ideally, every people in the world should have access to an H5N1 influenza vaccine within the time frame of the pandemic. Assuming a single-dose regimen, this would mean producing, distributing, and administering 6.5 billion doses in a 6-month period. But even if the aim is to guarantee 25% worldwide coverage, that is, ~1.6 billion doses, this would mean manufacturing 60% more doses than what is currently produced for seasonal flu every year (~1 billion[20]). This tremendous challenge can only be met if the technology chosen to produce the vaccine is easy to scale up at a controlled cost. The first consideration is the volume required to manufacture the active product in the vaccine. In the case of egg-based vaccines, billions of healthy eggs would have to be available in a very short period. If in a normal situation such figures are already daunting, during an influenza pandemic, when chicken might also face health risks, this requirement is close to unpractical. Manufacturing systems in which the reassorted viral strain or the recombinant viral vector has to replicate in mammalian cell cultivated in large-scale bioreactors will also have a hard time in meeting scale.[20] A significant problem is the low productivity per liter that is characteristic of mammalian cell culture. The volumetric capacity required to produce billions of vaccine doses in less than 6 months will clearly not be available worldwide. In theory, the scale challenge will be met more easily by insect and microbial cell platforms, not only because volumetric productivities are typically higher but also because they are easier to scale.[25,32] For example, production yields of HA in insect cells have been claimed to be 7–10 times higher than with traditional mammalian cell line methods.[25] Some authors have also suggested that existing facilities used to produce antibiotics and recombinant proteins could be adapted to produce DNA vaccines in *E. coli*.[32]

The adequateness of DNA vaccines in terms of scale can be illustrated by assuming a best-case scenario wherein a single shot of a 10 μg DNA vaccine is used. The delivery of this amount of DNA via bombardment of gold particles was shown to be sufficient to elicit serum HA inhibition antibody responses

TABLE 9.2. Comparative Scalability of Different Pandemic Influenza Vaccine Platforms

Platform	Amount per Dose* (μg HA or DNA)	Amount/Egg or mL† (μg HA or DNA)	Required Capacity‡ (million eggs or m³)
Eggs	15	15§	1600
MDCK cells	15	12	4000
Insect cells	15	70	686
DNA vaccine	10	1000	32

Calculations assume a 25% worldwide coverage, that is, 1.6 billion doses of a single-shot vaccine.
*Fifteen microgram HA/dose are typical in flu vaccines[20] and 10 μg DNA/dose has led to protective antibody titers in a phase 1 trial.[29]
†Estimates made on the basis of literature data for eggs,[20] MDCK cells,[26] insect cells,[34] and DNA.[33]
‡Assumes a 50% yield in the downstream processing associated with the nonegg platforms.
§Amount after purification.

in a human study.[29] Thus, in order to guarantee 25% world coverage (1.6 billion doses), only 16 kg of plasmid DNA would have to be produced. If we further consider that fermentation yields of the order of 1 kg/m³ are becoming routine (see Chapter 13)[33] and that a 50% yield on the downstream processing is feasible, 32 m³ of cell culture would suffice to meet the demand! If one compares this with influenza vaccines containing a typical 15 μg HA/dose and produced by eggs (15 μg purified HA/egg[20]), MDCK cells (12 μg HA/mL of microcarrier culture[26]), and insect cells (70 μg HA/mL suspension culture[34]), the order-of-magnitude difference in manufacturing scale becomes evident (Table 9.2). Furthermore, the scale of DNA vaccine manufacturing would still be comparable to the best alternative (insect cells) if, by efficacy reasons, amounts of plasmid DNA per dose 20-fold higher than the 10 μg assumed become necessary.

9.2.5.3 Biocontainment

Although the pathogenicity of the viral strains used to produce inactivated and live attenuated vaccines in eggs or mammalian cell lines will be attenuated relatively to the pandemic H5N1 strain, risks to the environment will not be inexistent. This means that facilities have to be designed with a biosafety level adequate to fully contain the vaccine strains within the manufacturing space. Such requisites add complexity to the design, layout, and operation of the facility, not to mention increased costs. On the contrary, these stringent biosafety measures will not be required if vaccines based on recombinant antigens, VLPs, or plasmid DNA are selected.[25]

9.2.5.4 Cost

One of the decisive factors for selecting a pandemic influenza vaccine manufacturing platform is cost. This parameter is intricately linked to the three criteria described above. The superiority of DNA vaccines in terms of speed, scalability, and biocontainment renders them one of the best platforms in this aspect. Some estimates say that a DNA vaccine for influenza could be produced at a cost of US$9 per dose.[30] Still, due consideration should be given to the costs that might be incurred with the delivery system selected. For example, the selection of a gene gun approach to administer the DNA vaccine would bring with it the costs associated with the gold particles, holding cartridge, and device used[29] (see Chapter 6).

9.2.6 Pitfalls of Influenza DNA Vaccines

Like in the case of so many other human DNA vaccines, the first and most significant problem that has to be solved is to guarantee that a pandemic influenza DNA vaccine is effective, that is, that it confers some degree of protection to the immunized people. If this obstacle is overtaken before a pandemic hits its peak, and if sufficient doses are made available, millions of people worldwide could be immunized with DNA. Some critics have pointed that there will be safety risks associated with this type of indiscriminate mass immunization. The argument is that all results warranting safety would have been obtained from trials in a limited number of individuals, and that it could be dangerous to immunize so many people in such a short period of time with a type of vaccine (i.e., DNA vaccine) that has no track record.[30] This uncertainty and the associated fear of liability suits if anything goes wrong, could also bar manufacturers from investing in the development of a vaccine with a use essentially limited to the pandemic period.[30]

9.2.7 Putting DNA Vaccines to the Test: The H1N1 Pandemic of 2009

In the Spring of 2009, and at a time when everybody was watching carefully for the possible emergence of a highly pathogenic H5N1 influenza virus capable of warranting human-to-human transmission, an outbreak of an influenza-like respiratory illness in Mexico triggered alerts by the Centers for Disease Control (CDC) and the WHO.[2] The culprit was rapidly identified as an H1N1 influenza A virus of swine origin, which probably resulted from the reassortment of circulating swine, avian, and human viruses.[2] The disease was thus named influenza A/H1N1. Most of the infections recorded during the first 2 months since the outbreak were sufficiently mild not to require hospitalization of the afflicted individuals, who were essentially younger people under the age of 25 years.[35] Unfortunately, 2% of the cases developed into a severe illness, which typically involved a very rapid progression to life-threatening pneumonia. The biggest toll was taken on adults between the ages of 30 and 50 years.[35] This pattern emulates the one observed during the 1918–1919 H1N1 pandemic and is significantly different from that seen during epidemics of seasonal influenza, when most deaths occur in elderly people. The H1N1 virus spread so rapidly over the globe that the WHO was compelled to declare a pandemic on June 11[35] (Figure 9.5), less than 3 months after the first disease outbreak notice had been issued on April 24. As of July 6, 2009, 135 countries and overseas territories reported a total of 94,512 laboratory-confirmed cases

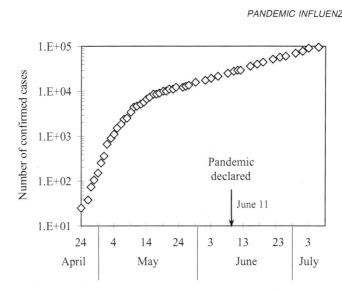

Development of Vical's H1 DNA vaccine

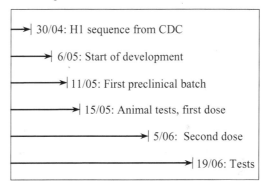

Figure 9.5 *Temporal evolution of the global number of laboratory-confirmed cases of the 2009 pandemic influenza A/H1N1. The graphic on the top of the figure was constructed with data provided by the WHO during the period spanning from the first outbreak notice (April 24) to the last detailed update provided (July 6). From this date on, on account of the rapid spreading of the disease, the WHO stopped counting individual cases. The bottom chart depicts the development of an H1 DNA vaccine undertaken by Vical Inc. (based on information provided in news releases issued by the company[40–42]).*

of pandemic H1N1, including 429 deaths.[36] By this time, the exponential increase in the number of cases prompted the WHO to recommend the most afflicted countries to stop trying to account and to confirm all cases through laboratory testing.[37] According to the WHO, the dissemination of the new H1N1 worldwide was unprecedented since in past pandemics, more than 6 months had been required for the virus to spread to the same geographic extent.[37] Fortunately, and as a result of the efforts developed in the previous years in anticipation of an H5N1 pandemic, the international community was not caught off guard since an adequate surveillance and response system had been mounted in many countries. In spite of its explosive nature, it became apparent in early 2010 that the H1N1 pandemic was not as severe as initially feared. As a consequence, the WHO, health officials, and pharmaceutical companies were eventually accused of having overrated the situation. By May 2, 2010, over 18,000 deaths had been reported worldwide, with more than 214 countries with laboratory-confirmed cases.[38]

As soon as the pandemic potential of the new H1N1 strain became apparent, major relevant stakeholders worldwide, and most notably the large vaccine manufacturers, started congregating efforts with the goal of developing an effective vaccine. Although a strong focus was placed by manufacturers in developing vaccines for production in eggs and cell-based platforms, at least two companies that are active in the plasmid biopharmaceutical area (see Chapter 8, Section 8.5), Vical Inc. (San Diego, California) and Inovio Biomedical Corporation (San Diego, California), initiated programs to develop DNA vaccines against H1N1 influenza.[39,40] In this regard, it is instructive to review the information available regarding the pace of development of Vical's prototype since this illustrates very well the speed with which a DNA vaccine can be developed (Figure 9.5).[40–42] The progress in the development of the vaccine is schematically shown on the bottom part of Figure 9.5 and in parallel with the graphic, which depicts the evolution of the number of laboratory-confirmed cases worldwide. According to the news release documents issued by the company, a collaborative H1N1 vaccine development program with the U.S. Naval Medical Research Center started in the beginning of May.[40] As a first step, and on the basis of the gene sequence provided by the CDC for the selected A/H1N1 influenza strain on April 30, a prototype DNA vaccine containing the H1 HA was constructed. A first preclinical batch of research-grade material was then produced on May 11, and two parallel immunogenicity studies in animals started on May 15, around 1 month before the declaration of the pandemic status by the WHO[42] (Figure 9.5). The vaccine, which is formulated with Vical's patented Vaxfectin® adjuvant, was administered in groups of mice and rabbits according to a standard pandemic influenza vaccination regimen, with a first dose on day 0 and a second one on day 21.[41] An analysis of animal sera collected 2 weeks after the second dose showed that the prototype vaccine had the potential to provide protection against the H1N1 virus in 100% of the animals.[41] Thus, vaccine production and successful immunogenicity testing in animals was completed very rapidly, making the company ready to advance to human clinical trials in less than 2 months. In the subsequent months, however, and probably due to the lack of track record and absence of funding, the development of DNA vaccines was overtaken by conventional, egg-based vaccines, with the first doses of the latter becoming available to the general population by October. It was only in October 1 that Vical announced that the U.S. Navy awarded the company $1.25 million to support large-scale good manufacturing practice (GMP) vaccine manufacturing and related clinical and regulatory preparations for a clinical trial.[43] In May 2010, the company reported the initiation of a double-blind, placebo-controlled phase 1 trial at a U.S. clinical site. According to a news release, the 30 or so healthy volunteers enrolled in the trial are randomized into vaccine or placebo groups; the vaccine is administered on days 0 and 21; and immunogenicity is evaluated during the subsequent 6 months.[44]

9.3 CLI

9.3.1 Introduction

The narrowing or blocking of arteries due to atherosclerosis results in the impairment of blood supply (i.e., ischemia), which ultimately leads to damage of the neighboring tissue due to lack of nutrients and oxygen. The ischemia of the lower extremities and of the heart originates from the medical conditions known as peripheral arterial disease and myocardial ischemia, respectively.[45] The most severe manifestation of peripheral arterial disease, known as CLI, is characterized primarily by a burning/aching pain in the feet and toes while resting and by skin ulcers or sores that do not heal and eventually result in gangrene. CLI develops in approximately 500–1000 people per million every year,[46] and in the United States alone, the incidence of the disease is 125,000–250,000 patients/year.[47] Currently, there are no drugs available capable of altering the course of the disease.[46] The only therapeutic alternative is to treat CLI by revascularization of the lower extremities, either through open bypass surgery or endovascular techniques, as long as the extent and distribution of the disease remains anatomically restricted. Unfortunately, the success of revascularization is limited, and almost 40% of patients with CLI require amputation of the affected limb within 1 year. The annual mortality rate for CLI exceeds 20%. Furthermore, approximately 95% of the patients with ischemic gangrene and 80% of those with rest pain die within a 10-year period.[47] This scenario underscores the fact that there is an unmet need for a noninvasive and efficient therapeutic alternative to conventional vascularization procedures to improve blood supply to the affected limbs of CLI patients. Therapeutic angiogenesis, a strategy that seeks to improve blood supply by promoting the formation of new blood vessels in the ischemic tissues, could be one of such alternatives. The technique relies on the delivery of growth factors that control the structure and functioning of blood vessels to the affected tissues. As we will see next, plasmids can play a decisive role in this context.

9.3.2 Therapeutic Angiogenesis

Angiogenesis is fundamental in reproduction, development, and wound repair. The deregulation of blood vessel formation can also lead to either excessive or insufficient blood vessel growth and thus contributes to the pathogenesis of diseases like blindness, cancer, rheumatoid arthritis, and heart, brain, and limb ischemia, to name a few.[48-50] The postnatal formation of a new vascular network involves the proliferation and migration of differentiated endothelial cells (ECs), the major components of capillary vessels, from pre-existing blood vessels. In the embryo, these ECs differentiate from angioblasts, whereas in adults, they differentiate from a series of progenitor cells found in the bone marrow.[49] Building a vascular network is a multistep process that starts with the activation of ECs by an angiogenic stimulus (Figure 9.6). One of the most

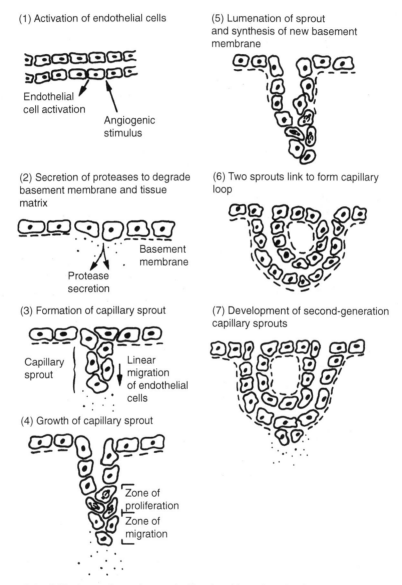

Figure 9.6 *Critical steps in angiogenesis. Reprinted from Annals of the Rheumatic Diseases, 51, Colville-Nash P, Scott D. Angiogenesis and rheumatoid arthritis: pathogenic and therapeutic implications, 919-925, Copyright 1992,[68] with permission from BMJ Publishing Group Ltd.*

important stimuli is hypoxia, that is, the lack of oxygen in the surrounding tissue (other metabolic stimuli include low pH and hypoglycemia[51]). This condition sets off a series of hypoxia-inducible transcription factors (HIFs) that, in turn, upregulate a number of angiogenic genes, of which the vascular endothelial growth factor (VEGF) is probably the most important. VEGF acts mainly by activating mitosis of vascular ECs, that is, by encouraging them to divide. This triggers a series of events, which comprise the enzymatic degradation of the basement membrane of the parental vessel, the migration and proliferation of some ECs with the subsequent formation and growth of capillary sprouts, and finally the formation and maturation of a complete capillary tube[48] (Figure 9.6). The overall angiogenic process is complex and highly regulated, and depends on the concerted and synergistic action of a number of soluble factors and inhibitors. The most prominent and clinically relevant among these so-called angiogenic growth factors are VEGF, the fibroblast growth factor (FGF) and hepatocyte growth factor (HGF).[46] Among other functions, FGFs stimulate the proliferation of a variety of cell types, including ECs. As for HGF, it is involved in the regulation of multiple genes that control key actions of the angiogenic process, including cell migration, proliferation, protease production, invasion, and organization into capillary-like tubes.

By working in concert, the different growth factors can turn angiogenesis on or off, depending on the momentary requirements of our bodies. If the underlying mechanisms and interplay between these growth factors are understood, one could aim to control angiogenesis and explore its potential for therapeutic purposes. Of course, such an intervention calls for a clear understanding of the molecular, genetic, and cellular mechanisms of vessel growth and of the target disease. As described in the previous section, in CLI, the blocking of arteries deprive the surrounding tissue from bulk blood flow, rendering it ischemic. Many times, the body attempts to counteract this by enlarging the collateral vessels that are interconnected to the arterial systems and thus restores at least a part of the flow.[49] This process of endogenous angiogenesis, however, is usually insufficient to fully overcome ischemia.[51] The rationale behind the therapeutic angiogenesis of CLI patients is simply to stimulate and accelerate this process of formation of new collateral vessels by delivering the appropriate angiogenic factors to the affected sites, and thus to improve tissue oxygenation and perfusion.

Three options are available when considering angiogenesis for the therapy of CLI and other cardiovascular diseases. In a first case, the angiogenic growth factors are produced exogenously via recombinant DNA technology and then are administered to the affected tissues.[52] Although therapeutic effects have been obtained with this strategy, a sustained angiogenic effect may be difficult to obtain due to the short half-life (a few minutes) of recombinant growth factors in circulation or in the tissues.[53] Cell-based therapies have also been considered as a means of achieving safe and effective therapeutic angiogenesis. For example, one could transplant CLI patients with autologous bone marrow mononuclear cells and thus take advantage of their natural ability to supply endothelial progenitor cells and to secrete various angiogenic factors as a means of promoting angiogenesis.[54] A third and final alternative is to adopt a gene therapy approach in which the genes that code for the target growth factors are locally delivered via an adequate vector. The ideal vector should enter the target cells and mediate the subsequent expression of the transgene for an amount of time sufficient to yield a clinical effect. Although viral vectors have been used to induce functionally significant angiogenesis,[55,56] a significant amount of attention has been devoted to the use of plasmid vectors to improve blood supply to ischemic limbs.[47,57–59] This focus is due in part to the fact that plasmids are well tolerated and present a superior safety profile when compared to viral vectors.[46] Another reason for this preference is probably related to the fact that nonintegrative expression of the angiogenic genes has been shown to be sufficient to promote the growth of blood vessels. The transient nature of plasmid-mediated gene expression is thus well suited for therapeutic angiogenesis in CLI patients. Although lipids and polymers can be used as delivery adjuvants, naked plasmids have been the favorite option in CLI trials. As for the administration route, local intramuscular injection has prevailed over other options like catheter-mediated intravascular injection.

9.3.3 Plasmid-Mediated Angiogenesis for CLI

The majority of human trials conducted to investigate the potential (i.e., safety and efficacy) of plasmid-mediated therapeutic angiogenesis in CLI have focused on the delivery of three main growth factors: VEGF,[60,61] FGF,[52,62] and HGF[47]. The clinical trials typically involve the randomization of the eligible CLI patients into plasmid or placebo groups. Single or repeated intramuscular injections of the target plasmid biopharmaceutical (usually naked) or of the placebo in the limbs of the patients are then performed. The typical single dose used in most studies contains between 0.5 to 4.0 mg of plasmid. The effect of the treatment is subsequently evaluated by monitoring clinical (mortality, amputation, ulcer healing, and pain) and hemodynamic (e.g., transcutaneous oxygen tension, toe pressure, and ankle brachial index) end points. Safety is also carefully considered in these studies since complications and side effects (e.g., retinopathy) associated with the diffusion of angiogenic factors and similar to the ones observed in animal models could be expected.[46] Although by now a substantial number of clinical trials have been completed, we will highlight only a few of them, particularly those that have moved to, or past, phase 2.

Many studies have attempted to determine the ability of the VEGF gene to induce therapeutic angiogenesis in CLI patients.[57,58,60,61] Generically, all studies conclude that administration of plasmids coding for VEGF, either by intramuscular injection or by catheter-mediated infusion, is safe and well tolerated. As for the efficacy of the treatment, meaningful improvements in some end points are typically found, which suggest that there is a therapeutic benefit associated with the procedure. In a recent trial, for example, improved wound healing and reduced hemodynamic insufficiency have been demonstrated after local, intramuscular injection of a VEGF-carrying plasmid. However, no significant amputation reduction was observed in the same study.[60] In another randomized, placebo-controlled, double-blind phase 2 trial, the VEGF-coding plasmid was encapsulated in liposomes and administered in the lower-limb arteries by catheter-mediated infusion after angioplasty (i.e., the mechanic widening of narrowed or obstructed blood vessels).[61] With this procedure, the plasmid is released into the blood stream and a more extensive distribution of the transgene in the affected limb, with the concomitant transfection of distal vascular endothelium, is obtained as compared with intramuscular delivery. Although VEGF transfer increased vascularity, no statistically significant improvements in the clinical outcome were detected relative to the control groups.[61]

The safety and efficacy of a plasmid biopharmaceutical coding for FGF has been evaluated in a series of phase 1[62] and phase 2[52] trials involving 51 and 125 CLI patients, respectively. Both studies concluded that single or repeated intramuscular injections of the plasmid were well tolerated up to a maximum dose of 16 mg. Furthermore, the phase 2 study showed that the use of the FGF plasmid reduced the risk of amputation by twofold when compared with the placebo injections.[52] A trend toward reduced death rate and time of death was also detected in patients who had received the plasmid. However, the improvements in ulcer healing were similar in the two groups.[52]

Intramuscular injection of a plasmid coding for recombinant HGF, an angiogenic protein that is underexpressed in the limbs of CLI patients, has been shown to induce robust collateral formation of new blood vessels in animal models of CLI[47] and of other ischemic diseases.[63] Building on these observations, the Japan-based company AnGes (Osaka, Japan) has sponsored a series of clinical trials designed to assess the safety of intramuscular injections of a plasmid coding for HGF into the limbs of CLI patients and to determine whether this strategy results in increased limb perfusion.[47,64] Results from a phase 1/2 trial showed that three intramuscular injections of doses up to 4 mg HGF plasmid were safe and well tolerated, and suggested a favorable effect on limb perfusion. A subsequent phase 3 randomized, placebo-controlled, double-blind study conducted in Japan with 40 CLI patients showed a 70.4% improvement of rest pain or ischemic ulcer size in patients who received 8 mg (4 mg × 2) plasmid as compared with 30.4% in a placebo group.[65] This has prompted the company to submit a new drug application (NDA) to the competent authorities in Japan[66,67] and to initiate an equivalent phase 3 program in the United States.

9.4 CONCLUSIONS

In spite of the vast amount of research and clinical investigations of the past years, the usefulness and value of plasmid biopharmaceuticals in the context of human disease management still remains to be demonstrated. The slow progress, however, has not deterred the enthusiasts in their defense of plasmid-based gene transfer as a possible solution to unmet medical needs and challenges to come. The two case studies described in this chapter, pandemic influenza and CLI, illustrate very well why in some cases a plasmid biopharmaceutical approach could be valuable. In the first situation, the short response time that humankind will have to face the inevitable pandemic influenza requires the swift development and deployment of millions of doses of vaccines. Thus, the effectiveness of response will depend on the rapidity with which the pandemic strain is identified and incorporated in a candidate product, and the vaccine is manufactured, formulated, and released. Among the different vaccination platforms available, DNA vaccines are probably the one that will best face the challenges of speed, scalability, and cost. Thus, although the consequences and impact of a pandemic influenza are likely to be tremendous, such an event may well constitute an opportunity for DNA vaccines to unfold and demonstrate their full potential. The first months of the 2009 influenza A/H1N1 pandemic confirmed this to some extent, since at least one DNA vaccine prototype was produced and successfully tested in animals for immunogenicity in less than 2 months.

The epidemic proportions of complex cardiovascular diseases in modern-day societies are creating urgency among the different stakeholders for the development of successful, long-term pharmacological treatments that could thwart the associated morbidity and mortality. CLI constitutes a paradigmatic case of a cardiovascular disease that has both high societal and individual costs, and for which there is a lack of adequate treatment. The delivery of genes coding for angiogenic factors via plasmids is one of most promising options under study to promote the revascularization of the ischemic limbs of CLI patients. So far, clinical trials involving plasmid administration have shown both safety and some clinical efficacy. In one case, a NDA has even been submitted in the aftermath of a phase 3 trial. Thus, a plasmid coding for an angiogenic factor might well be the first plasmid biopharmaceutical for human use to receive marketing approval.

REFERENCES

1. World Health Organization. *Avian influenza: Assessing the pandemic threat*. Geneva: World Health Organization, 2005.

2. Neumann G, Noda T, Kawaoka Y. Emergence and pandemic potential of swine-origin H1N1 influenza virus. *Nature*. 2009;459:931–939.

3. Subbarao K, Murphy BR, Fauci AS. Development of effective vaccines against pandemic influenza. *Immunity*. 2006;24:5–9.

4. Gerdil C. Using the strains and getting the vaccine licensed—A vaccine manufacturer's view. *Development of Biologicals (Basel)*. 2003;115:17–21.

5. Crosby A. Influenza: In the grip of the grippe. In: Kiple KF, ed. *Plague, pox and pestilence*. London: Weidenfeld & Nicolson, 1997:148–153.

6. Oldstone MBA. Influenza virus, the plague that may return. In: Oldstone MBA, ed. *Viruses, plagues and history*. Oxford: Oxford University Press, 1998:172–186.

7. Luke CJ, Subbarao K. Vaccines for pandemic influenza. *Emerging Infectious Diseases*. 2006;12:66–72.

8. Smallman-Raynor M, Cliff AD. The geographical spread of avian influenza A (H5N1): Panzootic transmission (December 2003–May 2006), pandemic potential, and implications. *Annals of the Association of American Geographers*. 2008;98: 553–582.

9. Subbarao K, Klimov A, Katz J, et al. Characterization of an avian influenza A (H5N1) virus isolated from a child with fatal respiratory illness. *Science*. 1998;279: 393–396.

10. World Health Organization. Cumulative number of confirmed human cases of avian influenza A/(H5N1) reported to WHO. 2010. Available at: http://www.who.int/ csr/disease/avian_influenza/country/cases_table_2010_05_06/en/index.html. Accessed May 11, 2010.

11. Nicita A. *Avian Influenza and the poultry trade. Policy Research Working Paper 4551*. Washington, DC: The World Bank, 2008.

12. Uyeki TM. Global epidemiology of human infections with highly pathogenic avian influenza A (H5N1) viruses. *Respirology*. 2008;13:S2–S9.

13. Daems R, Del Giudice G, Rappuoli R. Anticipating crisis: Towards a pandemic flu vaccination strategy through alignment of public health and industrial policy. *Vaccine*. 2005;23:5732–5742.

14. McKibbin W, Sidorenko A. *Global macroeconomic consequences of pandemic influenza*. Sidney: Lowy Institute for International Policy, 2006.

15. Ryan F. *Virus X*. London: Harper Collins Publishers, 1998.

16. Brahmbhatt M. *Economic impacts of avian influenza propagation*. Washington, DC: World Bank, 2006.

17. Fedson DS. Pandemic influenza: A potential role for statins in treatment and pro-phylaxis. *Clinical Infectious Diseases*. 2006;43:199–205.

18. Ilyinskii PO, Thoidis G, Shneider AM. Development of a vaccine against pandemic influenza viruses: Current status and perspectives. *International Reviews in Immunology*. 2008;27:392–426.

19. Gerdil C. The annual production cycle for influenza vaccine. *Vaccine*. 2003; 21:1776–1779.

20. Ulmer JB, Valley U, Rappuoli R. Vaccine manufacturing: Challenges and solutions. *Nature Biotechnology*. 2006;24:1377–1383.

21. PowderMed. *Pandemic influenza and biothreat preparedness: Role of PMED™ DNA vaccines*. Oxford: Oxford PharmaGenesis, 2005.

22. Thomas A, Guldager N, Hermansen K. Pandemic flu preparedness: A manufactur-ing perspective. *Biopharm International*. 2007;August:46–55.

23. Davis AR, Bos T, Ueda M, Nayak DP, Dowbenko D, Compans RW. Immune response to human influenza virus hemagglutinin expressed in *Escherichia coli*. *Gene*. 1983;21:273–284.

24. Shoji Y, Bi H, Musiychuk K, et al. Plant-derived hemagglutinin protects ferrets against challenge infection with the A/Indonesia/05/05 strain of avian influenza. *Vaccine*. 2009;27:1087–1092.

25. Robinson JM. An alternative to the scale-up and distribution of pandemic influenza vaccine. *Biopharm International*. 2009 (Suppl);20:12–20.

26. Hu AY, Weng TC, Tseng YF, et al. Microcarrier-based MDCK cell culture system for the production of influenza H5N1 vaccines. *Vaccine*. 2008;26:5736–5740.

27. Hoelscher MA, Garg S, Bangari DS, et al. Development of adenoviral-vector-based pandemic influenza vaccine against antigenically distinct human H5N1 strains in mice. *Lancet*. 2006;367:475–481.

28. Chen Z, Yoshikawa T, Kadowaki S, et al. Protection and antibody responses in different strains of mouse immunized with plasmid DNAs encoding influenza virus haemagglutinin, neuraminidase and nucleoprotein. *Journal of General Virology*. 1999;80(Pt 10):2559–2564.

29. Drape RJ, Macklin MD, Barr LJ, Jones S, Haynes JR, Dean HJ. Epidermal DNA vaccine for influenza is immunogenic in humans. *Vaccine*. 2006;24:4475–4481.

30. Margaronis S. An influenza pandemic vaccine strategy. www.Influenza-Pandemic. com, 2006.

31. Forde GM. Rapid-response vaccines-does DNA offer a solution? *Nature Biotechnology*. 2005;23:1059–1062.

32. Hoare M, Levy MS, Bracewell DG, et al. Bioprocess engineering issues that would be faced in producing a DNA vaccine at up to $100 \, m^3$ fermentation scale for an influenza pandemic. *Biotechnology Progress*. 2005;21:1577–1592.

33. Carnes AE, Williams JA. Plasmid DNA manufacturing technology. *Recent Patents on Biotechnology*. 2007;1:151–166.

34. Nwe N, He Q, Damrongwatanapokin S, et al. Expression of hemagglutinin protein from the avian influenza virus H5N1 in a baculovirus/insect cell system significantly enhanced by suspension culture. *BMC Microbiology*. 2006;6:16.

35. Chan M. World now at the start of 2009 influenza pandemic. Statement to the press: World Health Organization; 2009.

36. World Health Organization. Pandemic (H1N1) 2009—Update 58. Available at: http://www.who.int/csr/don/2009_07_06/en/index.html. Accessed July 6, 2009.

37. World Health Organization. Changes in reporting requirements for pandemic (H1N1) 2009 virus infection. Pandemic (H1N1) 2009 briefing note 3 (revised). Available at: http://www.who.int/csr/disease/swineflu/notes/h1n1_surveillance_20090710/en/index. html. Accessed July 13, 2009.

38. World Health Organization. Pandemic (H1N1) 2009—Update 99. Available at: http://www.who.int/csr/don/2010_05_07/en/index.html. Accessed May 11, 2010.

39. Inovio Biomedical. Inovio Biomedical H1N1 influenza DNA vaccines demonstrate 100% responses against swine flu in vaccinated pigs (news release). San Diego, CA, July 13, 2009.

40. Vical Inc. Vical and U.S. Navy to expedite development of H1N1 pandemic influenza (swine flu) vaccine (news release). San Diego, CA, May 6, 2009.

41. Vical Inc. Vical H1 influenza vaccine delivers robust preclinical results with 100% response (news release). San Diego, CA, June 30, 2009.

42. Vical Inc. Vical advances H1N1 pandemic influenza (swine flu) vaccine (news release). San Diego, CA, May 21, 2009.

43. Vical Inc. U.S. Navy to fund Vical's H1N1 pandemic influenza (swine flu) vaccine (news release). San Diego, CA, October 1, 2009.

44. Vical Inc. Vical begins phase 1 trial of DNA vaccine against H1N1 pandemic influenza (news release). San Diego, CA, May 5, 2010.

45. Dishart KL, Work LM, Denby L, Baker AH. Gene therapy for cardiovascular disease. *Journal of Biomedicine and Biotechnology*. 2003;2003:138–148.

46. Bobek V, Taltynov O, Pinterova D, Kolostova K. Gene therapy of the ischemic lower limb—Therapeutic angiogenesis. *Vascular Pharmacology*. 2006;44:395–405.

47. Powell RJ, Simons M, Mendelsohn FO, et al. Results of a double-blind, placebo-controlled study to assess the safety of intramuscular injection of hepatocyte growth factor plasmid to improve limb perfusion in patients with critical limb ischemia. *Circulation*. 2008;118:58–65.

48. Colville-Nash PR, Willoughby DA. Growth factors in angiogenesis: Current interest and therapeutic potential. *Molecular Medicine Today*. 1997;3:14–23.

49. Carmeliet P. Angiogenesis in health and disease. *Nature Medicine*. 2003;9: 653–660.

50. Folkman J, Shing Y. Angiogenesis. *The Journal of Biological Chemistry*. 1992; 267:10931–10934.

51. Rissanen TT, Vajanto I, Ylä-Herttuala S. Gene therapy for therapeutic angiogenesis in critically ischaemic lower limb—On the way to the clinic. *European Journal of Clinical Investigation*. 2001;31:651–666.

52. Nikol S, Baumgartner I, Van Belle E, et al. Therapeutic angiogenesis with intramuscular NV1FGF improves amputation-free survival in patients with critical limb ischemia. *Molecular Therapy*. 2008;16:972–978.

53. Takeshita S, Pu LQ, Stein LA, et al. Intramuscular administration of vascular endothelial growth factor induces dose-dependent collateral artery augmentation in a rabbit model of chronic limb ischemia. *Circulation*. 1994;90:II228–II234.

54. Tateishi-Yuyama E, Matsubara H, Murohara T, et al. Therapeutic angiogenesis for patients with limb ischaemia by autologous transplantation of bone-marrow cells: A pilot study and a randomised controlled trial. *Lancet*. 2002;360:427–435.

55. Mohler ER, 3rd, Rajagopalan S, Olin JW, et al. Adenoviral-mediated gene transfer of vascular endothelial growth factor in critical limb ischemia: Safety results from a phase I trial. *Vascular Medicine*. 2003;8:9–13.

56. Pinkenburg O, Pfosser A, Hinkel R, et al. Recombinant adeno-associated virus-based gene transfer of cathelicidin induces therapeutic neovascularization preferentially via potent collateral growth. *Human Gene Therapy*. 2009;20:159–167.

57. Isner JM, Pieczek A, Schainfeld R, et al. Clinical evidence of angiogenesis after arterial gene transfer of phVEGF165 in patient with ischaemic limb. *Lancet*. 1996;348:370–374.

58. Baumgartner I, Pieczek A, Manor O, et al. Constitutive expression of phVEGF165 after intramuscular gene transfer promotes collateral vessel development in patients with critical limb ischemia. *Circulation*. 1998;97:1114–1123.

59. Simovic D, Isner JM, Ropper AH, Pieczek A, Weinberg DH. Improvement in chronic ischemic neuropathy after intramuscular phVEGF165 gene transfer in patients with critical limb ischemia. *Archives of Neurology*. 2001;58:761–768.

60. Kusumanto YH, van Weel V, Mulder NH, et al. Treatment with intramuscular vascular endothelial growth factor gene compared with placebo for patients with diabetes mellitus and critical limb ischemia: A double-blind randomized trial. *Human Gene Therapy*. 2006;17:683–691.

61. Makinen K, Manninen H, Hedman M, et al. Increased vascularity detected by digital subtraction angiography after VEGF gene transfer to human lower limb artery: A randomized, placebo-controlled, double-blinded phase II study. *Molecular Therapy.* 2002;6:127–133.

62. Comerota AJ, Throm RC, Miller KA, et al. Naked plasmid DNA encoding fibroblast growth factor type 1 for the treatment of end-stage unreconstructible lower extremity ischemia: Preliminary results of a phase I trial. *Journal of Vascular Surgery.* 2002;35:930–936.

63. Aoki M, Morishita R, Taniyama Y, et al. Angiogenesis induced by hepatocyte growth factor in non-infarcted myocardium and infarcted myocardium: Up-regulation of essential transcription factor for angiogenesis, ets. *Gene Therapy.* 2000;7:417–427.

64. Morishita R, Aoki M, Hashiya N, et al. Safety evaluation of clinical gene therapy using hepatocyte growth factor to treat peripheral arterial disease. *Hypertension.* 2004;44:203–209.

65. AnGes MG, Inc. Announcement of results of phase III clinical trials of HGF gene therapy in Japan (news release). Osaka, Japan, June 14, 2007.

66. Kim S, Peng Z, Kaneda Y. Current status of gene therapy in Asia. *Molecular Therapy.* 2008;16:237–243.

67. AnGes MG, Inc. AnGes submits NDA for HGF gene therapy (news release). Osaka, Japan, March 28, 2008.

68. Colville-Nash P, Scott D. Angiogenesis and rheumatoid arthritis: Pathogenic and therapeutic implications. *Annals of the Rheumatic Diseases.* 1992;51:919–925.

10

Veterinary Case Studies: West Nile, Infectious Hematopoietic Necrosis, and Melanoma

10.1 INTRODUCTION

Veterinary DNA vaccines were the first plasmid biopharmaceuticals to hit the marketplace, even though, as some may argue, they have had a reduced impact so far. Nevertheless, these veterinary vaccines constitute some of the first proofs of concept and proofs of value to emerge from the area of plasmid biopharmaceuticals. The handful of pioneering products that led the way, together with their development and associated circumstances, constitutes an interesting set of case studies from which a number of lessons can be extracted. In this chapter, three specific cases will be described and analyzed in some detail. The first situation refers to the vaccination of endangered California condors against West Nile virus (WNV), which took place in the years 2003 and 2004. Although the prototype DNA vaccine used then had not received formal approval and was not marketed as a bird DNA vaccine, the story illustrates particularly well one of the most acclaimed advantages of DNA vaccines, that is, the speed of development and deployment in case of an emergency. The condors involved in the experiment also deserve the honor of being

Plasmid Biopharmaceuticals: Basics, Applications, and Manufacturing, First Edition.
Duarte Miguel F. Prazeres.
© 2011 John Wiley & Sons, Inc. Published 2011 by John Wiley & Sons, Inc.

recognized as the first animals immunized with a DNA vaccine to be deliberately released into the environment. As a second case study, the development of a DNA vaccine against the causative virus of the infectious hematopoietic necrosis (IHN), which affects farmed Atlantic salmon, is described. A distinctive feature of this DNA vaccine when compared with the others examined in this chapter is that it is intended to be used in animals that are destined for human consumption. A special focus will be put in this case on describing the safety issues and environmental risks that inevitably surrounded the licensing of this product in 2005. In the third part of the chapter, the development of a canine malignant melanoma (CMM) DNA vaccine is examined. This case is especially interesting not only due to the intrinsic therapeutic value of the plasmid biopharmaceutical in question but also because a similar DNA vaccine is being developed by the same team for use in humans. It thus serves as a perfect example of comparative oncology, a discipline that attempts to translate the knowledge and therapies generated from studies of naturally occurring cancers in animals into humans.[1]

10.2 WNV AND CALIFORNIA CONDORS

10.2.1 The New York Outbreak of WNV

In late August 1999, a number of human cases of infectious neurological disease associated with muscle weakness emerged in New York City. Throughout a crisis that lasted approximately 2 months, a total of 59 patients were hospitalized and diagnosed with encephalitis (i.e., an inflammation of the brain) or meningitis (i.e., an inflammation of the membrane around the brain and the spinal cord).[2] The clinical symptoms reported included fever in most cases, but also weakness, nausea, vomiting, headache, and altered mental status. Seven patients eventually died in the aftermath of the crisis. The first tests performed on the cerebrospinal fluid of the afflicted patients initially suggested that a virus could be the causative agent. Simultaneously, an environmental investigation into the neighborhoods where most of the cases had clustered revealed the presence of larvae and breeding sites of mosquitoes of the *Culex* species.[2] This evidence further pointed to an arbovirus (i.e., an arthropod-borne virus) as the culprit. The outbreak was initially attributed to St. Louis encephalitis virus, a member of the Flaviviridae family that is common in North America, when enzyme-linked immunosorbent assay (ELISA) tests for the corresponding antibodies yielded positive.[2] Meanwhile, parallel investigations on the cocurrent and unexpected death of a substantial number of birds in the New York area resulted in the isolation of WNV from bird tissue specimens.[3,4] This finding shifted the focus of the investigations of the human cases away from St. Louis virus. Eventually, a genomic sequence identical to the ones found in the affected birds was detected in a specimen from a human case, confirming West Nile infection as the cause of the encephalitis and meningitis cases.[5]

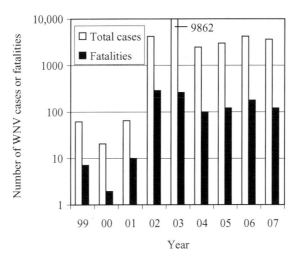

Figure 10.1 *Human cases of West Nile virus activity in the United States from 1999 to 2007. The cases reported include meningitis, encephalitis, and mild fever. The figure was constructed on the basis of data provided by the Division of Vector-Borne Infectious Diseases of the Centers for Disease Control and Prevention (information accessed from http://www.cdc.gov/ncidod/ dvbid/westnile/surv&control.htm on September 1, 2008).*

The 1999 northeastern U.S. outbreak was the first time WNV was ever detected in the Western Hemisphere.[3] Although the epidemic initially clustered around the New York City area, it subsequently spread westward throughout most of North America, the Caribbean islands, and portions of Central America.[6] Statistics, surveillance, and control data from the Centers for Disease Control and Prevention (CDC)* show that human WNV activity in the United States peaked in the 2002 and 2003 seasons (Figure 10.1). The total number of severe (meningitis and encephalitis) and mild (fever) human cases of WNV infection reached ~27,603 by the end of 2007. During the 1999–2007 period, close to 1100 human fatalities were attributed to WNV.

In 2004, positive cases of WNV in birds had been detected in virtually all the states of the United States (Figure 10.2). In the specific case of California, the virus is thought to have entered the state carried by migratory birds flying from Mexico. The velocity at which the virus spread was particularly compelling in the case of California, where the number of WNV-positive birds soared from 96 in 2003 to 3232 in 2004. This increased the Californian share of total cases reported in the United States from 0.8% to 44.0%.[7] Like in many other cases in which viruses invaded new geographic areas (e.g., Japanese encephalitis in Australia), the incursion of WNV in the new continent is probably a result of increasing global commerce and travel, as well as of climate change.[8] Apart from affecting a significant number of humans, the WNV epidemic

---

* CDC, Division of Vector-Borne Infectious Diseases. Information accessed from http:// www.cdc.gov/ncidod/dvbid/westnile/surv&control.htm, on September 1, 2008.

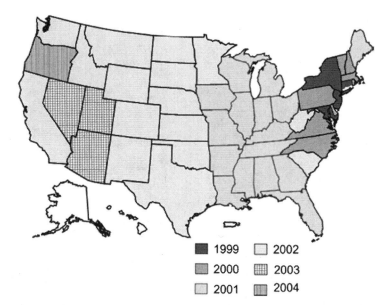

Figure 10.2 *States that reported positive tests for West Nile virus by year of first reporting, 1999–2004. Reprinted from Ornithological Monographs, 60, McLean R. West Nile virus in North American birds, 44-64, Copyright 2006,[7] with permission from the American Ornithologists' Union.*

spread among a large number of bird species and mammals. The national surveillance system, which was put in place in the United States from 1999 to 2004, enabled the identification of WNV in close to 48,000 birds from 294 species.[7] Although the infection affected mostly American crows, birds as various as flamingos, ducks, parrots, cormorants, and vultures were infected. WNV infection has also been detected in approximately 30 species of mammals, including bats, squirrels, dogs, and cats.[9] Horses, an animal species with high commercial value, were also affected by the virus, with 20 and 23 cases reported in 1999 and 2000, respectively.[10]

10.2.2 West Nile Virus

West Nile virus is a flavivirus from the Flaviviridae family, which also includes the viruses that cause St. Louis and Japanese encephalitis, as well as yellow and dengue fever. Attempts to diagnose infections caused by these viruses are often complicated by the close antigenic relationships among the members of the family and the inherent cross-reactions in ELISA-type tests.[8] This cross-reactivity explains the positive results for the St. Louis virus initially obtained when specimens from patients of the New York epidemic were tested. Originally isolated from a human patient from the West Nile region of Uganda in 1937, the geographic distribution of WNV includes Europe, Africa, Middle East, and Western Asia. The virus is transmitted from host to host mostly through mosquitoes from the Culex family, but also from the Aedes, Anopheles,

Minomyia, and Mansonia families.[11,12] Birds are the primary reservoir for WNV, but isolations from mammals, reptiles, and amphibians have all been reported.[7] Unlike birds, mammals are considered to be "dead-end" hosts. This means that the amount of circulating virus in their blood is not sufficient to infect subsequent biting mosquitoes, as is usual in birds. WNV can also pass from host to host without the intervention of mosquitoes. Known transmission routes in humans include blood transfusions, organ transplants, breast feeding, and occupational activities which involve the manipulation of infected animals or specimens.[9] Prey-to-predator transmission has also been documented, for instance, in the case of raptors feeding on infected mice.[13]

WNV affects the central nervous system, causing encephalitis or meningitis, which can result in paralysis or death. The traditional WNV strains circulating in the areas mentioned above did not cause significant outbreaks of disease in humans or birds.[7] From the mid-1990s on, however, both the frequency and severity of WNV disease in humans and birds has increased significantly.[8] The strain responsible for the New York epidemic (NY99) was found to be particularly virulent. Furthermore, and when compared with the introduction of other flavivirus in new continents, the easiness of spread of WNV throughout the American continent was uncharacteristic of mosquito-borne viruses.[9]

Like other flaviviruses, WNV is characterized by an icosahedral, protein capsid (30–35 nm), which contains a single-stranded, positive-sense RNA[11]. This viral capsid is further enclosed in an envelope of host cell membranes.[8] The diameter of the approximately spherical full virion is around 50 nm. The genome is 11,029 nucleotides (nt) and contains a single open reading frame (ORF) of 10,301 nt, which encodes seven nonstructural proteins (NS1, NS2a, NS2b, NS3, NS4a, NS4b, and NS5) and three structural proteins (C, prM/M, and E).[11] The seven nonstructural proteins are likely to be directly or indirectly involved in viral RNA synthesis. The C protein is the key component of the nucleocapsid, whereas E and M are integral membrane proteins.[11] The majority of the neutralizing antibodies elicited in flavivirus-infected hosts are directed to epitopes in the viral envelope E-glycoprotein, making this the most immunologically important protein and thus a potential and logical candidate antigen for a vaccine. Although the exact mechanisms underlying West Nile virus pathogenesis are still unclear, experimental evidence indicates that the virus capsid protein (C) has a prominent role in the induction of cell apoptosis and tissue inflammation.[14] Among others, the inflammation of brain and spinal cord tissue (i.e., meningoencephalitis) is especially serious since it can potentially lead to death.

10.2.3 Condors at Risk

The California condor (*Gymnogyps californianus*) is a rare and endangered species which inhabits the North American continent and whose range used to extend across the entire United States. These giant birds weigh around 10 kg, can have a wingspan of up to 9.5 ft, and feed exclusively on large animal carcasses. As a consequence of anthropogenic factors (mainly shooting and lead poisoning), the numbers of California condors in the wild declined substantially during the nineteenth and twentieth centuries.[15] The species was listed as endangered in 1967 by the U.S. Fish and Wildlife Service and has since been at the brink of extinction. The last free-flying individual was eventually captured in 1987.[15] Subsequently, protection and captive breeding programs started at the San Diego Wild Animal Park and the Los Angeles Zoo where captive condor flocks had been established. These programs contributed to an increase of the population from a mere 22 individuals in 1982, to ~100 in 1996[15] and more than 200 in early 2003, many of which have been reintroduced in the wild. In spite of this success, the WNV epidemic that hit the continent in 1999 and recurred in subsequent years cast a shadow over the future of the California condor. The concerns that the still small population of condors could be irreversibly affected were grounded not only on the large number of different bird species (>300) infected and killed by WNV but also by the possibility of oral transmission of the virus due to the scavenger behavior of condors.[6,16]

The fears that WNV infection could be lethal to California condors, together with the endangered status of the species, prompted officials at the U.S. CDC and the Los Angeles Zoo to expedite the inoculation of the entire population of birds with an experimental DNA vaccine. Although at the time an inactivated WNV vaccine for horses was commercially available from Fort Dodge Laboratories (Fort Dodge, Iowa), this option was discarded since no humoral responses were detected following the experimental vaccination of Chilean flamingos and red-tailed hawks.[17] The failure of this vaccine was partially attributed to potential alterations of the surface antigens of the virus during the inactivation process used to eliminate virulence.[17] The use of a DNA vaccine in 2003 preceded the formal approval by the Food and Drug Administration (FDA) of the first two DNA vaccines ever, a milestone event that would take place 2 years later. The first of such vaccines, which was licensed in July 2005 to Fort Dodge Laboratories (see Chapter 8, Section 8.4.2), was designed precisely to protect horses against West Nile virus.[18] The promising results obtained with a prototype version of this vaccine in 2001, which was found to protect both mice and horses from virus challenges,[19] encouraged the use of a derived version in condors.[6] The excellent safety profile of DNA vaccines, which had then been demonstrated by numerous animal studies, also convinced officials to use the prototype in condors.[18]

The DNA vaccine tested in horses in 2001 (pCBWN) codes for the premembrane/membrane (prM) and envelope (E) glycoproteins of WNV[19] (Figure 10.3). A transmembrane signal peptide from the Japanese encephalitis virus was cloned upstream of the WNV prM-E gene cassette in order to ensure a correct processing of the antigenic proteins. Cells transformed *in vitro* with this plasmid were able to express and secrete high levels of both proteins.[19] The effectiveness of this DNA vaccine in birds was first demonstrated in an experimental study with fish crows, which showed complete protection of individuals inoculated by intramuscular injection from a subsequent challenge

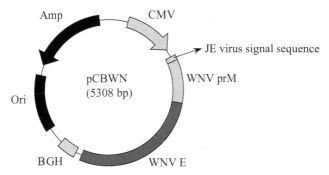

Figure 10.3 *Map of the pCBWN DNA vaccine (adapted from Davis et al.[19]). The vaccine was originally designed to protect horses from WNV infection. A derived version was eventually constructed by replacing the ampicillin resistance gene with a kanamycin resistance gene and was used to immunize the entire population of the California condor.[6]*

with WNV[20]. In the case of the condor immunization study/experiment, the ampicillin resistance gene in the pCBWN construct (Figure 10.3) was replaced with a kanamycin resistance gene, yielding the 5300-bp pVWN DNA vaccine prototype. The pVWN plasmid was then produced both by the CDC laboratories (Division of Vector Borne Infectious Diseases, National Center for Infectious Diseases, Fort Collins, Colorado)[6] and by the company Aldevron (Fargo, North Dakota).[21] The CDC vaccine material was produced in *E.coli* XL-1 Blue cells, a strain commercialized by Stratagene (La Jolla, California). However, scientists at Aldevron decided to use *E.coli* K-12 in order to minimize instability problems observed during *in vivo* expansion of the plasmid, which led to high amounts of genomic DNA, nonsupercoiled isoforms, and an extra piece of DNA[21]. The purification methods used in both cases were also different. At the CDC research laboratories, plasmid DNA material was purified on the basis of the EndoFree plasmid Giga kit marketed by QIAGEN Inc. (Valencia, California),[6] whereas at Aldevron, the downstream process featured alkaline lysis, a proprietary clarification step and a final ion pair, reversed-phase chromatography step with a Perfluorosorb S resin from Prometic Life Sciences (Montreal, Canada) (see Chapter 17, Section 17.2.6.3 for further details on this chromatographic step).[21] The plasmid produced by the Aldevron process was found to meet and exceed current good manufacturing practice (cGMP) lot release specifications, namely in regard to the final amount of impurities (<2% gDNA, <1% RNA, <2% protein, <100 EU/mg) and percentage of supercoiled isoform (>95%).[21] The diverse production and purification methodologies used by the CDC and Aldevron illustrate very well the way research laboratories and companies approach the manufacturing of plasmid material for trials. While research laboratories typically resort to well-established protocols and commercial kits to expedite the generation of the material needed, companies prefer to rely on the use of scalable procedures developed in-house and amenable to validation.

The purified plasmid DNA in phosphate buffered saline (PBS) produced at the CDC and Aldevron was formulated with 1% aluminum phosphate gel. The total amount of plasmid DNA in the final 1 mL doses was 500 µg, and the vaccines were administered by intramuscular injection into the leg muscle of the condors.[6] Although two doses given 3 weeks apart were selected as the ideal vaccination regimen, this was essentially only possible in the case of captive birds. Most of the condors living in the wild, on the other hand, received a single shot upon capture due to the unfeasibility of recapturing them at the right time for a second dose.[6] Pilot experiments conducted in captive California and Andean condors at the Los Angeles zoo not only showed excellent humoral responses but also a complete absence of acute side effects. In view of these preliminary safety and efficacy data, the vaccination was extended to captive and field-released condors, eventually covering the entire population by the end of 2004.[6]

The first set of results of the vaccination of the California condors, which was published recently, prompted the authors of the article to state that "The prospective vaccination of the entire population of California condors before the arrival of West Nile virus has thus potentially saved this endangered species from subsequent lethal West Nile virus encephalitis, and possible extinction."[6] This cautious, but nevertheless bold, claim is supported by the analysis of protective antibodies in prevaccine (193 individuals) and post vaccine (167 individuals) sera of condors, which showed that close to 90% of the condors seroconverted. The study also revealed unusual increases in neutralizing antibodies and the presence of detectable antibodies against the nonstructural WNV protein NS1 (which is not coded for in the vaccine) in some individuals. Taken together, these serological results were interpreted as the first ever evidence of the natural infection of condors with WNV. The documentation of the death of two young condors in 2005 due to WNV infection further confirmed this.[6]

10.2.4 Final Remarks

Even though the full extent of a hypothetic WNV infection of California condors in the wild remains unknown, hints of the birds' vulnerability have surfaced recently.[6] This evidence supports the initial fears that the rare and endangered California condors would be wiped out if WNV were to hit California (as it eventually did in 2004), as well as the decision to vaccinate the entire population with an experimental DNA vaccine. This preemptive vaccination is believed to have saved the endangered population of condors from subsequent infections with the natural WNV, which circulated during the 2004 and subsequent seasons. The immunization of California condors with a DNA vaccine against WNV is emblematic not only because condors were the first animals immunized with DNA to be deliberately released into the environment but also due to the favorable outcome of the experiment. And, even though a prototype vaccine had already been tested, the speed of development and deployment of the DNA vaccine in face of the potential emergency is noteworthy. Finally, the follow-up and study of the vaccinated individuals are still expected to generate important insights for the development of other veterinary and human DNA vaccines.

10.3 IHN AND THE ATLANTIC SALMON

10.3.1 Salmon Farming and the Infectious Hematopoietic Necrosis Virus (IHNV)

Today, many fish species are cultivated in farms specifically for human consumption. One of the most popular of such species is the Atlantic salmon (*Salmo salar*), a member of the Salmonidae family, which lives in the Atlantic Ocean and in the adjacent rivers that flow into it.[22] Apart from its organoleptic characteristics, the Atlantic salmon is a highly valued commodity in human nutrition due to the health benefits associated with the high levels of (n-3) highly unsaturated fatty acids that are found in its oily flesh. The increasing demand for salmon, together with the decline in the wild stocks, has contributed to fostering the development of aquaculture production. In 2007, the total amount of farmed salmon produced both in the native geographic regions (Norway, Canada, and Scotland) and beyond, in countries like Chile and Australia, exceeded 1.2 million metric tons.[22] Most Atlantic salmon populations lay and hatch their eggs in freshwater, migrating later on to the ocean for feeding. The implementation of salmon aquaculture thus requires the production of juvenile salmon in freshwater and then their transfer to marine salmon farms for further growth. These farms are usually located in bays and in other semi-sheltered coastal areas. Here the salmons are typically held captive in large, floating mesh cages, but nevertheless exposed to the surrounding environment. This means that nutrients, dejects, chemicals (e.g., antibiotics and pesticides), viruses, and parasites can transfer in and out of the cages.[22] The morphological, physiological, and genetic conditions of salmon produced in aquaculture farms, as well as their behavior, competitive ability, and breeding characteristics, are significantly different from those observed in wild salmon.[22] As a consequence, any farmed salmon escaping from a cage represents a competitor that can potentially displace the native, wild populations and can contribute to their decline. The negative impacts of escaped salmon in those regions where the Atlantic salmon is an exotic species (e.g., ecological interactions and genetic variation due to interbreeding) are thus one of the key problems associated with their large-scale production in marine mesh cages. Although these cages provide a certain degree of confinement, the number of fish escaping through "trickle" losses (i.e., leakage of smaller individuals through the nets) or as a result of storms is of the order of millions of individuals per year.[22] As we will see in Section 10.3.3, this difficulty in keeping farmed salmon out from the wild constitutes an important issue when pondering the potential impact of large-scale immunization practices.

One of the most important threats faced by aquaculture companies involved in salmon farming is an acute, systemic, infectious disease characterized by the necrosis of hematopoietic tissues of the fish. Other clinical signs include abdominal distension, severe hemorrhaging in the viscera, as well as bloody ascites and pale gills.[23] IHN was first noted in aquacultured salmon in the early 1990s and ever since, several outbreaks have been described among Canadian farm sites.[23–25] The causative agent of the disease is an RNA virus of the Rhabdoviridae family, which is endemic both in wild and cultured salmonid fish throughout the Pacific Northwest (from Alaska to northern California). The virus has also been found in continental Europe and in Asian countries. The linear single-stranded, negative-sense RNA genome of the IHN virus (IHNV) contains approximately 11,000 nt. This genome specifies six mRNA segments that encode two matrix proteins (M1 and M2), three structural proteins (RNA polymerase [L], envelope glycoprotein [G], and nucleocapsid protein [N]), and a nonstructural protein (NV). Morphologically, the virus presents itself in the shape of a bullet with protruding G-protein spikes.[26] The virus from infected fish is shed in the secretions (e.g., urine and feces) and subsequently dispersed in the surrounding water. These virus particles are then transmitted to healthy fish which share the same tank or mesh cage by entering through the base of the fins.[27] The mortality among populations exposed to the virus is especially high in the smaller fish, usually reaching over 70% and sometimes up to 90%.[23] The economic losses associated with IHN have significantly affected a number of aquaculture companies. For example, the 2001–2003 outbreaks, which occurred in Western Canada and affected 36 farm sites, led to a loss of approximately C$200 million in sales.[24,25] The economic threat posed by IHN to the salmon industry and the fact that no efficacious treatments were available thus became the drivers for the development of an effective vaccine. Furthermore, and as will be described next, it constituted an excellent opportunity for DNA vaccine technology to prove its worth.

10.3.2 The Apex-IHN DNA Vaccine

The challenge of developing a safe and effective DNA vaccine to protect farm-raised salmon against IHN was undertaken by the Canadian company Aqua Health, Ltd., an affiliate of Novartis Animal Health (Victoria, Canada). The DNA vaccine was approved by the Canadian Food Inspection Agency (CFIA) in July 2005, entering the market with the trade name Apex-IHN. Together with the West Nile virus vaccine for horses alluded to in the previous section, the Apex-IHN vaccine became one of the first to obtain licensure[25] (see Chapter 1, Section 1.3.6). The pathway to approval of this vaccine is described in detail by its promoters in a recent review.[25]

The fact that the majority of the neutralizing antibodies in IHNV-infected fish are directed toward the 59-kDa G protein made this a logical candidate antigen to include in a DNA vaccine.[28] This was confirmed in earlier experiments by immunizing rainbow trout with a DNA vaccine harboring the

G protein.[29] The results conclusively showed that the expression of this antigen induced protective neutralizing antibodies while conferring significant protection against an ulterior challenge with the live virus. At the same time, the use of other viral proteins (N, M1, M2, and NV) failed to induce a similar level of protective immunity.[29] The Apex-IHN vaccine was thus constructed by cloning the G-protein gene of IHNV in a plasmid backbone, yielding plasmid pUK-inhG[30]. Other elements in this plasmid included a bovine growth hormone polyadenylation signal, a cytomegalovirus (CMV) immediate early promoter–enhancer, and a selection marker.[25] Once purified to meet established quality standards, the plasmid DNA construct is formulated in a sterile saline solution with no adjuvants and at a concentration of 200 µg/mL.[24] The effectiveness of the Apex-IHN vaccine was demonstrated in large-scale, prelicensure field trials, which involved the intramuscular injection of 1000 salmon with 10 µg of the vaccine.[25] A first assessment of the outcome of the experiment was made 4 months after immunization by challenging 200 individuals in each of the vaccinated and control groups with live virus. The mortality among the immunized salmon was close to 29%, whereas only 1% of unvaccinated control individuals were able to survive. Furthermore, neutralizing antibodies were detected on half of the vaccinated fish. Similar levels of survival were obtained among vaccinated fish when challenges were performed at 8, 12, and 17 months after immunization, indicating that the vaccine was able to provide a long-lasting protection.[25] On the basis of these field trials, the manufacturer instructs users to immobilize healthy fish (>30 g) by anesthesia and then to inject intramuscularly a single 0.05 mL dose of the vaccine (10 µg plasmid) in the area close to the dorsal fin.*

Experiments performed with other fish species have confirmed this ability of DNA vaccines expressing the G protein to offer durable protection against IHNV.[31] This is illustrated, for example, in Figure 10.4, which displays the kinetics of the cumulative percent mortality (CPM) in rainbow trout immunized by intramuscular injection with 0.1 µg of a plasmid DNA vaccine encoding the IHNV G protein after a challenge with live IHNV at 25 months postvaccination.[31] The results show that 1 month after the challenge, the mortality among the immunized salmon was around 30%, whereas it reached almost 95% among nonimmunized salmon. The fact that the protective immunity provided a significant degree of protection 2 years after vaccination is impressive and constitutes one of the most striking features of fish DNA vaccines for IHNV[31]. Although reasons for the high effectiveness of the Apex-IHN DNA vaccine and of other G-protein-based DNA vaccines in salmon remain to be determined, some hypotheses were put forward to explain it. First, the high efficacy could be attributable to the type of antigen used, since DNA vaccines encoding other glycoproteins from fish rhabdoviruses have shown a similar ability to induce protective immunity in different fish hosts (e.g., carp, flounder).[32] This favorable antigenicity of glycoproteins is supported

* Available and accessed from http://www.drugs.com/vet/apex-ihn-can.html on September 9, 2009.

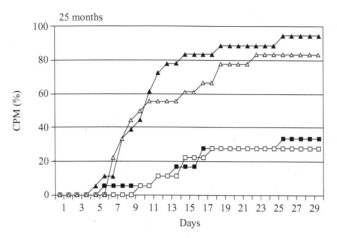

Figure 10.4 *Cumulative percent mortality (CPM) in rainbow trout (25 per group) immunized by intramuscular injection with 0.1 µg of a plasmid DNA vaccine encoding the IHNV G protein (squares) or with a mock plasmid vaccine (triangles) after a challenge with live IHNV at 25 months after vaccination. The experiments were performed in duplicate (group 1: open symbols, group 2: closed symbols). Reprinted from Vaccine, 24, Kurath G, Garver KA, Corbeil S, Elliott DG, Anderson ED, LaPatra SE. Protective immunity and lack of histopathological damage two years after DNA vaccination against infectious hematopoietic necrosis virus in trout, 345-354, Copyright 2006,[31] with permission from Elsevier.*

by the fact that fish DNA vaccines designed to elicit protection against other viruses have produced poorer results. The excellent results obtained, which have hardly been paralleled by mammalian DNA vaccines, may also be related to specific characteristics of the immune system in fish.[25,32] Finally, another hypothesis suggests that higher levels of the G-protein antigen are produced in salmon because enzymatic degradation of plasmid and mRNA is decreased in cold-blooded animals.[25,32]

10.3.3 Safety Issues and Environmental Risks

10.3.3.1 Introduction

It is clear from the review published recently by the promoters of the Apex-IHN DNA vaccine that safety concerns had to be tackled and investigated throughout the process, which eventually led to the approval of the product.[25] The willingness of the regulatory body responsible for the approval of the vaccine in Canada, the CFIA, to share with the public the information gathered on "the molecular and biological characteristics of the recombinant vaccine, target animal and non-target animal safety, human safety, environmental considerations and risk mitigation measures prepared" is also a good indication of the importance devoted to the safety issues that surround the use of DNA vaccines.[30] Although the safety and environmental risks associated with the veterinary use of a plasmid biopharmaceutical were presented in general terms in the last section of Chapter 7, in closing this discussion of the IHN case study, the available published data concerning the impact of the Apex-IHN DNA vaccine on the vaccinated specie, humans, and the environment are reviewed.

10.3.3.2 Persistence, Biodistribution, and Integration

One of the critical issues examined concerns the fate of the DNA vaccine once it is injected in fish. Although a fraction of the plasmid DNA is degraded locally at the injection site, other portions of it may gain access to the circulatory system and may thus be distributed to other tissues and organs.[33] Other plasmid molecules may also reach the organs and tissues by migration of cells harboring the plasmid from the injection site. An adequate knowledge of this distribution and persistence is important not only because the immunized fish will eventually be consumed by humans but also to determine if integration in the fish genome (hence germline transmission) is a likely event. This would open up the possibility for vertical transmission, not only in populations of captive fish but also, and perhaps more importantly, among populations of wild salmon. The issue of whether sequences of the DNA vaccine integrate into the fish genome is also extremely important since in the majority of countries, this fact would constitute a proof that a genetically modified organism (GMO) had been created. As was described in Chapter 7 (Section 7.5), the impact of such a GMO label in the marketing and consumer acceptance of the immunized farmed salmon would be very important, especially in regions such as the European Union.

In the case of the Apex-IHN vaccine, the experiments designed and conducted to determine how long and where exactly the plasmid and derived sequences persist in the immunized fish involved the injection of fish in a test group with a 2× dose of the DNA vaccine (i.e., 20 µg). Subsequently, samples from the gonads, liver, spleen, kidney, and intestines were collected at different time points postimmunization.[25] Following DNA extraction from these tissues, a quantitative polymerase chain reaction (PCR) assay was performed to look for the presence of sequences specific to the plasmid. The results were all negative with the exception of some liver samples examined 1 day postinjection. The examination of muscle close to the injection site also showed that the plasmid copy number decreased 99.5% within the first month postimmunization. Furthermore, after 2 months, only 0.01% of the initially injected plasmid could be detected.[25] These figures clearly show that the quantities of persisting plasmid are insignificant when compared with the levels of the host genomic DNA[30]. On the basis of these and other experiments, the likelihood of integration was determined to be negligible and substantially lower when compared with the probability of a spontaneous mutation.[25]

10.3.3.3 Human and Salmon Safety

The results described above indicate that the amounts of plasmid DNA in harvested salmon hardly constitute a hazard to human health. Even if some DNA fragments remain in the flesh of the immunized fish, it is more than likely that they will be readily degraded in the gastrointestinal tract upon ingestion.[30]

Another risk to human health that was evaluated by the CFIA regarded the possibility of self-administration of the vaccine by the operators in charge of the immunization procedure. On the basis of data reported by Aqua Health, Ltd., which showed that no such accidents occurred during the administration of 6.1 million doses in field trials, the probability of self-injection was considered extremely low. Even if such an accident might occur, experiments conducted by the company in mice showed that no adverse events could be associated with the injection of up to 10 times the recommended dose.[30] These results, together with other characteristics of the vaccine (e.g., nonpathogenic, no adjuvants, and small amount per dose) and with the current clinical experience, caused the CFIA to conclude in their assessment that "the widespread use of the vaccine is not expected to have any public health significance."[30]

The safety of the Apex-IHN vaccine to the salmon was supported on the basis of the safety trials and field studies conducted by the company, which showed no adverse reactions in fish following the administration of around 6.6 million doses and no genome integration. Further reassurance can also be found in the literature since there is currently an extensive amount of data showing that DNA vaccines are safe to fish.[30]

A series of safety precautions are associated with the use of the Apex-IHN vaccine.* For example, there is a specific recommendation stating that the vaccine should not be administered within 60 days before slaughter. This time period should be sufficient to allow the majority of the vaccine to be cleared from the system of the fish, thus minimizing the possibility of horizontal transfer to humans. A remark is also made regarding the possibility of an accidental injection of the operator. In this case, the recommendation is that the affected area should be cleaned with water and disinfectant, and that medical attention should be sought if infection develops. A final recommendation urges users to destroy unused vaccines by incineration.

10.3.3.4 Environmental Risks
Finally, one of the most critical questions surrounding the widespread use of the Apex-IHN DNA vaccine in farmed salmon has to do with the potential consequences caused by the escape of immunized fish. As was described above, the potential impact of the millions of farmed salmon that escape their cages every year over wild populations is very large. On top of this, the possibility that the escaping fish might host fragments of the Apex-IHN DNA vaccine (either in the tissues, cells, or integrated in the genome) and distribute them into the environment was an added concern for the promoters, regulatory authorities,[30] and other stakeholders.[33-35] Even if it was possible to prevent the escape of immunized salmon altogether, the semi-open cage systems used to farm salmon are clearly not an efficacious environmental barrier. For example, if the intestinal aerobic microbial flora that inhabits the fish gut is able to uptake plasmid sequences,[36] transformed microbes could easily access the

---

* Available and accessed from http://www.drugs.com/vet/apex-ihn-can.html on September 9, 2009.

external environment through shedding and dispersion across the mesh of the marine cages. Additionally, small fish could enter the cage and feed on any dead salmon.

Since the field studies described above (Section 10.3.3.2) discarded the possibility of integration of sequences from the vaccine in the fish genome, vertical integration to wild salmon through breeding is highly unlikely. Horizontal transmission to different phyla could also occur if the DNA vaccines or fragments thereof persist in the cells and tissues of the immunized animals. Other nontarget species could then contact with the extraneous DNA, for example, if they feed on the immunized animals. However, the results from the persistence and biodistribution described above, together with the fact that the vaccine is administered to salmon in an artificial tank several days before the fish are transferred to sea cages, provide a guarantee that any residual amounts of the vaccine will be negligible.[30]

The shedding of DNA from the salmon would constitute another possible exit route for the vaccine to reach the environment and other species.[33–35] This release of the vaccine from the fish is more likely to occur within the first week after immunization. According to the CFIA, Aqua Health provided sufficient evidence demonstrating that the vaccine is not shed from the immunized fish while they are kept in the artificial tanks prior to sea transfer. Furthermore, all effluent water from these tanks is mandatorily treated before being discharged into the environment.

The possibility of transformation of microbes in the intestines of salmon with fragments of the DNA vaccine was investigated in an experiment that looked for the resistance of microorganisms collected from the feces of vaccinated and control salmon to kanamycin, the selective antibiotic marker of the vaccine. Although resistance to kanamycin was detected, the study concluded that this was either innate or acquired, and was not due to transfer of the gene sequence from the vaccine.[36] An additional reassurance comes with the fact that *E. coli*, the production host used to manufacture the vaccine, is usually not found in the flora of salmon.[30]

In spite of the possibilities for the spread of the Apex-IHN DNA vaccine into the environment that were enumerated above, the results from the persistence, biodistribution, and integration studies, together with other safety trials, have led the CFIA to declare that "The risk to the environment is considered negligible."[30]

10.3.4 Final Remarks

The projected increase in the worldwide fish consumption, together with the fact that the wild populations of many fish species are drastically decreasing, has increased the attractiveness of the aquaculture market. One of the keys to the economic success of this business is the ability to maintain the health of the farmed captive fish. The availability of vaccines will undoubtedly play a key role in preventing many fish diseases. This scenario, together with the fact that many DNA fish vaccines have shown an efficacy that is yet without equal in human or mammalian veterinary medicine, provides an excellent ground for the development of commercial DNA vaccines. The case of Aqua Health's DNA vaccine against IHNV in Atlantic salmon constitutes an excellent example of the potential of DNA vaccines. First of all, a safe and highly efficacious product was licensed and introduced in the market in record time. Second, around 10 million doses of vaccine continue to be sold in Canada every year, at a cost of US$0.4 per dose, amounting to an annual volume of sales of the order of US$4 million (K. Salonious, Aqua Health R&D, pers. comm.). This clearly shows that there is a market for DNA vaccines. Finally, and in spite of the favorable outcome of the safety studies, it should be kept in mind that there are still some limitations and uncertainties when it comes to determining exactly what is the fate of DNA vaccines administered to fish, and thus what are the consequences to the ecosystem.[34,35] Thus, and in order to improve our understanding of these issues, a careful and continued monitoring should be carried out, as recommended by regulatory authorities.[30]

10.4 CMM

10.4.1 Melanoma as a Case for Comparative Oncology

CMM is a highly aggressive and frequently metastatic neoplasm that occurs spontaneously in the oral cavity, nail bed, foot pad, and mucocutaneous junction.[37,38] CMM can readily metastasize to the lymph nodes, liver, lung, and kidney and accounts for approximately 4% of all tumors diagnosed in dogs.[39] Like its human counterpart, CMM is a disease of older individuals.[38] The best treatment option for CMM is surgical extirpation, provided that distant metastatic disease is not present. Radiation therapy is a common solution when it is not possible to remove the tumor or if it has metastatized to local lymph nodes. The use of chemotherapy with agents like carboplastin or cisplatin is usually reserved for melanomas that have a moderate to high metastatic propensity. Unfortunately, melanoma is often resistant to chemotherapy.[38]

As is the case with other naturally occurring cancers in dogs and humans, CMM shares a number of similarities with advanced human melanoma, including tumor genetics, molecular targets, histological appearance, and biological behavior. Additionally, both are initially treated with local therapies like surgery and/or radiation therapy. Chemotherapy is used alike in canine and human melanoma, but with low response rates, which range from 8% to 28%, and little evidence of improvements in survival.[37,39] The likeness between the two diseases, together with the strong anatomical, physiological, and genetic similarities between the two species, offers an excellent opportunity to study the disease and to evaluate and develop alternative therapeutic methodologies.[1] For instance, the similarities among many of the gene families associated with cancer are significantly closer between humans and dogs as compared with humans and mice, the ubiquitous animal model of human disease in many research laboratories.[1] The large number of dogs diagnosed and treated with cancer every year also provides researchers with a large pool of potentially useful research subjects. The veterinary care services (practitioners and hospitals) for pet animals, which are in place in most of the first world countries, further constitute an excellent network of infrastructures for the control of clinical trials.[1] The technologies available in many of the veterinary centers include sophisticated diagnostic capabilities and imaging modalities (e.g., magnetic resonance imaging and computerized tomography) and advanced therapeutic options (e.g., nuclear medicine and radiation therapy), which are particularly valuable in the case of cancer.[1] Dog melanoma thus constitutes an excellent target to perform comparative oncology, an approach that aims to translate the knowledge and therapies generated from studies of naturally occurring cancers in animals into humans.[1]

The life span of dogs with melanomas that have gone beyond the initial stages and that are treated with conventional therapies typically varies between 1 and 5 months. This outcome is rather disappointing, and it is clear that alternatives to the treatment of melanoma should be pursued.[38] One such alternative relies on mobilizing the patient's immune system with the goal of eliciting antitumor responses via antibodies and T cells that mediate tumor regression and rejection.[40] This so-called cancer immunotherapy is thought to be particularly promising in those cases where patients have minimal residual disease. Different immunotherapy strategies have been pursued including, among others, the use of autologous tumor cells, gene-modified tumor cells, or peptide-based vaccines.[41] A number of research groups are also actively involved in the development of DNA vaccines for the treatment of human melanoma. One of the most promising products under development is Allovectin-7® (see Chapter 8, Section 8.5), a DNA vaccine designed by Vical Inc. (San Diego, California),[42,43] which is currently being tested in patients with recurrent metastatic melanoma in the context of phase 3 clinical trials (www.clinicaltrials.gov; identifier: NCT00395070). Another melanoma DNA vaccine project is being carried out consistently by Drs. Jedd Wolchok and Alan Houghton of the Memorial Sloan–Kettering Cancer Center (MSKCC) in New York.[44–47] Although focusing on human melanoma, the research carried out by this group served as the groundwork for the collaborative development of a canine melanoma DNA vaccine with Dr. Philip Bergman at the Animal Medical Center (AMC) in New York.[37,39,41] The development and evaluation of this vaccine and the codevelopment of its human analogue, which will be described next, constitutes an excellent illustration of the potential of translating biomedical research from dogs to human patients.

10.4.2 Xenogeneic DNA Vaccines for Melanoma

In order to stimulate an effective antimelanoma immunity, researchers at MSKCC have designed DNA vaccines with genes that express immunogenic melanoma-associated antigens in the target tissues. The focus had been specifically on melanoma differentiation antigens of the tyrosinase family (e.g., gp75/tyrosinase-related protein1 [TRP-1], TRP-2, and gp100/pMel-17). Tyrosinase is a glycoprotein normally expressed by cells of melanocytic origin, which is involved in the rate-limiting step of melanin synthesis from tyrosine. Such differentiation antigens, and particularly those that are involved in synthesis of pigment, are expressed homogeneously by most melanoma specimens. They are also the most prevalent antigens recognized by $CD8^+$ T cells from melanoma patients.[47] The restricted, tissue-specific expression of tyrosinase and other related proteins is an additional characteristic that makes them adequate antigens for the immunotherapy of melanoma.[41]

Given that most tumor antigens are also expressed on normal tissues, one of the problems associated with cancer DNA vaccines is host immune tolerance/ignorance due to poor immunogenicity of "self" antigens. This makes it difficult to induce immunity against a tissue-specific differentiation antigen on cancer cells. One way to circumvent this obstacle is to use DNA coding for a xenogeneic antigen that is homologous to the cancer antigen. Compelling results on mouse models have supported this hypothesis. For instance, although immunization of mice is ineffective when DNA coding for mouse melanosomal differentiation antigens (e.g., gp100) is used, replacing them by xenogeneic (e.g., human) genes leads to specific antibodies and T-cell responses.[44,45] This difference in the immunologic response is striking since the amino acid homology between mouse and human tyrosinase (huTyr) is very significant. The explanation for the results probably lies in the small differences in the epitopes of mouse and human antigens that improve recognition by major histocompatibility complex (MHC) class I or the T-cell receptor.[41]

10.4.3   Clinical Trials in Dogs

Following an inquiry by Dr. Philip Bergman from the AMC, an opportunity emerged to extrapolate the xenogeneic model to CMM. A first pilot clinical trial was thus set up and conducted at the AMC in 2000 in order to determine the safety and efficacy of xenogeneic DNA immunization of dogs with melanoma.[39,48] In this specific trial, the gene coding for huTyr, a protein with an 87.5% amino acid homology with canine tyrosinase, was cloned into an adequate DNA vaccine vector.[39] Nine dogs with confirmed spontaneous melanoma were enrolled in the trial and were separated in groups of three. Each group was treated with a total of four intramuscular vaccinations given 2 weeks apart and with doses of 100, 500, or 1500 µg DNA. Delivery was accomplished with the carbon dioxide-powered jet device Biojector 2000 (Bioject Medical Technologies, Inc., Tualatin, Oregon; see Chapter 6, Section 6.2.3). Based on clinical antitumor responses and remarkably prolonged median survival times of 389 days of the enrolled dogs when compared to historical controls that report survival times of 1–5 months with conventional therapies, the xenogeneic huTyr DNA vaccination was evaluated as potentially efficacious. Furthermore, the lack of systemic toxicity and minimal local toxicity demonstrated the safety of the DNA vaccine approach.[39] Subsequent investigations showed that the huTyr antigen was able to induce antibodies capable of cross-reacting with canine tyrosinase in three of the nine dogs, an important finding that suggests the overcoming of canine immune ignorance or tolerance.[41] An analysis of the survival of dogs further suggested an association between the positive antibody responses in these three dogs and their long-term survival (Figure 10.4). However, this effect was not statistically significant, given the small sample size involved.[41]

Subsequent animal studies of xenogeneic DNA vaccinations at the AMC involved the treatment of approximately 170 dogs with malignant melanoma.[37] Apart from huTyr, genes for murine GP75 (muGP75), murine tyrosinase (muTyr), and murine tyrosinase + human granulocyte macrophage colony-stimulating factor (muTyr/huGM-CSF) were also tested. In these studies, the treatment was fixed at a total of four intramuscular vaccinations given 2 weeks apart with the Biojector 2000 jet delivery device. The amounts of DNA vaccine per dose administered were varied, among subgroups of dogs, between 50 and 1500 µg. The median survival times for all dogs treated with huTyr, muGP75, and muTyr were 389, 153, and 224 days, respectively. Furthermore, the combination of muTyr/HuGM-CSF was found to improve the efficacy of muTyr or huGM-CSF alone. Essentially, no toxicity was observed.[37]

10.4.4   Licensing

Following some of the trials in dogs, licensing rights to the DNA vaccine were granted by the MSKCC and AMC to Merial, Inc. (Athens, Georgia), a company that specializes in animal health, which subsequently completed the industrialization and regulatory requirements for licensure. On March 22, 2007, a conditional U.S. Veterinary Biological Product License valid for 1 year was finally issued by the Animal and Plant Health Inspection Service (APHIS) to Merial for the manufacture and distribution of the DNA vaccine (product code 9240.D0).[48,49] According to U.S. regulations (9 CFR Part 102), conditional licenses may be issued to meet an emergency situation, limited market, local situation, or special circumstance. In the case of the canine melanoma DNA vaccine, the responsible authorities in the notice communicating the issuance of the license stated that "The special circumstance addressed here is the need for a product to treat dogs with stage II or stage III oral melanoma in which local disease control has been achieved."[49] The license was issued on the basis of safety data and a reasonable expectation of efficacy, but also on the assumption that Merial would complete efficacy studies and conduct further work to support full marketing approval. This supplementary data was gathered in the years that followed. More specifically, Merial performed a study where 58 dogs with stage II or stage III oral melanoma underwent surgery and were then treated with the DNA vaccine with four bi-weekly doses and booster administrations every six months.[50] The survival times of dogs treated with the vaccine were found to be significantly higher when compared with controls treated with surgery alone.[50] As a result, the U.S. Department of Agriculture granted full licensure to the vaccine, which received the trade name ONCEPT™ in January 2010.[50] This constituted an important landmark, since at that time no other therapeutic vaccine (whether DNA-based or not) had ever been approved for the treatment of cancer in either animals or humans. The vaccine is made available in packages with four 0.4 mL doses (Figure 10.5) and is to be administered with a needle-free transdermal device.[50]

10.4.5 Human Trials

The significant clinical responses observed in dogs vaccinated with the xeno-geneic tyrosinase DNA vaccine, together with their prolonged survival, urged researchers at MSKCC to conduct equivalent trials in human melanoma patients.[46,47] The first report on one of these clinical experiments has been published recently.[47] The major goals of this trial were to compare the safety and the therapeutic effect of DNA vaccines encoding either huTyr or mouse tyrosinase (muTyr) in patients with advanced-stage melanoma. The 18 subjects enrolled in the study were randomized into two groups and received a total of six injections of DNA vaccine (3 huTyr + 3 muTyr). According to the crossover design selected for the study, patients in one group were first primed with huTyr vaccine and then boosted with the muTyr vaccine, whereas in the other group, this scheme was reversed. Within each group, patients were further separated into three different dose cohorts (100, 500, and 1500 µg). As in the case of the dog trials, immunizations were given intramuscularly with the Biojector 2000 jet injection device. No significant side effects were developed by patients following injection of the DNA vaccines. Furthermore, the level of anti-DNA antibodies throughout the treatment was kept constant, even in those patients who received the highest doses. T-cell responses were detected in seven patients, independently of the dose or sequence of injection

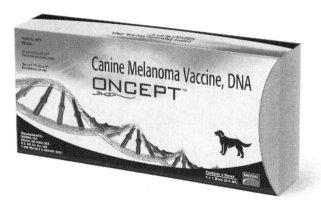

Figure 10.5 *ONCEPT™, the canine melanoma DNA vaccine co-developed by MSKCC, AMC, and Merial, was the first therapeutic plasmid biopharmaceutical to receive full approval from regulatory authorities on January 10, 2010. (©Merial Limited. All rights reserved. Reprinted with permission.)*

of the huTyr and muTyr vaccines. However, no antibody responses against tyrosinase were measured. Although the trial was not designed to demonstrate the therapeutic activity of tyrosinase DNA vaccines and patient selection may have resulted in skewing, the survival data reported compare favorably with historical data on the mean survival of melanoma patients. According to the authors, this study was the first to demonstrate the induction of T-cell responses to a self-antigen using xenogeneic DNA. Furthermore, it also showed that xenogeneic DNA vaccines can prime immune responses to self-antigens.[46,47]

10.4.6 Final Remarks

The xenogeneic melanoma DNA vaccine project led by MSKCC and AMC resulted in the first licensing of a therapeutic plasmid biopharmaceutical, a canine melanoma DNA vaccine. The introduction of such a truly novel product to the market is clearly an event to be highlighted, not only because of the promises it holds but also because of the questions that the use of DNA as a drug raises. For example, the Environmental Risk Management Authority (ERMA) in New Zealand received an inquiry from someone who was seeking to know "whether the vaccination of her dog (*Canis familiaris*) with the Canine Melanoma Vaccine (manufactured by Merial) would make that animal a GMO."[51] On the basis of evidence that showed that the likelihood for the vaccine to replicate within the vaccinated dog or integrate into its genome is highly improbable, the ERMA ruled that the vaccinated animal is not a GMO and is therefore not a new organism. This outcome can be considered favorable since it is likely to increase the user acceptance of the new plasmid biopharmaceuticals. However, it also illustrates very well the type of interrogations and worries that will be raised by the general public once more products arrive in the market.

10.5 CONCLUSIONS

The three cases examined in this chapter describe some of the most successful and impactful plasmid biopharmaceuticals as yet. In the case of the California condors, the value associated with the WNV DNA vaccine is unquestionable, even though it is not possible to put a price tag on saving a species from extinction. For aquaculture companies, the availability of a cheap DNA vaccine to protect farmed salmon against the deadly IHNV infection fulfills an unmet need and significantly contributes to minimize one of the most prominent risks faced by the industry in recent years. As for the canine melanoma DNA vaccine, a substantial number of pet owners will definitely be willing to pay the cost of the full treatment. For companies, the melanoma vaccine further shows that the possibility of return on investment is a reality. Finally, the codevelopment of this veterinary product with a human equivalent also illustrates the value of the two-species approach. But perhaps the real worth of these three DNA vaccines lies on the lessons and insights that have been gained throughout the process of their development, use, and licensing, and on the demonstration that there is a place in the market for successful plasmid biopharmaceuticals.

REFERENCES

1. Paoloni M, Khanna C. Translation of new cancer treatments from pet dogs to humans. *Nature Reviews in Cancer.* 2008;8:147–156.

2. Nash D, Mostashari F, Fine A, et al. The outbreak of West Nile virus infection in the New York City area in 1999. *New England Journal of Medicine.* 2001;344: 1807–1814.

3. Lanciotti RS, Roehrig JT, Deubel V, et al. Origin of the West Nile virus responsible for an outbreak of encephalitis in the northeastern United States. *Science.* 1999;286:2333–2337.

4. Anderson JF, Andreadis TG, Vossbrinck CR, et al. Isolation of West Nile virus from mosquitoes, crows, and a Cooper's hawk in Connecticut. *Science.* 1999;286: 2331–2333.

5. Jia XY, Briese T, Jordan I, et al. Genetic analysis of West Nile New York 1999 encephalitis virus. *Lancet.* 1999;354:1971–1972.

6. Chang GJ, Davis BS, Stringfield C, Lutz C. Prospective immunization of the endangered California condors (*Gymnogyps californianus*) protects this species from lethal West Nile virus infection. *Vaccine.* 2007;25:2325–2330.

7. McLean R. West Nile virus in North American birds. *Ornithological Monographs.* 2006;60:44–64.

8. Petersen LR, Roehrig JT. West Nile virus: A reemerging global pathogen. *Emerging Infectious Diseases.* 2001;7:611–613.

9. National Audubon Society. *West Nile virus: The virus.* New York: National Audubon Society, 2005.

10. Trock SC, Meade BJ, Glaser AL, et al. West Nile virus outbreak among horses in New York State, 1999 and 2000. *Emerging Infectious Diseases.* 2001;7:745–747.

11. Brinton MA. The molecular biology of West Nile virus: A new invader of the Western Hemisphere. *Annual Reviews in Microbiology.* 2002;56:371–402.

12. Komar N, Langevin S, Hinten S, et al. Experimental infection of North American birds with the New York 1999 strain of West Nile virus. *Emerging Infectious Diseases.* 2003;9:311–322.

13. Nemeth N, Gould D, Bowen R, Komar N. Natural and experimental West Nile virus infection in five raptor species. *Journal of Wildlife Disease.* 2006;42:1–13.

14. Yang JS, Ramanathan MP, Muthumani K, et al. Induction of inflammation by West Nile virus capsid through the caspase-9 apoptotic pathway. *Emerging Infectious Diseases.* 2002;8:1379–1384.

15. Kiff LF, Mesta RI, Wallace MP. *California condor recovery plan.* Portland, OR: U.S. Fish and Wildlife Service, 1996.

16. DNA vaccine deployed for endangered condors. *Nature Biotechnology.* 2003;21:11.

17. Nusbaum KE, Wright JC, Johnston WB, et al. Absence of humoral response in flamingos and red-tailed hawks to experimental vaccination with a killed West Nile virus vaccine. *Avian Disease.* 2003;47:750–752.

18. Powell K. DNA vaccines-back in the saddle again? *Nature Biotechnology.* 2004;22: 799–801.

19. Davis BS, Chang GJ, Cropp B, et al. West Nile virus recombinant DNA vaccine protects mouse and horse from virus challenge and expresses *in vitro* a noninfectious recombinant antigen that can be used in enzyme-linked immunosorbent assays. *Journal of Virology.* 2001;75:4040–4047.

20. Turell MJ, Bunning M, Ludwig GV, et al. DNA vaccine for West Nile virus infection in fish crows (*Corvus ossifragus*). *Emerging Infectious Diseases.* 2003;9:1077–1081.

21. Ballantyne J, Klocke D, Smiley L. *Production of a West Nile virus DNA vaccine using PerfluorosorbS.* Fargo, ND: Aldevron, 2004.

22. Thorstad EB, Fleming IA, McGinnity P, Soto D, Wennevik V, Whoriskey F. *Incidence and impacts of escaped farmed Atlantic salmon* Salmo salar *in nature. NINA Special Report 36*: World Wildlife Fund, 2008.

23. Saksida S. *Investigation of the 2001–2003 IHN epizootic in farmed Atlantic Salmon in British Columbia.* Prepared for the British Columbia Ministry of Agriculture, Fisheries and Food and the British Columbia Salmon Farmers Association; 2003.

24. Simard NC. The road to licensure of a DNA vaccine for Atlantic salmon. Paper presented at the Workshop on Genetic Vaccines—Benefit and Challenges, November 24–25, 2008, Oslo.

25. Salonius K, Simard N, Harland R, Ulmer JB. The road to licensure of a DNA vaccine. *Current Opinion in Investigational Drugs.* 2007;8:635–641.

26. Schutze H, Enzmann PJ, Kuchling R, Mundt E, Niemann H, Mettenleiter TC. Complete genomic sequence of the fish rhabdovirus infectious haematopoietic necrosis virus. *Journal of General Virology.* 1995;76(Pt 10):2519–2527.

27. Harmache A, LeBerre M, Droineau S, Giovannini M, Bremont M. Bioluminescence imaging of live infected salmonids reveals that the fin bases are the major portal of entry for Novirhabdovirus. *Journal of Virology.* 2006;80:3655–3659.

28. Huang C, Chien MS, Landolt M, Batts W, Winton J. Mapping the neutralizing epitopes on the glycoprotein of infectious haematopoietic necrosis virus, a fish rhabdovirus. *Journal of General Virology.* 1996;77(Pt 12):3033–3040.

29. Corbeil S, Lapatra SE, Anderson ED, et al. Evaluation of the protective immunogenicity of the N, P, M, NV and G proteins of infectious hematopoietic necrosis virus in rainbow trout *Oncorhynchus mykiss* using DNA vaccines. *Diseases of Aquatic Organisms.* 1999;39:29–36.

30. Canadian Food Inspection Agency, Veterinary Biologics Section, Animal Health and Production Division. Environmental assessment for licensing infectious haematopoietic necrosis virus vaccine, DNA vaccine in Canada. Ottawa, July 5, 2005.

31. Kurath G, Garver KA, Corbeil S, Elliott DG, Anderson ED, LaPatra SE. Protective immunity and lack of histopathological damage two years after DNA vaccination against infectious hematopoietic necrosis virus in trout. *Vaccine.* 2006;24:345–354.

32. Kurath G. Overview of recent DNA vaccine development for fish. *Development of Biologicals.* 2005;121:201–213.

33. Tonheim TC, Bøgwald J, Dalmo RA. What happens to the DNA vaccine in fish? A review of current knowledge. *Fish & Shellfish Immunology*. 2008;25:1–18.

34. Gillund F, Kjolberg KA, von Krauss MK, Myhr AI. Do uncertainty analyses reveal uncertainties? Using the introduction of DNA vaccines to aquaculture as a case. *Science of the Total Environment*. 2008;407:185–196.

35. Gillund F, Dalmo R, Tonheim TC, Seternes T, Myhr AI. DNA vaccination in aquaculture—Expert judgments of impacts on environment and fish health. *Aquaculture*. 2008;284:25–34.

36. Simard NC, Moores D. DNA vaccines and environmental safety. Paper presented at the 31st Eastern Fish Health Workshop, March 31–April 4, 2006, Mount Pleasant.

37. Bergman PJ, Camps-Palau MA, McKnight JA, et al. Development of a xenogeneic DNA vaccine program for canine malignant melanoma at the Animal Medical Center. *Vaccine*. 2006;24:4582–4585.

38. Bergman PJ. Canine oral melanoma. *Clinical Techniques in Small Animal Practice*. 2007;22:55–60.

39. Bergman PJ, McKnight J, Novosad A, et al. Long-term survival of dogs with advanced malignant melanoma after DNA vaccination with xenogeneic human tyrosinase: A phase I trial. *Clinical Cancer Research*. 2003;9:1284–1290.

40. Chapman PB. Melanoma vaccines. *Seminars in Oncology*. 2007;34:516–523.

41. Liao JC, Gregor P, Wolchok JD, et al. Vaccination with human tyrosinase DNA induces antibody responses in dogs with advanced melanoma. *Cancer Immunology*. 2006;6:8. Available at: http://www.cancerimmunity.org/v6p8/060308.htm.

42. Galanis E. Technology evaluation: Allovectin-7, Vical. *Current Opinion in Molecular Therapy*. 2002;4:80–87.

43. Gonzalez R, Hutchins L, Nemunaitis J, Atkins M, Schwarzenberger PO. Phase 2 trial of Allovectin-7 in advanced metastatic melanoma. *Melanoma Research*. 2006;16:521–526.

44. Bowne WB, Srinivasan R, Wolchok JD, et al. Coupling and uncoupling of tumor immunity and autoimmunity. *Journal of Experimental Medicine*. 1999;190: 1717–1722.

45. Weber LW, Bowne WB, Wolchok JD, et al. Tumor immunity and autoimmunity induced by immunization with homologous DNA. *Journal of Clinical Investigation*. 1998;102:1258–1264.

46. Wolchok J, Chapman PB, Houghton AN, et al. *MSKCC therapeutic/diagnostic protocol: Injection of AJCC Stage IIB, IIC, III and IV melanoma patients with mouse gp100 DNA–A pilot study to compare intramuscular jet injection with particle mediated delivery*. New York: Memorial Sloan–Kettering Cancer Center, 2007 2005. IRB#: 06-113A(2).

47. Wolchok JD, Yuan J, Houghton AN, et al. Safety and immunogenicity of tyrosinase DNA vaccines in patients with melanoma. *Molecular Therapy*. 2007;15: 2044–2050.

48. Merial Limited. USDA grants conditional approval for first therapeutic vaccine to treat cancer (news release). Duluth, MN, March 26, 2007.

49. Hill RE. *Issuance of a conditional license for canine melanoma vaccine, DNA (Center for Veterinary Biologics notice No. 07-03)*. Ames, IA: Animal and Plant Health Inspection Service, 2007.

50. Merial Limited. *ONCEPT^{TM} canine melanoma vaccine, DNA now fully licensed by USDA (news release)*. Duluth, MN, January 10, 2010.

51. Environmental Risk Management Authority. To determine whether a dog vaccinated with the canine melanoma vaccine is a new organism (Application Number: S2608008, ERMA New Zealand Evaluation and Review Report). Wellington, 2008.

Part III

Manufacturing

11

Good Manufacturing Practice and Validation

11.1 INTRODUCTION

The passage of the Pure Food and Drug Act in the United States in 1906 led directly to the creation of the Food and Drug Administration (FDA), the first citizen protection agency of the U.S. federal government.[1] At a time when deception, fraud, and adulteration were common expedients used by merchants and businessmen taken over by moneymaking fever, the goal of this pioneering law was to ensure that commercial enterprises would provide consumers with unadulterated, uncontaminated food and potent and safe medicines.[1] However, and despite its good intentions, the 1906 law had too many loopholes and, in most instances, failed to protect citizens from the more aggressive business interests.[1] The inability of the law to prevent disasters like the mass poisoning caused by the elixir sulfanilamide in the United States in 1937 led to its replacement by the *Food, Drug, and Cosmetic Act*, which was signed by Franklin Roosevelt on June 15, 1938.[1] The 1938 act constituted a landmark, most noticeably because it was the first law ever to require companies to check their drugs for safety and to submit the corresponding data to the FDA before commercialization. From then on, the whole process by which medicines were ultimately brought to the public changed radically. New drugs were no longer concocted by amateurs but had rather to be discovered and developed on the basis of a rational scientific approach and experimentation.

Plasmid Biopharmaceuticals: Basics, Applications, and Manufacturing, First Edition.
Duarte Miguel F. Prazeres.
© 2011 John Wiley & Sons, Inc. Published 2011 by John Wiley & Sons, Inc.

This constituted a radical departure from the past and was one of the key drivers in the creation of the modern pharmaceutical industry.

11.2 THE QUALITY TRIPOD

The discovery, development, and commercialization of any medicinal product intended to be used as a therapeutic agent in humans is a long, multistage process (Figure 11.1). Once the decision to proceed with the development of a particular product is made, usually on the basis of solid scientific evidence established by basic and applied research findings, a series of activities ensues, which includes the conceptualization of the product, process development, preclinical testing, clinical trials, and large-scale manufacturing. The successful completion of each of these stages contributes to add value to the product, hence the name "value chain," which is often used to describe the spectrum of activities that are carried out during the development of a medicinal product.

The drug/biological development and commercialization stages are subject to different types of legislative controls that have been put in place by governments and their regulatory agencies in order to guarantee that those products sold to and used by the general public are safe and effective.[2] The quality that is inherent to these two attributes (i.e., safety and effectiveness) must be present throughout the preclinical testing, clinical trials, and manufacturing stages of the value chain (Figure 11.1). Each of these three stages is controlled by a set of rules or regulations that have the power of law behind them and together form a "quality tripod" (Figure 11.2).[2] The first of these regulations,

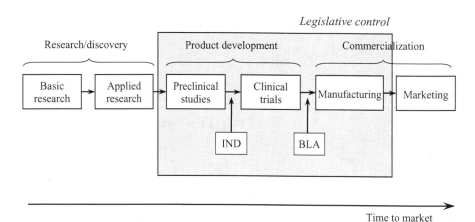

Figure 11.1 *The discovery, development, and commercialization of medicinal products for therapeutic use in humans. The gray box identifies those stages that are subject to legislative controls. The duration of each stage will vary from product to product. BLA, biologics license application; IND, investigational new drug.*

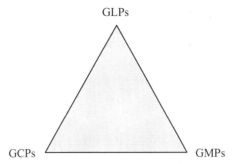

Figure 11.2 *The quality tripod: assuring the safety and efficacy of drugs and biologics. Preclinical testing, clinical trials, and large-scale manufacturing are controlled by the good laboratory practice (GLPs), good clinical practice (GCPs), and good manufacturing practice (GMPs) rules, respectively.*

known as good laboratory practice (GLP), contains the minimum requirements for the planning, conduct, and reporting of nonclinical safety and efficacy studies carried out with a medicinal product in the laboratory and in experimental animal models. The main goal of GLPs is to ensure the quality, integrity, and reliability of the study data while simultaneously reducing the likelihood that experiments have to be repeated later on.[3] In the end, the observance of GLPs will guarantee that the potential safety and efficacy of products is demonstrated on the basis of high quality and scientifically sound preclinical studies.[4] The use of GLP in European Union (EU) member states is governed by the European Directive 2004/10/EC, whereas in the United States, they can be found in Part 58 ("Good Laboratory Practice for Nonclinical Laboratory Studies") of Title 21 of the *Code of Federal Regulations* (CFR). Development of a product can be suspended by the FDA if GLPs are not adhered to.[5]

Clinical trials on medicinal products for human use are also controlled, namely, by a set of rules known as good clinical practice (GCP).[6] GCPs are "internationally recognized ethical and scientific quality requirements which must be observed for designing, conducting, recording and reporting clinical trials that involve the participation of human subjects."[7] The strict observation of GCPs by any individual, company, institution, or organization (i.e., any sponsor) that conducts, manages, or finances clinical trials should offer a guarantee that "the rights, safety and well-being of trials subjects are protected, and that the results of the trials are credible."[7] GCP is especially important in the context of conceptually and radically new therapeutic strategies like gene therapy, which may not be totally free from potential side effects.[8] For instance, in the case of the ornithine transcarbamylase (OTC) gene therapy death described in Chapter 1 (Section 1.1.4), doubts were raised over whether the letter and spirit of GCPs had been violated by the responsible researchers and their institutions. In its final allegation on the case, the U.S. Department of Justice concluded that the trial should have been halted prior to the accident on the basis of toxic reactions in humans, and that the lead investigators had misrepresented the clinical findings to the NIH and FDA, the institutions overseeing the study.[9]

Although necessary, the demonstration of the safety and efficacy of a specific medicinal product, which is supported by the results of the preclinical testing and clinical trials performed under GLP and GCP, respectively, is not sufficient. In order for the quality of a medicinal product to be guaranteed with a very high degree of assurance, its manufacturing process must comply with a third set of regulatory requirements known as good manufacturing practice (GMPs). The principle underlying GMPs is that in order to get new products approved by regulatory agencies, "The holder of a manufacturing authorization must manufacture medicinal products so as to ensure that they are fit for their intended use, comply with the requirements of the Marketing Authorization, and do not place patients at risk due to inadequate safety, quality or efficacy."[10] This goal calls for the implementation of a quality assurance (QA) system that incorporates GMPs, a set of rules that deals essentially with the production and quality control (QC) of a drug or biologic. Such GMPs were elaborated on the basis of three fundamental QA principles:[2]

(1) Quality, safety, and effectiveness must be designed and built into a product.
(2) Quality cannot be inspected or tested into a finished product.
(3) Each step of the manufacturing process must be controlled to maximize the likelihood that the finished product will be acceptable.

It should be stressed that GMPs must be observed not only during regular manufacturing of products that have received marketing authorization but also while preparing material that is intended for the different phases of human clinical trials (Figure 11.1).

The first GMP regulations were developed in the United States. Following their publication in 1963, a series of updates, reassessments, and revisions have been made over the years so that the rules reflect the latest technological and scientific knowledge.[11] For this reason, they are sometimes referred to as the "current" good manufacturing practice (cGMPs) rules.[2] Similar regulations have been issued by other countries, including the EU, Canada, Australia, and Japan. In the United States, the text of the GMP regulations can be found in Sections 210[12] and 211[13] of Title 21 of the CFR. Specific regulations for biologics, hence for plasmid biopharmaceuticals, can be found in Section 600 of the same code.[14] In the EU, the principles and guidelines of GMP for medicinal products for human use were laid down by the Commission Directive 91/356/EEC of June 13, 1991.[15] The same GMP requirements also apply to the manufacture of veterinary medicinal products, as arranged in the similar Commission Directive 91/412/EEC of July 23, 1991.[16] The full text of the GMP rules has been published by the European Union Drug Review Agency (EUDRA).[10] In Canada, the GMP regulations are codified in the *Food and Drug Act* Part C,

Division 2, Sections C.02.001–030, whereas in Japan, the regulations are specified in Ordinance No. 31, 1980, of the Ministry of Health and Welfare (MHW).[2] The World Health Organization (WHO) has also published reports describing the general manufacturing requirements contained in GMP for pharmaceutical[17] and biological[18] products. Attempts at harmonizing the regulatory requirements pertaining to medicinal products (including GMPs) were initiated in 1990 with the establishment of the International Conference on Harmonization (ICH), a project that brings together the regulatory authorities and experts from the pharmaceutical industries of Europe, Japan, and the United States. The specific topic of GMP requirements has been formalized in a document entitled "Good Manufacturing Practice Guide for Active Pharmaceutical Ingredients."[19]

The GMP requirements are enforced by regulatory agencies like the FDA, the European Medicines Agency (EMA), and the Canadian Health Products and Food Branch Inspectorate (HPFBI). These agencies check for GMP compliance by conducting inspections of manufacturing facilities, reviewing documents, and performing random tests of products. Many times, the inspection activities of regulatory agencies are extended abroad to exporting companies.[20] In the United States, if the methods or facilities used to manufacture a drug or a biologic do not conform to or are not operated in conformity with cGMPs, the product in question is deemed adulterated. Similar strictness is found within the EU where legal action can be taken against the persons responsible for manufacturing in case of noncompliance.[11]

11.3 GMPs

A possible definition of GMP states that "Good Manufacturing Practice is that part of Quality Assurance which ensures that products are consistently produced and controlled to the quality standards appropriate to their intended use and as required by the Marketing Authorization or product specification."[10] GMPs should be viewed more as a set of minimum requirements[12] issued in the context of a QA philosophy rather than a strict list of rules that companies must obey blindly. Actually, not all requirements that need to be followed are clearly written in the GMPs, and thus it is the responsibility of manufacturers to actively do their best to guarantee the quality of their products.[20] Although the range of topics addressed by GMPs may vary slightly from country to country, they generally cover topics such as personnel, premises and equipment, documentation, production, QC, validation, contract manufacturing and analysis, complaints and product recalls, and self-inspection. A brief description of some of the aspects covered in those topics is provided next, which is essentially based on an overview of the European,[10,15] U.S., and harmonized GMPs.[12,13,19] The reader should examine the original documents and specialized literature (e.g., see Kanarek[2]) for a more detailed and comprehensive description of GMPs.

11.3.1 Personnel

The manufacturing of medicinal products and the assurance of their quality depend on the existence of qualified and experienced people in a number sufficient to carry out all tasks involved. The existence of an organization chart and the unambiguous definition of the duties, responsibilities, and authority involved are vital aspects in this context. GMPs identify as key persons the heads of production and of QC. The latter is especially important, given the power he/she has to approve or reject (1) all materials used in the manufacture, packaging, and labeling of the product and (2) finished products.[2] The QC head should also ensure the accuracy of all production and testing records. The success of a facility will, to a large extent, depend on the level of its personnel, who should have the education, experience, and training adequate for the tasks ascribed to them.[20] Continued training, with an emphasis on the theory and practice of QA and GMP, is essential and should be provided by the manufacturer according to the specific duties assigned to the personnel. The establishment of hygiene programs, including methods related to the health, hygiene, and clothing of personnel, is another important aspect to be looked upon.[11] Health surveillance of personnel, including detailed medical examination and tests, is usually required on an annual basis. Persons who have a condition that can be adverse to the product should be excluded from the production areas.[21]

11.3.2 Premises and Equipment

GMPs stress that operations used to manufacture medicinal products should be carried out in adequately located, designed, constructed, and maintained premises. The same requirements apply to the equipment used throughout the entire processing. The key driver during the layout, design, and operation of a facility and associated equipment is the minimization of the occurrence of process errors and contamination. Contamination can be broadly defined as "any material, substance or energy that adversely affects the product or the process."[22] Particulate contamination includes, for instance, metal particles from equipment, rubber particles from stoppers, fibers from wipes or clothing, or glass debris from broken vials. The control and reduction of the number of these particles in the manufacturing environment is extremely important since many of them act as carriers of bacteria and viruses. The sources for these microbes include personnel, water, air, surfaces, and equipment.

Contamination issues are particularly relevant when manufacturing parenterals, that is, products that are to be administered by injection through intravenous, intramuscular, or other routes. In these cases, the possibility of product contamination with bacteria or viruses should be minimized in order to guarantee the required sterility of the parenteral. This is especially important when terminal sterilization of products at the end of the process is not feasible (e.g., due to product degradation). In this case, aseptic conditions should be adopted

TABLE 11.1. Classification of Clean Rooms According to the FDA and International Standard ISO 14644-1

Description		Maximum Number of Particles per Cubic Meter
ISO 14644-1	FDA	
ISO Class 5	Class 100	3,520
ISO Class 6	Class 1000	35,200
ISO Class 7	Class 10000	352,000
ISO Class 8	Class 100000	3,520,000

Source: Adapted from del Valle.[23]

throughout the process.[23] The best way to prevent product contamination with particles and associated microbes is to reduce their number in the air by operating within rooms with a high level of cleanliness. Such a *clean room* may be defined as "a room in which the concentration of airborne particles is controlled, and which is constructed and used in a manner to minimize the introduction, generation and retention of particles inside the room, and in which other relevant parameters, for example, temperature, humidity, and pressure, are controlled as necessary."[23] Clean rooms are typically classified into classes (in the United States), grades (in the EU), or ISO (International Organization for Standardization) classes, according to the number of 0.1- to 5.0-μm particles/m^3 of air (Table 11.1). The level of cleanliness of the different clean room classes can be best judged by comparing the particle numbers shown in Table 11.1 for the different clean room classes, with a typical untreated air, which contains, on average, 4×10^7 particles of size 0.5μm and larger per cubic meter.[23]

Although operating an entire manufacturing facility under the most stringent conditions would ensure product sterility, this is usually not necessary, apart from being too expensive. Alternatively, the class of the clean room should be chosen on the basis of the contamination risks associated with the specific operations that are going to be performed there. For instance, an ISO 8 (Class 100000) room could be adopted for fermentation and an ISO 7 (Class 10000) for downstream processing, whereas ISO 5 (Class 100) rooms are mandatory in critical areas, that is, those areas where the product is, or could be, directly exposed to the environment such as during aseptic filling.[22,23]

Systems combining air handling units and high-efficiency particulate air (HEPA) filters are used to provide an air supply that is cleaner than that required.[23] The air typically enters a room through HEPA filters installed in the ceiling and exits through air ducts strategically located at the floor level behind equipment/operations that may generate particles.[24] The airflow rate and direction should be such that any particles generated during operation are swept away smoothly while nonturbulent air passes through the room. ISO 6 (Class 1000) and ISO 7 (Class 10000) clean rooms typically use airflow rates equal to 120 and 60 air changes (AC)/h, respectively.[24]

Other issues that have to be addressed when constructing a clean room include the characteristics of the floor, ceiling, and wall surfaces (smooth, hard, and easily cleanable); the use of air-locks and pass-throughs as the entry point of materials and equipment; the use of negative or positive pressure to control airflow when doors are opened; and the existence of systems for monitoring and controlling environmental conditions such as temperature and humidity.[13,15] Particle generation during processing should also be minimized by adopting a series of measures. Since more than 95% of contamination comes from personnel, specific emphasis should be put on their health, hygiene, and clothing (see Section 11.3.1). Different types of clothing will be required depending on the air grade of the room where the personnel will be working. Additionally, wristwatches, jewelry, and cosmetics, which can shed particles, should not be used in clean areas.[10] Cleaning (i.e., the removal of particulate matter) and sanitization (i.e., the removal, destruction, or inactivation of microorganisms) of the rooms prior to and after processing is also crucial. This should be done according to validated procedures (see Section 11.4), using adequate materials, equipment, supplies, and techniques by dedicated and trained personnel.[22,25,26] Logbooks are typically used to document every cleaning and sanitization step that has been carried out (see Section 11.3.3).

Contamination can also be minimized by orderly placing clean rooms, equipment, and materials, and by adequately designing the flow of the different materials and personnel through the manufacturing building. This requires the definition of sufficiently sized areas for specific operations, for example, storage, processing, packaging, labeling, and quarantine. Clean rooms of different ISO classes should be placed in such a way that differential pressures can be delivered to ensure that a gradient of airflow runs from the cleaner to the dirtier spaces (Figure 11.3). The exception to this rule includes rooms

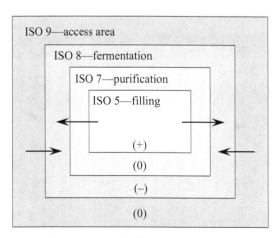

Figure 11.3 *Placement of clean rooms of different ISO classes within a facility dedicated to the manufacturing of biologics. The direction of the airflow indicated by the arrows is imposed by the differential pressurization of rooms. The air flows from the cleaner (ISO 5, filling) to the dirtier (ISO 8, fermentation) spaces. This case assumes that containment of the biological material is required, and thus the pressure in the fermentation room is lower than the pressure in the access area. Symbols indicate negative (–), normal (0), and positive (+) pressures.*

where biosafety containment is mandatory (e.g., if biohazardous material is involved), in which case negative pressure must be ensured.[23] For instance, rooms used for bacterial fermentation with recombinant *Escherichia coli* are typically maintained at negative pressure, whereas purification areas are usually positively pressured. In some cases, localized containment can be achieved in a positively pressurized room by working within adequate safety cabinets. The use of a negative "sink" area is also a means of providing containment between adjacent rooms.[27] Air locks with adequate air pressures are often used to separate individual rooms. The flow of personnel, components, product, and waste through the production areas is usually unidirectional. This means that rooms have separate entrances and exits. An efficient way of transporting materials between adjacent rooms is via pass-throughs.[21] These units feature interlocking doors that help maintain the clean room seal and offer protection against possible airborne contamination from loss of pressure.

Whenever possible, equipment should be designed, chosen, and installed so that (1) it can be moved outside clean rooms for repair and planned maintenance, (2) it is easily and thoroughly cleaned according to validated procedures, (3) it is not a source of contamination, (4) risks and errors are prevented, and (5) it does not present any hazard to the product. The qualification of the different equipment items prior to the start of routine manufacturing is a mandatory validation task (see Section 11.4.2).

11.3.3 Documentation

One of the requisites that is ubiquitous throughout the whole GMP is the need to write down and document material specifications, product specifications, standard operating procedures (SOPs), and batch manufacturing records, as well as keep equipment and facility logbooks, validation protocols, calibration files, and personal education and training records.[21,28] Such documents and records should be comprehensive, legible, error free, and up to date, so that it may be possible to trace back the manufacture of a particular batch in case an adverse event takes place. Additionally, such documents must be approved, signed, and dated by appropriate and authorized persons (e.g., the QC head), and all must be available for inspection purposes.[11] The strict adherence to the instructions written in SOPs and other documents will ensure compliance with most of the topics covered in GMP rules.[2] Furthermore, the adequacy and safety of any electronic data processing and storage systems should be validated (see Section 11.4) in order to ensure that there is a very low risk of loss of or damage to information when using such systems.[11] The strictness on documentation is such that as far as inspecting authorities are concerned, activities that have not been recorded have not been performed.[29]

11.3.4 Production

Production operations are at the heart of a manufacturing plant. GMP considerations on this topic usually contain recommendations on issues like prevention of cross contamination in production, starting raw materials, packaging materials and operations, and processing operations.[10] The risks associated with accidental cross contamination of products (especially parenterals) can be avoided and minimized by taking appropriate technical and organizational measures. As seen previously, this includes operation in an adequately clean environment, which is supplied with an appropriate amount of sufficiently treated air, adequate gowning of healthy personnel, and adoption of effective cleaning and sanitization procedures. A strong emphasis is also put by GMPs on the quality of starting raw materials. These should be purchased by knowledgeable staff and only from approved and qualified suppliers. The processes used by suppliers to manufacture raw materials should be scrutinized as an extra guarantee. This is particularly important in those cases (e.g., bovine-derived materials) where risks have been identified which are associated with their direct incorporation into products or use in manufacturing[30] (see Section 11.5.3). Materials should be transported and delivered in adequately labeled and appropriate containers, and stored in dedicated areas. Only those materials that have been tested and released by the QC unit should be used. Similar attention should be paid to packing materials, including labels.

Only those materials and documents[30] that are required for a particular operation should be taken into the production area. The rooms and equipment should be cleaned adequately[30] in advance of the operation. Only the minimum number of workers required should be present, and their movement should be controlled and methodical to reduce the possibility of particle and microorganism shedding. The manufacturing process, and chiefly those steps that have been identified as critical, should be validated (see Section 11.4) before starting routine production of material which is intended for commercialization.

11.3.5 QC

Given the philosophy inherent to GMPs, the existence of a QC department is mandatory. Headed by a qualified person, adequately staffed (see Section 11.3.1) and equipped, the mission of this department is to test intermediate and finished products, as well as containers, labeling, and raw and packaging materials, in order to check that they conform to the respective specifications. The QC department should also review the entire production process used to manufacture any lot prior to its release for sale or distribution by analyzing the corresponding record, in order to ensure that no errors have occurred. The QC department is further responsible for retaining samples of each batch of finished products and of starting materials (excluding solvents, gases, and water). These should be readily available if required by competent authorities. Additional responsibilities of the unit include the review and approval of written documents like specifications, SOPs, and protocols; the conduction of internal quality and compliance audits; and the certification of subcontractors and suppliers.[20] Overall, the QC unit has the prerogative to approve or reject any products manufactured, processed, packed, or held under contract by another company.[13,15]

11.3.6 Contract Manufacturing and Analysis

The contracting out of specific manufacturing operations or QC analysis is possible, provided that a number of arrangements are made, including the contractual definition of the responsibilities of the two parties and the observation of the principles and guidelines of GMPs by the contract acceptor. Additionally, the contract acceptor shall not subcontract any portion of the work and should be ready to accommodate any inspection of its premises and operations carried out by competent authorities.

11.4 VALIDATION

11.4.1 Introduction

Validation is one of the cornerstone provisions of cGMPs. This topic has been introduced into GMPs as an extra requirement to ensure the consistent manufacturing of products with the required quality at the lowest possible cost.[31] According to a well-known definition, validation is "the process of establishing documentary evidence that provides a high degree of assurance that any product, process, activity, procedure, system, equipment, or software used in the control and manufacture consistently performs to or meets its predetermined specifications." From this definition, it is clear that almost every activity within a manufacturing plant is prone to validation. Typical procedures and topics within a manufacturing process that are subject to validation include facilities, equipment, computers, cleaning, sterilization, measuring, dispensing, weighing, filling, labeling, and packing, apart from the unit operation steps and associated analytical methods themselves.[31,32] Specific attention should be focused on any aspect of the process where variability is known to occur—in these cases, the validation process will contribute to identification, understanding, and control of the sources of variability.[32,33] In the end, manufacturers will be asked by regulatory authorities to provide documents demonstrating that the processes and methods that have a significant effect in final product quality have been validated.

11.4.2 Qualification

Validation calls for the *qualification* of (1) the facility; (2) critical support systems like heating, ventilation, and air conditioning (HVAC), water, compressed air and gases, and air filtration; and (3) equipment.[31] In any case, the first step of the process involves demonstrating and documenting that the design selected complies with GMP (design qualification [DQ]). The subsequent qualification process usually encompasses three phases, which take place after the facility has been built and the systems and equipment have been put in place. The first step is installation qualification (IQ), a process that can be defined as "the documented verification that the facilities, systems, and equipment, as installed or modified, comply with the approved design and the manufacturer's recommendations." IQ should include, among others, (1) the installation and checking of equipment, piping, services, and instrumentation according to updated engineering drawings and specifications; (2) the collection of supplier operating and working instructions and maintenance requirements; (3) gathering of calibration requirements; and (4) the verification of materials of construction.

Following the IQ phase, the facilities, systems, and equipment, as installed or modified, are verified to confirm that they perform as intended throughout the anticipated operating ranges. This so-called operational qualification (OQ) verification must be documented adequately, and includes (1) tests that have been developed from knowledge of processes, systems, and equipment and (2) tests to include a condition or a set of conditions encompassing upper and lower operating limits, sometimes referred to as "worst case" conditions. Once OQ has been successfully completed, the facilities, systems, and equipment can be formally released. The final step in the qualification process is performance qualification (PQ). Documented evidence must now be produced, which verify that "the facilities, systems, and equipment, as connected together, can perform effectively and reproducibly, based on the approved process method and product specification." PQ, which in some cases may be performed together with OQ, involves the execution of tests (1) with production materials, qualified substitutes, or simulated product, which have been developed from the knowledge of the process and the facilities, systems, or equipment and (2) under conditions that cover upper and lower operating limits.

The qualification of a manufacturing facility and associated systems and equipment is a costly activity, which may account for as much as 75% of the overall money spent in validation, as opposed to process validation.[34]

11.4.3 Process Validation

Once the facilities, systems, and equipment to be used in manufacturing have been qualified and analytical testing methods have been validated, documented evidence has to be generated to show that the process, when operated within established parameters, can effectively and reproducibly produce the target medicinal product within the predetermined specifications. This so-called *process validation* usually starts during the development phase (*prospective validation*), before the marketing of the new product or of a product being made under a revised process, with a risk assessment of the process and of those individual steps that may lead to critical situations. The understanding of the potential risks associated with the host organism, raw materials, processing materials, product-related impurities, and specific process steps is of utmost importance during prospective validation. The manufacturing process should be designed so as to mitigate those risks or avoid them altogether.[35] If a critical situation or process step is identified, a scientific study (i.e., a validation trial) is adequately designed and carried out to prove that that particular step performs consistently from batch to batch and is under control. The experiments in these studies should be performed using upper and lower processing limits of the selected test variables, particularly those that pose the greatest chance of process or product failure compared to ideal conditions. An adequate number of replicate experiments should be performed to demonstrate reproducibility and to measure variability among successive runs. A typical outcome of such a validation study will be the determination of critical process variables and corresponding acceptable limits, and the setup of appropriate in-process controls.[31] If the results of the trial fail to meet the criteria set, then the corresponding process step should be modified and retested until it can be considered to be validated.[2]

Once the process is defined, a series of technical batches of the final product, preferably of the same size as the intended industrial scale batches, may be produced under routine conditions to test and control the process and associated equipment and facility under realistic manufacturing conditions. The number of process runs carried out and observations made should be sufficient to allow the normal extent of variation and trends to be established and to provide sufficient data for evaluation. The process is generally considered validated once three consecutive batches/runs within the finally agreed on parameters have been obtained. If, for whatever reason, it is not possible to complete a validation program before the commercialization, processes may be validated during routine production of a product intended for sale (*concurrent validation*). This involves the comprehensive monitoring of at least three consecutive batches. The results obtained during this early phase can be used to fine-tune specifications.[2] Processes used for some time to manufacture a product that has been marketed should also be validated based upon accumulated manufacturing, testing, and control batch data (*retrospective validation*). This historical data include rejects or rework occurrences; yields; physical, chemical, biological, and microbiological test results; process deviations; product complaints; and stability test results.[31] Typically, data from 10 to 30 consecutive batches that are representative of all batches made during the review period (including failed runs) should be sufficient to assess and demonstrate process consistency. Retained samples may be retested to obtain further data. This periodic revalidation constitutes an extra guarantee that processes and procedures remain capable of achieving their intended results.[10]

Overall, validation results in a better understanding of all steps in a given process and of the causes of variation. Apart from contributing to the overall assurance of product quality, a natural consequence of validation studies is almost inevitably the optimization of the process, reduction in the number of failed batches, and an overall reduction in total production costs.[31] An important requirement in this topic is the need for a formal, documented validation of any new manufacturing step or important modification of an established process. The rationale for this is that any change in a process can alter the safety and effectiveness profile, rendering the product inconsistent with the product made in earlier batches and evaluated in clinical trials.[28] This imperative often bars manufacturers from introducing even the slight changes into their processes.

11.5 GUIDELINES PERTAINING TO PLASMID BIOPHARMACEUTICALS

GMPs are broad-ranging guidelines that cover all medicinal products for human use. In addition to them, regulatory agencies publish additional guidelines, which are specific to certain categories of products (e.g., blood derivatives and vaccines), procedures (e.g., xenotransplantation), and principles (e.g., validation). Like GMPs, these guidelines are issued to ensure the safety and efficacy of the products being manufactured, but unlike GMPs, manufacturers are not legally bound to follow them, although this is obviously advantageous.[36] Thus, guidelines are not regulations and rather represent issues that the regulatory agencies believe should be considered by manufacturers and sponsors.[37]

A number of guidelines have been issued by the FDA, EMA, ICH, and WHO that deal with preclinical, clinical, manufacturing, and safety issues relevant to the development of gene therapy products and DNA vaccines (Table 11.2). Some of these guidelines are directed at the whole range of gene therapy products,[37,38] including cells that have been modified *ex vivo* and recombinant viruses and plasmids that have been engineered to safely deliver transgenes. Separate documents are also available that specifically cover the use of DNA vaccines to prevent infectious diseases.[39,40] In either case, the EMA and FDA guidelines cover issues like production, quality and control testing, preclinical safety, and clinical efficacy and safety. Those aspects that relate to preclinical and clinical safety and efficacy were dealt with in detail in Chapter 7, whereas the QC of plasmids is examined in Chapter 12. In this section, I will focus exclusively on the guidance that is provided regarding those aspects that are related to the construction and manufacturing of plasmids. The guidelines advise manufacturers to gather a set of data and information regarding their plasmid product in order to ensure adequate safety. Such information, which is described in detail in the different guidance documents, is summarized next.

TABLE 11.2. Guidelines Issued by the Food and Drug Administration (FDA), European Medicines Agency (EMA), and World Health Organization (WHO) That Deal with PreClinical, Clinical, Manufacturing, and Safety Issues Relevant to the Development of Gene Therapy Products and DNA Vaccines

Entity	Title of Guidance Document	Year
FDA	*Guidance for Industry: Guidance for Human Somatic Cell Therapy and Gene Therapy*[37]	1998
FDA	*Guidance for Industry: Considerations for Plasmid DNA Vaccines for Infectious Disease Indications*[40]	2007
EMA	*Note for Guidance on Quality and Pre-clinical and Clinical Aspects of Gene Transfer Medicinal Products*[38]	2001
EMA	*Concept Paper on Guidance for DNA Vaccines*[39]	2007
WHO	*Guidelines for Assuring the Quality and Nonclinical Safety Evaluation of DNA Vaccines*[62]	1998

11.5.1 Plasmid Construction and Characterization

Plasmids should be generated from cloned and well-characterized constructs, and information regarding these constructs and the development of the final plasmid should be available.[37,38,41] This may include, for instance, a description of any plasmid used to prepare the final product and the identification of key regulatory elements such as promoters, enhancers, and selection markers. The origin of the transgene, the rationale behind its use, and details of biological properties, for example, function or antigenicity, should also be described in detail.[38] A judicious selection of the elements that will form the final plasmid during the design phase is critical in order to avoid instability problems. For instance, sequences like direct repeats, which are known to mediate recombination events, homologous sequences, which are conducive to recombination in the target recipient, retroviral-like long terminal repeats, oncogenes,[41] and homopurine tracts, which are likely to drive the formation of intramolecular triplexes, should be avoided whenever possible. Sequencing of the whole vector or, when not feasible, of appropriate segments such as the transgene and flanking regions, should be performed.[41] Specific attention should be directed toward particular sites within the plasmid which might be vulnerable to alteration during manipulation. Restriction mapping also provides helpful characterization information. Guidelines also make it very clear that specific antibiotic selection markers should be avoided due to the associated risks of hypersensitivity and spread of antibiotic resistance.[37,38] The use of such markers also comes with a cost with regard to process validation (see Section 11.4).

11.5.2 Producer Cells

For the sake of process and product consistency, every plasmid batch should be manufactured from the exact same cell source. This means that stocks of producer *E. coli* cells should be handled adequately by a formal cell banking system. The generation and characterization of the master cell banks (MCBs), working cell banks (WCBs), and producer cells, which lie at the heart of such systems, are the subject of recommendations in the FDA[37], EMA,[38] and WHO[41] guidance documents (see Chapter 13, Section 13.2.4). Basically, the origin, form, storage conditions, use, and expected duration must be described for all banks. The MCB is generated under full cGMP conditions from selected clones and will typically consist of approximately 200 vials containing a homogeneous suspension of the transformed bacterial cells. One of the MCB vials is then used to produce a WCB of around 200 vials. Each of these vials will serve as the starting inoculum for each production batch. A new WCB is constructed every time the previous bank has been emptied, and thus approximately 40,000 batches can be generated from the original MCB[42]. Appropriate genotypic and phenotypic features should be identified, which can form a basis for identification. The sequence of the plasmid once hosted, as well as the viability of the cell–plasmid system under storage and recovery conditions, should also be established at the stage of MCB and WCB characterization.[41] Both banks must be shown to be free from extraneous biological agents.

11.5.3 Materials Used during Manufacturing

The guidelines stress the fact that the safety and efficacy of plasmid products can be affected by the different materials that are used during manufacturing. Clear statements are made on the need to avoid the use of highly toxic chemicals such as ethidium bromide and beta-lactam antibiotics such as penicillin, which are known to cause hypersensitivity reactions. The use of materials of bovine origin should also be considered carefully, given the risk of transmission of animal-derived infections like bovine spongiform encephalopathy (BSE). These and other components "should be clearly identified and a qualification program with set specifications should be established for each component to determine its acceptability for use during the manufacturing process."[37] All materials that may persist in the final product must be removed, and their residual amounts must be shown by adequate tests to be below prespecified limits.

11.5.4 Manufacturing

The European and WHO guidelines draw some considerations on the production and purification of plasmid vectors, stressing the need for (1) a detailed description of the methods and procedures used, (2) the identification of relevant in-process controls, (3) the establishment of rejection criteria, and (4) validation studies (see Section 11.4) that demonstrate the clearance capacity of each purification step and ensure reproducibility and consistency. For instance, the plasmid copy number, the degree of retention of plasmid in the producer cells, and restriction mapping of the plasmid are some of the characteristics that should be inspected at the end of the production cycle.[41] The ability of the downstream processing train to remove host-related impurities such as RNA, genomic DNA, proteins, and irreversibly denatured plasmids, as well as process-related impurities such as antibiotics, should be investigated thoroughly. The removal of lipopolysaccharides (i.e., endotoxins) is underscored as a task in need of special attention.[38]

11.5.5 Characterization of Bulk Purified Plasmid

The bulk plasmid material obtained from each production batch and before formulation should be characterized in terms of identity, purity, potency, and stability. A series of tests and methodologies should be in place to allow such characterization to take place on a routine basis. The FDA, EMA, and WHO documents (Table 11.2) offer extensive guidance on this subject, which is described in detail in Chapter 12.

11.6 ISSUES ON THE VALIDATION OF PLASMID MANUFACTURING

Bioprocess engineers involved in the development and implementation of plasmid manufacturing are recurrently faced with a number of problems and aspects that are likely to constrain validation. Examination of some of these issues is worthwhile at this stage.

11.6.1 Toxic Materials

Although this is usually a starting point for the learning neophyte, it is clearly unwise to develop a process on the basis of the traditional methods used by molecular biologists, especially those that resort to dangerous and hazardous materials.[37,38] The need to eliminate these materials from the final product and the validation efforts required to demonstrate consistent removal run after run should bar process engineers from using them. And even if this can be successfully accomplished, regulators are not likely to accept their use in view of the overall philosophy of GMPs, which is clearly in favor of the use of low-risk materials. The use of solvents, for instance, is often critical to the success of specific steps in pharmaceutical manufacturing. However, since not all solvents are alike in terms of their toxicity, their use should be judiciously considered beforehand. A guideline document from the ICH suggests the classification of solvents into three classes according to the possible risk they present to human health.[43] This risk is usually assessed in terms of the "permitted daily exposure" (PDE), which is basically a measure of the pharmaceutically acceptable intake of residual solvents.[43] PDE figures can be converted into concentration limits using the product mass administered daily. Solvents, which are known human carcinogens, strongly suspected human carcinogens, or environmental hazards, compose class 1, and their use should be avoided altogether. Class 2 incorporates those solvents that are associated with less severe toxicity and, as such, their use in manufacturing should be avoided. Those solvents that can be regarded as less toxic and of lower risk to human health are grouped in class 3. Ideally, manufacturing processes should use only solvents from this class. The classification just described implies that the solvents used should be removed consistently throughout the process so that their residual amount in the final product is acceptable. As a rough guideline, the concentration limits for residual solvents in a pharmaceutical product are usually lower than 10, 1000, and 5000 ppm for class 1, class 2, and class 3 members, respectively.[43]

The use of solvents like phenol, chloroform, acetonitrile, ethanol, and isopropanol is widespread in the purification of plasmids at laboratorial scale. Phenol and chloroform, for instance, are used to extract RNA and proteins from lysates. However, since they are class 1 (phenol) and class 2 (chloroform) solvents,[43] their use should be avoided when producing plasmid biopharmaceuticals. Acetonitrile is often found in the composition of eluents used for the purification of plasmids by reverse-phase chromatography.[44] The use of this class 2 solvent should be either limited, or else its residual amount should be guaranteed to be lower than 410 ppm[43]. The use of ethanol and isopropanol as plasmid precipitating agents, on the other hand, does not raise particular concerns in terms of toxicity since they are both class 3 solvents.[43] However, their use at large scale is likely to require the implementation of safety measures such as the design of explosion-proof facilities or the use of appropriate protection masks.[45]

11.6.2 Selection Markers

A number of validation issues usually arise in connection with the selection markers that are often encountered in plasmids when antibiotic selection is used during production in *E. coli* hosts. Regulatory agencies recommend that penicillin and other beta-lactam antibiotics be avoided during cell culture since some patients may be prone to serious hypersensitivity reactions. Also, markers that confer resistance to clinically relevant antibiotics should not be used since plasmids may transform the patient's microflora and thus may spread antibiotic resistance genes.[37,38,46] This means that if such antibiotics are used nevertheless, their residual amount in the final product should be quantitated and shown to be below an acceptable limit. Furthermore, a validation study is likely to be required to ensure that the downstream processing train is able to consistently remove the antibiotic independently of any process variability. In this context, the adoption of strategies that avoid the use of such selection markers would minimize the need for validation later on during process development. Examples of such strategies include the use of nonantibiotic-based markers, which select and maintain plasmids by a repressor titration mechanism[47] (see Chapter 13).

11.6.3 RNase

One of the materials that is commonly found in plasmid isolation laboratory-scale protocols is the enzyme RNase. The popularity of its use stems from the

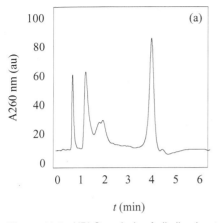
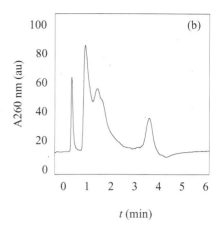

Figure 11.4 *HPLC analysis of alkaline lysates, which were prepared with (a) and without (b) RNase. The smaller amount of high-molecular-weight RNA impurities (peak at 3.5-4.0 min) in the case of RNase pretreatment is readily apparent from the chromatogram in (b). Plasmid DNA elutes at 0.7 min and low molecular weight RNA between 1.0 and 3.0 min.*

excellent removal of host *E. coli* RNA that can be achieved by enzymatic degradation, which is unmatched by any other procedure. This is clearly illustrated in Figure 11.4, which compares the high-performance liquid chromatography (HPLC) analysis of alkaline lysates which were prepared with and without RNase. The smaller amount of high-molecular-weight RNA (peak at 3.5–4.0 min) obtained in the first case as a result of the RNase activity is readily apparent from the chromatograms. In spite of this, since the majority of commercially available RNase is of bovine origin, the concern for the use of this enzyme in plasmid processing is recurrent. The reasons for this concern are essentially due to the theoretical risk of transmission of animal-derived infections, and most noticeably of transmissible spongiform encephalopathies (TSEs), such as BSE, which have been associated with human cases of the variant form of the Creutzfeldt–Jakobs disease in the United Kingdom[30]. This concern has been expressed by the Center for Biologics Evaluation and Research (CBER), the FDA body responsible for the regulation of biologic products, in a series of documents,[48] including letters to manufacturers requesting that "manufacturers of biologic products provide information regarding the source(s) and control of any bovine- or ovine-derived material(s) used in preparing products to be administered to humans for prophylaxis, therapy, or diagnosis."[49] This covers not only materials that are directly incorporated into products but also any materials used in manufacturing (e.g., enzymes, cell culture components, and chromatographic media). It should be the responsibility of the manufacturers to take whatever steps are necessary to ensure that materials derived from all species of animals born, raised, or slaughtered in countries where BSE is known to exist, or in countries where it may exist, are not used in the manufacture of FDA-regulated products intended for administration to humans. Although this means that RNase batches (or any other animal-derived substance) produced according to the FDA recommendations by certified manufacturers from countries where BSE occurrence is unlikely or highly unlikely are admissible,[30] an RNase-free process would clearly be preferable from a regulatory and validation standpoint.

An alternative to bovine-derived RNase would be to use recombinant RNase.[50] This solution is likely to be adopted by manufacturers in the near future, but only if the costs associated with RNase production can be brought down to acceptable levels. Another strategy relies on the use of a modified *E. coli* strain, which contains a bovine RNase A expression cassette integrated into the chromosome (see also Chapter 13, Section 13.2.2). The RNase A, which is expressed in the periplasm, is released during plasmid isolation by alkaline lysis, hydrolyzing the bulk of the host RNA. The residual endogenous RNase activity of *E. coli* following cell lysis can also be harnessed to hydrolyze RNA[51]. The consistency of these two approaches, however, may be difficult to prove.

11.6.4 Alkaline Lysis

Validation concerns are also usually associated with the alkaline lysis of the host *E. coli* cells for plasmid release (see Chapter 15, Section 15.3.2). This operation, which is as extensively used at process scale as it is at the laboratory bench, has been systematically identified by researchers as a process step that is particularly difficult to reproduce at laboratory scale.[52–54] Such variability is intimately linked to the nature of the cell breakage process, which involves the sequential addition of an alkaline (pH 12) and an acidic (pH 5) solution (see Chapter 15, Section 15.3.2). An adequate mixing should be provided upon addition of each solution and during the subsequent incubation periods. This mixing should be efficient enough to rapidly homogenize the contents and to avoid deleterious pH extremes, which are known to denature plasmid DNA, but also sufficiently gentle to avoid fragmentation of the released *E. coli* genomic DNA. The process is further complicated due to the transient nature of the viscosity and properties of the non-Newtonian lysates generated. The contact time and the solid–liquid separation, which is needed to separate the mass of precipitated material, are other critical parameters. The difficulty in guaranteeing the consistency of alkaline lysis increases as the scale increases. One way to avoid this, as practiced by renowned manufacturers of plasmid material at pilot scale, would be to split the cell suspension into smaller batches, and thus keep the scale of lysis small and independent of the fermentation scale. However, there is clearly a limit to this approach. All in all, parameters such as plasmid yield, cell breakage yield, and impurity profile obtained after alkaline lysis can vary significantly from batch to batch, even when cells from the same lot are lysed. At process scale, and above a certain degree, this variability will be unacceptable, given the likelihood of affecting the subsequent purification steps.

Strictly from a prospective validation point of view, one might argue that alkaline lysis should be dismissed in advance as a process step in plasmid manufacturing. However, few alternatives have been proposed to alkaline lysis that could rival its efficiency, particularly with respect to the removal of genomic DNA. For this reason, the variability and lack of reproducibility of alkaline lysis becomes acceptable. Thus, many manufacturers and a significant number of researchers have developed processes that rely on the rather unreliable alkaline lysis for cell breakage[54–57] (see Section 15.3.2).

11.7 GMP FACILITIES FOR PLASMID PRODUCTION

The design, equipping, start-up, and validation of a full GMP facility is a mammoth endeavor, which requires huge financial and human resources.[58–60] The description and analysis of this intricate process is out of the scope of this chapter. In this section, I will give a brief overview of some of the basic requirements and features that are likely to be considered when designing a small, academic-type facility for the production of small amounts of GMP plasmid DNA.

Researchers in academia are sometimes faced with the prospect of conducting early phase trials, once positive results have been obtained with their target plasmid products in preclinical and animal studies. Such phase 1 or early phase 2 clinical human trials must use GMP-grade plasmids, which have to be manufactured either in-house or by a third party, under a manufacturing contract. In both these cases, GMP compliance is less stringent than if products and facilities are intended for market approval.[28] The costs associated with the subcontracting of the manufacturing of such small quantities can be extremely high, on the order of £188–£419 (approximately US$376–US$838) per milligram of plasmid DNA, as described in a recent report by the U.K. Department of Health.[61] Thus, institutions with limited financial resources, which anticipate a recurrent need for plasmids, may rather choose to adapt existing research facilities and adopt GMP concepts and specific guidelines to produce their own material. This approach has been reported recently by Przybylowski and coworkers, who describe the production of clinical-grade plasmid DNA for human phase 1 clinical trials and large animal clinical studies in a small production facility set up and operated in the context of their research center, the Memorial Sloan–Kettering Cancer Center (MSKCC).[57] The plasmid material is claimed to be produced under cGMPs using a process/facility that simultaneously avoids unnecessary investments, insolvable difficulties, or exorbitantly high processing costs. In the following paragraphs, a critical analysis of the report of Przybylowski et al. is made, which is supplemented with considerations regarding the design of GMP facilities and plasmid manufacturing.

The Gene Transfer and Somatic Cell Engineering Facility of the MSKCC is composed of a dedicated 72-ft^2 clean room (Class 10000) equipped with a Class 100 biosafety cabinet and an adjacent 24-ft^2 gowning room (Figure 11.5). Other supporting areas include a pregowning room, a quarantine storage room, a release storage room, and a final product storage room[57]. Although

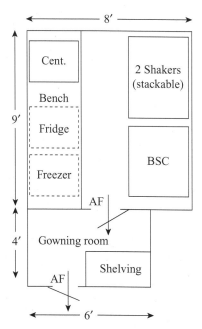

Figure 11.5 *Schematic diagram of the Gene Transfer and Somatic Cell Engineering facility of the Memorial Sloan–Kettering Cancer Center (MSKCC), used to produce clinical grade plasmid DNA for phase I trials. The facility is composed of a dedicated 72 ft² clean room (Class 10000), equipped with a Class 100 biosafety cabinet (BSC) and an adjacent 24 ft² gowning room. Personnel and materials enter the production facility through a single entrance. The air-flow (AF) is indicated on the schematic diagram of the production. Reprinted from Vaccine, 25, Przybylowski M, Bartido S, Borquez–Ojeda O, Sadelain M, Riviere I. Production of clinical-grade plasmid DNA for human phase I clinical trials and large animal clinical studies, 5013–5024, Copyright 2007,[57] with permission from Elsevier.*

the authors do not give these details, HEPA filters are likely installed in the ceiling of the rooms. Typically, the air delivered will pass through the rooms once, exiting via air ducts installed at the floor level. Walls are probably made with materials adequate for clean rooms (e.g., welded vinyl and wall boards coated with epoxy), with coving at the ceiling, floor, and corners.[28,59] The production room is unlikely to contain water, sinks, or drains, since these would constitute a potential source for aerosols (e.g., formed by running water striking the sink) and contaminants (e.g., from the sewer adjacent to the drain).[28,59]

The layout and design adopted for the clean room and gowning room are intended to facilitate cleaning and decontamination operations. One specific feature used for this purpose is a single entrance/exit for materials and personnel.[57] Although a one-entrance, one-exit layout would be more in accordance with GMPs, this departure from the philosophy is probably accommodated by regulatory agencies at such an early stage of trials. The authors state that the RNase-based process they use for plasmid manufacturing does not involve significantly biohazardous material.[57] Thus, containment of the production areas is not required, and the air handling system is rather balanced and controlled to ensure that positive pressure drives air out of the production clean room into the gowning room when the door is opened. The two doors separating the gowning room from the production area and from the general corridor are probably electronically interlocked. This guarantees that only one door is opened at a time and thus prevents the inadvertent flows of air and contaminants.[28] The presterilized pharmaceutical gowning typically used by GMP personnel includes a head cover with integral shoulder hood, mask, jumpsuit, gloves, and shoe covers. It should be used only once and then cleaned and sterilized before the next use.[28,59] Disposable versions may be preferable in such a small facility, which is unlikely to have adequate laundry services for cleaning gowning.

Apart from the biosafety cabinet, the clean room is equipped with a centrifuge, a refrigerator, a $-20°C$ freezer, and two stackable bacterial shakers, which are dedicated to cell culture. For each fermentation run, 22 (2 L) shake flasks with 560 mL of media are used. According to the authors, this rather unusual and suboptimal "large-scale" cell culture system was selected in order to avoid the cumbersome validation of the sterilization in place (SIP) that is required under GMPs when working with bioreactors.[57] Such testing usually involves the placement of thermocouples attached with spore strips (in the case of the vessel headspace) or glass vials containing spore suspensions (liquid material) in 10–12 of the locations in the bioreactor reckoned hardest to sterilize. SIP cycles are then performed, and the death rate of spores is determined in order to test and validate the sterilization procedure.[34] Although the use of shake flasks may be fully justifiable in an academic environment where financial resources are typically scarce, such an option is rather poor from a bioprocessing point of view and would hardly be taken in an industrial context.

The operation in itself is performed according to the philosophy of GMPs. A significant emphasis is put in the cleaning and decontamination of areas, internal surfaces and auxiliary parts of equipment using approved cleaning agents (e.g., 70% isopropanol), and validated procedures. The authors stress that cleaning and waste disposal are performed according to the SOPs. The attention given to the observance of GMP can also be judged by the materials and reagents used during processing, which include medical-grade plastics, ultrapure sterile buffers acquired from certified vendors, water for injection, and sterile microtubes.[57] In light of the theoretical risk of transmission of animal-derived infections, the concern for the use of RNase from bovine origin is obvious. Thus, and even though the origin and purity of the RNase used is certified by the manufacturer, the authors understand and defend that an RNase-free process would be preferable from a regulatory standpoint.[57]

The results of the operation of the MSKCC facility reported by the authors show that every fermentation run (12 L medium) delivers 60 g of bacterial paste. After recovery and purification, which are carried out by sequentially performing alkaline lysis, filtration, chromatography, isopropanol precipitation, and sterile filtration, around 70 mg of pure plasmid can be obtained. Three times more plasmid can be obtained by performing three serial fermentation runs and then by pooling the bacterial pastes prior to recovery and purification.[57] Although suitable for producing phase 1 and phase 2 material, this academic facility is likely inadequate for later-stage trials or initial commercial production. In this case, either construction of a new facility or subcontracting will be required.[28]

11.8 CONCLUDING REMARKS

The whole GMP philosophy, documentation, and jargon are viewed by many people in academia as daunting. Also, the costs associated with GMPs are more than often considered as an insurmountable barrier to compliance. These notions are deeply rooted in the minds of some academics involved in bioprocess engineering, who often dismiss GMPs from their worries. However, it is a fact that a fraction of the GMP (and GLP) rules and recommendations could be observed by academic research laboratories with minimum effort and investment. Such an incorporation of the GMP philosophy into the practices, products, and processes developed by research scientists and engineers would add quality and credibility to their work while facilitating and smoothing interactions with industrial partners. While academics can ignore them and live with it, failure to comply with GMPs in an industrial setting is not an option since it directly translates into loss of business. Although many critics assume that regulations entail only costs while simultaneously delaying the approval of potentially life-saving medicines, this rather superficial analysis typically does not factor in the gains in innovation associated with validation by companies pressed to a higher standard by regulations.[1] Furthermore, and although many manufacturers have probably been saved from mistakes and lawsuits by the rules, the trouble avoided by GMPs remains to be quantified.

REFERENCES

1. Hilts P. *Protecting America's health: The FDA, business and one hundred years of regulation.* Chapel Hill, NC: The University of North Carolina Press, 2003.
2. Kanarek AD. *A guide to good manufacturing practice.* Westborough, MA: D&MD, 2001.
3. Abad X, Bosch A, Navarro C. Implementation of good laboratory practice in a university research unit. *Quality Assurance Journal.* 2005;9:304–311.
4. Baldeshwiler A. History of FDA good laboratory practices. *Quality Assurance Journal.* 2003;7:157–161.
5. Rosin LJ. Regulatory affairs: If you didn't write it down, it didn't happen. *BioProcess International.* 2006;4:16–23.
6. European Medicines Agency. ICH Topic E 6 (R1). Guideline for good clinical practice (CPMP/ICH/135/95). London, July 2002.
7. European Union. Directive 2001/20/EC of April 4, 2001 on the approximation of the laws, regulations and administrative provisions of the member states relating

to the implementation of good clinical practice on medicinal product for human use. (OJ No L 121 of 1.5.2001, p.34), 2001.

8. Cohen-Haguenauer O. Gene therapy: Regulatory issues and international approaches to regulation. *Current Opinion in Biotechnology.* 1997;8:361–369.

9. Couzin J, Kaiser J. Gene therapy. As Gelsinger case ends, gene therapy suffers another blow. *Science.* 2005;307:1028.

10. European Union, Drug Review Agency. Good manufacturing practices. In: *The rules governing medicinal products in the European Union,* Vol. 4. Luxembourg: Office for Official Publications of the European Communities, 1998.

11. Grazal J, Earl D. EU and FDA GMP regulations: Overview and comparison. *Quality Assurance Journal.* 1997;2:55–60.

12. United States Code of Federal Regulations. Part 210—Current good manufacturing practice in manufacturing, processing, packing, or holding of drugs: General. 21 CFR 210, 1998.

13. United States Code of Federal Regulations. Part 211—Current good manufacturing practice in manufacturing for finished pharmaceuticals. 21 CFR 210, 1998.

14. United States Code of Federal Regulations. Part 600—Biological products: General. 21 CFR 600, 1998.

15. European Union. Commission Directive 91/356/EEC of June 13, 1991 laying down the principles and guidelines of good manufacturing practice for medicinal products for human use. (OJ No L 193 of 17.7.1991, p.30), 1991.

16. European Union. Commission Directive 91/412/EEC of July 23, 1991 laying down the principles and guidelines of good manufacturing practice for veterinary medicinal products. (OJ No L 228 of 17.8.1991, p.70). 1991.

17. World Health Organization. Good manufacturing practices for pharmaceutical products. WHO Expert Committee on Specifications for Pharmaceutical Preparations: Thirty-Second Report. Vol. Annex 1 (WHO Technical Report Series, No. 823). Geneva, 1992.

18. World Health Organization. Good manufacturing practices for biological products. WHO Expert Committee on Specifications for Pharmaceutical Preparations: Forty-Second Report. Vol Annex 1 (WHO Technical Report Series, No. 822). Geneva, 1992.

19. European Medicines Agency. ICH Topic Q 7. Note for guidance on good manufacturing practice for active pharmaceutical ingredients (CPMP/ICH/4106/00). London, November 10, 2000.

20. Vesper J. So what are GMPs, anyway? *BioProcess International.* 2003;1(February):24–26. 28–29.

21. Webster H. Compliance issues for the contract manufacturing of cGMP gene therapy products. *Quality Assurance Journal.* 1997;2:135–140.

22. Dixon A. Cleaning and sanitization of clean rooms and materials. In: Carleton F, Agalloco J, eds. *Validation of pharmaceutical processes—Sterile products.* New York: Marcel Dekker, 1999:645–668.

23. del Valle M. Keeping clean rooms compliant. *Pharmaceutical Technology Europe.* 2006;18:47–52.

24. Straker M. Clean rooms and air handling systems—Design for compliance. *Pharmaceutical Technology Europe.* 2005;17:14–20.

25. Kuhne W, Zöllner K. Recommendations for successful quality assurance of production of bulk drug substances for non-viral gene therapy. *Quality Assurance Journal.* 1997;2:129–133.

26. Möller AL. Clean room technologies of the 1990s. *Medical Device Technology.* 1992;3:24–33.

27. Boyd J. Facilities for large-scale production of vectors under GMP conditions. In: Meager A, ed. *Gene therapy technologies, applications and regulations.* Chichester: John Wiley & Sons, 1999:383–400.

28. Tolbert W, Merchant B, Taylor J, Pergolizzi R. Designing an initial gene therapy manufacturing faciltiy. *BioPharm.* 1996;November:32–40.

29. Doblhoff-Dier O, Bliem R. Quality control and assurance from the development to the production of biopharmaceuticals. *Trends Biotechnology.* 1999;17:266–270.

30. Berger CN, Le Donne P, Windemann H. Use of substances of animal origin in pharmaceutics and compliance with the TSE-risk guideline—A market survey. *Biologicals.* 2005;33:1–7.

31. Kieffer R, Nally J. Why validation? Carleton F, Agalloco J, eds. *Validation of pharmaceutical processes—Sterile products.* New York: Marcel Dekker, 1999:1–16.

32. Sofer G. Validation of biotechnology products and processes. *Current Opinion in Biotechnology.* 1995;6:230–234.

33. United States Food and Drug Administration. *Guideline on general principles of process validation.* Rockville, MD: FDA, 1987.

34. Junker B. Technical evaluation of the potential for streamlining of equipment validation for fermentation applications. *Biotechnology and Bioengineering.* 2001; 74:49–61.

35. Sofer G, Ahnfelt M. Validation: Advances in the validation of chromatographic processes. *BioPharm.* 2007;February:20–25.

36. Steel M, Roessler B. Compliance with good manufacturing practices for facilities engaged in vector production, cell isolation, and genetic manipulations. *Current Opinion in Biotechnology.* 1999;10:29–297.

37. United States Food and Drug Administration. *Guidance for industry: Guidance for human somatic cell therapy and gene therapy.* Rockville, MD: FDA, 1998.

38. European Medicines Evaluation Agency. ICH Topic Q6b. Note for guidance on quality, pre-clinical and clinical aspects of gene transfer medicinal products (Doc. Ref. CPMP/BWP/3088/99). London, April 24, 2001.

39. European Medicines Evaluation Agency. Concept paper on guidance for DNA vaccines (Doc. Ref. EMEA/CHMP/308136/2007). London, July 16, 2007.

40. United States Food and Drug Administration. *Guidance for industry: Considerations for plasmid DNA vaccines for preventive infectious disease indications.* Rockville, MD: FDA, 2007.

41. World Health Organization. WHO guidelines for assuring the quality of DNA vacines. *Biologicals.* 1998;26:205–212.

42. Schleef M, Schorr J. Plasmid DNA for clinical phase I and II studies. In: Walden P, Trefzer U, Sterry W, eds. *Gene therapy of cancer.* Vol. 451. New York: Springer-Verlag, 1998:481–486.

43. European Medicines Agency. ICH Topic Q 3 C (R3). Note for guidance on impurities: Residual solvents (CPMP/ICH/283/95). London, March 1997.

44. Lee AL, Sagar S, inventors; Merck & Co., Inc., assignee. Method for large scale plasmid purification. U.S. Patent 6,197,553, March 6, 2002.

45. Marquet M, Horn NA, Meek JA. Process development for the manufacture of plasmid DNA vectors for use in gene therapy. *BioPharm*. 1995;September:6–37.

46. Glenting J, Wessels S. Ensuring safety of DNA vaccines. *Microbial Cell Factories*. 2005;4:26.

47. Cranenburgh RM, Hanak JA, Williams SG, Sherratt DJ. *Escherichia coli* strains that allow antibiotic-free plasmid selection and maintenance by repressor titration. *Nucleic Acids Research*. 2001;29:E26.

48. United States Food and Drug Administration. *Draft of points to consider in the characterization of cell lines used to produce biologicals*. Rockville, MD: FDA, 1993.

49. Quinnan GV. *Letter to the manufacturers of biological products*. Bethesda, MD: Center for Biologics Evaluation and Research, FDA, 1991.

50. Voss C, Lindau D, Flaschel E. Production of recombinant RNase Ba and its application in downstream processing of plasmid DNA for pharmaceutical use. *Biotechnology Progress*. 2006;22:737–744.

51. Monteiro GA, Ferreira GNM, Cabral JMS, Prazeres DMF. Analysis and use of endogenous nuclease activities in *Escherichia coli* lysates during the primary isolation of plasmids for gene therapy. *Biotechnology and Bioengineering*. 1999;66:189–194.

52. Prazeres DMF, Ferreira GNM, Monteiro GA, Cooney CL, Cabral JMS. Large-scale production of pharmaceutical-grade plasmid DNA for gene therapy: Problems and bottlenecks. *Trends in Biotechnology*. 1999;17:169–174.

53. Clemson M, Kelly WJ. Optimizing alkaline lysis for DNA plasmid recovery. *Biotechnology and Applied Biochemistry*. 2003;37:235–244.

54. Urthaler J, Ascher C, Wohrer H, Necina R. Automated alkaline lysis for industrial scale cGMP production of pharmaceutical grade plasmid-DNA. *Journal of Biotechnology*. 2007;128:132–149.

55. Diogo MM, Queiroz JA, Monteiro GA, Martins SA, Ferreira GNM, Prazeres DMF. Purification of a cystic fibrosis plasmid vector for gene therapy using hydrophobic interaction chromatography. *Biotechnology and Bioengineering*. 2000;68:576–583.

56. Stadler J, Lemmens R, Nyhammar T. Plasmid DNA purification. *The Journal of Gene Medicine*. 2004;6(Suppl 1):S54–S66.

57. Przybylowski M, Bartido S, Borquez-Ojeda O, Sadelain M, Riviere I. Production of clinical-grade plasmid DNA for human phase I clinical trials and large animal clinical studies. *Vaccine*. 2007;25:5013–5024.

58. Lias R, Ruddy K. Case study of a clinical -scale CGMP biopharmaceutical production facility. Part one: Site selection. *BioProcess International*. 2005;3(June):6–19.

59. Lias R, Perry S. Case study of a clinical-scale CGMP production facility. Part two: Facility design. *BioProcess International*. 2006;4(June):12–18.

60. Perry S, Greiner-Powell D. Case study of a clinical-scale CGMP production facility. Part three: Equipping, start-up and validation. *BioProcess International*. 2007; 5(June):14–20.

61. Watson R. *The vector directory: An analysis of international GMP gene therapy vector capacity and capability*. London: U.K. Department of Health, 2007.

62. World Health Organization. Guidelines for assuring the quality and nonclinical safety evaluation of DNA vaccines. Vol. Annex 1 (WHO Technical Report Series, No. 941). Geneva; 2007.

12

Product Specifications and Quality Control

12.1 INTRODUCTION

The discovery that plasmids could be used as gene carriers in gene therapy and DNA vaccination, and the subsequent preclinical and clinical development of these molecules, has given rise to a new class of medicinal agents.[1] In view of their physical and chemical structure, and of the biological nature of the source materials and manufacturing process used to prepare them, such plasmids can be classified unequivocally as biologics or biopharmaceuticals.[1] As is the case for many other biologics, plasmid products are characterized by an inherent variability in their composition, stability, and potency. In view of this variability, an extensive characterization of the products obtained at the end of manufacturing is imperative in order to demonstrate that a given plasmid biopharmaceutical lot (1) is consistent in terms of its composition, (2) exhibits long-term physical-chemical and biological stability, and (3) is essentially free of impurities (e.g., genomic DNA [gDNA], lipopolysaccharides [LPSs], RNA, and proteins) and adventitious contaminants (e.g., microorganisms and bacteriophages).[1] Such a thorough description of a plasmid biopharmaceutical candidate is a crucial activity, both during product development, when smaller amounts of material are prepared for preclinical and clinical trials, and during commercialization, when larger quantities are manufactured on a routine basis (see Chapter 3). During the initial phases of trials, for

Plasmid Biopharmaceuticals: Basics, Applications, and Manufacturing, First Edition.
Duarte Miguel F. Prazeres.
© 2011 John Wiley & Sons, Inc. Published 2011 by John Wiley & Sons, Inc.

example, the information gathered regarding the product quality is important to assess any safety risks associated with the manufacturing process or with the product itself. On top of this, and when product is being prepared for late-stage clinical trials, preliminary evidence regarding the consistency of the manufacturing process and its validation should be generated. Finally, and once a product has been approved and is manufactured on a routine basis, the inspection of its quality is a regulatory imperative. One of the keys to the characterization efforts just described is the installation of a quality control (QC) laboratory. Among other tasks, the QC laboratory is responsible for setting up, establishing, and validating a series of analytical techniques, procedures, and methodologies. This is a crucial task that should be planned in advance and undertaken as soon as possible in the product/process development track. Apart from aiding the clinical development, this will also allow a tight control of plasmid quality to take place on a routine basis once manufacturing of a product for marketing purposes becomes a reality. The analytical methodologies used to characterize plasmid DNA vectors should be susceptible to validation; that is, it should be possible to establish documentary evidence that they consistently perform as they should regarding precision, sensitivity, robustness, and statistical accuracy.[2-4] Once established, the QC laboratory is called to perform analysis in a number of different instances (Figure 12.1). During routine operation, for example, the analysis of samples

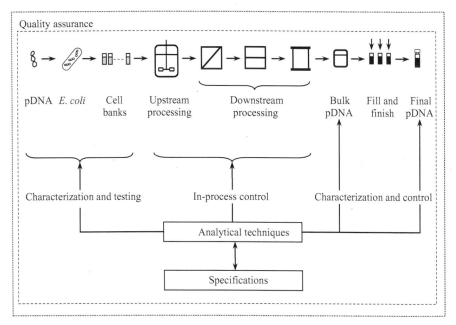

Figure 12.1 *The role of analytical techniques in the manufacturing of plasmid biopharmaceuticals.*

collected at different points in the process is fundamental since it allows a firm control of the performance of the different unit operations used. The data collected also contribute to the "writing" of the history of each manufacturing batch, a set of information that is essential from a good manufacturing practice (GMP) point of view (Chapter 11). Furthermore, if deviations from the expected values are observed during the course of process monitoring, corrective actions can be taken that can salvage a batch which would otherwise fail. Analytical techniques also play a determinant role in validation studies and in the establishment of acceptance criteria for critical manufacturing steps. Additionally, the bulk plasmid obtained from each production batch and before formulation should be rigorously characterized in terms of identity, purity, potency, and stability, and the output figures compared with predefined specifications. The characterization of the finished formulated plasmid product, which in many cases can contain excipients and/or adjuvants, is also imperative.[5] Finally, since the molecular conformation of plasmids, hence their biological activity (potency), may be particularly sensitive to factors such as temperature, oxidation, ionic content, shear stress, and light,[6] a correct evaluation of product stability using convenient analytical techniques should be performed. Other important roles for analytical techniques and the QC laboratory in the context of plasmid manufacturing are, for example, the analysis of source materials, the assessment of the impact of changes in the processes, and the validation of individual process steps and cleaning procedures (see Chapter 11). This chapter presents the key specifications that are usually set in advance for plasmid biopharmaceuticals, together with the analytical methodologies recommended and commonly used to check compliance. A number of the analytical techniques used in this context have been described in detail in Chapter 5, which dealt with the analytical characterization of plasmids. However, here, the focus is directed at the usefulness of those techniques from a QC perspective. Additionally, a review is made of the technologies used to detect and quantify impurities and contaminants and to determine potency.

12.2 SPECIFICATIONS

One of the core concepts hovering over GMPs is that of quality assurance, as described in Chapter 11. Among other attributes, quality assurance is a means of guaranteeing the excellence, security, and dependability of the manufacturing process or of its product.[7] As described above, quality assurance relies heavily on the monitoring of the performance of the process, as well as on the assessment of the end-product quality.[8–11] While analytical results obtained during monitoring are judged against expected values from historical records, in the latter case, they are compared with pre-established specifications. Such specifications can be defined as a list of tests, references to analytical procedures, and appropriate acceptance criteria.[12] These acceptance criteria may be numerical limits, ranges, or other types of measures that are associated with the tests described. A product is said to conform to a particular specification if it meets the acceptance criteria when tested according to the reference analytical procedures. Specifications are thus critical quality standards that are proposed and justified by the manufacturer and approved by regulatory authorities as conditions of approval.[12]

The exact set of final specifications of a plasmid biopharmaceutical will usually depend on its intended therapeutic use. While specifications regarding items like identity, homogeneity, and impurity levels can be established in advance, others such as concentration and potency may have to be defined by the sponsor during preclinical and clinical trials.[13] Regulatory agencies such as the Food and Drug Administration (FDA) and the European Medicines Agency (EMA) in the European Union[5,14–17] issue important recommendations, guidelines, and quality standards in this regard. Table 12.1 lists a series of test items, specifications, and acceptance criteria that are commonly used to control the final quality of a bulk plasmid product that is meant for medical application.[18–20] The analytical techniques that can or should be used to check if the acceptance criteria are met are also listed in the table. These techniques are varied and include chemical, physical, and biological methods. Some of the analytical techniques and methodologies listed (e.g., high-performance liquid chromatography [HPLC] and gel electrophoresis) are important not only to control the final product quality but also to assess the performance/consistency of the different unit operations used throughout the downstream processing, as described earlier.

The first part of Table 12.1 contains information regarding the plasmid molecule and the plasmid solution. The specifications found here deal with issues such as the appearance of the solution, identity, homogeneity, concentration, and potency. Many of the techniques associated with these specifications have been described in detail in Chapter 5. The second part of the table deals with the residual impurities that one is more likely to find in the final product, that is, with the major components of the *Escherichia coli* host: proteins, RNA, gDNA, and LPS. According to FDA recommendations, the maximum level of DNA, RNA, and proteins should be preferably lower than 1% (impurity weight/plasmid weight), whereas the amount of endotoxins should not exceed 40 endotoxin units (EU)/mg of plasmid.[5] An observation of the table shows that other authors/companies have adopted specifications that are less stringent than these ones. This pre-establishment of a degree of impurity in a plasmid product that is higher than the ones recommended by regulatory agencies might be acceptable, provided that an adequate justification is presented by the sponsor.[15]

12.3   TEST ITEMS AND ANALYTICAL TECHNIQUES

As described in the previous section, a plasmid product is typically characterized by a number of different test items (Table 12.1) that can be determined

TABLE 12.1. Typical Specifications and Acceptance Criteria for Plasmid DNA Products and Analytical Techniques Used to Assess Them

Test Item	Specification/Acceptance Criteria	Analytical Method
Plasmid		
Appearance	Clear, colorless solution	Visual inspection
Identity	Conformance to plasmid DNA map	Multiple restriction enzyme mapping
	Sequence homology	Sequencing, PCR
	Retention time identical to standard[20]	HPLC
Homogeneity	≥90% supercoiled form[20]	Agarose gel electrophoresis + densitometry, HPLC, and capillary electrophoresis with laser-induced fluorescence (LIF)
Concentration	According to application	Absorbance at 260 nm, HPLC, fluorescence, agarose gel electrophoresis + densitometry, and capillary electrophoresis with LIF
Potency	According to application	Cell transfection
Impurities		
Purity	A260/A280 = 1.80–1.95[20]	Absorbance at 260 and 280 nm
Proteins	Not detectable <0.01 µg/dose <5 µg/mL[20] <0.2%,[116] 1.0%[5]	Colorimetric assays (Biuret, Lowry, bicinchoninic acid [BCA], and Coomassie blue) and sodium dodecyl sulfate–polyacrylamide gel electrophoresis (SDS-PAGE)
RNA	Not detectable <0.3%,[116] 1.0%,[5] 4.0%[20]	0.8% Agarose gel and Northern blots
gDNA	<0.01 µg/dose <0.4%,[116] 1%,[5] 5%[20]	Hybridization blots, real-time PCR, and fluorescence
Endotoxins	<5-EU/kg body weight <0.0002-EU/µg plasmid,[116] 0.01-EU/µg plasmid,[20] 0.04-EU/µg plasmid[5]	*Limulus* ameobocyte lysate (LAL) assay
Bioburden	0 colony-forming units[20]	Total viable count

Source: Based on information from Sofer and Hagel,[3] the United States Food and Drug Administration,[5] Horn et al.,[18] Quaak et al.,[20] and Hebel et al.[116]

using different chemical, biochemical, and physical assays. In the following sections, the rationales that lead to the selection and inclusion of these items in the QC of plasmid biopharmaceuticals are discussed. The analytical techniques more often used to determine the measures associated with those items are also described briefly.

12.3.1 Identity

During the production of plasmid DNA in *E. coli* hosts, structural changes such as deletions, insertions, and recombination events may occur with certain plasmids and host strains.[21] Additionally, if more than one plasmid DNA vector is manipulated in a plant or laboratory environment, sample mix-up and cross contamination are events that are likely to occur.[22] Thus, the identity of the plasmid DNA molecule obtained at the end of the manufacturing process or laboratorial isolation procedure must be assessed in order to confirm that the target product has been effectively obtained.[15] The analytical tests used to check identity should be highly specific for the target molecule and should be based on unique aspects of its molecular structure.[4] Some of them are described next.

12.3.1.1 *Restriction Mapping*

Restriction mapping with multiple enzymes is a recommended test for checking plasmid DNA identity.[9,19,22] Besides contributing to confirm the identity of a plasmid, mapping also provides a good estimate of the plasmid size.[6] Typically, the plasmid is digested to completion with different restriction enzymes, and the size of restriction fragments is determined after separation by agarose or polyacrylamide gel electrophoresis (PAGE). The exact set of restriction enzymes selected to perform the task should include a combination of enzymes that cut the plasmid once with enzymes that cut the plasmid more frequently.[19] A comparison of the restriction "fingerprint" obtained with the target plasmid map will then enable a positive or negative identification. Although the restriction fragments could also be analyzed by capillary electrophoresis[23] or HPLC, agarose electrophoresis is clearly the method of choice in most laboratories.

12.3.1.2 *Sequencing*

Plasmid identity can also be checked by determining the complete nucleotide sequence of both DNA strands.[22] The sequence of the therapeutic transgene and of the associated eukaryotic regulatory elements is especially important in this regard.[19] DNA sequencing can be carried out by a number of different procedures that resort either to chemical or enzymatic cleavage.[24] Recent improvements to this key analytical technique include the coupling of high-performance separation techniques such as capillary electrophoresis,[25] the use of highly sensitive detection methods such as mass spectrometry[26] or single-photon detection,[27] and automation using robotic workstations.[28]

12.3.1.3 *Polymerase Chain Reaction (PCR)*

A given plasmid can be identified with PCR using primers designed to amplify defined regions of the molecule. By using one or several appropriate pairs of primers (multiplex PCR) and then analyzing the PCR mixture by agarose gel electrophoresis, the plasmid can be easily identified by checking for DNA bands with the correct size. The PCR products can be further purified from the gel and sent for sequencing. In the limit, the whole plasmid sequence can be covered by PCR amplification if larger sets of primers are designed.[20]

12.3.2 Concentration

The determination of plasmid DNA mass in pure (final product) and impure (process samples) preparations is an important task. Although quantification of total plasmid DNA in pure solutions is relatively easy to accomplish, mass estimation in impure process streams requires the separation of impurities and contaminants from plasmid molecules before a quantitative detection can be made. Some of the analytical techniques commonly used in the context of plasmid quantification are described next.

12.3.2.1 Spectrophotometry

The amount of plasmid DNA in pure preparations can be estimated by measuring the maximum DNA absorbance at 260 nm ($A260$) in a spectrophotometer.[29] The method is relatively accurate, reproducible, and fast when applied to moderately diluted or concentrated pure preparations (0.5–15.0 μg/mL). The plasmid DNA concentration in microgram per milliter is obtained by multiplying the absorption reading by a factor of 50 ($\varepsilon = 0.02$ mL/(μg cm). Erroneous readings can be produced if the solutions are not pure or if they contain particulate material in suspension (e.g., poorly resuspended plasmid DNA precipitates). Although relatively simple, UV absorbance at 260 nm is extremely important since in many cases it is used to determine the concentration of DNA in plasmid standards used to construct calibration curves associated with other methods, such as HPLC and electrophoresis. The usefulness of the absorbance method in this context, however, is decidedly dependent on the availability of highly pure standards, since impurities commonly found in plasmid preparations such as nucleotides, single-stranded nucleic acids, and proteins can contribute significantly to the absorbance signal.

12.3.2.2 Fluorescence

A high-sensitivity quantification of plasmid DNA (<0.5 μg/mL) can be accomplished by using fluorescent dyes that bind specifically to double-stranded DNA, usually by intercalation between consecutive base pairs[30,31] (see Chapter 5, Section 5.2.1). In order to be suitable for detection, the dye in case should have a low intrinsic fluorescence when unbound, but should become intensely fluorescent when bound to plasmid DNA. An important property of such DNA-dye complexes is that their fluorescence emission intensity must be a linear function of the number of intercalated dye molecules. A number of commonly used intercalating dyes have been described in Chapter 5, which include ethidium bromide,[32] PicoGreen,[33] Sybr-Gold,[34]

TABLE 12.2. Major Characteristics of DNA Intercalating Dyes

Fluorescent Dye	λ_{ex} (nm)	λ_{em} (nm)	ε (1/(cm M))	FE (fold)	Sensitivity (pg/mL)
Ethidium bromide[117]	270	605	6,600	40	1,000
Hoechst 33258	350	450	46,000	100	1,000
PicoGreen[33]	480	520	70,000	>1,000	25
SYBR-Gold[34]	300/495	537	–	>1,000	–
YOYO-1[35]	457	510	84,000	3,200	500
TOTO-1[35]	488	530	112,000	1,100	500

The ability of these compounds to fluoresce brightly when bound can be explored to measure the concentration of plasmid DNA products in solution and also in agarose gels. For comparison, the determination of absorbance at 260 nm is characterized by DNA sensitivities of the order of 0.5 μg/mL (ε = 1/(cm M)). FE, fluorescence enhancement.

YOYO-1,[35] and TOTO-1.[35]* The major characteristics of these compounds are shown in Table 12.2. From the table, it is clear that PicoGreen, TOTO, and YOYO allow fluorescence detection and DNA quantification with picogram sensitivity. With PicoGreen, for example, concentrations as low as 25 pg/mL have been determined in pure samples with linearity extending up to 1 μg/mL. In spite of this sensitivity, fluorescence is seldom used with pure plasmid samples, since absorbance at 260 nm is usually sensitive enough to determine the typical concentration in plasmid products (0.5–2.0 μg/mL). On the other hand, the high selectivity of a dye such as PicoGreen toward double-stranded DNA makes it especially useful to quantify plasmid DNA in solutions containing host cell impurities and process-related contaminants.[36–38] The dye also binds to single-stranded nucleic acids, but since this is accompanied by an emission wavelength shift, contribution to the overall 520-nm signal is minimal.[33] Significant interference can only be caused by the presence of double-stranded DNA contaminants. However, since the DNA from the host cell is usually denatured during cell lysis (see Chapter 15), double-stranded gDNA is only present in trace amounts during processing. And, although the fluorescence signal may change in the presence of a number of other compounds such as salts, proteins, poly(ethylene glycol), and so on,[33] linearity remains unaffected. With PicoGreen, plasmid concentrations as low as 5 ng/mL have been measured in crude alkaline lysates and in solutions with high salt and poly(ethylene glycol) content.[38]

12.3.2.3 HPLC

HPLC is routinely used to assess plasmid mass (see Chapter 5, Section 5.6). The technique is especially valuable to quantify plasmid content in impure samples such as the ones that are collected during the course of downstream processing. The success of the particular HPLC mode chosen will depend on its ability to

* PicoGreen, Sybr-Gold, TOTO, and YOYO are trade names of dyes commercialized by Molecular Probes (Eugene, Oregon).

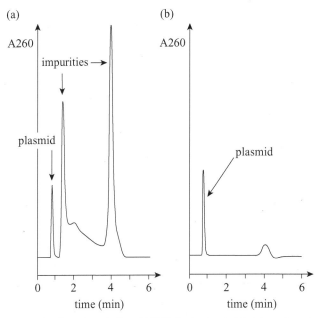

Figure 12.2 *Quantification of total plasmid DNA by hydrophobic interaction chromatography HPLC in (a) an impure plasmid DNA sample and in (b) a pure plasmid DNA sample.*

separate the plasmid from the remaining impurities, that is, RNA, gDNA, and proteins. Plasmid detection in HPLC-based methods is usually based on measurements of absorbance at 260 nm, with corresponding lower detection limits in the 0.5-μg/mL range. However, and similarly to what is currently done with capillary electrophoresis, the use of fluorescent intercalators and fluorescence detectors is likely to improve current sensitivity. Anion exchange and hydrophobic interaction are the most commonly used modes of separation in the HPLC of plasmid-containing samples (see Chapter 5, Section 5.6). Figure 12.2 shows an example of total (supercoiled + open circular + linear) plasmid DNA quantification in a cell lysate and in a final preparation using hydrophobic interaction HPLC. In both cases, the plasmid peak area can be transformed into a mass value, as long as an adequate calibration curve is available. Furthermore, in the case of the impure sample, information can be extracted from the chromatogram regarding the plasmid purity, for example, by computing the ratio of the plasmid peak area to the total area of all peaks.[39] Although it is obvious that some impurities may not elute from the column and that others may not be detected by UV absorbance at 260 nm, this "HPLC purity" is a convenient parameter especially in terms of process monitoring and control.[39]

12.3.2.4 *Electrophoresis*

The amount of plasmid DNA in a sample can be estimated following separation of the nucleic acids components by one-dimensional agarose gel electrophoresis (see Chapter 5, Section 5.3.1). The establishment of an electric field through a polyelectrolyte solution promotes the separation of the nucleic acid molecules during migration through the polymeric network of the gel. DNA and RNA are essentially separated on the basis of size or shape. After staining of the gel with ethidium bromide, the individual bands are visualized by transillumination with light of the adequate wavelength. A densitometry analysis is then performed on the plasmid bands, and the total mass is estimated with the aid of a calibration curve constructed with plasmid standards of known mass. As referred to above, the plasmid concentration in these standards is usually determined by measuring the absorbance at 260 nm. Although the linear range of quantification per band when using ethidium bromide is usually limited (50–250 ng/band[40]), the use of a staining reagent with better fluorescence enhancement properties like Sybr-Gold (Table 12.2) may improve this range to 0.5–300 ng/band.[41]

12.3.2.5 Capillary Electrophoresis

Capillary electrophoresis is a powerful DNA separation technique[42] which is becoming more often used to quantify plasmid DNA and its topoisomers[43–47] (see Chapter 5, Section 5.3.3). This analytical technique combines a high degree of resolution with a fast analysis time. Coated capillaries and elution with dilute polymer solutions (e.g., 0.1% w/w hydroxypropyl methylcellulose) are typically used.[44,46] Furthermore, if intercalating fluorescent dyes such as ethidium bromide,[43] YOYO,[45] or YO-PRO (Molecular Probes, Eugene, Oregon)[44] are combined with laser-induced fluorescence (LIF), the sensitivity can be improved tremendously and plasmid concentrations as low as 100 ng/mL can be determined.[44,46]

12.3.3 Homogeneity

12.3.3.1 Rationale

An inherent degree of structural heterogeneity occurs in plasmids due to the biosynthetic processes used by host cells to produce them[48]. The majority of plasmid DNA molecules isolated from cells such as *E. coli* adopt the plectonemically supercoiled interwound structure described in detail in Chapter 4 (Section 4.3). Nevertheless, a fraction of the population can also exist in a relaxed or open circular form. Other forms, such as knots, catenanes, and multimers, may also be present. Furthermore, the manufacturing process itself can also produce some heterogeneity due to the action of different agents (chemicals and enzymes)[49] and environmental conditions (shear stress and elevated temperatures), which originate denatured and linear variants.[50,51] Degradation during storage may also occur through a depurination and β-elimination process caused by free radical oxidation, which leads to the conversion of supercoiled to open circular forms.[6,52] The supercoiled conformation of a plasmid has been associated with a more efficient transfection of cells when compared to open circular forms (e.g., see Cupillard et al.[53] and Remaut et al.[54]). One hypothesis that has been put forward to explain this is that super-coiled plasmid isoforms are able to reach the perinuclear region of cells more efficiently than open circular and linear isoforms, and thus become more easily entrapped in the cell nuclei during division.[54] On the basis of the belief of the superiority of the supercoiled isoform in terms of biological activity, compa-nies and institutions usually set a lot release specification for the proportion of supercoiled plasmid DNA in the final product (e.g., >90% supercoiled[20]). Regulatory agencies also recommend an assessment of the homogeneity of size and structure (supercoiled vs. open circular vs. linear) of plasmid DNA in preparations intended for gene therapy or DNA vaccination.[15,22,55] For example, in a recent document, the FDA recommends that the supercoiled plasmid content in DNA vaccines should preferably be higher than 80%.[5] Arguments have been made against this specification since the supercoiled form is likely to be "nicked" and relaxed by shear associated with injection devices or plasma nucleases even before entering the target cells.[13] This has been sup-ported by some experimental evidence that indicates that the levels of plasmid DNA supercoiling do not significantly affect gene transfer.[56] Nevertheless, and since supercoiling plays an important role in cell physiology (e.g., in DNA replication, recombination, and transcription[57]), it is reasonable to suggest that most plasmid DNA-based products should be in the supercoiled form[6]. A number of different methods can be used to assess the heterogeneity of plasmid DNA products, as described next.

12.3.3.2 HPLC

Some HPLC columns can selectively separate plasmid DNA isoforms (super-coiled vs. open circular), thus providing a means to assess the heterogeneity of plasmid DNA preparations.[58–61] For example, the anion-exchange TSKgel DNA-NPR column from Toso-Bioscience (Tokyo, Japan) is able to produce a baseline resolution of open circular, supercoiled, and linear isoforms of a 6500-bp plasmid within 5 min, provided that an appropriate buffer and gradient slope are used.[41] Resolution of open circular and supercoiled isoforms is also achievable with hydrophobic interaction[60] and thiophilic affinity[61] analytical columns. In these cases, however, the separation is much slower.

12.3.3.3 Electrophoresis

The plasmid isoform distribution in a sample is usually monitored by perform-ing one-dimensional agarose gel electrophoresis. The more common super-coiled, open circular, and linear plasmid DNA structures have different migration patterns (see Chapter 5, Section 5.3) usually following the sequence supercoiled (faster), linear, and open circular (slower).[62] After staining with ethidium bromide, Sybr-Gold, or other intercalators, the individual isoforms are visualized by transillumination with UV light. With some plasmids, difficul-ties in attributing each band to the correct isoform may occur. The amount of each isoform is estimated by scanning the gels and performing densitometry on the individual bands. However, for this procedure to be accurate, a calibration should be made for each form, since the amount of ethidium bromide bound per mass of plasmid isoform may sometimes vary with the relative concentrations of dye and DNA[63,64] (see also Chapter 4, Section 4.3.5 and Chapter 5, Section 5.3.1). Another problem of the technique when it comes to determining the relative amounts of the different isoforms has to do with its limited effective linear range. This means that serial dilutions of the test sample and of the different isoform standards have to be made if a rigorous determination of the relative amounts of the isoforms is required.[41] The topoisomer distribution of bulk plasmids obtained at the end of manufacturing or of stored plasmid samples can also be determined using capillary electrophoresis, as described in Chapter 5 (Section 5.3.3). If adequate analytical conditions are selected, plasmid DNA topoisomers (supercoiled, open circular, and linear) and dimeric structures can be separated with baseline resolution within 35–40 min.[45,46] An example of an electropherogram of a plasmid sample is shown in Figure 5.6 (Chapter 5).

12.3.3.4 Fluorescence

A method to determine the percentage of the supercoiled form in plasmid DNA preparations has also been described, which takes advantage of the phenomena of reversible/irreversible denaturation of the analytes (supercoiled, open circular, and linear plasmids) and of the high specificity of the PicoGreen dye for double-stranded DNA.[36] According to this method, plasmid samples are incubated at 95°C for 4–5 min and then cooled by incubation on ice for 2 min. Next, samples are mixed with the PicoGreen reagent, and fluorescence enhancement is measured and compared with the enhancement produced by plasmid samples that were not subjected to thermal denaturation. During heating, a substantial number of hydrogen bonds between the complementary strands of the different topoisomers are broken and plasmid structure becomes altered. In the case of supercoiled plasmids, however, and since the incubation is very short, the molecules regain their native configuration and double strandedness when cooled down. They thus retain their ability to intercalate large amounts of the PicoGreen dye and thus produce a strong fluorescence enhancement. On the contrary, open circular (relaxed and nicked) and linear isoforms become irreversibly denatured and remain essentially singlestranded after cooling. They are thus unable to intercalate PicoGreen and display minimal fluorescence. The amount of supercoiled plasmid in a sample can thus be calculated by comparing the fluorescence of the ambient control with the fluorescence produced after thermal denaturation and cooling.[36] Although the method is claimed to be adequate for monitoring the quality of plasmid biopharmaceuticals, the literature shows that the traditional and more established agarose electrophoresis and HPLC methods are still preferred.

12.3.4 Purity

12.3.4.1 Impurities

Purity is a relative parameter. It compares the amount of plasmid DNA with the amount of compounds/entities other than the plasmid that are present in a sample. These compounds are either related to the product or to the process, in which case they are termed impurities, or may be adventitious, and are thus called contaminants. More specifically, an impurity may be defined as any component present in the biopharmaceutical which is not the desired product, a product-related substance (e.g., an adjuvant), or excipient (including buffer components). Process-related impurities are directly linked to the manufacturing process and may be derived from cell constituents (e.g., host cell proteins, RNA, and DNA), culture medium (e.g., antibiotics and media components), or downstream processing (e.g., column leachables, solvents, and mass-separating agents). Product-related impurities are molecular variants of the desired product (e.g., denatured plasmids and dimers) that do not have properties comparable to those of the desired product with respect to efficacy and safety. An adequate knowledge of the product and process means that impurities that are likely to be present in a final plasmid preparation are known beforehand. As for contaminants, it is obviously harder to predict which specific extraneous entity might compromise the end product. The assessment of impurities and contaminants can be performed either with a quantitative test or with a limit test for the impurity/contaminant in the sample. A quantitative test will yield an exact value, while limit tests assess whether an analyte is present in a sample below or above the lowest amount of analyte that can be detected (the detection limit).[4] In order to correctly assess the purity of a plasmid DNA product, the impurities and contaminants present should be identified and quantified. This constitutes a major challenge since impurities/contaminants may be present in very small amounts when compared with plasmid DNA. Furthermore, and if possible, the analytical tests used should be able to discriminate the target impurity (the analyte) from the other impurities and contaminants.[4] The ratio of absorbance at 260 nm to that at 280 nm is often used in research laboratories as a nonspecific indicator of DNA purity,[65] although the method was initially developed to assess nucleic acid contamination in protein preparations. A pure DNA sample usually presents a 260 nm/280 nm ratio between 1.8 and 2.0. The FDA also refers to this ratio as a purity indicator.[22] However, the validity of this procedure has been questioned,[65,66] and a full assessment of the purity of plasmid DNA preparations should not rely exclusively on this nonspecific methodology. Rather, tests should be developed and implemented to look for very specific impurities, as described next.

12.3.4.2 *Proteins*

E. coli, the host of choice for plasmid DNA production, contains around 4300 protein-coding genes.[67] More than 1100 of the proteins encoded in those genes have been recently identified by using high-pressure liquid chromatography–tandem mass spectrometry, which include proteins involved in protein synthesis, energy metabolism, and binding.[67,68] Given this diversity, the risks associated with the presence of trace amounts of some of these proteins in plasmid products should not be dismissed, and include the possible generation of immune responses and allergies, as well as the activation and development of biological reactions on the recipient that promote the production of cytokines, hormones, and/or antibodies.[69] The minimum immunogenic amount of protein depends on the specific protein and recipient. Immune responses have been reported with less than 1 ng of contaminating protein.[69] Standard colorimetric assays are recommended for the analysis of trace protein in plasmid DNA biopharmaceuticals.[70] Among them, the bicinchoninic acid (BCA) assay, a modification of the biuret reaction, has been used more frequently.[11,51,70,71] The working range of the BCA assay is 1–1000 µg/mL.[72] Proteins can also be monitored by silver staining PAGE either in native or denaturing conditions. The detection limit of this method is as low as 0.5 ng of protein/band.[69] Immunoassays (e.g., Western blots, enzyme-linked immunosorbent assays [ELISAs], and radio immune assays [RIAs]) can also be adapted whenever appropriate.[69,70,73] However, these assays require the generation of antibodies against a mixture of the host cell proteins (usually in goats or rabbits), a process that is costly and time-consuming. Furthermore, the FDA specifications for the final plasmid DNA preparation regarding contamination by proteins only require this impurity to be undetectable in final plasmid solutions by silver staining PAGE or BCA assays.[22,55]

12.3.4.3 gDNA

The presence of cellular DNA from continuous mammalian cell lines in recombinant therapeutic products has always presented a concern for regulatory agencies and developers of human biopharmaceuticals. The key worry here is that residual fragments of the foreign DNA can insert into the genome of the recipient, and eventually lead to the inactivation of tumor suppressor genes or the activation of oncogenes.[74–76] Based on the current state of knowledge, the WHO Expert Committee on Biological Standardization has concluded that a residual continuous cell line DNA level lower than 10 ng/dose of pure product is acceptable.[75] Since the risk posed by microbial (e.g., *E. coli*) DNA is smaller when compared with DNA from continuous mammalian cell lines, a specification for a gDNA content of 10 ng/dose of final plasmid product is more than acceptable. Current specifications for gDNA in plasmid products require the residual amount to be lower than 0.4–5.0% (see Table 12.1). Electrophoresis in agarose gels is probably the simplest method used to detect such residual gDNA. However, this methodology is unspecific and not sensitive enough to quantify the residual amounts of gDNA usually present in biopharmaceuticals. This is especially true in the case of plasmid biopharmaceuticals where gDNA impurities are actually made up of a multitude of differently sized fragments (from several hundreds of kilobase to less than 100 bp). Until recent years, Southern hybridization was the most common method for the quantitative detection of gDNA.[77] The procedure involves the denaturation of the nucleic acids in the test samples and the subsequent transfer onto solid supports such as nitrocellulose or nylon membranes, either by spotting or by using a dot-blot or slot-blot apparatus. After fixing the DNA, the blotted membrane is contacted with a solution that contains an oligonucleotide probe, which is specific for *E. coli* gDNA. This probe should be designed so as to look for sequences from multicopy genes that are characteristic of the *E. coli* genome, since in these cases, the probability of finding a fragment from the gene in the residual gDNA is increased.[78] The gene that codes for 16S ribosomal RNA is a good example of such a gene, since seven copies of it are present in the genome. The probes can be generated by enzymatic (e.g., PCR) or chemical methods and are typically labeled with a fluorophore or with an antigenic molecule like digoxigenin. In the first case, the hybrids formed on the membrane between the residual gDNA fragments on the plasmid sample and the probes are detected directly by fluorescence. In the second situation, the membranes must be first immersed in a solution of an anti-digoxigenin antibody that is conjugated to a reporter enzyme, for example, alkaline phosphatase or horseradish peroxidase. Upon a subsequent addition of a chemiluminescent or chromogenic substrate, a signal is generated, which can be detected by exposure of the membrane to photographic or X-ray film or by colorimetric analysis. Today, optical systems are typically used to capture an image of the fluorescent, chemiluminescent, or colored membranes. These images can then be subjected to scanning densitometry, and the intensity of the signal is compared to standards in order to perform a quantitative analysis.[69,79] Slot-blot assays are able to detect the complementary target sequence even in the presence of a large excess of noncomplementary targets. Apart from this high specificity, they are also sensitive enough to detect levels of the target nucleic acid sequence down to 1 pg.[77] Quantitative hybridization assays can also be performed by using microparticles instead of membranes. The assay is basically similar and involves denaturation of the DNA in the sample to be analyzed, adsorption onto the microparticles, hybridization with a labeled bacterial host-specific probe, and detection of hybrids.[80] For example, an assay that uses controlled pore glass microparticles and digoxigenin-labeled 16S rDNA probes has been developed that is able to detect gDNA in pure plasmid preparations at the 1% level, even in the presence of 1000-fold excess of noncomplementary target (i.e., the plasmid). The detection limit of this method was 1.4 pM of gDNA.[80] Among other advantages, microparticles offer large surface areas and exhibit excellent hybridization kinetics.

Hybridization assays are currently being substituted by faster and more sensitive methods like quantitative PCR[81,82] or real-time PCR.[83–85] These methods use sets of primers especially designed to amplify defined regions of the *E. coli* genome, for example, sequences of the 16S rRNA gene.[85] Due to the high sensitivity and low detection limits of these assays (1 pg of gDNA), interfering molecules that might be present can be diluted by several-fold. This makes it possible to use PCR detection of gDNA not only in a final bulk plasmid product, but also in crude process samples.[85] Although real-time PCR is a very sensitive and rapid method, it requires expensive and specific equipment—this normally impairs a broader use of the technique.

The methods described earlier may soon face the competition of new technologies like DNA microarrays or chips, in which hundreds to thousands of immobilized DNA probes are spotted or directly synthesized with a predetermined spatial arrangement on an impermeable, rigid, flat support such as glass (e.g., see the review by Huyghe et al.[86]). Usually, robots are required to place this large number of probes onto slides.[87] The nucleic acids in the samples must then be labeled (e.g., chemically or enzymatically) with an appropriate reporter molecule and placed over the probe spots to promote hybridization. After a series of stringent washes, the signal that results from hybridization at each spot is measured with an adequate scanner. Although high-density microarrays have been used in applications as varied as transcriptomics, single nucleotide polymorphism (SNP) analysis, and drug discovery,[86] with the current state of the microarray technology, it is easy to envision a microarray specific for the detection of residual *E. coli* gDNA in plasmid samples, where selected probes (e.g., for the 16S ribosomal RNA gene) are attached to specific sites in a chip. The costs that are currently associated with microarray technology, however, may constitute an important obstacle for routine use in an industrial manufacturing setting.

12.3.4.4 RNA

When compared with DNA, the presence of RNA in human therapeutics is usually considered a minor risk since insertion in the genome of the recipient is clearly not an issue. The current method of RNA detection is agarose gel electrophoresis.[3,18] Here, the absence of RNA bands in a 0.8% agarose gel is usually considered sufficient proof to demonstrate that the degree of contamination of the product is acceptable. Alternative methods to detect RNA are quite similar to the ones described above to detect gDNA and include Northern blot analysis, fluorescent dye-based technologies, and reverse transcription polymerase chain reaction (RT-PCR). All of these allow for a more sensitive quantification of RNA impurities to be carried out when compared with agarose electrophoresis. Northern hybridization or blotting is similar to the Southern procedure described above, with the exception that now the target molecule is RNA. And like Southern hybridization, the recognition between probe and target RNA, which is at the heart of Northern blotting, can also be implemented in the microarray format. Levels of RNA in plasmid samples of the order of 20 ng/mL can also be detected by using the RNA-specific fluorescent dye RiboGreen (Molecular Probes).[88] However, the method requires samples to be pretreated by a methodology that involves spermidine affinity precipitation of interfering DNA followed by an ethanol precipitation to concentrate RNA and to allow detection at lower concentrations.[88] The use of DNAse is another pretreatment strategy that could be used to reduce interference from DNA.[89] Although the method is rapid and easy to implement and to automate, the fact that RiboGreen can be subjected to interference from salts, ethylenediamine tetraacetic acid (EDTA), alcohols, and DNA[89] may preclude a more widespread utilization. Finally, RT-PCR is probably the most sensitive, accurate, and reproducible method available to quantify low concentrations of defined RNA sequences. Since RNA cannot be used as a template in PCR assays, a reverse transcriptase must first be used to transcribe the RNA analytes back to complementary DNA (cDNA). In the present context, specific primers for *E. coli* RNA should be used to prime this reverse transcriptase catalyzed reaction. Only then can the exponential amplification and quantification of cDNA, which are characteristic of quantitative PCR, take place.[90]

12.3.4.5 Lipopolysaccharides

Endotoxins from gram-negative bacteria like *E. coli* have a strong pyrogenic activity.[91] Chemically speaking, such endotoxins are LPS, the major constituents of the outer cell membrane of gram-negative bacteria (3–8% of the total dry weight).[91,92] LPS, which are released both by live and dead cells, have been recognized as a major cause of pyrogenic and acute immunoresponsive reactions induced after the administration of *E. coli*-derived products.[93] The detection and monitoring of LPS in a parenteral pharmaceutical such as plasmid DNA is therefore of utmost concern to regulatory agencies and manufacturers.[94] Even at the research stage, quantification of LPS in plasmid DNA products should be performed in order to ensure that *in vivo* tests with cells or animals are not biased.[95] LPS are negatively charged amphipathic molecules ($\approx 10\,kDa$ in *E. coli*) made of three general regions: the O-antigenic polysaccharide, the core oligosaccharide, and the hydrophobic, biologically active lipid A[92,96] (see Chapter 14, Section 14.2 and Figure 14.2). In response to LPS, the immune system releases molecular mediators such as interleukin-1, interleukin-6, and tumor necrosis factor α, which cause a biological response (e.g., changing metabolic functions, raising body temperature, triggering the coagulation cascade, modifying hemodynamics, and causing shock).[94,96] When compared to mice and other animal models, humans are especially sensitive to intravenous LPS challenges, requiring much smaller doses (250 times smaller) to produce a response.[97] The immunostimulatory properties of LPS are responsible for the toxic effect observed following parenteral administration.[97,98] However, these same properties are responsible for the beneficial adjuvant effects observed when residual amounts of LPS are combined with vaccines.[98] For example, a recent study has shown that the presence of higher LPS in a DNA vaccine formulation administered to mice by tattooing was associated with a higher cytotoxic T-lymphocyte response. Furthermore, and at the concentrations tested, LPS neither affected antigen expression nor induced systemic toxicity.[98]

The maximum level for intravenous application is set to 5-EU/kg body weight and hour (1 EU corresponds to 100–200 pg of endotoxin[96]). Various bioassays are available to measure endotoxins, such as the rabbit test, the *Limulus* amoebocyte lysate (LAL) assay, the chicken embryo lethality assay, and the galactosamine-primed mice lethality test.[96] The LAL assay is recommended by the FDA[22] and pharmacopeias[91] for the detection and quantification of gram-negative bacterial LPS. The assay, which is based on the immune defense system of the horseshoe crab (*Limulus polyphemus*), uses an aqueous extract of blood cells (the amoebocyte lysate) from this specie. *In vitro*, LPS molecules activate this isolated coagulation system, initiating a series of events that can be detected directly or indirectly. Currently, there are three variants of the LAL assay for LPS testing: the gel-clot method, the turbidimetric method, and the chromogenic method, all of which are approved by the United States[93] and European pharmacopeias.[91] In the gel-clot method, the LPS in the specimen activates the *Limulus* coagulation cascade in the amoebocyte lysate, originating insoluble products. As they form, these products coalesce, producing a gel that can be detected visually. The sensitivity of a given lysate lot is defined as the amount of LPS required to produce clots under standard conditions.[91] The gel-clot method is available both as a limit and as a semi-quantitative test.[91] Although it is the most accurate, the gel-clot method is time-consuming and is not prone to automation. In the chromogenic method, a colorless, artificial peptide substrate containing the *p*-nitroaniline (*p*NA) moiety is used. During the assay, the LPS present in the sample activates one of the enzymes of the coagulation system, which then cleaves *p*NA from the substrate. The amount of the yellow *p*NA product formed can then be continuously monitored by recording the absorbance at 405 nm. The LPS content in the sample can be related to the time needed to reach a particular absorbance value (kinetic chromogenic method) or to the absorbance value obtained after a fixed time (end-point chromogenic method).[91,93] In the turbidimetric method, the turbidity of the reaction mixture generated by the coalescence of the products formed upon mixing the lysate with the LPS-containing specimen is recorded.[93] As in the case of the chromogenic method, the turbidimetric method can be implemented in the kinetic or end-point modality.[91] The availability of automated systems for the chromogenic and the turbidimetric methods decreases the amount of time needed to perform the test.

12.3.4.6 *Solvents*

Organic volatile chemicals are commonly used in the manufacturing of pharmaceutical products. Based on current knowledge, such solvents can be classified into three categories: solvents to be avoided (class 1), solvents to be limited (class 2), and solvents with low toxic potential (class 3)[99] (see Chapter 11, Section 11.6.1). Although the majority of added solvents are removed throughout the process, traces of them are often a part of the end product. In spite of this inevitability, the end product should not contain a residual content higher than the permitted daily exposure (PDE), a parameter defined as the maximum acceptable intake per day of residual solvent in pharmaceutical products.[99] The solvents more likely to be found in processes used for the manufacturing of plasmid DNA belong to class 3 (e.g., acetic acid, ethanol, and isopropanol) or class 2 (e.g., acetonitrile).[100] The presence of residual amounts of these solvents in plasmid products is typically determined using chromatographic techniques such as gas chromatography or HPLC. Nonspecific methods such as loss on drying may also be admissible if only class 3 solvents are present.[99]

12.3.4.7 *Contaminants and Sterility*

Contaminants in a pharmaceutical product include all adventitiously introduced materials not intended to be part of the manufacturing process, such as
chemical and biochemical materials and/or microbial species.[15] According to
the FDA, a general safety test for the detection of extraneous toxic contaminants should be performed on biological products intended for administration
to humans.[101] Briefly, this would involve the administration of the product to
animals (e.g., guinea pigs and mice) and the monitoring and observation of
their health status for at least 7 days to look for unexpected responses.

Sterility tests are also mandatory to demonstrate that a specific plasmid
batch is free from microbial agents.[17] The membrane filtration method is the
sterility test recommended by pharmacopeias.[102,103] According to this procedure, products are filtered through a membrane with a nominal pore size not
greater than 0.45 μm in a closed system, after which the membrane is placed
in an appropriate growth media.[103] Two different media (e.g., soybean casein
digest medium and fluid thioglycollate) are commonly used since this increases
the range of microorganisms potentially detected.[102,103] The inoculated media
are then incubated at a temperature of 30–35°C for a test period of no fewer
than 14 days, after which it is examined visually. The presence of turbidity is a
strong evidence for the presence of viable cells in the plasmid product.[103]
Alternatively, the presence of viable cells could be tested by checking for the
presence of DNA or of other biomarkers. However, this would entail the
proper validation of the method.[102] One critical limitation of the membrane
filtration sterility test is, of course, that it will only detect those microorganisms
that are able to grow under the conditions used. All sterility tests should be
performed in clean-room facilities to minimize the occurrence of extraneous
contaminations.

12.3.5 Potency

12.3.5.1 *Potency Assays*

Potency is the quantitative measure of the ability or capacity of a given product
to elicit a specific effect.[104] This parameter is critical since it is the only one
that actually provides important information about the efficacy of individual
lots of a given plasmid biopharmaceutical. Therefore, potency assays (also
known as bioassays) should be selected, set up, and implemented during early
clinical development by taking into consideration the specificities of the therapeutic application, namely, the target disease, the proposed delivery methodology, the transgene product, and the biological response being sought.[15] The
existence of such assays is crucial to decide whether a specific production lot
can be released, to check for manufacturing consistency, and to control product
shelf stability.[104] In general, potency assays will evaluate the efficiency of gene
transfer, the level and stability of expression of the encoded transgene, and its
effects.[15] To meet these objectives, the appropriate cells or tissues must be
transfected with a specific amount of the plasmid, either *in vitro* or *in vivo*.

The advantages of *in vitro* assays over *in vivo* assays are obvious—in general, they are simpler, faster and more reproducible, and can be performed in larger numbers so that statistical significance is achieved more easily.

12.3.5.2 In Vitro Bioassays

In vitro measures of the transfection efficiency and of the corresponding level of gene expression are commonly used as indicators of potency, independently of the exact type of plasmid biopharmaceutical under analysis. These assays are basically designed to monitor transcription and/or translation of the gene(s) encoded in the plasmid[105] (Figure 12.3). The tests typically involve the cultivation of relevant cells in culture plates, and then the addition of a certain amount of the plasmid biopharmaceutical using the appropriate delivery methodology. Following incubation of the plates for a predetermined amount of time, the transfection efficiency is examined. Although it is possible to determine the average number of plasmid copies that were taken up by the

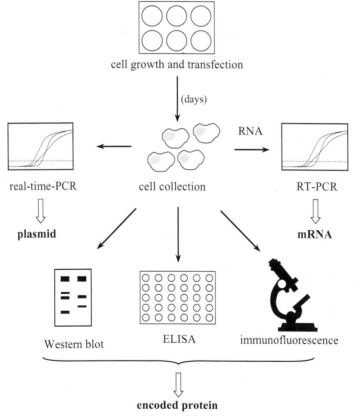

Figure 12.3 *Schematic representations of in vitro potency assays commonly used to characterize plasmid biopharmaceuticals. Following the delivery of the plasmid to cultured cells, the transfection efficiency can be gauged by measuring the amount of plasmid, transgene mRNA, and expressed gene product.*

cells, for instance, by using PCR-based tests (Figure 12.3)[106], it is much more relevant in terms of potency to determine the amount of transgene-specific messenger RNA (mRNA) in the transfected cells.[104] As described in the previous section, when the issue of the quantification of residual *E. coli* RNA was discussed, the most sensitive method available today to detect RNA is RT-PCR. For the purpose of measuring potency, an RT-PCR assay will require forward and reverse primers to be designed in such a way that they will only recognize the plasmid-derived, transgene-specific mRNA. RT-PCR reactions are then carried out by mixing these primers and assay reagents (e.g., reverse transcriptase and polymerase) with the total RNA extracted from the transfected cells. The number of PCR cycles (*Ct*) required to amplify the cDNA above a prespecified threshold value is then taken as a measure of potency. One should notice that a higher level of mRNA, hence a higher potency, should result in a lower *Ct* number. In principle, a dose range should be identified where *Ct* values correlate linearly with the plasmid concentration used in transfection, as illustrated in Figure 12.4.[104] With this methodology, the relative potency of a specific plasmid lot can be assessed by comparing results with the *Ct* values obtained when transfecting cells with a reference plasmid standard. An important advantage of this methodology has to do with the fact that in many cases, the *in vitro* transcriptional potency of plasmid DNA may correlate with the *in vivo* biological potency.[104] If this correlation can be demonstrated

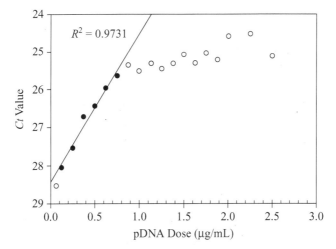

Figure 12.4 *Determination of DNA vaccine potency by quantification of transgene mRNA using reverse transcription polymerase chain reaction. The* in vitro *potency assays involve (1) the transfection of murine melanoma cells cultured in vitro with a given concentration of a bivalent human cytomegalovirus (CMV) DNA vaccine, (2) the lysis of cells and the extraction of total RNA, and (3) the analysis of transgene mRNA by RT-PCR. The figure shows a plot of the number of amplification cycles (Ct) as a function of the plasmid concentration and highlights the linear transfection dose range. Ct values are shown in reverse order to stress the fact that higher expression correlates with smaller Ct. Reprinted with kind permission from Springer Science+Business Media: Molecular Biotechnology, A TaqMan reverse transcription polymerase chain reaction (RT-PCR)* in vitro *potency assay for plasmid-based vaccine products, 40, 2008, 47-57, Mahajan R, Feher B, Jones B, et al., Figure 3.[104]*

and validated, transgene-specific mRNA levels can be used routinely as a surrogate for *in vivo* assays. This will result in significant cost and time savings.

Although it may be important to determine the amount of plasmid DNA and transgene mRNA in the cells after a certain time period, for example, by using real-time PCR and RT-PCR (Figure 12.3), respectively, the detected levels of either nucleic acid specie may not necessarily reflect the rate of protein expression. Thus, it is the presence of the expressed gene product that ultimately needs to be determined quantitatively. This can be done by resorting to antibody-based tests like immunofluorescence, Western blotting, or ELISA (Figure 12.3). An example of an immunofluorescence assay is shown in Figure 12.5. Here, a fluorescently labeled antibody that recognizes a plasmid-encoded transgene was added to cells previously cultured and transfected *in vitro* (Figure 12.5a), as well as to nontransfected control cells (Figure 12.5b).[107] Comparison of the images obtained with a fluorescence microscope clearly shows the presence of the transgene product in the test sample.[107] A disadvantage of this particular type of assay is that it might be difficult to extract quantitative information from such photographs.

While the levels of mRNA or of the transgene product provide a good indication of the transfection efficiency, they may not reflect the therapeutic activity of the expressed transgene. In some cases, however, *in vitro* assays can be developed to measure this activity much more directly. For example, if a plasmid product is developed to deliver a transgene that codes for a cytotoxic

(a)   (b)

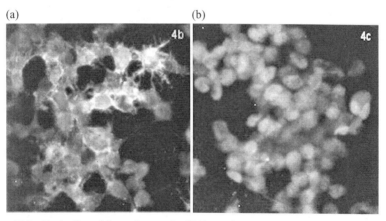

Figure 12.5 *Evaluation of the potency of a DNA vaccine against rabies by indirect immunofluorescence microscopy. A mouse D1 monoclonal antibody that recognizes the plasmid-encoded rabies virus glycoprotein was first added to (a) cells previously cultured and transfected in vitro and also to (b) nontransfected neuroblastoma cells. Then, an antimouse fluorescein isothiocyanate-conjugated secondary antibody was added to probe for the presence of the primary antibody. Comparison of the images obtained with a fluorescence microscope clearly shows the presence of the transgene product (increased fluorescence) in the test sample. Reprinted from Journal of Gene Medicine, 3, Diogo MM, Ribeiro S, Queiroz JA, et al. Production, purification and analysis of an experimental DNA vaccine against rabies, 577-584, Copyright 2001,[107] with permission from John Wiley & Sons.*

product, a cell growth assay can be implemented to determine the reduction in the amount of viable cells post-transfection as compared with a control of untreated cells.[108] Or if the transgene product is an enzyme, an enzymatic assay can be implemented to measure the corresponding activity.

12.3.5.3 In Vivo Bioassays

Although the results obtained with *in vitro* potency assays can in many cases be correlated with the therapeutic activity, *in vivo* assays of the biological potency of a plasmid biopharmaceutical are clearly preferable. These assays should use relevant animal models and should reflect the planned *in vivo* activity of the product whenever possible. In many situations, the measurement of serum levels of the transgene product, for example, by using ELISA tests, may be a sufficient indicator of the *in vivo* potency of the plasmid product,[109,110] whereas in others, more detailed tests may have to be used. In the case of DNA vaccines, for example, the ability of a specific plasmid lot to elicit an immune response should be tested by immunizing groups of animals with the target plasmid construct. The immunogenicity of the vaccine is then assessed by checking for (1) humoral and (2) cellular responses (Figure 12.6). In the first case, this assessment involves the determination of serum titers of antibodies against the encoded antigen using ELISA or Western blotting tests.[111,112] In either case, microtiter plates or membranes are coated with the antigenic protein and are then incubated with an appropriate dilution of the animal serum in order to allow antibodies elicited in response to the plasmid-encoded antigen to bind. A secondary antibody labeled with horseradish peroxidase is then used to check for the presence of and to quantify the bound immunoglobulins. Besides humoral responses, the cellular response elicited in response to DNA vaccination may also constitute an important indicator of potency. In this case, and since cytokines play an important role in acquired cell-mediated immune responses, bioassays that detect and quantify specific cytokines secreted by the antigen-specific T cells that are activated and proliferate upon immunization can be used as a measure of immunogenicity. Although ELISA assays are useful here, a key challenge, however, resides in the fact that cytokines are usually found in very low concentrations in biological fluids and are almost always bound to other proteins. One way to overcome this difficulty requires that specific cells (e.g., peripheral blood mononuclear cells) are isolated from the immunized animal and then stimulated *in vitro* to scale up cytokine production and secretion into culture supernatants.[113] However, the fact that this rather indirect methodology requires a secondary stimulation may not directly reflect the *in vivo* situation. Enzyme-linked immunospot (ELISPOT) assays (Figure 12.6) are especially useful in this context, since a key feature of the methodology is that cytokine-secreting cells can be identified *ex vivo* without the requirement for stimulation.[113,114] Thus, ELISPOT assays can be designed to determine the number of antigen-specific T cells in an immunized animal that secrete a given cytokine. For example, interferon γ-ELISPOT assays can be used to quantify functional CD8$^+$ T-cell

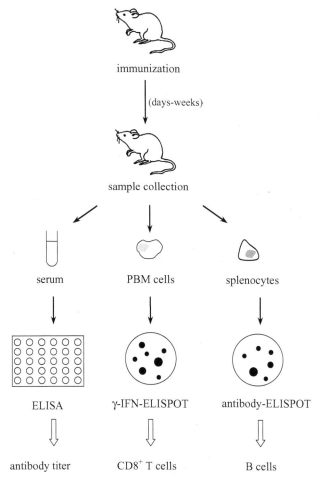

Figure 12.6 *Schematic representations of in vivo potency assays commonly used to characterize the immunogenicity of DNA vaccines. Following the delivery of the vaccine to the animal model, immunogenicity is assessed by checking for humoral and cellular responses. IFN, interferon; PBM, peripheral blood mononuclear.*

responses elicited by DNA vaccines.[114] In general, the ELISPOT method involves the coating of microtiter plates with a monoclonal antibody against the cytokine of interest and the subsequent addition of the test cells.[114] During the incubation period that follows, the cytokines that are secreted by a specific cell are captured locally by the coated antibody. Following cell removal and washing, the bound cytokines are recognized by a biotinylated secondary antibody, which is specific for the chosen cytokine. The captured cytokines can then be detected by adding an avidin-horseradish peroxidase conjugate alongside a precipitating substrate. This originates a dark blue spot that can be ascribed to a single cell.[113,114] The total number and individual size of spots generated in a plate can be then be counted manually or with an automatic reader. The number of spot-forming cells (i.e., the number of cells activated to secrete a specific cytokine) detected per million of cells can then be used as an indicator of the cellular response.[112] ELISPOT assays can also be used to detect the levels of B cells that secrete antibodies specific to the plasmid-encoded antigen and that are produced as a result of DNA immunization. In this particular case, B cells must be isolated from the spleens of vaccinated animals; the target antigen is used to coat microtiter plates, and a secondary antibody that recognizes the antibodies secreted by the B cells is used.[115]

12.4 CASE STUDY

In this final section, a published example of the QC performed on a bulk plasmid biopharmaceutical is presented to illustrate the typical results that might be obtained. The data presented here were extracted from a recent publication that describes the GMP production of a melanoma DNA vaccine.[20] The corresponding plasmid encodes a melanoma-associated epitope (MART-1) and an immunostimulatory sequence (the tetanus toxin fragment c), and is intended to be administered intradermally using a tattoo strategy. GMP batches of approximately 200 mg of plasmid were produced by growing *E. coli* in a 10-L bioreactor for 15 h up to an optical density at 600 nm (OD_{600}) of approximately 7. Plasmid recovery and purification were then accomplished by performing the following sequence of operations: cell recovery by tangential flow filtration, alkaline lysis, vacuum filtration, anion-exchange chromatography, tangential flow filtration, and, finally, sterile filtration. Further information on the fundamentals behind each of these unit operations can be found in Chapters 14–17. The quality of the bulk product obtained was then assessed by performing a series of tests (Table 12.3). The results show that the process used is able to consistently reduce host cell impurities to below the acceptable limits, batch after batch. When analyzed by sequencing and restriction mapping, the identity of the bulk plasmid obtained at the end of each of the six lots examined is also unquestionable (Table 12.3). However, discrepancies emerged in batch 4 when analyzing the plasmid topology by analytical anion-exchange HPLC. Here, and instead of the single peak that is characteristic of the super-coiled plasmid DNA isoform, a second peak was obtained, overlapping the supercoiled peak. Agarose electrophoresis further supported the idea that the extra peak corresponds to a plasmid molecule with an altered topology. This departure from the expected chromatographic profile and gel migration pattern was sufficient to reject the corresponding lot (Table 12.3).

12.5 CONCLUSIONS

The definition of the exact end-product specifications is an important part of the development of a plasmid biopharmaceutical and of the process used to

TABLE 12.3. Example of the Quality Control Performed on a Bulk Plasmid Biopharmaceutical

Test Item	Acceptance Criteria	Batch 1	Batch 2	Batch 3	Batch 4	Batch 5	Batch 6
Appearance	Clear, colorless solution	Conforms	Conforms	Conforms	Conforms	Conforms	Conforms
Sequencing	Conform reference	Conforms	Conforms	Conforms	Conforms	Conforms	Conforms
Identity (HPLC)	Rt identical to standard	Conforms	Conforms	Conforms	Twin peak	Conforms	Conforms
Identity (size, AGE)	3,395–4149 bp	3,700	3,728	3,756	3,785	3,756	3,609
Identity (restriction map)	Compares to theoretical	Conforms	Conforms	Conforms	Conforms	Conforms	Conforms
Homogeneity (HPLC)	≥90% supercoiled	98	90	91	88	94	96
Concentration (UV)	For information (mg/mL)	1.048	1.024	1.180	1.252	1.152	1.044
Purity (A260/A280)	1.80–1.95	1.86	1.88	1.83	1.84	1.84	1.87
Proteins (BCA)	<5 μg/mL	nd	nd	nd	nd	nd	nd
RNA (AGE)	<0.04 μg/μg plasmid	<4%	<4%	<4%	<4%	<4%	<4%
gDNA (AGE)	<0.05 μg/μg plasmid	<5%	<5%	<5%	<5%	<5%	<5%
Endotoxins (LAL)	<0.01 EU/μg plasmid	<2	<2	<2	<2	<2	<2
Total viable count	0 colony-forming units	0	0	0	0	0	0
Approved?	Complies to all test items	Yes	Yes	Yes	No	Yes	Yes

The table further illustrates that failure to comply with one of the pre-established test items results in batch rejection. Adapted from Quaak et al.[20]

nd, not detectable. AGE, agarose gel electrophoresis; Rt, retention time.

produce it. While some specifications may be set in advance on the basis of regulatory guidance, literature data, and experience, others have to be selected during preclinical and clinical development. Simultaneously, the analytical methodologies that will be used to check whether the final product is in compliance or not with those specifications have to be decided as well. These analytical methodologies are important not only to characterize the product in bulk and in its final formulation but also to monitor the product during manufacturing and to ensure a consistent production, as required by cGMP regulations. In the case of plasmids, sets of specifications have been suggested by regulatory agencies and have been adopted by companies which essentially deal with issues like the identity, homogeneity, concentration, and potency of the plasmid, and with the residual *E. coli* components one is more likely to find in the final product, such as proteins, RNA, gDNA, and LPS. A strict observation and adherence to the limits preset for all these parameters is a key requirement for the production of a high-quality and consistent product. Therefore, critical attention should be paid to this issue as soon as possible during the product/process development track.

REFERENCES

1. Meager A, Vocke T, Zimmermann G. The development of the regulatory process in Europe for biological medicines: How it affects gene therapy products. In: Meager A, ed. *Gene therapy technologies, applications and regulations—From laboratory to clinic.* Chichester: John Wiley & Sons, 1999.

2. Doblhoff-Dier O, Bliem R. Quality control and assurance from the development to the production of biopharmaceuticals. *Trends in Biotechnology.* 1999;17: 266–270.

3. Sofer G, Hagel L. *Handbook of process chromatography: A guide to optimization, scale-up and validation,* 1st ed. San Diego, CA: Academic Press, 1997.

4. *European Medicines Agency.* ICH Topic Q2(R1). Validation of analytical procedures: Text and methodology (CPMP/ICH/381/95). London, June 1995.

5. United States Food and Drug Administration. *Guidance for industry: Considerations for plasmid DNA vaccines for preventive infectious disease indications.* Rockville, MD: FDA, 2007.

6. Middaugh CR, Evans RK, Montgomery DL, Casimiro DR. Analysis of plasmid DNA from a pharmaceutical perspective. *Journal of Pharmaceutical Sciences.* 1998;87:130–146.

7. Kanarek AD. *A guide to good manufacturing practice.* Westborough, MA: D&MD, 2001.

8. Prazeres DMF, Monteiro GA, Ferreira GNM, Diogo MM, Ribeiro SC, Cabral JMS. Purification of plasmids for gene therapy and DNA vaccination. In: El-Gewely MR, ed. *Biotechnology Annual Review,* Vol. 7. Amsterdam: Elsevier, 2001:1–30.

9. Marquet M, Horn NA, Meek JA. Characterization of plasmid DNA vectors for use in human gene therapy, Part 1. *BioPharm.* 1997;May:42–50.

10. Marquet M, Horn NA, Meek JA. Characterization of plasmid DNA vectors for use in Human gene therapy, Part 2. *BioPharm*. 1997;June:40–45.

11. Schleef M. Issues of large-scale plasmid DNA manufacturing. In: Mountain A, Ney U, Schomburg D, eds. *Recombinant proteins, monoclonal antibodies and therapeutic genes*, Vol. 5a, 2nd ed. Weinheim: Wiley-VCH, 1999:443–469.

12. *European Medicines Agency*. ICH Topic Q6b. Note for guidance on specifications: Test procedures and acceptance criteria for biotechnological/Biological products (CPMP/ICH/365/96). London, 1999.

13. Prazeres DMF, Ferreira GNM, Monteiro GA, Cooney CL, Cabral JMS. Large-scale production of pharmaceutical-grade plasmid DNA for gene therapy: Problems and bottlenecks. *Trends in Biotechnology*. 1999;17:169–174.

14. *European Medicines Evaluation Agency*. Concept paper on guidance for DNA vaccines (Doc. Ref. EMEA/CHMP/308136/2007). London, July 16, 2007.

15. *European Medicines Evaluation Agency*. ICH Topic Q6b. Note for guidance on quality, pre-clinical and clinical aspects of gene transfer medicinal products (Doc. Ref. CPMP/BWP/3088/99). London, April 24, 2001.

16. United States Food and Drug Administration. *Guidance for industry: Guidance for human somatic cell therapy and gene therapy*. Rockville, MD: FDA, 1998.

17. World Health Organization. Guidelines for assuring the quality and nonclinical safety evaluation of DNA vaccines. Vol. Annex 1 (WHO Technical Report Series, No. 941). Geneva, 2007.

18. Horn NA, Meek JA, Budahazi G, Marquet M. Cancer gene therapy using plasmid DNA: Purification of DNA for human clinical trials. *Human Gene Therapy*. 1995;6:565–573.

19. Durland RH, Eastman EM. Manufacturing and quality control of plasmid-based gene expression systems. *Advanced Drug Delivery Reviews*. 1998;30:33–48.

20. Quaak SGL, Berg JH, Toebes M, et al. GMP production of pDERMATT for vaccination against melanoma in a phase I clinical trial. *European Journal of Pharmaceutics and Biopharmaceutics*. 2008;70:429–438.

21. Oliveira PH, Prather KJ, Prazeres DMF, Monteiro GA. Structural instability of plasmid biopharmaceuticals: Challenges and implications. *Trends in Biotechnology*. 2009;27:503–511.

22. United States Food and Drug Administration. *Addendum to the points to consider in human somatic cell and gene therapy (1991)*. Rockville, MD: FDA, 1996.

23. Maschke HE, Frenz J, Belenkii A, Karger BL, Hancock WS. Ultrasensitive plasmid mapping by high performance capillary electrophoresis. *Electrophoresis*. 1993;14: 509–514.

24. Franca LT, Carrilho E, Kist TB. A review of DNA sequencing techniques. *Quaterly Reviews in Biophysics*. 2002;35:169–200.

25. Azadan RJ, Fogleman JC, Danielson PB. Capillary electrophoresis sequencing: Maximum read length at minimal cost. *BioTechniques*. 2002;32:24–26. 28.

26. Taranenko NI, Allman SL, Golovlev VV, Taranenko NV, Isola NR, Chen CH. Sequencing DNA using mass spectrometry for ladder detection. *Nucleic Acids Research*. 1998;26:2488–2490.

27. Alaverdian L, Alaverdian S, Bilenko O, et al. A family of novel DNA sequencing instruments based on single-photon detection. *Electrophoresis*. 2002;23: 2804–2817.

28. Wilson RK, Yuen AS, Clark SM, Spence C, Arakelian P, Hood LE. Automation of dideoxynucleotide DNA sequencing reactions using a robotic workstation. *BioTechniques*. 1988;6:776–777, 781.

29. Heptinstall J, Rapley R. Spectophotometric analysis of nucleic acids. In: Rapley, R, ed. *The nucleic acid protocols handbook*. Totowa: Humana Press Inc., 2000: 57–60.

30. Rye H, Yue S, Wemmer D, et al. Stable fluorescent complexes of double-stranded DNA with bis-intercalating asymmetric cyanine dyes: Properties and applications. *Nucleic Acids Research*. 1992;20:2803–2812.

31. Yue ST, Haugland RP, inventors; Molecular Probes, Inc., assignee. Dimers of unsymmetrical cyanine dyes containing pyridinium moieties. U.S. patent 5410030. 4/1995, 1995.

32. LePecq JB, Paoletti C. A fluorescent complex between ethidium bromide and nucleic acids. Physical-chemical characterization. *Journal of Molecular Biology*. 1967;27:87–106.

33. Singer VL, Jones LJ, Yue ST, Haugland RP. Characterization of PicoGreen reagent and development of a fluorescence- based solution assay for double-stranded DNA quantitation. *Analytical Biochemistry*. 1997;249:228–238.

34. Tuma RS, Beaudet MP, Jin X, et al. Characterization of SYBR Gold nucleic acid gel stain: A dye optimized for use with 300-nm ultraviolet transilluminators. *Analytical Biochemisty*. 1999;268:278–288.

35. Hirons GT, Fawcett JJ, Crissman HA. TOTO and YOYO: New very bright fluoro-chromes for DNA content analyses by flow cytometry. *Cytometry*. 1994;15: 129–140.

36. Levy MS, Lotfian P, O'Kennedy R, Lo-Yim MY, Shamlou PA. Quantitation of supercoiled circular content in plasmid DNA solutions using a fluorescence-based method. *Nucleic Acids Research*. 2000;28:E57.

37. Noites IS, O'Kennedy RD, Levy MS, Abidi N, Keshavarz-Moore E. Rapid quantitation and monitoring of plasmid DNA using an ultrasensitive DNA-binding dye. *Biotechnology and Bioengineering*. 1999;66:195–201.

38. Ribeiro SC, Monteiro GA, Martinho G, Cabral JMS, Prazeres DMF. Quantitation of plasmid DNA in aqueous two-phase systems by fluorescence analysis. *Biotechnology Letters*. 2000;22:1101–1104.

39. Diogo MM, Queiroz JA, Prazeres DMF. Assessment of purity and quantification of plasmid DNA in process solutions using high-performance hydrophobic inter-action chromatography. *Journal of Chromatography. A*. 2003;998:109–117.

40. Bautista D, Yagubi A, Roberts P. *DNA quantification by gel densitometry with Norgen DNA ladders*. Ontario: Norgen Biotek, 2009.

41. Molloy MJ, Hall VS, Bailey SI, Griffin KJ, Faulkner J, Uden M. Effective and robust plasmid topology analysis and the subsequent characterization of the plasmid isoforms thereby observed. *Nucleic Acids Research*. 2004;32:e129.

42. Slater GW, Kenward M, McCormick LC, Gauthier MG. The theory of DNA separation by capillary electrophoresis. *Current Opinion in Biotechnology*. 2003;14: 58–64.

43. Nackerdien Z, Morris S, Choquette S, Ramos B, Atha D. Analysis of laser-induced plasmic DNA photolysis by capillary electrophoresis. *Journal of Chromatography. B*. 1996;683:91–96.

44. Schmidt T, Friehs K, Flaschel E. Rapid determination of plasmid copy number. *Journal of Biotechnology*. 1996;49:219–229.

45. Schmidt T, Friehs K, Schleef M, Voss C, Flaschel E. Quantitative analysis of plasmid forms by agarose and capillary gel electrophoresis. *Analytical Biochemistry*. 1999;274:235–240.

46. Schmidt T, Friehs K, Schleef M, Voss C, Flaschel E. Assessing the homogeneity of plasmid DNA: An important step toward gene therapy. *P/ACE Setter Newsletter*. 2000;4:1–3.

47. Schleef M, Schmidt T, Flaschel E. Plasmid DNA for pharmaceutical applications. *Developments in Biologicals*. 2000;104:25–31.

48. Sinden RR. *DNA structure and function*. San Diego, CA: Academic Press, 1994.

49. Monteiro GA, Ferreira GNM, Cabral JMS, Prazeres DMF. Analysis and use of endonuclease activities in *Escherichia coli* lysates during the primary isolation of plasmids for gene therapy. *Biotechnology and Bioengineering*. 1999;66:189–194.

50. Diogo MM, Queiroz JA, Monteiro GA, Prazeres DMF. Separation and analysis of plasmid denatured forms using hydrophobic interaction chromatography. *Analytical Biochemistry*. 2000;275:122–124.

51. Prazeres DMF, Schluep T, Cooney CL. Preparative purification of supercoiled plasmid DNA using anion-exchange chromatography. *Journal of Chromatography. A*. 1998;806:31–45.

52. Evans RK, Xu Z, Bohannon KE, Wang B, Bruner MW, Volkin DB. Evaluation of degradation pathways for plasmid DNA in pharmaceutical formulations via accelerated stability studies. *Journal of Pharmaceutical Sciences*. 2000;89:76–87.

53. Cupillard L, Juillard V, Latour S, et al. Impact of plasmid supercoiling on the efficacy of a rabies DNA vaccine to protect cats. *Vaccine*. 2005;23:1910–1916.

54. Remaut K, Sanders NN, Fayazpour F, Demeester J, De Smedt SC. Influence of plasmid DNA topology on the transfection properties of DOTAP/DOPE lipoplexes. *Journal of Controlled Release*. 2006;115:335–343.

55. United States Food and Drug Administration. *Points to consider on plasmid DNA vaccines for preventive infectious disease indications*. Rockville, MD: FDA, 1996.

56. Bergan D, Galbraith T, Sloane DL. Gene transfer *in vitro* and *in vivo* by cationic lipids is not significantly affected by levels of supercoiling of a reporter plasmid. *Pharmaceutical Research*. 2000;17:967–973.

57. Summers DK. *The biology of plasmids*. Oxford, UK: Blackwell Science Ltd, 1996.

58. Onishi Y, Azuma Y, Kizaki H. An assay method for DNA topoisomerase activity based on separation of relaxed DNA from supercoiled DNA using high-performance liquid chromatography. *Analytical Biochemistry*. 1993;210:63–68.

59. Thompson JA. A review of high performance liquid chromatography in nucleic acids research III. Isolation, purification, and analysis of supercoiled plasmid DNA. *Biochromatography*. 1986;1:68–80.

60. Iuliano S, Fisher JR, Chen M, Kelly WJ. Rapid analysis of a plasmid by hydrophobic-interaction chromatography with a non-porous resin. *Journal of Chromatography. A*. 2002;972:77–86.

61. Bennemo M, Blom H, Emilsson A, Lemmens R. A chromatographic method for determination of supercoiled plasmid DNA concentration in complex solutions. *Journal of Chromatography. B*. 2009;877:2530–2536.

62. Viovy J-L. Electrophoresis of DNA and other polyelectrolytes: Physical mechanisms. *Reviews of Modern Physics*. 2000;72:813–872.

63. Projan SJ, Carleton S, Novick RP. Determination of plasmid copy number by fluorescence densitometry. *Plasmid*. 1983;9:182–190.

64. Shubsda MF, Goodisman J, Dabrowiak JC. Quantitation of ethidium-stained closed circular DNA in agarose gels. *Journal of Biochemistry and Biophysics Methods*. 1997;34:73–79.

65. Glasel JA. Validity of nucleic acid purities monitored by 260 nm/280 nm absorbance ratios. *BioTechniques*. 1995;18:62–63.

66. Laws GM, Adams SP. Measurement of 8-OHdG in DNA by HPLC/ECD: The importance of DNA purity. *BioTechniques*. 1996;20:36–38.

67. Corbin RW, Paliy O, Yang F, et al. Toward a protein profile of *Escherichia coli*: Comparison to its transcription profile. *Proceedings of the National Academy of Sciences of the United States of America*. 2003;100:9232–9237.

68. Ishihama Y, Schmidt T, Rappsilber J, et al. Protein abundance profiling of the *Escherichia coli* cytosol. *BMC Genomics*. 2008;9:102.

69. Briggs J, Panfili PR. Quantitation of DNA and protein impurities in biopharmaceuticals. *Analytical Chemistry*. 1991;63:850–859.

70. Marquet M, Horn NA, Meek JA. Process development for the manufacture of plasmid DNA vectors for use in gene therapy. *BioPharm*. 1995;September:26–37.

71. Ferreira GNM, Cabral JMS, Prazeres DMF. Development of process flow sheets for the purification of plasmid vectors for gene therapy applications. *Biotechnology Progress*. 1999;15:725–731.

72. Ritter N, McEntire J. Determining protein concentration. Part 1: Methodology. *BioPharm*. 2002;April:12–22.

73. Rathore AS, Sobacke SE, Kocot TJ, Morgan DR, Dufield RL, Mozier NM. Analysis for residual host cell proteins and DNA in process streams of a recombinant protein product expressed in *Escherichia coli* cells. *Journal of Pharmaceutical and Biomedical Analysis*. 2003;32:1199–1211.

74. Nichols WW, Ledwith BJ, Manam SV, Troilo PJ. Potential DNA vaccine integration into host cell genome. *Annals of the New York Academy of Sciences*. 1995;772: 30–39.

75. World Health Organization. WHO requirements for the use of animal cells as *in vitro* substrates for the production of biologicals (Requirements for Biological Substances No. 50). *Biologicals*. 1998;26:175–193.

76. Doerfler W, Hohlweg U, Müller K, Remus R, Heller H, Hertz J. Foreign DNA integration—Perturbations of the genome—Oncogenesis. *Annals of the New York Academy of Sciences*. 2001;945:276–288.

77. DiPaolo B, Ji X, Venkat K. Validation of a chemiluminescent hybridization assay for quantitative determination of host cell DNA in clarified conditioned media. *BioPharm*. 1999;May:38–48.

78. Diogo MM, Queiroz JA, Monteiro GA, Martins SAM, Ferreira GNM, Prazeres DMF. Purification of a cystic fibrosis plasmid vector for gene therapy using hydrophobic interaction chromatography. *Biotechnology and Bioengineering*. 2000;68: 576–583.

79. Riggin A, Davis GC, Copman TL. Reassessing the control of residual DNA in biopharmaceuticals. *BioPharm*. 1996;October:36–41.

80. Martins SA, Prazeres DMF, Fonseca LP, Monteiro GA. Chemiluminescent bead-based hybridization assay for the detection of genomic DNA from *E. coli* in purified plasmid samples. *Analytical and Bioanalytical Chemistry*. 2008;391: 2179–2187.

81. Lahijani R, Duhon M, Lusby E, Betita H, Marquet M. Quantitation of host cell DNA contaminate in pharmaceutical-grade plasmid DNA using competitive polymerase chain reaction and enzyme-linked immunosorbent assay. *Human Gene Therapy*. 1998;9:1173–1180.

82. Gregory CA, Rigg GP, Illidge CM, Matthews RC. Quantification of *Escherichia coli* genomic DNA contamination in recombinant protein preparations by polymerase chain reaction and affinity-based collection. *Analytical Biochemistry*. 2001;296:114–121.

83. Smith GJ, 3rd, Helf M, Nesbet C, Betita HA, Meek J, Ferre F. Fast and accurate method for quantitating *E. coli* host-cell DNA contamination in plasmid DNA preparations. *BioTechniques*. 1999;26:518–522, 524, 526.

84. Vilalta A, Whitlow V, Martin T. Real-time PCR determination of *Escherichia coli* genomic DNA contamination in plasmid preparations. *Analytical Biochemistry*. 2002;301:151–153.

85. Martins SAM, Prazeres DMF, Cabral JMS, Monteiro GA. Comparison of real-time polymerase chain reaction and hybridization assays for the detection of *Escherichia coli* genomic DNA in process samples and pharmaceutical-grade plasmid DNA products. *Analytical Biochemistry*. 2003;322:127–129.

86. Huyghe A, Francois P, Schrenzel J. Characterization of microbial pathogens by DNA microarrays. *Infection, Genetics and Evolution*. 2009;9:987–995.

87. Southern E, Mir K, Shchepinov M. Molecular interactions on microarrays. *Nature Genetics*. 1999;21:5–9.

88. Murphy JC, Winters MA, Watson MP, Konz JO, Sagar SL. Monitoring of RNA clearance in a novel plasmid DNA purification process. *Biotechnology Progress*. 2005;21:1213–1219.

89. Jones LJ, Yue ST, Cheung CY, Singer VL. RNA quantitation by fluorescence-based solution assay: RiboGreen reagent characterization. *Analytical Biochemistry*. 1998;265:368–374.

90. Bustin SA. Absolute quantification of mRNA using real-time reverse transcription polymerase chain reaction assays. *Journal of Molecular Endocrinology*. 2000;25:169–193.

91. Council of Europe, Directorate for the Quality of Medicines & Healthcare. 2.6.14. Bacterial endotoxins. *European Pharmacopoeia*. 2008;1:182–189.

92. Hancock REW, Karunaratne DN, Bernegger-Egli C. Molecular organization and structural role of outer membrane macromolecules. In: Ghuysen J-M, Hakenbeck R, eds. *Bacterial cell wall*. Amsterdam: Elsevier, 1994:263–279.

93. Joiner TJ, Kraus PF, Kupiec TC. Comparison of endotoxin testing methods for pharmaceutical compounds. *International Journal of Pharmaceutical Compounding*. 2002;6:408–409.

94. Wicks IP, Howell ML, Hancock T, Kohsaka H, Olee T, Carson DA. Bacterial lipopolysaccharides copurifies with plasmid DNA: Implications for animal models and human gene therapy. *Human Gene Therapy*. 1995;6:317–323.

95. Butash KA, Natarajan P, Young A, Fox DK. Reexamination of the effect of endotoxin on cell proliferation and transfection efficiency. *BioTechniques*. 2000;29:610–614, 616, 618–619.

96. Petsch D, Anspach FB. Endotoxin removal from protein solutions. *Journal of Biotechnology*. 2000;76:97–119.

97. Copeland S, Warren HS, Lowry SF, Calvano SE, Remick D. Acute inflammatory response to endotoxin in mice and humans. *Clinical and Diagnostic Laboratory Immunology*. 2005;12:60–67.

98. van den Berg JH, Quaak SG, Beijnen JH, et al. Lipopolysaccharide contamination in intradermal DNA vaccination: Toxic impurity or adjuvant? *International Journal of Pharmaceutics*. 2010;390:32–36.

99. *European Medicines Agency*. ICH Topic Q 3 C (R3). Note for guidance on impurities: Residual solvents (CPMP/ICH/283/95). London, March 1997.

100. Prazeres DMF, Ferreira GNM. Design of flowsheets for the recovery and purification of plasmids for gene therapy and DNA vaccination. *Chemical Engineering and Processing*. 2004;43:609–624.

101. United States Code of Federal Regulations. PART 610—General Biological Products Standards. 21 CFR 610.

102. Sutton S. Validation of alternative microbiology methods for product testing quantitative and qualitative assays. *Pharmaceutical Technology*. 2005;29:118–122.

103. Council of Europe, Directorate for the Quality of Medicines & Healthcare. 2.6.1. Sterility. *European Pharmacopoeia*. 2008;1:3919–3922.

104. Mahajan R, Feher B, Jones B, et al. A TaqMan reverse transcription polymerase chain reaction (RT-PCR) *in vitro* potency assay for plasmid-based vaccine products. *Molecular Biotechnology*. 2008;40:47–57.

105. Cai Y, Rodriguez S, Hebel H. DNA vaccine manufacture: Scale and quality. *Expert Reviews in Vaccines*. 2009;8:1277–1291.

106. Carapuça E, Azzoni AR, Prazeres DMF, Monteiro GA, Mergulhão FJM. Time-course determination of plasmid content in eukaryotic and prokaryotic cells using real-time PCR. *Molecular Biotechnology*. 2007;37:120–126.

107. Diogo MM, Ribeiro S, Queiroz JA, et al. Production, purification and analysis of an experimental DNA vaccine against rabies. *The Journal of Gene Medicine*. 2001;3:577–584.

108. Kim C-K, Choi E-J, Choi S-H, Park J-S, Haider KH, Ahnc WS. Enhanced p53 gene transfer to human ovarian cancer cells using the cationic nonviral vector, DDC. *Gynecologic Oncology*. 2003;90:265–272.

109. Fewell JG, MacLaughlin F, Mehta V, et al. Gene therapy for the treatment of hemophilia B using PINC-formulated plasmid delivered to muscle with electroporation. *Molecular Therapy*. 2001;3:574–583.

110. Sebestyén MG, Hegge JO, Noble MA, Lewis DL, Herweijer H, Wolff JA. Progress toward a nonviral gene therapy protocol for the treatment of anemia. *Human Gene Therapy*. 2007;18:269–285.

111. Rainczuk A, Scorza T, Spithill TW, Smooker PM. A bicistronic DNA vaccine containing apical membrane antigen 1 and merozoite surface protein 4/5 can prime humoral and cellular immune responses and partially protect mice against virulent *Plasmodium chabaudi adami* DS malaria. *Infection and Immunity*. 2004;72:5565–5573.

112. Xin K-Q, Jounai N, Someya K, et al. Prime-boost vaccination with plasmid DNA and a chimeric adenovirus type 5 vector with type 35 fiber induces protective immunity against HIV. *Gene Therapy.* 2005;12:1769–1777.

113. Ozenci V, Kouwenhoven M, Press R, Link H, Huang YM. IL-12 elispot assays to detect and enumerate IL-12 secreting cells. *Cytokine.* 2000;12:1218–1224.

114. Cox JH, Ferrari G, Janetzki S. Measurement of cytokine release at the single cell level using the ELISPOT assay. *Methods.* 2006;38:274–282.

115. Ramanathan MP, Kutzler MA, Kuo YC, et al. Coimmunization with an optimized IL15 plasmid adjuvant enhances humoral immunity via stimulating B cells induced by genetically engineered DNA vaccines expressing consensus JEV and WNV E DIII. *Vaccine.* 2009;27:4370–4380.

116. Hebel H, Attra H, Khan A, Draghia-Akli R. Successful parallel development and integration of a plasmid-based biologic, container/closure system and electrokinetic delivery device. *Vaccine.* 2006;24:4607–4614.

117. Bonasera V, Alberti S, Sacchetti A. Protocol for high-sensitivity/long linear-range spectrofluorimetric DNA quantification using ethidium bromide. *BioTechniques.* 2007;43:173–174, 176.

13

Cell Culture

13.1 INTRODUCTION

Cell culture is at the center of a plasmid manufacturing process (see Chapter 12, Figure 12.1). The goal of this critical upstream processing stage is to generate large amounts of plasmid-containing cells that will then proceed to the downstream processing stage, where a train of unit operations is set to isolate and purify bulk plasmid according to pre-established specifications (see Chapter 12, Section 12.2). The fastest and most efficient way of producing large amounts of plasmid DNA material is to promote its replication in *Escherichia coli*. However, before *E. coli* is routinely cultured to amplify the target plasmid, a strain has to be chosen or developed and high-production clones must be carefully selected and isolated. The best clone is then used to establish master cell banks (MCBs) and working cell banks (WCBs), which contain stocks of vials of the plasmid-bearing cells. In observance with good manufacturing practices (GMPs), rigorous quality control is mandatory during this stage (see Chapter 11, Section 11.5.2). Every vial in the banks should hold virtually the same material, generated by the selected clone. The cultivation strategy used to amplify the plasmid should then be designed to maximize the volumetric productivity. Important tasks that need to be carried out in this context are the selection of the composition of the growth medium, the setup of the most adequate operating variables (e.g., pH, dissolved oxygen and stirring rate, and

Plasmid Biopharmaceuticals: Basics, Applications, and Manufacturing, First Edition.
Duarte Miguel F. Prazeres.
© 2011 John Wiley & Sons, Inc. Published 2011 by John Wiley & Sons, Inc.

temperature), and the establishment of the cultivation strategy (e.g., feeding rates in fed-batch operations and temperature shifts in the case of temperature-sensitive plasmids). The combination of an optimized cultivation strategy and medium composition with a high-copy number plasmid and a healthy plasmid can ultimately lead to volumetric plasmid yields of the order of 1000–2000 mg/L.[1] The first section of this chapter is devoted to the plasmid producer organism, E. coli, and to the preparative steps that must be taken before starting the cultivation of the cell culture strain, clone selection, and cell banking. In the second section of the chapter, a number of aspects such as the selection of growth media, the preparation of the inoculum, and the operational strategies used to carry out the cell culture are examined and discussed in detail. The focus is placed on those procedures and processes that have been the most successful when it comes to producing large amounts of plasmid DNA per culture volume (milligram per liter) and per dry cell weight (DCW) (milligram per gram).

13.2   PREPARING FOR CELL CULTURE

13.2.1   *E. coli*

The range of hosts used to amplify plasmid DNA is essentially restricted to *E. coli*, even though other bacteria, in principle, could be used. This would, of course, require the introduction of specific modifications in the plasmid backbone, namely, on the origin of replication. For example, some suggestions have been made regarding the possibility of using gram-positive bacteria like *Lactococcus lactis*, which lacks the highly immunogenic lipopolysaccharides (LPS) characteristic of *E. coli* (see Chapter 14, Section 14.2). Although this would be advantageous from a safety and downstream processing point of view, this avenue of research has not been actively pursued, probably because of the lower plasmid productivity associated with *L. lactis*,[2] and thus *E. coli* remains the workhorse of plasmid production.

   E. coli is a multifaceted microorganism that belongs to a group of fast-growing, gram-negative, rod-shaped bacteria known as Enterobacteriaceae. Other prominent members of this family include *Salmonella*, *Klebsiella*, and *Serratia*.[3] The typical *E. coli* rods have a diameter of 0.5 μm, a length of roughly 2 μm, and a cell volume of 0.6–0.7 μm^3 (Figure 13.1).[4] The average weight of a single cell is approximately 1 pg (10^{-12} g), with water accounting for about 70% of this mass.[5] As a rule, *E. coli* will grow optimally under aerobic conditions and at temperatures around 37°C. The doubling time in the exponential phase can vary anywhere from 20 min to several hours, depending on the composition of the growth medium. If fully supplied with the most adequate nutrients, *E. coli* cells will grow at their maximum rate ($\mu \approx 1.73\,h^{-1}$).[6] One of the features of such an ultrafast growth is that the cells complete one division within a time span (~24 min) that is smaller than the time required for the replication the

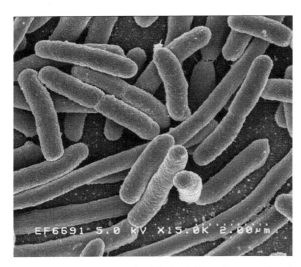

Figure 13.1 *Scanning electron micrograph of* Escherichia coli, *grown in culture and adhered to a cover slip. Source: http://en.wikipedia.org/wiki/Image:EscherichiaColi_NIAID.jpg); Rocky Mountain Laboratories, National Institute of Allergy and Infectious Diseases [NIAID], National Institutes of Health [NIH].*

TABLE 13.1. Composition of an Average *E. coli* B/r Cell as a Function of Growth Rate

μ (h^{-1})	t_D (min)	Cell (fg)	Protein (fg)	RNA (fg)	Genomes (Number)	gDNA* (fg)
0.42	99	198	100	20	1.6	8.1
0.69	60	308	156	39	1.8	9.1
1.04	40	483	234	77	2.3	11.7
1.39	30	691	340	132	3.0	15.2
1.73	24	915	450	211	3.8	19.3

*Calculated on the basis of the number of genomes and assuming that the average weight of one base pair in the 4,630,221-bp-long genome of *E. coli*[3] is 660 g/mol (see Chapter 4, Section 4.2). t_D, doubling time.
Source: Data taken from Cox.[8]

genome.[6] This apparent paradox is explained by the fact that such fast-growing bacteria are able to initiate a round of genome replication before the previous round is completed. As a result, newborn cells have more than one genome equivalent.[7] The size and composition of *E. coli* cells in a culture depend on the strain, the growth rate, and the phase of growth.[7,8] For example, an increase in the growth rate of *E. coli* B/r at 37°C (brought about by changes in media composition) is accompanied by an exponential increase in the cell mass and volume, and in the RNA, gDNA, and protein content (see Table 13.1). However, the magnitude of the increase of the mass of the cell and of the total protein is different when compared to gDNA and RNA—whereas the protein mass per DCW remains roughly constant, gDNA concentration decreases (even though more genomes per cell are present), while RNA concentration increases[8] (see Figure 13.2). More detailed information on the typical chemical

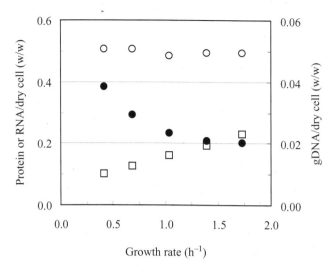

Figure 13.2 *Concentration of protein (○), gDNA (●), and RNA (□) in an average E. coli B/r cell as a function of growth rate (constructed on the basis of data taken from Cox[8]).*

composition of an *E. coli* strain B/r growing at 37°C in an aerobic glucose minimal medium, with a mass doubling time of 40 min ($\mu \approx 1.0\,h^{-1}$), is given and discussed in detail in Chapter 14 (Section 14.2, Table 14.1, and Figure 14.1).

E. coli is ubiquitous in most life science laboratories and one can aptly say that modern biotechnology has strived on its "shoulders." For example, molecular biology relies on *E. coli* for a variety of procedures, including the construction of DNA libraries, plasmid-based DNA manipulations, and protein expression, to name but a few. And, although nowadays there are a whole range of alternative expression systems available, the large-scale production of recombinant proteins of the early days would have not been possible without *E. coli*. For example, somatostatin, the first recombinant protein produced in a laboratory, and insulin, the first recombinant protein to receive market approval, were expressed in the cytoplasm of *E. coli*. The reasons for the predominance of this rather simple bacterium in the realm of molecular biologists and biotechnologists have been expressed most adequately by Neidhardt in the massive treatise Escherichia coli *and* Salmonella: *Cellular and Molecular Biology*:[9] "The popularity of *E. coli* […] derives from a mix of convenient properties, historical accident, and the force of knowledge begetting knowledge."[3] The remarkable ability of *E. coli* to grow and divide rapidly and efficiently under a wide range of conditions is an example of the convenient properties alluded to by Neidhardt. The fact that *E. coli* cells can be coaxed into delivering high plasmid yields constitutes an additional advantage in the context of this book. Two examples of the earlier knowledge mentioned in the above quotation are the germinal studies of Monod on the physiology of bacterial growth and the discovery by Joshua Lederberg of the genetic exchange mechanism of conjugation.[3] Nowadays, the genomes of different *E.*

coli strains like the popular K-12[10] and derivatives thereof, such as DH10B,[11] with their ca. 4300 genes, have been fully sequenced. Furthermore, functional information has been assigned to 87% of *E. coli* K-12 proteins,[12] and more than 80% of the metabolic pathways of the bacterium are known. Comprehensive databases like the EcoCyc (http://EcoCyc.org/) are also available, which provide a wealth of useful information on the biology of *E. coli*, including the description of all known genes, proteins, pathways, and molecular interactions.[13] In short, the molecular architecture, metabolism, general physiology, and genetics of *E. coli* constitute a very well-known and -researched subject. Since a description of all these aspects is clearly out of the scope of this chapter, the reader should consult the specialized literature, for example, the *Escherichia coli* and *Salmonella* treatise mentioned above, for an in-depth coverage of the subject.[9] In this chapter, we are rather more interested in the specific utilization of *E. coli* cells as microbial factories for the production of large amounts of plasmid DNA. Only with the advent of plasmid biopharmaceuticals has this topic deserved a more focused attention since plasmid productivity has never been an issue in the case of molecular biology applications. In that context, it was then, and still is today, usually sufficient to grow cells into the exponential phase and up to an optical density at 600 nm (OD_{600}) of 1.0–2.0 using 100–200 mL of media in an Erlenmeyer flask incubated at 37°C and shaken by orbital motion. In these cases, and although the corresponding plasmid concentrations depend on the plasmid type and size, as well as on the growth media used, typical values of volumetric productivity for high-copy number plasmids are found within the 1- to 100-mg/L range.[14,15] While growing plasmid-harboring *E. coli* cells in small-volume shake flasks is a trivial task even for the nonprofessional researcher, the cultivation of large amounts of cells with the purpose of producing kilogram quantities of plasmid DNA for clinical development or marketing purposes is a wholly different matter. Now, productivity and cost issues make it imperative to grow cells up to densities of the order of hundreds of grams per liter and target volumetric plasmid concentrations around and above 1000 mg/L. The scale at which cells are grown will depend on factors like the annual plasmid production envisaged (see Chapter 3, Section 3.3.2), but highly demanding applications may require production batches of the order of hundreds of cubic meters.

13.2.2 Strain Selection

The selection of the *E. coli* strain used for the large-scale production of the target plasmid is very important since the choice made can potentially affect the performance of the entire manufacturing process, including parameters such as plasmid productivity and quality. Clearly, the selected strain should be able to grow to high cell densities while delivering high plasmid yields. Furthermore, the strain should produce a highly homogeneous and stable supercoiled plasmid. Other desirable characteristics include compatibility with the subsequent downstream processing. For example, strains that produce large amounts of carbohydrates, such as HB101 and its derivatives (e.g., the JM100 series), may potentially interfere with some purification operations, and thus their use should be carefully considered.[14,16] Apart from the inherent phenotypic and genotypic characteristics of the strain, the overall performance of the production system will also depend on factors like plasmid size and copy number,[17-19] medium composition,[20] and operating conditions. In the case of these last factors, it is important to select not only the best pH, temperature, oxygen concentration, and so on, but also to decide whether a batch or a fed-batch strategy is more adequate.[21,22] The expression of plasmid-borne marker genes for selection purposes (e.g., coding for antibiotics) can also have a detrimental effect on plasmid replication and cell growth due to the metabolic burden with which they are associated.[23,24] Since the ideal strain will depend on all of these factors,[14] it is hard to predict a priori which strain is best suited for the replication of a particular plasmid. Rather, an empirical approach is probably the correct way to select the most adequate host strain. Even so, one should bear in mind that laboratory results obtained with a given strain grown in a shake flask may not translate directly to process scale.[15,25] An example of such a study was published recently, in which the effect of the genotype of 17 different strains on both plasmid quality and quantity was examined.[15] The extensive amount of data gathered indicated, for instance, that the specific plasmid yields per unit of optical density at 600 nm varied anywhere from 0.14 to 2.91 mg/(L·OD$_{600}$) for the case of a 5900-bp plasmid, and from 0.06 to 0.95 mg/(L·OD$_{600}$) for the case of a 20,000-bp plasmid. Furthermore, the amount of supercoiled plasmid isolated from the different strains varied from 0% to 100%! Although 17 different strains were thoroughly evaluated in that study, one of the final conclusions drawn by the authors could not be more blunt: "this study demonstrates that it is not possible to look at the genotype of the strain and draw accurate conclusions about the productivity and quality of the plasmid DNA produced in that strain."[15] In spite of this, it is important to be aware of the genotypic characteristics of the strains that dominate the large-scale plasmid production scene.

13.2.2.1 Common Strains
A variety of *E. coli* strains have been used to produce plasmids, namely, DH5α,[22,26-28] DH10B,[29,30] HB101,[21] JM108,[31] JM109,[20] and TOP10F'.[32] All of these strains were constructed by mutating *E. coli* K-12, a very well-characterized strain that presents a biosafety profile adequate for biotechnology applications.[15] Most of the specific mutations found on the strains listed above were introduced essentially with cloning or protein expression in mind. As it happens, some of these mutations also favor plasmid amplification (see Table 13.2). For example, and with the exception of HB101, all strains listed earlier have mutations in the *recA* and *endA* genes. In the first case, the disruption of the *recA* gene hampers the expression of a protein that plays a key role in homologous recombination and SOS response to DNA damage.[33] This mutation decreases the probability of plasmid recombination events (dele-

TABLE 13.2. *E. coli* Strains Commonly Used to Amplify
Plasmid DNA and Some of Their Most Relevant Mutations

Strain	*recA*	*endA*	*relA*	*gyrA*
BL21	No	No	No	No
DH5α	Yes	Yes	Yes	Yes
DH10B	Yes	Yes	No	No
HB101	Yes	No	No	No
JM108, JM109	Yes	Yes	Yes	Yes
TOP10F'	Yes	Yes	No	No

tions, multimerization, etc.) and should provide for a more homogeneous plasmid product. However, it also reduces cell viability.[14] In the second case, the elimination of the *endA*-encoded endonuclease 1, a periplasmic enzyme that cleaves within duplex DNA, reduces the likelihood of plasmid degradation inside the living cell and during lysis. The usefulness of *endA* and *recA* mutations can be better appreciated on the basis of a recent report that describes the adaptation of *E. coli* BL21, a strain commonly used in recombinant protein production, to plasmid production.[34] The BL21 strain has a number of desirable features that could prove advantageous in the context of plasmid production: It is less sensitive to growth conditions than strains like JM109 or DH5α, it grows to higher densities, and it is not sensitive to high-glucose concentration and produces less acetate due to its active glyoxylate shunt and anaplerotic pathways.[34] However, BL21 is not capable of producing large amounts of stable plasmid DNA since its *recA* and *endA* genes are intact. Hence a BL21-derived strain was constructed by mutating those genes. On a side-by-side comparison with DH5α, the new strain performed better when using both glucose and glycerol as the carbon source. In the case of glycerol, for instance, and when using a fed-batch fermentation mode, BL21 *recA⁻/endA⁻* cells grew to a higher optical density (OD_{600} nm ~190) and the volumetric productivity increased twofold, up to 2 g/L.[34] This is one of the highest volumetric productivities ever reported in the context of plasmid production. Furthermore, neither the structure nor the biological activity of the final plasmid product were affected by the new producer host when compared to the control DH5α.[34]

Mutations in *relA*, a gene that codes for guanosine tetraphosphate (ppGpp) synthetase I, an enzyme responsible for the synthesis of ppGpp, are also shared by JM108 and DH5α strains.[31] The usefulness of this mutation can be explained as follows. When amino acid starvation is imposed on strains with an intact *relA* gene, high concentrations of ppGpp lead to the inhibition of RNA and mRNA synthesis, and consequently to the inhibition of the replication of CoE1-like plasmids.[35,36] However, in strains with a mutated *relA* gene, this so-called stringent response becomes relaxed, and as a consequence, amino acid starvation can be used to impose a very slow growth rate without negatively affecting plasmid amplification.

While disruption of the *recA*, *endA*, and *relA* genes is advantageous from a plasmid production point of view, other mutations, on the other hand, may constitute an inconvenience. For instance, mutations in *gyrA*, the gene that codes for subunit A of gyrase,[13] can be found in DH5α and JM108 strains. Since gyrase carries out the ATP-dependent supercoiling of DNA, mutations in *gyrA* could originate plasmids with an altered supercoiling degree.[14] Nevertheless, such strains are often used for large-scale plasmid production with good results.[26,31] Most strains mentioned are also F⁻ (with the exception of TOP10F') and λ⁻, meaning that the conjugative low-copy number F plasmid and the λ bacteriophage are absent.[14] Since both the F factor and the λ bacteriophage have negative effects on plasmid replication and cell health, F⁻ and λ⁻ are preferred genotypes for plasmid-producing strains.[36]

13.2.2.2 Specific Strains

In some cases, precise modifications are introduced in the *E. coli* strains to provide for a specific feature. For example, the need to avoid antibiotic resistance markers (see Chapter 11, Section 11.6.2) has pushed the development of alternative, antibiotic-free selection systems. One of the strategies used, auxotrophy complementation, relies on mutating an essential gene in the *E. coli* host that renders cell growth dependent on the presence of the native gene in the plasmid. Examples of such essential genes include those required for the production of essential amino acids like alanine.[37] For this approach to be successful, however, the growth medium used to cultivate the cells must be devoid of the amino acid in question. Host genes have also been rendered thermosensitive while the wild type gene was placed in the plasmid. The ability of these cells to strive at temperatures that would otherwise be lethal is thus dependent on the presence of the plasmid.[38] In another example, the gene *infA* that codes for the translation initiation factor 1 (IF1) was deleted in the *E. coli* genome and was cloned in the plasmid. Again, the survival of the strain became totally dependent on the maintenance of the plasmid.[39]

The selection systems described above have a number of disadvantages.[24] First, the selective gene product can leak into the media from plasmid-bearing cells, thus enabling plasmid-free segregants to grow. Additionally, since the expression of a plasmid-borne gene is mandatory for the system to work, a metabolic burden is imposed on the cells, and thus biomass and plasmid productivity are likely to decrease. Cryptic expression of the selectable marker gene in the target, eukaryotic, recipient cells is also a cause for concern. These disadvantages have prompted the development of repressor titration systems that do not require the presence of plasmid-borne genes for selection.[24] In these cases, an essential gene in the chromosome is placed under the control of a given operator/promoter system, which can only be derepressed by the presence of a plasmid. As a paradigmatic example of this strategy, a gene that codes for a given antibiotic is placed in the chromosome under the action of the *lac* promoter/operator.[24] In the absence of the appropriate inducer (e.g., isopropyl β-D-1-thiogalactopyranoside [IPTG]), the *lac* repressor (LacI) protein acquires a three-dimensional structure that enables it to bind to two out of three possible operators (e.g., O_1 and O_3) in the *lac* operon (see Chapter 17, Section 17.2.8.3 and Figure 17.8a). Consequently, RNA polymerase is prevented from initiating transcription and the expression of the essential gene product is repressed. As an outcome of these molecular events, the strain is not able to grow in the medium containing the antibiotic. However, if the strain is transformed with a high-copy number plasmid containing O_1 and O_3 operator sequences, the LacI repressor is titrated away from the operator in the chromosome. In other words, as a result of the molar excess of plasmid over chromosomal genomes, the LacI repressor binds competitively to the plasmid and not to the operator, thus allowing for the expression of the gene product. Hence, growth in an antibiotic-containing medium becomes possible only for those cells that harbor the plasmid.[24]

Antibiotic-free selection systems based on RNA have also been developed. As a recent example of such a system, consider the integration of the *sacB* gene (from *Bacillus subtilis*) in the genome of an *E. coli* DH5α strain and its constitutive expression under the control of an RNA-IN promoter and leader.[40] The synthesis of the *sacB* product, the enzyme levansucrase, leads to the death of the bacteria when sucrose is added to the growth medium. This toxicity is thought to arise from the periplasmic accumulation of the high-molecular-weight fructose polymers formed by the levansucrase-catalyzed breakdown of sucrose.[41] As a second component of the system, plasmid backbones are modified to incorporate and express a 150-bp antisense RNA-OUT regulator that hybridizes to the RNA-IN promoter that drives *sacB* expression. If these plasmids are transformed into the modified strain, the expression of levansucrase is repressed and the lethal effect of sucrose can be avoided. In other words, only those cells that harbor the plasmid can strive in a sucrose-containing medium. The usefulness of such sucrose-selectable plasmid vectors and strains for large-scale manufacturing purposes has been successfully demonstrated in a fed-batch cell culture process that yielded 1213 mg plasmid/L.[40]

The development of strains that express recombinant bovine pancreatic RNase constitutes another example of strain specialization for plasmid production.[42] The goal underlying the integration of the RNase A expression cassette into the host genome is to provide for a means to degrade RNA without having to resort to an external animal-derived RNase, a procedure that is a cause for regulatory concerns (see Chapter 11, Section 11.6.3). In this case, the use of a secretion signal directs the RNase to the periplasm of *E. coli* during growth, which prevents the enzyme from degrading the cytoplasmic RNA during the normal cell functioning. The RNase only starts degrading RNA when the cell content is released during lysis[42] (see Chapter 15). *E. coli* strains with a reduced genome (up to 15% reduction) were also engineered by removing nonessential genes and sequences, including recombinogenic or mobile DNA and cryptic virulence genes.[43] As suggested by Carnes and Williams, such strains may eventually find application in plasmid production.[1]

13.2.3 Clone Selection

E. coli cells within a given culture are not all alike. Indeed, during the course of growth and division, *E. coli* cells assume different shapes, sizes, and chemical compositions. The need for bacteria to cope with environmental changes that might challenge their survival constitutes the most important biological reason behind this variability.[44] This will not be dealt with in detail here. Rather, what is important to realize is that the spreading of a few microliters of a transformation mixture in a selective agar plate is likely to originate clones with very different plasmid productivities, particularly when measured in fed-batch processes.[45,46] For instance, one report refers that the percentage of "high-producing" clones originating from a single transformation event can be as low as 0.1%.[46] This picture makes it clear that even after the best strain has been chosen and the target plasmid has been constructed, a careful selection is mandatory to identify the high producers in a population where low producers predominate.[31,46] This means that a very high number of clones should be screened in order to find the best candidates for plasmid production and cell banking. This issue of clone heterogeneity and selection was examined and described in detail by Chartrain and coworkers in their patent application (WO 2005/078115[45]). One important observation made was the recognition that clonal variants could be identified by observing phenotypic variations among the different colonies in a plate. In the specific case described, clonal isolates of a DH5α strain with the potential for high plasmid production formed gray-colored, irregularly shaped, flat, and translucent colonies in blood agar. On the contrary, the majority of cells in a transformed DH5α population originated distinct white, circular colonies in the same blood agar. A series of experiments further showed that the gray and white colonies were phenotypic variants of the same strain and that the gray phenotype exhibited a slight growth advantage over the white phenotype.[45] Most importantly, however, subsequent isolation of plasmid from those colonies enabled the identification of a direct correlation between the gray phenotype of the transformed cells and plasmid productivity—gray clonal isolates were 20-fold more productive when compared with white clonal isolates.[45] The switching of the white to gray phenotype is likely to occur due to the differential expression of a number of genes as a consequence of plasmid presence. It is in fact known that the presence of plasmids can impact the *E. coli* host and its physiology by imposing perturbations in DNA transactions (replication, transcription, and translation),[47] impacting on cell metabolism[18,48] and increasing ATP utilization in connection with the expression of antibiotic resistance genes.[49] Although the exact reasons for clonal heterogeneity among *E. coli* transformants are not fully clear, the emergence of individuals with different growth and productivity characteristics can result from mutations induced by the DNA transformation process itself or from environmental stresses during cultivation.[45] For instance, the low plasmid productivities of some clonal subtypes of *E. coli* described by Prather et al. were linked to the presence of IS1 insertional mutations in the genomes of low producers.[46] These mutations were absent from the genomes of high producers and nontransformed cells.

13.2.4 Cell Banking

Every plasmid batch should be manufactured from the exact same cell source to ensure the consistency and reproducibility of both the process and the product. This GMP imperative (see Chapter 11, Section 11.5.2) calls for the generation and storage of appropriate stocks of the selected producer clone. The best way to maintain the viability and plasmid retention of these stocks over time is probably to resort to cryogenic storage. The ultimate goal is that the cells in these vials last the life of the product.[50] A two-tiered cell banking system is used for this purpose, which consists of a first-level MCB and a second-level WCB[14] (see Figure 13.3). As a first step, a single colony selected as described earlier is used to grow an MCB. Following growth at ca. 37°C, the culture prepared from the selected clone is supplemented with 10–15% of an adequate cryoprotectant (e.g., glycerol and dimethyl sulfoxide [DMSO]) and aliquoted into cryovials. These cryovials (a typical MCB will contain approximately 200 vials) should be placed in adequate containers or racks and then cooled down to –80°C at approximately 1°C/min to minimize the cellular damage and to maximize viability.[51] Liquid nitrogen tanks are typically used for longer-term storage. The vials in the MCB provide the seed stock for the generation of the second-level WCB. One MCB vial is used to grow cells and

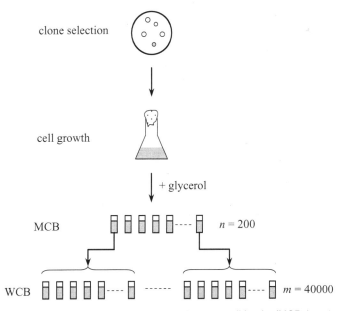

Figure 13.3 Clone selection and establishment of master cell banks (MCBs) and working cell banks (WCBs).

to construct a new WCB (around 200 vials) every time the previous WCB has been emptied. Each vial in these WCBs will constitute the starting inoculum for a single production batch. Approximately 40,000 batches can be generated from the original MCB,[52] all of which originated from a single, highly characterized and high-producing clone. As seen in Chapter 11 (Section 11.5.2), WCBs and MCBs are the subject of specific attention and recommendations by the Food and Drug Administration (FDA),[53] the European Medicines Agency (EMA),[54] and the World Health Organization (WHO).[55] For instance, extensive characterization of the culture used to generate the MCB in terms of strain and plasmid identity, percentage of plasmid-free cells, and absence of contaminating microorganisms is mandatory.

The stability of the cryopreserved vials in the MCB should be tested regularly in order to demonstrate the integrity of the bacterial host–plasmid system.[56] Cell viability can be assessed by monitoring the ability of a given amount of frozen material to generate the same number of colonies on non-selective agar plates over time.[50] Next, the ability of the colonies to grow on antibiotic-containing plates should be tested in order to determine plasmid retention. This crucial parameter is expressed as the ratio of the number of colonies that grow under selective conditions to the number of colonies that grow under nonselective conditions.[50] A 100% retention would indicate the absence of plasmid-free cells and hence a highly stable stock. Plasmid structural stability should also be assessed. Experience shows that both cell viability and plasmid retention can be maintained over extended periods of time given that MCBs are properly selected, frozen, and stored. For instance, in one of the more complete studies on the subject, a series of MCBs cryogenically frozen and stored at −80°C for long-term preservation showed stable viability and consistently high plasmid retention rates over periods of up to 11 years.[50] The lower viability and plasmid retention observed in a few MCBs were ascribed to poor selection of the initial colonies. In these cases, however, resistant clones could be rescued by resorting to high levels of antibiotic.[57]

13.3 CELL CULTURE

13.3.1 Introduction

The goal of the cell culture step is straightforward—to produce large amounts of high-quality plasmid DNA as rapidly as possible and at the lowest cost. In this context, the maximization of the volumetric plasmid yield (milligram per liter) is of course important, since this directly translates into smaller culture volumes for a given production target. Additionally, it is also desirable to maximize the specific plasmid yield (milligram per gram) because a higher proportion of plasmid relative to the other cell contents should, in principle, correlate to an easier downstream processing.[1] One of the keys to meeting these objectives is obviously the selection of the strain, as we have seen in

Section 13.2.2. Additionally, it is imperative to use plasmids with a replication origin conducive to high copy numbers. The plasmid backbones used to develop plasmid biopharmaceuticals usually contain derivatives of the ColE1 origin of replication (*ori*) that have been engineered specifically to provide for stable, high copy numbers in *E. coli* hosts. For example, the pUC plasmids have a G to A point mutation in *ori* relative to the widely used pBR322 cloning vector that affects the initiation of DNA replication, leading to copy numbers of the order of 400–500 copies per cell.[29] Furthermore, the copy numbers in such pUC-based plasmids are temperature sensitive, increasing several-fold when temperatures are raised from 20°C to 42–45°C.[58] A good illustration of the combined effect of the G to A point mutation with the upshift in temperature in plasmid productivity is given by Lahijani et al., as briefly described next.[29] First, the incorporation of the mutation in a low-copy number pBR322-derived plasmid led to a 10-fold increase in plasmid yield when cultures were grown at 35°C. Furthermore, an additional increase in both volumetric and specific plasmid yields was obtained as the growth temperature was shifted from 37°C to 42 or 45°C. Finally, excellent volumetric yields of the order of 220 mg/L were obtained when cells hosting the mutated plasmid were grown in a fed-batch fermentation with a 37–42°C shift at mid-log phase.[29]

Although the maximization of the number of plasmid copies within a single cell is highly desirable, it is important to stress that the presence of plasmid molecules usually leads to a deterioration of growth rates and biomass yield. This deleterious effect is expected to be more significant the higher the intracellular plasmid content is. The major reason for such an impact on cell metabolism has to do with the increase in the utilization of resources (nutrients, metabolites, enzymes, and energy) which are required for plasmid replication.[59] For example, the glycolysis, the tricarboxylic acid (TC) cycle, and the pentose phosphate (PP) pathways are among some of the metabolic pathways affected, with plasmid presence mediating subtle changes in the net expression of some of the genes involved.[18,48] This extra metabolic burden is even more significant when plasmid-borne marker genes such as those providing for antibiotic resistance are expressed due to the associated synthesis of the ATP required.[23,24,49,60] As an illustration of this latter point, in one situation, the expression product of a plasmid-borne kanamycin resistance gene was found to account for 18% of the cell protein of the host strain.[49]

Several reports in the specialized literature have shown that there is an inverse relation between the specific growth rate of ColE1/pMB1-derived plasmid-bearing *E. coli* cells and the intracellular plasmid concentration.[21,59,61] This behavior is probably related to the specific regulatory mechanisms that are involved in the control of plasmid replication. In plasmids of the ColE1 family, the frequency of events associated with replication initiation are negatively controlled via the interaction of two RNA molecules, RNAI and RNAII, and the 63-amino acid-long RNA one modulator (Rom) protein.[62] It has been suggested that the activities of the RNAI and RNAII promoters and the efficiency of plasmid replication by RNAI inhibition are somehow controlled by the growth rate.[61] Additionally, the effects of bacterial growth rate over plasmid replication should also be interpreted by acknowledging the fact that key cellular factors such as the abundance of ribosomes and RNA polymerases are directly linked to cell growth.[63] One corollary of the growth rate/plasmid content inverse correlation that is relevant from a plasmid production point of view is that reduced specific growth rates should be used during cultivation of *E. coli* in order to foster plasmid amplification. Besides improving plasmid accumulation, an additional advantage of this option is that segregational instability, that is, the loss of plasmid copies due to uneven segregation at cell division, is minimized under conditions that favor slow growth.[59] The implementation of such low rates (i.e., $\mu < 0.3\,h^{-1}$) can be accomplished, for example, by decreasing the temperature (e.g., to 30°C) and using carbon sources that are consumed at lower rates (e.g., glycerol) and/or by resorting to the controlled addition of limiting nutrients during a fed-batch fermentation.[1]

As described earlier in this chapter, the strain used to replicate a given plasmid, the composition of the growth/production media, and the exact conditions (e.g., temperature, pH, and aeration) used during the course of the cell culture operation can affect the quality of the plasmid as well as the overall composition of the host cell. This means that the challenges imposed on the downstream processing may be more or less demanding depending on the specific design of the cell culture step. To start with, changes in the composition, and hence in the strength of the cell wall, are likely to affect the susceptibility of cells to lysis. For example, the usual shifts to higher temperatures used to boost plasmid replication may compel cells into synthesizing lipidic membranes that are less fluid and thus affect cell lysis characteristics. Additionally, cells are likely to be more susceptible to lysis if fermentations are run in conditions conducive to *E. coli* filamentation, since this process is associated with modifications in the cell wall composition.[25] Changes in the intracellular distribution of cell components will also affect the profile of impurities that are encountered by the different unit operations used to purify the plasmid. For example, the simple extension of a batch fermentation past the exponential phase and into the stationary phase can lead to an increase of the ratio of plasmid DNA to intracellular RNA after cell lysis of up to twofold.[64]

13.3.2 Inoculum Preparation

Large-scale production bioreactors of up to $100\,m^3$ are typically inoculated with an adequate volume (1–5%) of a suspension of the producer recombinant *E. coli* cells. This inoculum material is prepared by a sequential expansion process, which starts with a frozen vial from the WCB (Figure 13.4). The cells in this vial are grown in a shake flask to reach a certain biomass and physiological status before being transferred to production. If a small bioreactor is to be used for plasmid production, a single seed stage may be sufficient. However, if large bioreactors are required, multiple seed stages with shake flasks and smaller bioreactors of increasing volume may be necessary until an amount

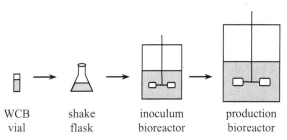

Figure 13.4 Schematic representation of a three-stage inoculum train. A vial from the WCB is used as the starting point for a sequence of E. coli cultures of increasing volume, where each new culture is inoculated with material generated from the previous one.

of microbial suspension sufficient to inoculate the production bioreactor is obtained. The succession of flask-to-flask and then of bioreactor-to-bioreactor transfers of microbial suspensions must be performed under sterilizing conditions to decrease the probability of contamination. The train can be prepared in a continuous operation, whereby actively growing cells are transferred successively from stage to stage. Alternatively, cell stocks can be collected at a specific point in the train and adequately frozen. The train development may then be resumed at a later time using the frozen material as seed. The development of such an "inoculum train" is an important part of the process given the impact that the quality of the seed material may have on the ensuing production fermentation.[26,65] Okonkowski et al. examined and discussed this issue in detail in the specific case of plasmid DNA production.[26] In their study, parameters that were varied during inoculum preparation included the number of stages, the cell concentration, and the cell status (thawed vs. actively dividing). The viability of a one-stage configuration was demonstrated and deemed preferable from a process economics point of view.[26] A further advantage of a configuration with a reduced number of stages is the decrease of the probability of contamination.

13.3.3 Media Composition

The composition of the media used to grow plasmid-producing *E. coli* cells is critical to obtaining high plasmid yields, high cell densities, and the desired product quality. The basic nutrients in the media—carbon, nitrogen, and mineral sources—should be able to promote growth and sustain biomass while providing the key components for plasmid amplification. Apart from their appropriateness for the goal at hand, nutrients should also be selected on the basis of their cost, availability, lot consistency, and impact on the downstream processing. Chemically defined and semidefined media are often preferred to complex media, since many times, it is rather difficult to guarantee consistency with the latter due to variability in the quality of components. Additionally, defined media are amenable to thorough analytical characterization, are relatively inexpensive, and can be prepared rather easily.[27] The media used to support the production of plasmids is usually developed on the basis of literature data, past experience, and optimization studies. The carbon source is indispensable to fuel the reactions required both for the synthesis of precursor metabolites and key components (e.g., lipids, carbohydrates, and nucleotides) and for the generation of energy as ATP or its equivalent.[20] The growth rate and specific yield of *E. coli* will depend on the specific carbon source used. Although glucose is always an obvious choice when designing defined and semidefined media, it displays inhibitory effects at high concentration as a result of acetate accumulation. For this reason, glycerol (e.g., 10–50 g/L) is often a preferred carbon source when growing *E. coli* for plasmid production,[25,27,29] even though it is not metabolized by cells as efficiently as is glucose. Actually, this may turn out to be an advantage since it contributes to reducing the maximum specific growth rate during the initial stages, a feature that is usually desirable since it is conducive to plasmid amplification and minimizes growth rate-dependent plasmid instability,[27,66] as seen in Section 13.3.1. The nitrogen required by cells to synthesize proteins, RNA, DNA, and plasmid DNA can be provided by an array of organic (e.g., peptone, yeast extract, soy extract, monosodium glutamate, and amino acids) and inorganic (e.g., ammonium salts such as $(NH_4)_2SO_4$ and NH_4Cl) compounds.[20] Complex nitrogen sources like yeast and soy extracts also bring with them important components for cell metabolism such as vitamins, trace metals, and alternative carbon sources. Defined mixtures of purified amino acids can also be used as a source of nitrogen.[20] However, a careful selection of constituents should be made since the presence of certain amino acids has been linked to segregational instability of plasmids.[20] Nitrogen-containing precursors for plasmid DNA synthesis, such as nucleotides, can also be added to the production media.

Bacteria need different types of minerals and trace metals to grow and strive, and for this reason, fermentation media should be formulated with various quantities of potassium, sulfur, magnesium, phosphorous, calcium, cobalt, copper, manganese, iron, molybdenum, zinc, and so on.[66] Some of these components may be especially relevant from a plasmid production point of view. For example, the presence of large amounts of magnesium ions (e.g., 80 mM Mg_2SO_4) on the fermentation media has been shown to correlate with an excellent homogeneity of supercoiled isoforms.[67] The addition of Mg^{2+} from an external source may also be expected to improve specific plasmid yields.[25] The beneficial effects of Mg^{2+} over plasmid topology and yields are probably associated with the ability of Mg^{2+} cations to compact plasmids via the shielding of phosphates in the DNA backbone. As a result of this improved compaction, the cell-carrying capacity of plasmid DNA would increase, as would the protection against endonuclease degradation.[25]

13.3.4 Production Fermentation

The quantitative data on plasmid fermentation that are available in the literature can be grouped into two categories according to the yields reported: (1)

TABLE 13.3. Examples of High-Yield Plasmid Production Processes

Strain	Plasmid	Media	Temperature (°C)	OD_{600}	pDNA (mg/L)	pDNA (mg/L·OD_{600})	Reference
DH10B	VCL1005G/A	SD	37→42	60	220	3.7	Lahijani et al.[29]
DH5α	pVRC5737Ap	SD	37	141	991	7.0	Phue et al.[34]
DH5α	gWiz GFP	SD	30→42	97	1070	11.0	Carnes et al.[25]
DH5α-derived	na	na	37→42	92	1213	~13	Luke et al.[40]
DH5α	pNTC7264-hmPA-EGFP	SD	37→42	86	1497	17.4	Carnes et al.[25]
DH5α	derivative of pV1Jns	D	37	90	1600	17.8	Listner et al.[27]
BL21 recA⁻	pVRC5737Ap	SD	37	187	1923	10.3	Phue et al.[34]
DH5α	pNTCUltra1	SD	30→42	~100	2130	~21	Williams et al.[73]

D, defined; SD, semidefined; na, not available.

low-moderate yield laboratorial-scale fermentations and (2) high-yield preindustrial fermentations. In the first category, we find an assortment of cultivation strategies, media compositions, cell strains, and plasmids, which lead to volumetric plasmid yields lower than 250 mg/L.[20,22,29,30,64,68,69] These studies have contributed significant findings and have provided important clues for the design and establishment of plasmid fermentation operations. Nevertheless, and although many manufacturing processes rely on plasmid yields below the 250 mg/L, the eventual marketing of plasmid biopharmaceuticals and the consequent industrialization of their production are both likely to drive the industry to develop processes capable of delivering yields higher than 500 mg/L.[1] This, however, is not an easy task, as can be judged by the scarce number of reports that describe methods that have surpassed that mark (see Table 13.3).

In a number of cases reported in the literature, the morphology of the plasmid-producing cells changed significantly, departing from the usual 2- to 5-μm-long rods and growing into >40-μm-long, healthy-looking aseptate filaments with regularly spaced nucleoids[25,70] (see Figure 13.5). Such an extensive filamentation of rod-shaped cells occurs as a result of an inhibition of cell septation and division, a mechanism that requires the participation of about a dozen temperature-sensitive proteins.[71] In general, filamentation is a survival strategy tactic used by bacteria to evade predators (e.g., immune cells and predatory protists) and to counteract the deleterious effects of stress. For example, when exposed to an antibiotic, cells will grow into a filamentary shape as result of the partial inhibition of cell wall synthesis.[72] In the case of the cultivation of plasmid-bearing cells described by Carnes et al.[25] and Silva et al.,[70] it is not clear whether filamentation is a direct result of the use of high temperatures of 37–42°C,[25] a consequence of the increased metabolic burden

(a)   (b)

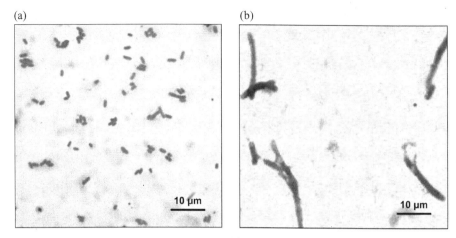

Figure 13.5   *Filamentation of* E. coli *cells. These optical microscopy images show plasmid-harboring* E. coli *DH5α cells grown in semi-defined media (30 g/l glycerol, 20 g/l tryptone) at 30°C (a) and 37°C (b). Cells were collected at late log phase and stained with safranin. The dramatic effect of temperature over cell morphology is readily visible. Reprinted from Journal of Microbiology and Biotechnology, 19, Silva F, Passarinha L, Sousa F, Queiroz JA, Domingues FC. Influence of growth conditions on plasmid DNA production, 1408–1414, Copyright 2009,[70] with permission from the Korean Society for Microbiology and Biotechnology.*

associated with plasmid amplification,[70] or both. Furthermore, the presence of antibiotics in the media used could also partially account for the phenomenon, even though resistance is conferred by the hosted plasmids. Independent of what the causative agent is, the experience shows that inhibition of cell division leads to growth arrest and ultimately to the lysis of the filaments.[25] Therefore, strategies should be devised to avoid the viability loss which is associated with filamentation.

In order to tackle the problem of growth arrest, Carnes and coworkers have devised as strategy whereby a lower temperature of 30°C is used during the initial stages of the cell cultivation process.[25] This minimizes the number of copies of temperature-sensitive plasmids (e.g., those with pUC replication origins) within the cells and thus allows for cell growth and division to proceed under reduced metabolic load conditions. Once the biomass concentration has reached a predetermined level (e.g., $OD_{600} \approx 40$–60), the temperature is increased to 37 or 42°C to boost plasmid copy number. With this strategy, cells can grow up to very high densities ($OD_{600} > 100$) without losing viability or growing into filaments. When this differential temperature strategy is combined with an exponential feeding of the media, a broth with both high cell densities ($OD_{600} \sim 86$) and plasmid concentration (~1500 mg/L) is obtained after only 41 h[25] (see Figure 13.6). In the example shown in Figure 13.6, the effect of the temperature shift on the specific yields of plasmid is clearly seen, with levels increasing almost ninefold from less than $2 \, mg/(L \cdot OD_{600})$ during growth at 30°C to ~18 mg/(L·OD_{600}) at the end of the cultivation.

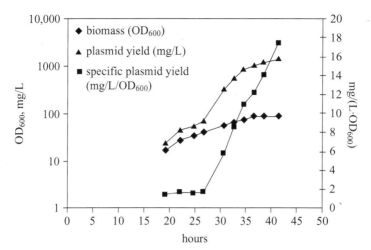

Figure 13.6 *High-yield production of plasmid DNA by inducible fed-batch cultivation of* E. coli *cells. The temperature is maintained at 30°C during the initial phases of growth (OD$_{600}$ 40, t= 25 h) and then shifted to 42°C to boost plasmid copy number. After 15 h, nutrients were supplemented at an exponential feed rate during the rest of fermentation. Reprinted with permission, from Carnes AE, Hodgson CP, Williams JA., 2006, Inducible* Escherichia coli *fermentation for increased plasmid DNA production,* Biotechnology and Applied Biochemistry, *45; 155–166.[25] © Portland Press Limited.*

In the remaining part of this section, a brief overview of the plasmid yields obtained in high-yield processes that have been reported in the literature is given (see Table 13.3). In the comparisons and discussion that follow, the results obtained by Lahijani et al.,[29] which were mentioned in Section 13.3.1, are used as a point of reference. The volumetric and specific plasmid yields obtained in the high-yield processes listed in Table 13.3 vary from 991 to 2130 mg/L and from 7 to 20 mg/(L·OD$_{600}$), respectively. These figures are substantially larger when compared with the reference case, and illustrate perfectly well the magnitude of the improvements that can be obtained when optimizing processes from the laboratory scale to a preindustrial scale. It is interesting to observe that there is no direct correlation between the maximum cell density obtained and the volumetric and specific plasmid yields. For example, in five of the examples listed in Table 13.3, the final OD$_{600}$ was around 100, but the volumetric plasmid yield varied from ~1000 to ~2100 mg/L. The lack of correlation is related to the fact that different plasmids, strains, and culture conditions are used.

13.4 CONCLUSIONS

Today, the best way to produce large amounts of a given plasmid biopharmaceutical is to promote its *in vivo* amplification in *E. coli*. The success of this endeavor depends on a first set of important activities, which include strain and plasmid backbone selection, assessment of producer clones, and the generation of WCBs and MCBs. As a result of a series of developments that have taken place in recent years (e.g., the engineering of new strains and plasmids and the development of specific media formulations and fermentation strategies), it is now possible to prepare cell cultures with high cell content (i.e., approximately 55 g of DCW/L) and plasmid concentrations (1600–2200 mg/L).[1,25,27,73] These highly concentrated and plasmid-rich broths constitute the starting material for the downstream processing stage, which is set at isolating and purifying plasmids with quality attributes compatible with their final medical/veterinary application. The challenges associated with the downstream processing are the subject of the coming chapters.

REFERENCES

1. Carnes AE, Williams JA. Plasmid DNA manufacturing technology. *Recent Patents on Biotechnology*. 2007;1:151–166.

2. Glenting J, Wessels S. Ensuring safety of DNA vaccines. *Microbial Cell Factories*. 2005;4:26.

3. Neidhardt FC. The enteric bacterial cell and the age of bacteria. In: Neidhardt FC, ed. *Escherichia coli and Salmonella: Cellular and molecular biology*, Vol. 1, 2nd ed. Washington, DC: ASM Press, 1996:1–3.

4. Kubitschek HE. Cell volume increase in *Escherichia coli* after shifts to richer media. *Journal of Bacteriology*. 1990;172:94–101.

5. Neidhardt FC, Umbarger HE. Chemical composition of *Escherichia coli*. In: Neidhardt, FC, ed. *Escherichia coli and Salmonella: Cellular and molecular biology*, Vol. 1, 2nd ed. Washington, DC: ASM Press, 1996:13–16.

6. Cox RA. Correlation of the rate of protein synthesis and the third power of the RNA: Protein ratio in *Escherichia coli* and *Mycobacterium tuberculosis*. *Microbiology*. 2003;149:729–737.

7. Bremer H, Dennis PP. Modulation of chemical composition and other parameters of the cell growth rate. In: Neidhardt FC, ed. *Escherichia coli and Salmonella: Cellular and molecular biology*, Vol. 1, 2nd ed. Washington, DC: ASM Press, 1996:1553–1568.

8. Cox RA. Quantitative relationships for specific growth rates and macromolecular compositions of *Mycobacterium tuberculosis*, *Streptomyces coelicolor* A3(2) and *Escherichia coli* B/r: An integrative theoretical approach. *Microbiology*. 2004; 150:1413–1426.

9. Neidhardt FC. *Escherichia coli and Salmonella: Cellular and molecular biology*, 2nd ed. Washington, DC: ASM Press, 1996.

10. Blattner FR, Plunkett G, Bloch CA, et al. The complete genome sequence of *Escherichia coli* K-12. *Science*. 1997;277:1453–1462.

11. Durfee T, Nelson R, Baldwin S, et al. The complete genome sequence of *Escherichia coli* DH10B: Insights into the biology of a laboratory workhorse. *Journal of Bacteriology*. 2008;190:2597–2606.

12. Serres MH, Goswami S, Riley M. GenProtEC: An updated and improved analysis of functions of *Escherichia coli* K-12 proteins. *Nucleic Acids Research*. 2004;32: D300–D302.

13. Keseler IM, Collado-Vides J, Gama-Castro S, et al. EcoCyc: A comprehensive database resource for *Escherichia coli*. *Nucleic Acids Research*. 2005;33:D334–D337.

14. Eastman EM, Durland RH. Manufacturing and quality control of plasmid-based gene expression systems. *Advanced Drug Delivery Reviews*. 1998;30:33–48.

15. Yau SY, Keshavarz-Moore E, Ward J. Host strain influences on supercoiled plasmid DNA production in *Escherichia coli*: Implications for efficient design of large-scale processes. *Biotechnology and Bioengineering*. 2008;101:529–544.

16. QIAGEN. *QIAGEN Plasmid purification handbook*, 3rd ed. Hilden: QIAGEN GmbH, 2005.

17. Cheah UE, Weigand WA, Stark BC. Effects of recombinant plasmid size on cellular processes in *Escherichia coli*. *Plasmid*. 1987;18:127–134.

18. Mason CA, Bailey JE. Effects of plasmid presence on growth and enzyme activity of *Escherichia coli* DH5α. *Applied Microbiology and Biotechnology*. 1989;32: 54–60.

19. Warnes A, Stephenson JR. The insertion of large pieces of foreign genetic material reduces the stability of bacterial plasmids. *Plasmid*. 1986;16:116–123.

20. Wang Z, Le G, Shi Y, Wegrzyn G. Medium design for plasmid DNA production based on stoichiometric model. *Process Biochemistry*. 2001;36:1085–1093.

21. Reinikainen P, Korpela K, Nissinen V, Olkku J, Söderlund H, Markkanen P. *Escherichia coli* plasmid production in fermenter. *Biotechnology and Bioengineering*. 1989;33:386–393.

22. O'Kennedy RD, Ward JM, Keshavarz-Moore E. Effects of fermentation strategy on the characteristics of plasmid DNA production. *Biotechnology and Applied Biochemistry*. 2003;37:83–90.

23. Bentley WE, Mirjalili N, Andersen DC, Davis RH, Kompala DS. Plasmid-encoded protein: The principal factor in the "metabolic burden" associated with recombinant bacteria. *Biotechnology and Bioengineering*. 1990;35:668–681.

24. Williams SG, Cranenburgh RM, Weiss AME, Wrighton CJ, Sherratt DJ, Hanak JAJ. Repressor titration: A novel system for selection and stable maintenance of recombinant plasmids. *Nucleic Acids Research*. 1998;26:2120–2124.

25. Carnes AE, Hodgson CP, Williams JA. Inducible *Escherichia coli* fermentation for increased plasmid DNA production. *Biotechnology and Applied Biochemistry*. 2006;45:155–166.

26. Okonkowski J, Kizer-Bentley L, Listner K, Robinson D, Chartrain M. Development of a robust, versatile, and scalable inoculum train for the production of a DNA vaccine. *Biotechnology Progress*. 2005;21:1038–1047.

27. Listner K, Bentley L, Okonkowski J, et al. Development of a highly productive and scalable plasmid DNA production platform. *Biotechnology Progress*. 2006;22: 1335–1345.

28. O'Mahony K, Freitag R, Hilbrig F, Muller P, Schumacher I. Strategies for high titre plasmid DNA production in *Escherichia coli* DH5α. *Process Biochemistry*. 2007;42: 1039–1049.

29. Lahijani R, Hulley G, Soriano G, Horn NA, Marquet M. High-yield production of pBR322-derived plasmids intended for human gene therapy by employing a temperature-controllable point mutation. *Human Gene Therapy*. 1996;7: 1971–1980.

30. Chen W, Graham C, Ciccarelli RB. Automated fed-batch fermentation with feedback controls based on dissolved oxygen (DO) and pH for production of DNA vaccines. *Journal of Industrial Microbiology & Biotechnology*. 1997;18:43–48.

31. Huber H, Pacher C, Necina R, Kollmann F, Reinisch C., inventors; Boheringer Ingelheim, assignee. Methods for producing plasmid DNA on a manufacturing scale by fermentation of the *Escherichia coli* K-12 strain JM108. U.S. patent WO 2005/098002, 2005.

32. Diogo MM, Ribeiro SC, Queiroz JA, et al. Production, purification and analysis of an experimental DNA vaccine against rabies. *Journal of Gene Medicine*. 2001;3: 577–584.

33. Courcelle J, Hanawalt PC. RecA-dependent recovery of arrested DNA replication forks. *Annual Reviews in Genetics*. 2003;37:611–646.

34. Phue JN, Lee SJ, Trinh L, Shiloach J. Modified *Escherichia coli* B (BL21), a superior producer of plasmid DNA compared with *Escherichia coli* K (DH5α). *Biotechnology and Bioengineering*. 2008;101:831–836.

35. Wegrzyn G. Replication of plasmids during bacterial response to amino acid starvation. *Plasmid*. 1999;41:1–16.

36. Wang Z, Yuan Z, Hengge UR. Processing of plasmid DNA with ColE1-like replication origin. *Plasmid*. 2004;51:149–161.

37. Wang MD, Buckley L, Berg CM. Cloning of genes that suppress an *Escherichia coli* K-12 alanine auxotroph when present in multicopy plasmids. *Journal of Bacteriology*. 1987;169:5610–5614.

38. Skogman SG, Nilsson J. Temperature dependent retention of a tryptophan-operon-bearing plasmid in *E. coli*. *Gene*. 1984;31:117–122.

39. Hägg P, Pohl JW, Abdulkarim F, Isaksson LA. A host/plasmid system that is not dependent on antibiotics and antibiotic resistance genes for stable plasmid maintenance in *Escherichia coli*. *Journal of Biotechnology*. 2004;111:17–30.

40. Luke J, Carnes AE, Hodgson CP, Williams JA. Improved antibiotic-free DNA vaccine vectors utilizing a novel RNA based plasmid selection system. *Vaccine*. 2009;27:6454–6459.

41. Reyrat JM, Pelicic V, Gicquel B, Rappuoli R. Counterselectable markers: Untapped tools for bacterial genetics and pathogenesis. *Infection and Immunity*. 1998;66: 4011–4017.

42. Cooke GD, Cranenburgh RM, Hanak JA, Dunnill P, Thatcher DR, Ward JM. Purification of essentially RNA free plasmid DNA using a modified *Escherichia coli* host strain expressing ribonuclease A. *Journal of Biotechnology*. 2001;85: 297–304.

43. Posfai G, Plunkett G 3rd, Feher T, et al. Emergent properties of reduced-genome *Escherichia coli*. *Science*. 2006;312:1044–1046.

44. Koch AL. Similarities and differences of individual bacteria within a clone. In: Neidhardt FC, ed. Escherichia coli *and* Salmonella: *Cellular and molecular biology*, Vol. 2, 2nd ed. Washington, DC: ASM Press, 1996:1640–1671.

45. Chartrain M, Bentley LK, Krulewicz BA, Listner KM, Sun W-J, Lee CB, inventors; Merck & Co., Inc., assignee. Process for large scale production of plasmid DNA by *E. coli* fermentation. U.S. patent WO 2005/078115, 2005.

46. Prather KL, Edmonds MC, Herod JW. Identification and characterization of IS1 transposition in plasmid amplification mutants of *E. coli* clones producing DNA vaccines. *Applied Microbiology and Biotechnology*. 2006;73:815–826.

47. Diaz Ricci J, Hernandez ME. Plasmid effects on *Escherichia coli* metabolism. *Critical Reviews in Biotechnology*. 2000;20:79–108.

48. Wang Z, Xiang L, Shao J, Wegrzyn A, Wegrzyn G. Effects of the presence of ColE1 plasmid DNA in *Escherichia coli* on the host cell metabolism. *Microbial Cell Factories*. 2006;5:34.

49. Rozkov A, Avignone-Rossa CA, Ertl PF, et al. Characterization of the metabolic burden on *Escherichia coli* DH1 cells imposed by the presence of a plasmid containing a gene therapy sequence. *Biotechnology and Bioengineering*. 2004;88: 909–915.

50. Koenig GL. Viability of and plasmid retention in frozen recombinant *Escherichia coli* over time: A ten-year prospective study. *Applied and Environmental Microbiology*. 2003;69:6605–6609.

51. Simione FP, Jr. Key issues relating to the genetic stability and preservation of cells and cell banks. *Journal of Parenteral Science and Technology*. 1992;46:226–232.

52. Schleef M, Schorr J. Plasmid DNA for clinical phase I and II studies. In: Walden P, Trefzer U, Sterry W, Farzaneh F, eds. *Gene therapy of cancer*, Vol. 451. New York: Springer-Verlag, 1998:481–486.

53. United States Food and Drug Administration. *Guidance for industry: Guidance for human somatic cell therapy and gene therapy*. Rockville, MD: FDA, 1998.

54. European Medicines Evaluation Agency. ICH Topic Q6b. Note for guidance on quality, pre-clinical and clinical aspects of gene transfer medicinal products (CPMP/BWP/3088/99). London, April 24, 2001.

55. World Health Organization. WHO guidelines for assuring the quality of DNA vacines. *Biologicals*. 1998;26:205–212.

56. Duncan PA. Characterization of microbial seeds used in the manufacture of biopharmaceuticals. *BioProcess International*. 2003;1:58–62.

57. Wright AD, Crease TJ. Detection of "lost" plasmids from *Escherichia coli* using excess ampicillin. *Analytical Biochemisty*. 1996;236:181–182.

58. Miki T, Yasukochi T, Nagatani H, et al. Construction of a plasmid vector for the regulatable high level expression of eukaryotic genes in *Escherichia coli*: An application to overproduction of chicken lysozyme. *Protein Engineering*. 1987;1: 327–332.

59. Satyagal VN, Agrawal P. A generalized model of plasmid replication. *Biotechnology and Bioengineering*. 1985;33:1135–1144.

60. Cunningham DS, Koepsel RR, Ataai MM, Domach MM. Factors affecting plasmid production in *Escherichia coli* from a resource allocation standpoint. *Microbial Cell Factories*. 2009;8:27.

61. Lin-Chao S, Bremer H. Effect of the bacterial growth rate on replication control of plasmid pBR322 in *Escherichia coli*. *Molecular and General Genetics*. 1986;203: 143–149.

62. Castagnoli L, Scarpa M, Kokkinidis M, Banner DW, Tsernoglou D, Cesareni G. Genetic and structural analysis of the ColE1 Rop (Rom) protein. *The EMBO Journal.* 1989;8:621–629.

63. Klumpp S, Zhang Z, Hwa T. Growth rate-dependent global effects on gene expression in bacteria. *Cell.* 2009;139:1366–1375.

64. Passarinha L, Diogo MM, Queiroz JA, Monteiro GA, Fonseca LP, Prazeres DMF. Production of ColE1 type plasmid by *Escherichia coli* DH5α cultured under non-selective conditions. *Journal of Microbiology and Biotechnology.* 2006;16:20–24.

65. Ignova M, Montague GA, Ward AC, Glassey J. Fermentation seed quality analysis with self-organising neural networks. *Biotechnology and Bioengineering.* 1999;64: 82–91.

66. Carnes AE. Fermentation design for the manufacture of therapeutic plasmid DNA. *BioProcess International.* 2005;October:36–44.

67. Schmidt T, Friehs K, Flaschel E, Schleef M. inventors; QIAGEN GmbH, assignee. Method for the isolation of ccc plasmid DNA. U.S. patent 6,664,078, 2003.

68. Chen W, inventor; American Home Products Corporation, assignee. Automated high-yield fermentation of plasmid DNA in *Escherichia coli*. U.S. patent 5,955,323, 1999.

69. Rozkov A, Larsson B, Gillstrom S, Bjornestedt R, Schmidt SR. Large-scale production of endotoxin-free plasmids for transient expression in mammalian cell culture. *Biotechnology and Bioengineering.* 2008;99:557–566.

70. Silva F, Passarinha L, Sousa F, Queiroz JA, Domingues FC. Influence of growth conditions on plasmid DNA production. *Journal of Microbiology and Biotechnology.* 2009;19:1408–1414.

71. Arends SJ, Weiss DS. Inhibiting cell division in *Escherichia coli* has little if any effect on gene expression. *Journal of Bacteriology.* 2004;186:880–884.

72. Burdett ID, Murray RG. Septum formation in *Escherichia coli*: Characterization of septal structure and the effects of antibiotics on cell division. *Journal of Bacteriology.* 1974;119:303–324.

73. Williams JA, Carnes AE, Hodgson CP. Plasmid DNA vaccine vector design: Impact on efficacy, safety and upstream production. *Biotechnology Advances.* 2009;27: 353–370.

14

An Overview of Downstream Processing

14.1 INTRODUCTION

Downstream processing is arguably the most challenging stage of biopharmaceutical manufacturing. The goal of the different activities that one can find within this part of a bioprocess is to isolate and purify the target molecule up to a point where the pre-established end-product specifications are met. In the case of plasmid biopharmaceuticals, the starting material for the downstream processing is the plasmid-containing biomass obtained at the end of cell culture. As we have seen in the previous chapter, *Escherichia coli* fermentations have been optimized and automated to deliver broths with high cell densities and plasmid concentrations. Specifically, by resorting to growth media with semidefined compositions and to cultivation strategies like fed-batch feeding and temperature shifts, optical densities at 600 nm (OD_{600}) of 100 and more (i.e., approximately 55 g of dry cell weight (DCW)/L) and volumetric plasmid productivities of up to 1600–2200 mg/L can be obtained at an industrial scale[1–3] (see Chapter 13, Table 13.3). In line with the case of other biopharmaceuticals, the different unit operations that make up the full downstream processing train can be broadly grouped into three different stages: primary isolation, intermediate recovery, and final purification. Ideally, the overall process should have a limited number of high-yield steps, so that processing costs and complexity are reduced.[4] Also, and as described in Chapter 11, the

Plasmid Biopharmaceuticals: Basics, Applications, and Manufacturing, First Edition.
Duarte Miguel F. Prazeres.
© 2011 John Wiley & Sons, Inc. Published 2011 by John Wiley & Sons, Inc.

process should preferably make use of reagents that are considered a priori as safe by regulatory agencies. For example, compounds that have received the Food and Drug Administration (FDA) food ingredient classification known as "generally regarded as safe (GRAS)" may, in principle, be used throughout manufacturing without a need for thorough evaluation since they have been already assessed and labeled as safe ingredients in many products. The selection of this type of safe reagents will facilitate both validation and regulatory approval. Furthermore, lengthy operations and processes should be avoided in order to cut costs from overhead, amortization of equipment, and direct labor charges. All in all, designing a downstream process for the purification of a plasmid biopharmaceutical requires a deep understanding of the different options available.

14.2 THE CHEMICAL COMPOSITION OF *E. coli*

A number of the separation challenges encountered in the downstream processing of plasmid biopharmaceuticals are related to the structural nature of plasmids, whereas others have to do more with the fact that *E. coli*-derived impurities and plasmids share a number of physical-chemical properties and characteristics. As such, it goes without saying that the design and establishment of a plasmid downstream processing scheme calls for a clear understanding and knowledge of the characteristics and distribution of the major components of *E. coli*. As we have seen in the previous chapter, the size and composition of *E. coli* cells in a culture depend on the strain and on its metabolic status (i.e., on its growth rate).[5,6] This variation and heterogeneity of growing cell populations mean that the outcome of a downstream process will depend on the manner by which the starting plasmid-containing cells were cultured and grown. It also stresses the need to consistently halt fermentation and harvest cells at the same time instant from batch to batch. An accurate inventory of the molecules that can be found in the *E. coli* strain B/r is provided by Neidhardt and Umbarger[7] (Table 14.1). The figures reported refer to the chemical composition of a typical cell in a population in "balanced growth" at 37°C and in an aerobic glucose minimal medium, with a mass doubling time of 40 min ($\mu \approx 1.0\,h^{-1}$).[7] The term balanced growth is used to describe the steady state during which every extensive property of the culture increases in the same proportion and the exponential growth rate is constant.[7] Although *E. coli* B/r is not commonly used for plasmid production, the data presented can probably be extrapolated and considered representative of other *E. coli* strains like K-12 and its derivatives (e.g., DH5α).

E. coli cells are essentially rod-shaped (see Chapter 13, Figure 13.1), with a diameter of 0.5 μm, a length of roughly 2 μm, and a cell volume of 0.6–0.7 μm³.[8] The average weight of the typical cell is approximately 1 pg (10^{-12} g), with water accounting for around 70% of this mass.[7] The distribution of the components that make up the remaining 0.3 pg of DCW is listed in Table 14.1 and is also

TABLE 14.1. Chemical Composition of an Average *E. coli* B/r Cell in a Population in Balanced Growth at 37°C in an Aerobic Glucose Minimal Medium with a Mass Doubling Time of 40 min ($\mu \approx 1.0\,h^{-1}$)

Components	% Total Dry Weight	Mass/Cell (10^{-15} g)	MW (Da)	Molecules/ Cell	Number of Different Molecules
Protein	55.0	156.0	4×10^4	2,350,000	1850
RNA	20.5	58.0	–	–	–
23S rRNA		31.0	1×10^6	18,700	1
16S rRNA		15.5	5×10^5	18,700	1
5S rRNA		1.2	3.9×10^4	18,700	1
tRNA		8.2	2.5×10^4	198,000	60
mRNA		2.3	1×10^6	1380	600
gDNA	3.1	8.8	2.5×10^9	2.1	1
Lipid	9.1	25.9	7.1×10^2	22,000,000	
LPS	3.4	9.7	4.1×10^3	1,430,000	1
Peptidoglycan	2.5	7.1		1	1
Glycogen	2.5	7.1	1×10^6	4300	1
Metabolites, cofactors, and ions	3.5	9.9	–	–	–

Source: Adapted from Neidhardt and Umbarger.[7]

shown in Figure 14.1 in a more schematic form. The first observation is probably the realization that proteins and RNA are the major constituents of *E. coli*, making up 55 and 21% of the DCW, respectively. Ribosomal RNA (rRNA) represents the most important fraction of RNA (82%), followed by transfer RNA (tRNA, 14%) and finally messenger RNA (mRNA, 4%). Lipids also constitute a significant fraction (9%) of the DCW, whereas genomic DNA (gDNA) and lipopolysaccharides (LPSs) at 3% each are relatively unimportant on a mass basis.

Apart from the weight distribution of each class of components in the cell, it is also important to recognize that there is a large variability within each category, both in terms of the individual components and of their masses. For instance, *E. coli* contains around 4300 genes that code for proteins involved in tasks as diverse as protein synthesis, energy metabolism, and binding. More than 1100 of those encoded proteins have been recently identified by using high-pressure liquid chromatography–tandem mass spectrometry.[9,10] Thus, the number of molecules from different protein species in an *E. coli* cell in a given moment is huge, and may totalize more than 2 million. The mass of these proteins, which are globular for the most part, falls within the 10- to 200-kDa range, averaging 40 kDa.[11] As for their electrostatic characteristics, most *E. coli* proteins possess pI values in the 4.3–6.0 range.[11]

The heterogeneity that is found in *E. coli* proteins is partially mirrored by mRNA—approximately 600 different mRNA molecules are estimated to exist in a certain moment and in a given cell (Table 14.1). Despite this, the chemical differences among the different mRNA species are not as striking as the ones found in proteins, simply because only four types of bases are found within

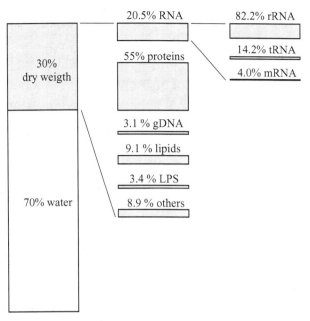

Figure 14.1 *Schematic representation of the distribution of the molecular components that make up a typical plasmid-free* E. coli *cell. The average weight is approximately 1 pg, that is, 10^{-12} g (from Neidhardt and Umbarger[7]). The plasmid content in transformed* E. coli *cells should be expected to account for 0.5–5.0% of the dry cell weight and is strongly dependent on the plasmid type, growth conditions, and growth phase. gDNA, genomic DNA; LPS, lipopolysaccharide; mRNA, messenger RNA; rRNA, ribosomal RNA; tRNA, transfer RNA.*

RNA (the modified bases typical of tRNA are excluded here from this consideration). The three RNA components (5S, 16S, and 23S rRNA) of the average 17,700 ribosomes found in each *E. coli* cell, on the other hand, are unique entities. As for tRNA, a total of 60 different species have been identified, which totalize close to 200,000 individual molecules. When compared with proteins, molecules such as mRNA, 23S rRNA, and 16S rRNA are larger on average, with masses of the order of 500–1000 kDa (Table 14.1). tRNA, the most abundant RNA species, however, has an average mass similar to the average *E. coli* protein. The single gDNA species, which can be found at an average of two molecules per cell, is the largest molecular entity in *E. coli* cells. With more than 4.6 million base pairs[12] and a mass of around 3 GDa, it dwarfs all other components in comparison (Table 14.1). RNA and gDNA are chemically identical to plasmids and, for this reason, are especially difficult to clear from plasmid-containing streams.

The inner and outer cell membranes of *E. coli* are essentially made of phospholipids and LPSs. LPSs deserve a special attention given the potential that they have to generate severe adverse reactions, like pyrogenic and immune-responsive reactions at very low concentrations, if they enter the bloodstream of patients. Thus, the downstream processing of *E. coli*-derived pharmaceutical products, particularly those that are intended for intravenous applications, must be designed to remove LPSs below a threshold level established by regulatory agencies (see Chapter 12, Section 12.3.4.5).[13] LPSs are the prevalent constituents of the outer cell membrane of gram-negative bacteria like *E. coli*, making up approximately three-quarters of the bacterial surface.[14] These molecules are important not only to confer organization and stability to the membrane but also to mediate interactions with the exterior.[14] *E. coli* cells are constantly releasing LPS into the surrounding environment during growth, division, and death. Chemically, LPSs are negatively charged amphipathic molecules ($\approx$10–20 kDa) made of three general regions: (1) an O-antigenic polysaccharide, (2) a core oligosaccharide, and (3) a hydrophobic, biologically active lipid called lipid A[14,15] (Figure 14.2). Despite their low size of approximately 10–20 kDa, LPS monomers have the ability to form highly stable aggregates such as micelles (300–1000 kDa) and vesicles (>1000 kDa). The LPSs in these aggregates are maintained together via the formation of hydrophobic interactions between adjacent alkyl chains and the establishment of bridges between phosphate groups and divalent cations such as Mg^{2+} and Ca^{2+}.[14] Thus, agents capable of destroying those interactions such as detergents (e.g., sodium dodecyl sulfate [SDS]) and chelators (e.g., ethylenediamine tetraacetic acid [EDTA]) will drive the disassembly of the aggregates into LPS monomers.

A plasmid-producing *E. coli* cell is expected to have an average composition close to the one described. However, since the presence of a plasmid imposes a metabolic burden on cells,[16,17] one should keep in mind that the relative levels of many host cell proteins and ribosome components are likely to change during the course of cell doubling and plasmid replication.[18] As for the plasmid content, and although the exact proportion will depend on the plasmid type, growth conditions, and growth phase, it should be expected to account for 0.5–5.0% of the DCW[2] (Chapter 13). This means that plasmid content on a mass basis is roughly on par with the gDNA, LPS, and mRNA content.

14.3 THE CHALLENGES OF PLASMID DOWNSTREAM PROCESSING

The train of unit operations in the downstream processing of plasmid biopharmaceuticals has to be arranged in such a manner as to remove the impurities associated with the producer organism down to the acceptable residual levels set in the product specifications (see Chapter 12, Section 12.2). This undertaking carries with it several challenges, most of which are determined by the diversity and specific characteristics of the *E. coli*-derived solutes described in the previous section. To start with, plasmids are extremely large (2000–10,000 bp, 1320–6600 kDa, micron sized) and structurally unusual when compared with proteins (see Chapter 4, Section 4.3). With their large size, plasmids

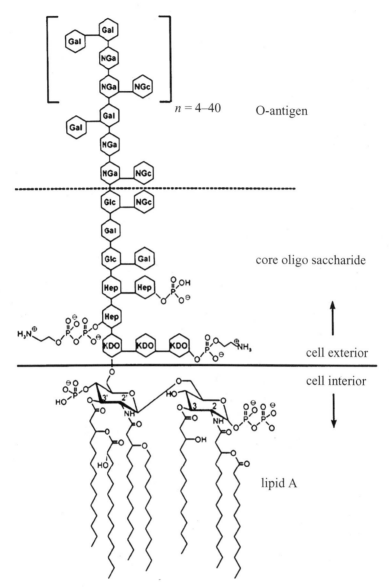

Figure 14.2 *The basic structure of the lipopolysaccharide molecule from* E. coli *O111:B4. Hep, L-glycero-D-manno-heptose; Gal, galactose; Glc, glucose; KDO, 2-keto-3-deoxyoctonic acid; NGa, N-acetyl-galactosamine; NGc, N-acetyl-glucosamine. Reprinted from Journal of Biotechnology, 76, Petsch D, Anspach FB. Endotoxin removal from protein solutions, 97–119, Copyright 2000,[14] with permission from Elsevier.*

have difficulty in accessing many of the pores of processing materials like membranes, chromatographic beads, and monoliths and are characterized by very small diffusion coefficients ($\sim 10^{-8}$ cm^2/s). These are two of the major reasons behind the notorious mass transfer and capacity limitations that are encountered especially in adsorptive unit operations like fixed-bed and membrane chromatography (see Chapter 17, Section 17.2.2). In the past years, attempts to overcome these limitations have focused on the tailoring of materials specifically to handle very large biomolecules, rather than trying to adapt conventional beads and membranes to plasmid processing.

The tightly twisted structure that is characteristic of the most effective (in biological terms) supercoiled topoisomer also brings with it a number of challenges. First, supercoiled plasmids can be easily converted into open circular, linear, and denatured isoforms, if care is not taken to avoid the action of *E. coli* nucleases or the use of excessive shear rates during processing. This means, for example, that the preferred supercoiled topoisomers may coexist with the less desirable open circular isoforms. Given that the current regulatory thinking favors the definition of a specification setting a minimum percentage of supercoiled isoforms (e.g., >90%; see Chapter 12, Section 12.3.3) in the final plasmid product, this means that unit operations have to be inserted in some processes with the specific goal of resolving the two isoforms. This separation, however, is not a trivial one to carry out, especially at a process scale.

But the separation challenges encountered during the downstream processing owe as much to the awkward structure and large size of plasmids as to the fact that most *E. coli*-derived impurities share a number of properties with them. For example, the polyanionic RNA and gDNA molecules and fragments, and the positively charged LPS, are expected to behave to some extent in a similar fashion to plasmids when faced with cationic surfaces (e.g., anion-exchange beads, membranes, or monoliths) and mass-separating agents (e.g., cationic surfactants), or when exposed to salt solutions. Likewise, some RNA species and gDNA fragments that arise during the course of processing have molecular weights that are comparable to those of plasmids (Figure 14.3). These similarities can compromise the selectivity of operations that attempt to explore charge (e.g., anion-exchange chromatography) and size (e.g., size exclusion and tangential flow filtration) differences for separation purposes. The net result is that plasmids and *E. coli* impurities are likely to compete and

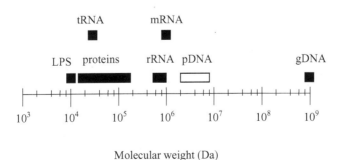

Molecular weight (Da)

Figure 14.3 *Overview of the range of molecular weight of the typical plasmid DNA molecules used medically (2000–10,000 bp, 1320–6600 kDa) and of the key* E. coli *components. gDNA, genomic DNA; LPS, lipopolysaccharide; mRNA, messenger RNA; pDNA, plasmid DNA; rRNA, ribosomal RNA; tRNA, transfer RNA.*

copurify with each other in the context of many of those unit operations. One of the solutions to these problems is of course to focus on those physical-chemical properties that differ the most between plasmids and impurities. One of such properties is hydrophobicity. The differences found here are intimately linked to the fact that plasmids are essentially double stranded, while RNA and fragmented gDNA are, for the most part, single stranded. This offers the possibility to explore interactions with and between exposed bases for separation purposes, as is the case, for example, when using hydrophobic interaction chromatography (see Chapter 17, Section 17.2.6). Another way to circumvent the similarity conundrum is to somehow act upon the biomolecules so as to change their size and charge density. This can be done, for example, by using enzymes that degrade RNA into smaller fragments, by selectively denaturing double-stranded gDNA impurities, or by adding chemicals to the environment that have the ability to compact plasmids into small globules.

The intracellular nature of plasmids renders lysis of *E. coli* cells inevitable. The generation and handling of lysates is a task with many challenges, as can be testified by anyone who has ever attempted to perform an alkaline or heat lysis at the bench scale. Although the specific challenges may vary according to the specific lysis methodology used, as will be described in detail in Chapter 15, some of them should be enumerated here briefly: (1) efficient release of intracellular components, (2) thorough and fast mixing of chemicals with cells, (3) minimization of shear degradation of gDNA, (4) non-Newtonian properties of viscous lysates, (5) separation of debris and precipitated impurities, and (6) minimization of thermal, shear, and enzymatic denaturation of plasmids in lysates. A correct addressing of these primary isolation challenges is probably the best guarantee for the success of a plasmid downstream process.

14.4 HEURISTICS

The downstream processing experience accumulated over the years with different bioproducts and biopharmaceuticals, both in academia and industry, can be crystallized into a handful of rules of thumb or heuristics.[19,20] These guidelines are helpful when considering the initial design and drafting of different process alternatives and, as such, are given in Table 14.2. Much of the know-how expressed in these heuristics is common sense. For example, the first heuristic, which states "Remove the most plentiful impurities first," can be interpreted as an instruction to separate cells from the surrounding liquid medium after cell culture. Water would thus qualify as the "most plentiful impurity." If one accepts this classification of the solvent water as "impurity," it is obvious that it is also one of the easiest impurities to remove. Thus, cell/medium separation also complies with the second heuristic: "Remove the easiest to remove impurities first." This said, and among other things, the first unit operations of many processes are designed to concentrate (i.e., to remove

TABLE 14.2. Heuristics for Setting Up a Plasmid Recovery and Purification Flow Sheet[19,20]

1	Remove the most plentiful impurities first (i.e., separate cells from the culture medium first).
2	Remove the easiest to remove impurities first (i.e., separate cells from the culture medium first).
3	Make the most difficult and most expensive separations last (i.e., push chromatography toward the end of the downstream processing).
4	Select processes that make use of the greatest differences in the properties of the product and impurities (i.e., separate large from small, cationic from anionic, hydrophilic from hydrophobic, etc.).
5	Select processes that exploit different separation driving forces (i.e., do not use the same unit operation in a row).
6	Just because it works in the laboratory does not mean it is right for the factory (i.e., contextualize the process).

water) the target biological product. As a result, an almost universal characteristic of downstream processes is the fact that the volume of the process streams that flow through the different unit operations usually decreases toward the end of the process. A lower volume of a process stream will usually translate into lower equipment size and in smaller amounts of mass-separating agents, materials, and aids. The cost associated with a given unit operation will thus be smaller if that operation is located at the end of the downstream processing train. Thus, when choosing among different unit operations, it makes sense to position those that are inherently more expensive at the end of the process (heuristic 3). This high cost is typical of high-resolution separation operations like chromatography, which use tailor-made beads or monoliths that have to be replaced regularly as their performance wanes. The high sophistication of chromatographic supports is directly related to the fact that such materials are called upon to perform very difficult tasks like the separation of isoforms or variants of the biological product. To leave the most difficult separations to the end implies that the easiest should be performed first. Such easier separations are clearly those that explore the greatest differences in the properties of the product and impurities—hence, the fourth heuristic. Heuristic 5 states that the unit operations should be selected and sequenced in such a way that different separation driving forces are explored. Still, in certain processes, one can find some redundancy in the driving forces explored in different unit operations (see Chapter 18). The experienced biochemical engineer should recognize that the realities of a factory and of a research laboratory are completely different. Thus, care has to be exerted when developing a process solution of the basis of modifications or adaptations of laboratory protocols (heuristic 6), since many of these cannot be scaled up or use reagents that are unacceptable from a regulatory point of view (see Chapter 11, Section 11.6.1). Finally, simplicity is usually the key to a successful process. Stripping complexity out of a process should thus be an imperative.

14.5 CONCLUSIONS

The key starting points for the development of a downstream process for the purification of plasmid biopharmaceuticals are (1) an adequate knowledge of the properties of the target molecule and of the associated *E. coli* impurities, (2) an understanding of the major problems that are likely to be encountered, and (3) a familiarity with the downstream processing know-how and experience accumulated over the years. On these grounds, one can then start to examine the different unit operations that have actually been experimented and tested in the laboratory and at different process scales. Empowered by the critical examination of the characteristics, weaknesses, and strengths of the most important of those operations, biochemical engineers and scientists are more apt to optimize and modify them, generating better process alternatives. This is the subject of the upcoming chapters. By convenience, the three stages of the downstream processing are discussed individually: primary isolation (Chapter 15), intermediate recovery (Chapter 16), and final purification (Chapter 17). The information provided in those chapters is important not only to understand the different plasmid downstream processes that have been patented and published in the literature but also to suggest better combinations. This process synthesis activity is the subject of Chapter 18.

REFERENCES

1. Listner K, Bentley L, Okonkowski J, et al. Development of a highly productive and scalable plasmid DNA production platform. *Biotechnology Progress*. 2006;22: 1335–1345.
2. Carnes AE, Williams JA. Plasmid DNA manufacturing technology. *Recent Patents on Biotechnology*. 2007;1:151–166.
3. Williams JA, Carnes AE, Hodgson CP. Plasmid DNA vaccine vector design: Impact on efficacy, safety and upstream production. *Biotechnology Advances*. 2009;27: 353–370.
4. Knight P. Downstream processing. *Bio/technology*. 1989;7:777–782.
5. Cox RA. Quantitative relationships for specific growth rates and macromolecular compositions of *Mycobacterium tuberculosis*, *Streptomyces coelicolor* A3(2) and *Escherichia coli* B/r: An integrative theoretical approach. *Microbiology*. 2004;150: 1413–1426.
6. Bremer H, Dennis PP. Modulation of chemical composition and other parameters of the cell growth rate. In: Neidhardt FC, ed. *Escherichia coli and Salmonella: Cellular and molecular biology*, Vol. 1, 2nd ed. Washington, DC: ASM Press, 1996:1553–1568.
7. Neidhardt FC, Umbarger HE. Chemical composition of *Escherichia coli*. In: Neidhardt FC, ed. *Escherichia coli and Salmonella: Cellular and molecular biology*, Vol. 1, 2nd edn. Washington, DC: ASM Press, 1996:13–16.
8. Kubitschek HE. Cell volume increase in *Escherichia coli* after shifts to richer media. *Journal of Bacteriology*. 1990;172:94–101.

9. Ishihama Y, Schmidt T, Rappsilber J, et al. Protein abundance profiling of the *Escherichia coli* cytosol. *BMC Genomics*. 2008;9:102.

10. Corbin RW, Paliy O, Yang F, et al. Toward a protein profile of *Escherichia coli*: Comparison to its transcription profile. *Proceedings of the National Academy of Sciences of the United States of America*. 2003;100:9232–9237.

11. Andrews AT, Noble I, Keeratatipibul S, Asenjo JA. Physicochemical properties of the matrix proteins of three main culture vehicles. *Biotechnology and Bioengineering*. 1994;44:29–37.

12. Blattner FR, Plunkett GI, Bloch CA, et al. The complete genome sequence of *Escherichia coli* K-12. *Science*. 1997;277:1453–1462.

13. Joiner TJ, Kraus PF, Kupiec TC. Comparison of endotoxin testing methods for pharmaceutical compounds. *International Journal of Pharmaceutical Compounding*. 2002;6:408–409.

14. Petsch D, Anspach FB. Endotoxin removal from protein solutions. *Journal of Biotechnology*. 2000;76:97–119.

15. Hancock REW, Karunaratne DN, Bernegger-Egli C. Molecular organization and structural role of outer membrane macromolecules. In: Ghuysen J-M, Hakenbeck R, eds. *Bacterial cell wall*. Amsterdam: Elsevier, 1994:263–279.

16. Rozkov A, Avignone-Rossa CA, Ertl PF, et al. Characterization of the metabolic burden on *Escherichia coli* DH1 cells imposed by the presence of a plasmid containing a gene therapy sequence. *Biotechnology and Bioengineering*. 2004;88: 909–915.

17. Wang Z, Xiang L, Shao J, Wegrzyn A, Wegrzyn G. Effects of the presence of ColE1 plasmid DNA in *Escherichia coli* on the host cell metabolism. *Microbial Cell Factories*. 2006;5:34.

18. Birnbaum S, Bailey JE. Plasmid presence changes the relative levels of many host cell proteins and ribosome components in recombinant *Escherichia coli*. *Biotechnology and Bioengineering*. 1991;37:736–745.

19. Harrison RG, Todd PW, Rudge SR, Petrides D. Bioprocess design. In: Harrison RG, Todd PW, Rudge SR, Petrides D, eds. *Bioseparations Science and Engineering*. Oxford: Oxford University Press, 2003:319–372.

20. Wheelwright SM. Designing downstream processes for large-scale protein purification. *Bio/technology*. 1987;5:789–793.

15

Primary Isolation

15.1 INTRODUCTION

In the primary isolation stage, *Escherichia coli* cells are harvested from the fermentation broth and are disrupted by appropriate means in order to release plasmid DNA. During disruption, the whole range of host cell components (see Chapter 14, Table 14.1 and Figure 14.1) is released alongside the plasmid, producing a solution that is relatively diluted in plasmid (<5% of the cell dry weight) but loaded with impurities, such as cell debris and membranes, proteins, genomic DNA (gDNA), RNA, lipids, and lipopolysaccharides (LPSs). This process stream should then be adequately clarified in order to eliminate any cell debris or particulate material. In line with the recommendations of heuristic 1 (see Chapter 14, Table 14.2), top priority should be given here to the removal of both water and the most abundant impurities. The clarified lysate obtained at the end of the primary isolation will typically consist of a dilute plasmid solution (~50–250 μg/mL), where RNA stands out as the dominating impurity. In this chapter, the methodologies and processes commonly used to harvest and disrupt plasmid-producing cells are presented and critically reviewed.

Plasmid Biopharmaceuticals: Basics, Applications, and Manufacturing, First Edition.
Duarte Miguel F. Prazeres.
© 2011 John Wiley & Sons, Inc. Published 2011 by John Wiley & Sons, Inc.

15.2   CELL HARVESTING

The use of selected nutrients and optimized process strategies (e.g., fed-batch) can foster plasmid-containing *E. coli* cells to grow up to densities of more than 40 g of dry cell weight (DCW)/L (i.e., $OD_{600} > 140$) and to produce plasmids with volumetric productivities up to 1600–2200 mg/L,[1,2] as described in Chapter 13. The cultivation of cells is typically halted at mid to late exponential phase, since this usually corresponds to the highest plasmid titers. Nevertheless, the extension of the culture beyond the end of the exponential phase and well into the stationary phase has been proposed as a means of reducing the intracellular RNA content.[3] As a result of this strategy, the ratio of plasmid DNA to RNA measured after cell lysis can increase up to twofold. However, an extension of growth into the late phase is known to cause plasmid relaxation in some cases, even though this situation may be plasmid dependent.[4] Furthermore, the reproducibility and consistency of this strategy may render validation extremely difficult. Thus, the feasibility of this approach at an industrial scale might be questionable.

The goal of harvesting is to generate a concentrated cell paste from the culture broth by removing the large amounts of spent fermentation media. The broth is usually chilled to temperatures around or below 10°C in order to suspend the activity of nucleases, which might be detrimental to plasmid integrity. Harvesting operations are well established in the biotechnology industry and usually include centrifugation, tangential flow filtration (TFF), rotary drum filtration, and depth filtration. For small cells such as *E. coli* (1–2 μm), TFF is probably the most attractive option since cell recoveries close to 100% can be obtained if the right operating conditions are selected.[5] Furthermore, lower capital and operating costs are required compared with centrifugation.[6] TFF separates cells on the basis of size exclusion by using microfiltration membranes made of different materials (e.g., polyethersulfone, polyvinylidene fluoride, and cellulose), and with pore sizes ranging from 0.1 to 0.65 μm. These membranes can be casted with a planar or tubular shape and are commercially available as plate and frame, hollow fiber, or spiral wound modules. When using TFF, *E. coli* cells in a broth can be concentrated up to final concentrations of 200 g DCW/L.[7] The filtration system can then be used to wash and diafilter the cells with 5–10 diafiltration volumes of a buffer deemed appropriate for the subsequent lysis step.[8] A system with one recirculation pump and one permeation pump is usually used to maintain a constant permeation flux between 20 and 30 L/h/m^2 during the concentration and diafiltration process.[7] Since there is always a tendency for cells to foul the membranes, this requires a constant adjustment (i.e., increase) of the transmembrane pressure (TMP), especially during the concentration stage. The membrane area should be selected in combination with the hydraulic parameters (permeation flux and TMP) so that the operation time does not exceed a standard value of 3 h,[7] since subjecting cells to higher processing times may lead to an untimely, shear-induced disruption.

The perpendicular filtration of a high-cell density broth in a depth filter is not as feasible as filtration with tangential flow systems due to the formation of a dense and compressible filter cake of bacteria, which leads to a rapid decline in the filtration flux. However, this problem can be substantially obviated if a filter aid material like diatomaceous earth or bentonite (an aluminum phyllosilicate) is added in advance to the bacterial suspension. Upon filtration of the aid/cell suspension under pressure, a noncompressible filter cake forms, which contains the micron-sized particles of the filter aid and the bacteria. The structure of this filter cake improves the filtration flux dramatically, and depth filtration becomes possible. The process can be further improved if a precoat of the aid material is deposited over the filter prior to the filtration of the suspension.[9] However, it should be kept in mind that the industrial application of this strategy requires the use of less than 20 g of filter aid/L of broth and filtration flow rates in the 500–1500-L m^2/h range.[10] A process compatible with these recommendations has been recently proposed, which uses bentonite in combination with polyethyleneimine (PEI), a flocculent agent.[10] Although the process enables the capture of 100% of cells, it is restricted to the filtration of *E. coli* cultures with an $OD_{600} < 15$ (≈ 5.2 g DCW/L). This constitutes a severe limitation for depth filtration with aids since *E. coli* cell densities with values of OD_{600} larger than 100 are becoming routine in plasmid manufacturing (see Chapter 13).

Disk stack and solid bowl centrifuges with continuous feed can also be used to harvest *E. coli* cells at process scales. Nevertheless, care should be exerted when using such equipments since high stresses are usually present both during the admission of the cell broth to the centrifuge and during discharge of the concentrated cell paste. These stresses could lyse cells, irreversibly damage plasmid, and generate low-molecular-mass fragments of gDNA. For instance, a recent report shows that up to 40% of the supercoiled plasmid isoform can be lost as a consequence of the fast, intermittent discharge of cells from a disk stack centrifuge operating at high speeds, compared with solid bowl centrifuge.[11]

The cell paste/suspension obtained after harvest is many times stored under low temperatures for a number of days in order to decouple cell harvest from the subsequent unit operations. In one case, experimental data showed that there is no significant increase in the open circle or linear isoforms, or a detectable reduction in the yield of the supercoiled isoform when pellets are stored at +4 or −20°C for up to 3 or 12 weeks, respectively.[12] The only visible change, at least when assessed by agarose gel electrophoresis, was a slight reduction in high-molecular-weight RNA when cells were stored at +4°C for more than 1.5 weeks. In another report, however, supercoiled plasmid losses ranging between 10% and 20% were associated with the freeze/thawing of the cells.[11] As an alternative to storing at low temperatures, the cells can be diafiltered (in the case of harvesting by TFF) or resuspended (in the case of harvesting by centrifugation) directly in a buffer with a composition appropriate for the subsequent disruption step (e.g., 50 mM tris–HCl pH 8.0, 10 mM ethylenediamine tetraacetic acid [EDTA][8]). This buffer usually contains agents that have the ability to disrupt ionic and hydrogen bonds between peptidoglycan, lipids, and/or proteins of the *E. coli* cell envelope. For example, EDTA is often used as a chelating agent to remove divalent cations (mainly Ca^{2+} and Mg^{2+}) from the cell wall, outer membrane and plasma membrane. Apart from destabilizing the structure of the cell wall and thus facilitating lysis, EDTA contributes to reduce the activity of endogenous, Mg^{2+}-dependent nucleases, preventing plasmid degradation. Glucose or sucrose are often included in the resuspension buffer in amounts sufficient to render the solution isosmotic (e.g., 50 mM glucose) and thus to minimize cell breakage at this stage.[13] The volume of buffer used to suspend the cells is determined on the basis of the cell concentration required in the subsequent disruption step. Although this may vary, cell suspensions prior to lysis typically have concentrations on the 10- to 200-g/L range.[14–20] Once they are thoroughly suspended in the buffer of choice, cells can move on to the disruption step.

15.3 CELL DISRUPTION

15.3.1 Introduction

The aim of the cell disruption step is to break the three-layered envelope characteristic of the gram-negative *E. coli* and thus to release high amounts of supercoiled plasmid DNA into the surrounding media. The breakage of the inner plasma membrane, of the peptidoglycan cell wall, and of the outer membrane is accompanied by the release of intracellular components such as RNA, gDNA, LPS, and proteins (Chapter 14, Table 14.1). The most common methods used to disrupt *E. coli* cells and to release plasmids are chemical cell lysis and physical destruction via mechanical forces. For a number of reasons, cell disruption has received the honor of being the most critical and troublesome of all unit operations in the downstream processing of plasmids.[21] A first cause of concern is the shear and chemical sensitivity of plasmids and gDNA molecules.[22] An uncontrolled or poorly designed disruption step can both lead to (1) the loss of the supercoiled plasmid material and (2) an excessive fragmentation of gDNA. In the first case, global plasmid yields will become compromised early in the process, whereas the latter situation will increase the purification burden placed upon the subsequent unit operations. The large concentration of nucleic acids found during release may also originate process streams with high viscosity.[14] The complexity, uncertainty, and lack of consistency that surround *E. coli* lysis also complicate the process of validating these operations (see Chapter 11, Section 11.6.4). An important aspect to consider when selecting a method for cell disruption is that the conditions used in the cell culture step (e.g., host strain, media composition, temperature, pH, and aeration) may change the cell envelope composition, strength, and morphology in such a way as to significantly affect the chemical/mechanical susceptibility of the different layers (see Chapter 13).

15.3.2 Alkaline Lysis

The alkaline lysis of *E. coli* cells was originally described by Birnboim and Doly.[23] Throughout the years, and although other alternatives have been suggested (e.g., the boiling method[24]), alkaline lysis has remained, by large, the preferred method for plasmid isolation, both at the laboratorial and manufacturing scales, as judged by the more than 12,290 citations accumulated by the original article.* Alkaline lysis is designed to disrupt cells and to denature gDNA and proteins that are then precipitated together with cell debris and other impurities. The process is essentially a combination of three operations that are performed sequentially: lysis, neutralization, and clarification (Figure 15.1). These steps are described in detail next.

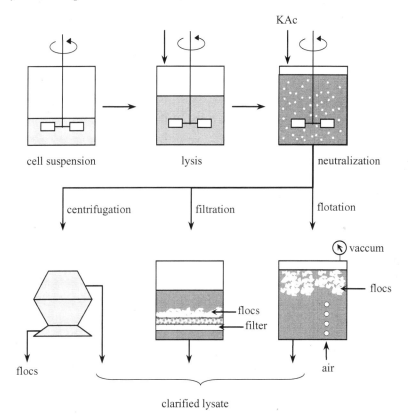

Figure 15.1 *The alkaline lysis process.* E. coli *cells are first contacted for a brief period of time (e.g., 10–15 min) with a mixture of a detergent (e.g., SDS) and an alkali (e.g., NaOH). The obtained lysate is then neutralized by adding a high salt/low pH solution (e.g., potassium acetate [KAc]). The resulting cell debris and flocs of precipitated impurities are typically removed with one of three possible options—centrifugation, dead-end filtration, and flotation. The performance of dead-end filtration can be improved by resorting to prefilters of adequate materials, and flotation can be induced and fostered by vacuum or gas sparging.*

* Figure taken from the ISI Web of Knowledge (http://isiwebofknowledge.com, accessed April 13, 2010).

15.3.2.1 Lysis

According to the original procedure, an alkaline solution of a detergent (e.g., 200 mM NaOH + 1% sodium dodecyl sulfate [SDS]) is added to the cell-containing solution, usually in a 1:1 volume ratio (Figure 15.1). NaOH and SDS are used in conjunction to break and solubilize cell membranes and to promote the irreversible denaturation of proteins and nucleic acids other than plasmids. The alkali raises the pH value, thus promoting the cleavage and irreversible separation of the complementary strands of gDNA (with the concomitant exposure of the hydrophobic bases). The complementary strands of the double-stranded plasmid DNA molecules are also separated as a result of the alkalinity of the medium. However, and as long as the pH is kept below 12.2–12.4, a certain number of nucleotides in the plasmid molecule always remain paired (Figure 15.2). These "anchor" base pairs will serve as nuclei for the complete renaturation of the plasmid back to its characteristic supercoiled structure during the subsequent neutralization step[25] (Figure 15.2). However, if the pH is higher than 12.5, the anchor base pairs may disrupt and translocate,

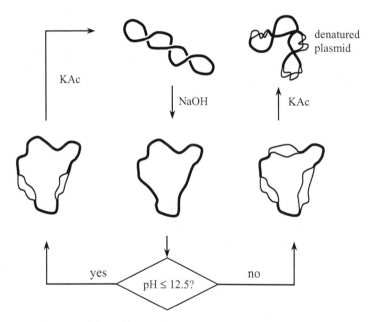

Figure 15.2 *The reversible and irreversible alkaline denaturation of plasmids. The addition of NaOH promotes the unwinding of the plasmid supercoils as well as the disruption of base pairs in the double helix. If the pH of the surrounding environment is controlled in the 12.0–12.5 range, base separation is restricted to a number of sites within the plasmid molecule. This makes it possible to reform the plasmid structure by decreasing the pH back to neutral or slightly acidic values. However, if the alkali increases pH past 12.5, base separation will predominate throughout the molecule, making it impossible to promote the refolding of the plasmid back to its original supercoiled structure.*

particularly if direct or inverted repeats are present, causing the plasmid to form incongruent complementary base pairs or cruciform loops upon neutralization. The result is an irreversibly denatured but nevertheless covalently closed plasmid molecule (Figure 15.2). Such alkali-denatured plasmids are usually compact and typically migrate faster than supercoiled plasmids in an agarose gel, originating the so-called ghost bands.[26–28] The lower ethidium bromide fluorescence intensity of such bands of denatured plasmid DNA when compared with the fluorescence of equal amounts of "native" supercoiled plasmid suggests a decrease in intercalation. In all likelihood, this is a direct consequence of the reduction in the amount of double "strandedness" that is brought about by partial denaturation of the molecule.[28] Atomic force microscopy (AFM) imaging of these alkali-denatured species has shown that although they retain a stable and circular supercoiled configuration, they present a shortened contour length and fewer supercoils (see Chapter 5, Figure 5.8). This decrease in the supercoiling degree could also explain the reduction in intercalation of ethidum bromide described earlier (see Chapter 4, Section 4.3.5.1). The AFM imaging has also revealed that the denatured molecules have a rough surface and inhomogeneous diameters with kinks and bulges, most likely due to the local unwinding of the DNA strands.[29] These single-stranded regions are probably richer in A•T duplexes than the remaining double-stranded regions, since the contribution of this type of base pairs to helix stability (e.g., via base stacking) is less important that the one provided by G•C base pairs[30] (see Chapter 4, Section 4.2.1). Depending on the base sequence, these single strands may fold back on themselves, forming irregular double-helical hairpin loops and other non-B-DNA secondary structures.

The different biological molecules that are freed from cells as lysis proceeds provide acid equivalents that partially neutralize and reduce the pH of the original mixture of cell suspension with NaOH/SDS lysis solution (~12.8). This means that the amount of cells initially present will dictate the time course of the pH during lysis. If few cells are present, the pH may remain above the 12.2–12.4 threshold and plasmid denaturation ensues, whereas too many cells may cause the pH to drop below the value required to guarantee full lysis.[28] A certain degree of control over the cell concentration should thus be exerted when performing alkaline lysis.

The detergent in the lysis solution solubilizes cell membranes by eliminating interfacial, noncovalent interactions between proteins and lipids. Although SDS is commonly used as the lysis detergent in laboratorial practice, its use presents some disadvantages from a manufacturing point of view, namely, due to its propensity to hydrolyze under alkaline conditions.[31] Detergents such as Tween® (a polysorbate), Triton® (a polyoxyethylene ether),[32,33] and alkyl dimethyl phosphine oxide (APO)[31] can be used alternatively. Although Tween and Triton are more common in a bioprocessing environment, the compatibility with good manufacturing practice (GMP) procedures that is associated with the defined nature and stability of APO on alkaline solutions has been especially highlighted as an important advantage of this alternative detergent.[31]

The mixing of the cell suspension and alkali solutions throughout the course of lysis is extremely important. First, the alkali solution must be added and mixed very rapidly, and in such a way as to guarantee the uniform distribution of pH around the critical range of 12.2–12.4 across the full volume. This homogenization process is complicated by the significant increase in the viscosity of the solution that accompanies the relatively fast disruption of cells (30–60 s for *E. coli* Dh5α grown in Luria broth[14,34]). This increase in viscosity, which peaks after 120–140 s at around 35–160 mPa·s, depending on the shear rate, is attributed to the denaturation of gDNA.[14,34] The viscoelastic properties displayed by the resulting lysate also makes the flow and handling of the material very difficult.[14,34] One of the problems associated with this viscoelasticity is, for example, the undesirable climbing of the lysate up the rotating rod or shaft of the mixing impeller, which is observed during the course of lysis, a phenomenon known as the Weissenburg effect.[35] During the first 1–3 min, gDNA becomes completely denatured, but the individual strands maintain a high molecular weight. Beyond this point, fragmentation of the denatured gDNA occurs due to shear associated with mixing. This is accompanied by a decline in viscosity until a "pseudo-equilibrium" value (<40 mPa·s) is reached at 500-s lysis time.[14,34] This fragmentation is undesirable since the resulting smaller gDNA fragments will be more difficult to remove in the subsequent precipitation and filtration steps. Thus, the agitation intensity should be low or reduced as soon as the majority of cells are lysed in order to maintain gDNA with the highest molecular weight possible. This decrease in agitation may also contribute to reduce shear degradation of plasmid molecules.[22] Unfortunately, gentle mixing further complicates the process because the use of low-shear stress conditions causes a shear-induced thickening of the material.[36] Also, the precipitation of cell impurities may be incomplete because a thorough mixing is difficult to achieve in a short time when using low-shear stirring.[37] A number of options have been described to accomplish the batch mixing of cell suspensions with alkaline/detergent solutions. For example, barred (rod) impellers propelled by high-torque motors could be an efficient solution to accomplish low-shear mixing across the wide range of viscosities found during alkaline lysis.[38] Helical, ribbon-type axial impellers commonly used in high-viscosity systems, which are able to provide low shear rates, may also be appropriate.[35]

Alkaline lysis is typically terminated after 5–10 min since after this time, few cells should remain intact. Furthermore, prolonging the operation will lead to fragmentation of gDNA, as previously described. Still, subjecting cells to alkaline lysis for extended times of up to 24 h may contribute to significantly reduce the amount of RNA, though at the expense of an irreversible denaturation of the supercoiled plasmid isoform.[12,32] This effect is clearly observed in the agarose gel shown in Figure 15.3, which displays the progression of the plasmid topoisomers and RNA species in an alkaline lysate during the course of an

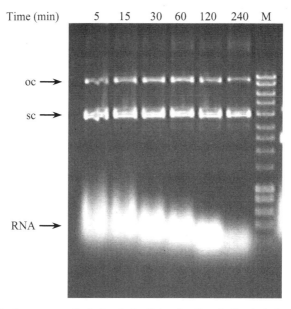

Figure 15.3 *The time course of alkaline lysis. Extending the alkaline lysis time past the usual 10–15 min contributes to the degradation of RNA. Although RNA is more susceptible to alkaline environments when compared with DNA, some plasmid degradation is also likely to occur, even though this might be plasmid dependent (reprinted with permission from Freitas et al.[12]). oc, open circular; sc, supercoiled; M, molecular weight marker. Reprinted with kind permission from Springer Science+Business Media: Molecular Biotechnology, On the stability of plasmid DNA vectors during cell culture and purification, 36, 2007, 151–158, Freitas SS, Azzoni AR, Santos JA, Monteiro GA, Prazeres DMF, Figure 3.[12]*

extended lysis. A densitometry analysis of the bands shows that approximately 40% of RNA is degraded after 24 h, whereas in comparison, a plasmid loss of 12–19% is observed.[12] In spite of this improvement in RNA clearance, alkaline lysis at process and laboratorial scales is seldom performed for more than 15 min.

In order to improve the control of the lysis procedure and to reduce its time sensitivity, suggestions have been made to replace the usual NaOH lysis solution with a buffer containing 0.5 M L-arginine and with pH values in the 11.4–12.0 range.[28] Under these conditions, plasmids are not exposed to the deleterious pH > 12.4, and the probability of denaturation is reduced. Furthermore, the buffering ability of arginine is claimed to compensate for variations in the cell concentration of the starting suspension. The yields obtained when arginine lysis is performed at pH values between 11.4 and 12.0 are comparable to those obtained by the original method, and the resulting plasmids are readily digested by restriction enzymes. Although this modified version of alkaline lysis has produced results at the mini prep scale, it has not been tested for large-scale plasmid isolation.[28]

15.3.2.2   *Neutralization*

Alkaline lysis is typically halted after 5–10 min by neutralizing the lysate with an acidic solution (Figure 15.1). A 5 M solution of chilled potassium acetate, prepared as an equimolar mixture of acetate salt and acetic acid, is the usual choice at process scale. Nevertheless, sodium, ammonium, and lithium acetate solutions should also work comparably well.[28] For example, a mixture of 1 M potassium acetate and 7 M ammonium acetate has been claimed to improve the clearance of RNA and gDNA impurities.[39] Neutralization with potassium phosphate is also effective. The key advantage associated with the use of this salt instead of potassium acetate is that after the addition of a certain amount of polyethylene glycol (PEG) to the neutralized lysate, it drives the formation of two aqueous phases. As described in Chapter 16 (Section 16.4.2), the partitioning of solutes between the two phases in these systems can then be explored to promote a first purification of plasmid.[40]

The neutralization solution, usually with a volume equal to the volume of the starting cell suspension, is added and carefully homogenized. During the short neutralization period of around 10 min, an ill-defined mass of solids with a gelatinous, cheeselike consistency is generated, which must be removed by low shear, solid–liquid unit operations. At this stage, the liquid phase presents itself with a characteristic golden yellow color. Upon neutralization, the lysate looses its viscoelastic properties and assumes a viscosity close to that of water. Neutralization and the ensuing separation of solids are key steps since large amounts of host cell impurities, including cell debris, denatured cytoplasmic and membrane-associated proteins, gDNA fragments anchored to cell wall remains, nucleic acids and potassium dodecyl sulfate precipitates are sequestered into these solids. The solid content in a crude lysate will of course depend on the cell concentration in the starting suspension prior to lysis. According to published data, a wet solid concentration of 65.1 g/L is obtained after neutralizing an alkaline lysate produced from a 120 g/L cell suspension.[41] As a rough rule, we can thus expect a solid content that is half of the starting cell concentration. Although a process time of around 10 min is commonly used during neutralization, longer times (up to 12 h) may improve precipitation.[39] As for the temperature, setting incubation at around 4–10°C is the preferred option on the account that a higher percentage of precipitation is obtained.[39]

15.3.2.3   *Clarification*

The separation of solids from the neutralized lysate is particularly difficult since a fraction of the solids floats while another sediments. Furthermore, the integrity of this rather fragile solid material should be maintained during separation in order to reduce dissociation of proteins, LPS, and gDNA fragments from cell debris and precipitates, and thus to minimize the release of those solutes into the clarified lysate.[17] This calls for the use of low-shear unit operations and for a careful handling of process streams. Although centrifugation is common at the laboratorial scale, the use of continuous centrifuges at the industrial scale is usually avoided since the high shear in the incoming liquid stream can break the precipitate material, both at the macroscopic and molecular levels. Additionally, centrifugation is a costly unit operation. Therefore, depth filtration techniques are the preferred option when it comes to clarifying crude alkaline lysates. Here, and in the simplest form, the lysate flows under the action of a pump or of gravity, through a filter with a pore size (~5–160 μm) adequate to retain cells debris, macroparticulate material and precipitates.[42] The filters can be made of materials like cellulose, polypropylene, polyester, or stainless steel.[42] These filters are available in a range of different formats, which include cloths,[41,42] flat sheets and membranes,[41,42] cartridges, and bags.[43] A commercial material often used to remove the gelatinous cell debris and precipitates[44,45] is Miracloth® (Calbiochem, San Diego, California), a white porous (22- to 25-μm pores) cloth composed of rayon polyester and an acrylic binder.

The efficiency of the filtration process in terms of plasmid yield, clarification, contamination of the filtrate with sheared gDNA, and filtration flow rate is highly dependent on the pore size and type of filter used, as described by Theodossiou et al. in their systematic study of the filtration of crude alkaline lysates.[42] After testing different filter types, the authors concluded that 99.4% of the solids in a lysate (~100 g wet solids/L) could be removed at an average filtration rate of 22.5 cm/h with a 5-μm pore diameter polypropylene cloth, although at the expense of a 33% plasmid loss. This loss was attributed to the trapping of plasmid in the liquid, which is commonly entrained in the cake and filter. Still, higher plasmid recoveries are probably possible if the dewatering of the retained material is improved.[42] The high content and gelatinous consistency of the solids in crude lysates usually leads to the formation of a compressible filter cake that produces a sharp decrease in the filtration flux and eventually clogs the filter.[42] This flux loss can be partially counteracted by increasing the filtration pressure during the course of filtration. Although plasmid DNA is relatively unaffected by this pressure increase, shearing of gDNA has been observed.[42] The loss of filtration flux and filter clogging can also be partially alleviated by layering filtration aids such as glass, silica gel, diatomaceous earth, aluminum oxides, and hydroxyapatite on top of the filter prior to clarification. The three-dimensional, noncompressible networks of solid particles formed by these aids contribute to retain solids, to extend throughput, to reduce back pressure, and to minimize shearing of solids and carryover of smaller particulates into the filtrate.[41,42,46] Additionally, some filter aids (e.g., diatomaceous earth) have the ability to adsorb soluble host impurities like RNA and LPS (see Chapter 16, Section 16.5) as the lysate flows through the filtration cake.[46] In order to take full advantage of this additional purification ability, it is important to guarantee that no plasmid is lost due to coadsorption and absorption to the filter cake, a problem that has been described in some cases.[42] The process of precoating a filter with a given aid may be difficult to reproduce, apart from the fact that it involves the use of valuable resources (labor and time). For this reason, some manufacturers (e.g., Sartorius, Germany) have developed disposable depth filters which already combine the filter with the aid material.

A number of authors have recognized that the performance of filtration can be improved significantly if the bulk of the solids is removed beforehand with a low-shear coarse operation.[41] This strategy relies on the aggregation of individual flocks to form a compressed flocculent phase that either settles on the bottom of the vessel or floats to the surface of the liquid. For example, a compact bed of floating material is formed if lysates are left to "age" in the neutralization tank for 1 h at 10°C.[41] The aggregation and flotation of the material can be further improved by promoting a low-shear mixing via the injection of air bubbles from the bottom the tank. Once the flocculent phase is floating, the plasmid-containing liquid is drained from underneath. Flotation experiments carried out at the 15-L scale have shown that the solid content in the drained liquid is 0.2 g/L, a figure that corresponds to a 99.7% reduction relatively to the crude lysate.[41] Flocculent phases can also be formed by subjecting neutralized lysates to vacuum conditions. According to a patented methodology, a reduction in pressure to a value that is 300–800 mbar lower than the atmospheric pressure drives the aggregation and flotation of a spatially highly compressed flocculent phase.[17] This process typically takes 5–10 min. Once all flakes have floated, the vacuum is released and phases can be separated by draining the liquid from the bottom of the vessel and through an outlet solid trap.[17] Although an increase in pressure will also produce a flocculent phase, the compact material will now sink rather than float. The low shear forces present during the formation of the flocculates, either by air injection or by pressure change, minimize the release of gDNA and LPS into the lysates. Furthermore, the small fraction of solids that might remain in the clarified lysates can be removed by filtration without the severe clogging effects observed when processing crude lysates. Also, since the amount of solids is substantially reduced, continuous centrifugation becomes an option for further clarification.

Although the exact figures will depend on the operating parameters and procedures used, the clearance capacity of a complete alkaline lysis disruption process can reach 98% for gDNA, 97% for proteins, and 98% for suspended solids.[47] This substantial purification is one of the key reasons for the domination of alkaline lysis over other alternative techniques when it comes to lysing *E. coli* cells for plasmid release.

15.3.2.4 *Continuous Flow Devices*

In spite of its advantages, the implementation of alkaline lysis at a process scale and in a GMP environment is faced with numerous challenges. The requirements for a rapid homogenization of alkali/detergent solutions with cells, together with the need to handle the precipitates very gently as denaturation of intracellular components proceeds, and the high content, sticky consistency, and fragile nature of the neutralized solids are major reasons for the lack of consistency and troublesome validation of alkaline lysis (see Chapter 11, Section 11.6.4). These challenges have been addressed through the design of different devices and apparatus that are capable of performing alkaline lysis of *E. coli* cells at large scale in a controlled and continuous manner.[18,19,37,39,48–50] A full system is typically constructed by combining pumps, valves, and fittings to assemble individual units dedicated to each of the substeps in the alkaline lysis process: lysis, neutralization, and clarification (Figure 15.1).

A common feature in many of the systems proposed is the presence of a low residence time mixer, where the cell suspension is contacted with the lysis solution for a very short period of time. For example, one option to improve low-shear mixing of cell suspensions, lysis, and neutralization solutions, which at the same time is scalable and allows a continuous flow-through process to be established, is to use static mixers.[18,39,48,49] These devices, which are common in the food, cosmetic, and pharmaceutical industry, are essentially composed of a series of motionless mixing elements (e.g., perpendicular plates) welded in supporting rods, which are positioned inside a tubular housing. The elements in this tube partially block the flow path of incoming streams, which are thus forced to split and divert, and hence mix. In the case of alkaline cell lysis, the strategy relies in the simultaneous pumping of the cell suspension and alkali/detergent solution through a first static mixer where cells are lysed and proteins and nucleic acids are denatured. The outcoming lysate is then further contacted with the neutralization solution in a second in-line static mixer. The resulting crude lysate with flocs of the precipitated material and cell debris must then be clarified adequately, for instance, by filtration, as described above. By using these mixing devices and by adjusting the individual flow rate velocity of the two incoming solutions together with the number of elements and mixer length, the reaction and mixing times can be controlled so as to maximize plasmid yields.[18] The use of tandem static mixers for cell lysis and neutralization can be further improved by injecting gas (e.g., N_2) bubbles at a controlled rate in the lysis solution, which enters the first mixer[49] (Figure 15.4a). As lysis proceeds in the first set of mixers, the small gas bubbles (~1 mm) get trapped in the cell wall fragments and thus provide sufficient buoyancy for the debris to float in the lysate. The air bubbles travel alongside the mixture into the next set of neutralization static mixers and similarly become entrained within the precipitate flocs as they form and aggregate. Upon collection of the crude lysate in a tank, the low-density solids rise as a consequence of the N_2 bubbles introduced earlier, leaving a clarified lysate beneath that is easily drained through a bottom port[49] (Figure 15.4a).

Alternatively, Hebel and coworkers have disclosed a lysis/neutralization setup and process that makes use of a high-shear, low residence time mixer, a holding coil, and a bubble-mixer chamber[37,50] (Figure 15.4b). The combination of high shear with a very short residence time of the order of 0.1–1.0 s in a suitable mixing device (e.g., a rotor/stator mixer) makes it possible to obtain a thorough and almost instantaneous homogenization of the cell suspension and lysis solution, without subjecting the released cell components to a prolonged, shear-induced denaturation. The mixture exiting the device is then pumped through a holding coil for a period of time sufficient to allow the lysis of all cells and the denaturation of proteins and nucleic acids. Contact times

(a)

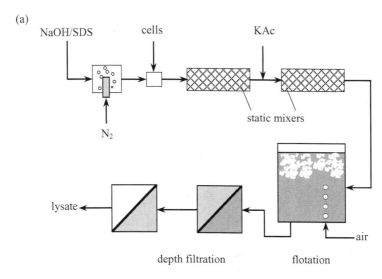

(b)

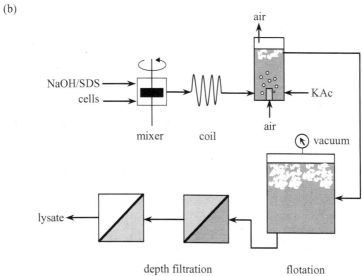

(c)

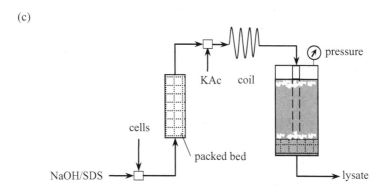

Figure 15.4 *Continuous flow alkaline lysis. Three examples of processes designed to perform continuous alkaline lysis of E. coli at a large scale are shown. In the first case,[49] (a) NaOH/SDS is injected with N_2 bubbles, mixed with cells and pumped through static mixers. The exiting lysate with trapped bubbles is then mixed with neutralization buffer and sent to a second set of mixers where precipitates form and aggregate. The resulting flocs are separated by vacuum-aided flotation in a tank, leaving a partially clarified lysate behind. Following drainage through a bottom port, the lysate is further clarified with depth filters (adapted from Au-Yeung and Bussey[49]). In the second case[37,50] (b), cells and NaOH/SDS are contacted in a high-shear, low residence time mixer. Following passage through a holding coil, the lysate is neutralized in an air-sparging bubble mixer and is sent to a tank where vacuum aids the flotation of flocs. The drained lysate is then clarified with depth filters (adapted from Hebel et al.[37,50]). In the last case[19] (c), cells and NaOH/SDS are mixed in a packed bed of glass beads and the exiting lysate is neutralized in a holding coil. The crude lysate is then clarified in a tank equipped with a bottom layer of packed glass beads, which retains the flocks but allows the clarified lysate to pass through and exit via a bottom port (adapted from Urthaler et al.[19]).*

←

of around 5 min are sufficient and can be controlled by an adequate preselection of the coil dimensions and flow rates. Finally, the lysate is directed to a bubble mixer where it is contacted with the neutralization solution. In this cylindrical device, mixing of the two entering solutions is promoted by the simultaneous pumping of compressed gas through a sintered sparger (Figure 15.4b). The collision of the entering bubble stream with the two liquid streams that takes place at the bottom of the device and their subsequent ascent through the column provides an efficient, but low-shear mixing, which is beneficial for the neutralization process. The crude neutralized lysate then exits the bubble column mixer from the top and is collected in a cooled (~15°C) tank where solid separation by flotation and/or settling of flocs with entrained air can be promoted by applying a vacuum, as described earlier.[37,50]

Another scalable setup that allows for continuous alkaline lysis/neutralization/clarification to take place is described by Urthaler et al.[19] Here, the continuous mixing of cell suspensions and lysis solutions is accomplished by pumping the two solutions through a column packed with 5-mm glass beads.[19] The residence time in this device, and hence the duration of lysis, can be controlled by adjusting the flow rates to the void volume of the packed column. The outcoming lysate is then continuously neutralized by promoting contact with a prechilled neutralization solution in a holding coil. Again, the duration of the operation is controlled via the flow rate and length of the coil. The crude lysate produced is continuously clarified in a tank that incorporates a 5-cm-deep retention layer made of packed glass beads (0.4–3.0 mm) in the bottom. This layer retains the flocks but allows clarified lysate to go through and to exit the tank via a bottom port.[19]

15.3.3 Heat-Induced Lysis

The combined action of enzymes, detergents, and high temperatures constitutes an interesting alternative for the large-scale disruption of *E. coli* cells

and plasmid release. This modality derives from the boiling lysis method originally developed by Holmes and Quigley for the rapid preparation of plasmids,
and typically encompasses a 30-s incubation of cells at temperatures around
95–100°C.[24] Although the method works well at the laboratory scale, the
implementation of the high-temperature batch incubation at a process scale
is clearly problematic, especially due to the difficulty in promoting the fast
heat transfer required across large volumes. In order to overcome this difficulty, flow-through devices and systems have been developed, much like in the
case of alkaline lysis, which allow for fast heat transfer and short lysis times.
In a typical process, cells are first suspended and incubated at 37°C in a buffer
containing 2% Triton X-100 and lysozyme. The lysozyme will damage bacterial
cell walls by catalyzing the hydrolysis of specific bonds within peptidoglycan
molecules, whereas the detergent contributes to solubilize cell membranes.
The goal of this initial pretreatment is to render cells more susceptible to heat,
so that temperatures lower than the original 100°C can be used.[51] The fra-
gilized cell suspension is then heated up to 70–77°C in a flow-through heat
exchanger.[51,52] This device consists basically of a stainless steel coil, which is
immersed in a constant high-temperature bath. Since the cell suspension entering the coil is usually not heated, a temperature gradient develops across the
coil length, which spans from room temperature up to high temperatures. Thus,
in order to maximize the performance of the lysis, a precise control of the
outlet temperature and residence time inside the coil is required. This is
accomplished by adjusting both the flow rate of the incoming cell slurry
according to the dimensions of the coil and the temperature of the external
bath. The high temperatures within the coil induce the lysis of the cells and
promote the precipitation of gDNA, proteins, and other debris while keeping
the plasmid in solution.[52] According to the literature, holding times of the
order of 20–60 s are sufficient to lyse cells completely.[51,52] An effective release
of plasmid is obtained alongside when using average temperatures in the
75–90°C range. However, the proportion of supercoiled plasmid in the isolated
plasmid material is higher at higher temperatures when compared with 75°C,
most likely as a result of the inactivation of nucleases.[51,52] The lysate exiting
the coil is then cooled down to room temperature to halt the lytic process by
flowing through a second coil, which is immersed in an ice water bath.[51,53] Cell
debris and precipitates are further separated by centrifugation or filtration.
The device enables a continuous and more reproducible processing when
compared with the usual batch alkaline lysis carried in tanks. Claims are also
made that this improved consistency of heat lysis renders validation easier. An
added advantage of heat lysis, when compared with alkaline lysis, has to do
with the fact that the initial suspension is not diluted further during the
process. This is not the case in alkaline lysis, where the addition of the lysis
and neutralization solutions typically increases the initial volume by threefold.
Thus, lysates produced by heat lysis are potentially more concentrated in
plasmid DNA.

15.3.4 Mechanical Lysis

Mechanical lysis by high-pressure homogenization and bead milling are the industry gold standard for releasing intracellular proteins from microbial cells. Other unit operations such as nebulization and microfluidization have also been gaining some momentum as possible alternatives. And at the laboratorial scale, sonication is still very practical and popular. In spite of this, the use of mechanical methods to break *E. coli* and to release plasmids is seldom described in the literature,[16,20,54] a fact that strongly suggests that mechanical disruption is not feasible in the plasmid production context. The major reason for this inadequacy is directly related to the fact that the high shear rates $(10^5–10^6 s^{-1})$ and hydrodynamic forces used to disrupt the *E. coli* cell envelope in such equipments are also able to break covalent bonds along the sugar–phosphate backbone of plasmids and other nucleic acid molecules.[20,55] This deleterious effect of shear is especially dramatic over plasmids since a single-strand break in one of the DNA strands is sufficient to cause the loss of the preferred supercoiled isoform. The forces exerted when a polymer molecule is subjected to a shear field increase with the end-to-end distance of the chain.[55] Accordingly, shear sensitivity and degradation are especially significant for plasmids that are larger than 5000 bp. Literature data support this claim—for example, experiments in which alkaline lysates containing 13,000-, 20,000-, and 29,000-bp plasmids were forced through a capillary tube $(0.2 \times 150 \text{ mm})$ show that at a shear rate of $4.8 \times 10^5 s^{-1}$ ($Re = 3525, 0.03 \text{ s}$ residence time), the supercoiled content decreased 20, 60, and 92%, respectively.[22] This dramatic effect of the plasmid molecular weight on the sensitivity to shear was also observed when alkaline lysates were subjected to a shear rate of $1.1 \times 10^6 s^{-1}$ in a small rotating disk shear device ($Re = 3525$)—after 20 s, the supercoiled content decreased 0, 25, and 99%, for the 13,000-, 20,000-, and 29,000-bp plasmids, respectively.[22] Another interesting result produced by the aforementioned study was the finding that the resistance of plasmids to shear in the rotating device was higher in solutions that had higher ionic strengths. However, this protective effect of ionic strength was not observed in the capillary rheometer. This fact constitutes an indication that the "quality" of the imposed shear is as important as its magnitude and duration in determining the stability of supercoiled plasmids.[22] The torsional strain introduced by supercoiling is thought to increase the susceptibility of supercoiled plasmids when compared to their relaxed counterparts.[55] In order to decrease the damage to plasmids, the key operating variables in a given device must be thus optimized and manipulated so that shear stress and contact times are reduced without affecting cell disruption yields.

The major difference between the different mechanical lysis methods when it comes to performance is related to the size of the *E. coli* fragments generated and to the denaturation imparted to the released impurities and target plasmid. The size of *E. coli* debris is important because it determines the easiness with which they can be removed further on from the lysate (e.g., by centrifugation or filtration). On the other hand, an excessive fragmentation of intracellular species such as gDNA down to sizes closer to the plasmid size will render subsequent purification more difficult. Although these aspects can be controlled to some extent by manipulating operating parameters and variables like residence time, flow rates, and pressure, it is ultimately the intrinsic characteristics and underlying mechanisms of the technique that determine the success of the operation. The most comprehensive study of mechanical disruption of *E. coli* for plasmid release was produced by Carlson and coworkers.[20] In this key article, the authors evaluate the performance of five different methods in terms of cell disruption yields and the recovery of a 10,400-bp plasmid. Sonication was very efficient in terms of *E. coli* disruption but extremely severe for plasmids. Although the power input used is important, short sonication operations (from 30 s to a few minutes) inevitably broke the released plasmid apart into small fragments.[20] Nebulization and homogenization were also no better than sonication. In the case of nebulization, an inert gas at high pressure is used to drive the cell suspension across a nozzle and thus to generate a mist. The atomized droplets in this stream are impacted onto a ceramic sphere and against the walls of the unit where shear forces break cells apart. Unfortunately, plasmids are also extensively degraded by this shear, and recoveries higher than 10% of intact plasmid are difficult to obtain, even when using the more amenable conditions.[20] In a homogenizer, a constant flow rate of the cell suspension is pumped at high pressure through a special valve designed with channels that accelerate the stream toward an impact wall. The hydrodynamic mechanisms responsible for cell breakage are several, including channel inlet pressure gradients, impingement forces, and postchannel turbulence.[56] Again, these forces and associated shear are also responsible for a substantial damage of plasmid molecules. With a single pass through a Gaulin homogenizer, cell breakage increased from 30% to 75%, when pressure was increased from 35 to 48 MPa, but only 30% of plasmid could be recovered in either case.[20] Still, a computational fluid dynamics study used to quantify the hydrodynamic forces in a homogenizer has suggested that plasmid yields can be improved by adopting an optimization strategy in which the operating pressure is adjusted to the solution viscosity.[56]

More encouraging results were obtained with microfluidization, a high shear technique developed in the last two decades, which is used for blending, mixing, homogenization, and cell disruption in the pharmaceutical and biotechnology industries.[57] Microfluidization uses an intensifier pump to feed process streams at pressures as high as 275 MPa into a fixed geometry interaction chamber. In the case of cell disruption applications, this interaction chamber consists of a system of rectangular (~100 μm height × 200 μm width) microchannels carved in a ceramic or diamond block, which split the incoming feed into two streams.[57] When an *E. coli* cell suspension is fed from a tank into such a chamber, the two separate streams accelerate to very high velocities, of the order of hundreds of meters per second. The two streams are then recombined at the end of the chamber and in front of a stationary impingement wall. This creates extremely high pressures and shear rates ($\sim10^6$–$10^7 s^{-1}$) that are orders of magnitude greater than the ones obtained by other mechanical means (e.g., $\sim10^5 s^{-1}$ for high-pressure homogenization). The intense energy ($\sim10^7$–$10^8 J/m^3$) that is concentrated in the streams is dissipated almost instantaneously at the point of impact, leading to disruption of cells and the release of intracellular contents. The exiting cell lysate is either collected in a reservoir or reintroduced in the chamber, depending on the yield of disruption obtained in face of the process specifications. The efficiency of microfluidization when it comes to disintegration of *E. coli* cells depends on the pressure and number of passages selected, and, to some extent, on the physiological state of the cells and strain used. For example, in the case of a 42.8 g DCW/L suspension of *E. coli* DH5α, a high-pressure system operating at 31 MPa leads to disruption yields of ~90 and ~100% when using two or five passages, whereas in a low-pressure system at 3.5 MPa, these figures drop to ~40 and ~60%, respectively.[16] The cell disintegrate obtained after a single passage of *E. coli* cells through a microfluidizer is characterized by a broad particle size distribution, with two peaks at 486 and 800 nm. These relatively large sizes of the debris translate into high separation degrees in the subsequent solid–liquid operation, whether centrifugation or microfiltration is used.[58] This improved separation is also partially explained by the fact that the extremely high shear forces at play in the interaction chamber degrade gDNA into smaller fragments to an extent that is higher when compared with alternative mechanical methods like high-pressure homogenization.[58] This effectively contributes to decrease the viscosity of the solution and hence facilitates solid–liquid separation. However, this shearing of gDNA is unwanted since it will clearly have a detrimental impact in subsequent purification steps.[58] Still, the degradation imparted to plasmid molecules when microfluidization is used to lyse cells is not as high as it might be expected since the residence time in the microchamber is extremely low, of the order of 25–40 ms.[59] For example, by using a single passage at 13.8 MPa, around 50% of plasmid DNA could be released from 75% of disrupted cells. The fact that microfluidization is very efficient when it comes to disrupting *E. coli*, together with the possibility of combining several interaction chambers with large pumps, makes the process scalable up to the industrial scale. Continuous disruption of *E. coli* with flow rates up to 3000 L/h is also possible.[57] Thus, if ways to minimize plasmid degradation can be devised, microfluidization could constitute an important alternative to the chemical lysis methods described in the previous section.

The best plasmid recoveries were obtained with bead mills. These flow-through devices consist of a chamber equipped with a series of impeller blades that are mounted in a rotating axis. A significant portion of the volume of the chamber (>50%) is filled with small (~0.5–1 mm) glass or steel beads, which are kept inside the equipment with the aid of adequate screens. During operation, the cell suspension is continuously fed through the chamber as the blades rotate at a given speed. The abrasion generated as cells contact with the beads and blades while passing through generates sufficient shear to fragment cells. Plasmid recoveries of 74%, of which 94% were in the supercoiled conformation, were obtained in bead mills with 50% cell disruption.[20] Unfortunately, and as usual, increases in cell disruption yields brought about by manipulation operating conditions led to a drop-off of the supercoiled plasmid recovery to less than 10%.

As we have seen above, the forces exerted when a plasmid molecule is subjected to a shear field increase with the length of the molecule. Accordingly, a reduction in the hydrodynamic size of plasmid translates directly into a lower shear-induced degradation. This means that the use of compaction agents like polylysine or spermidine can offer some protection against the damage generated during mechanical lysis. If the correct concentration of the agent in the starting cell suspension is used, the plasmid molecules collapse, forming aggregates that sediment alongside debris during centrifugation. The plasmid is then separated from the remaining solids by resolubilization with an adequate buffer. In one example representative of this strategy, *E. coli* cells were mixed with a compaction protection buffer containing 0.5% w/v Brij 58 and 15–30 mM spermidine at a ratio of 7–10 mL/g of wet cells.[54] The suspension was then subjected to a French press at 76 MPa. The results showed that plasmid compaction by spermidine resulted in a significant protection against shear. Furthermore, the compaction/protection effect also extended to gDNA, contributing to reduce the amount of its fragmentation. This may turn out to be an added benefit later on in the purification process since larger gDNA fragments are easier to clear from plasmid-containing solutions. The lysate is then subjected to centrifugation in order to separate the liquid and soluble solutes from the compaction-precipitated DNA and cell debris. In the subsequent step, the settled material is washed with a solution (50% ethanol, 600 mM NaCl with 10 mM EDTA) that strips spermidine from the insoluble plasmid. Finally, the plasmid is solubilized with an adequate buffer and is separated from the solid debris.[54]

15.3.5 Autolysis

The use of *E. coli* strains that have been genetically modified to undergo controlled self-lysis (i.e., autolysis) is another alternative available for plasmid release. Such recombinant strains contain genes under the control of inducible promoters that code for lytic proteins like endolysin, transglycosylase, or lysozyme. For example, a single copy of the bacteriophage λR endolysin can be integrated into the genome of *E. coli* strains in such a way that it replaces the tightly regulated araB gene.[60] As a consequence, the lytic gene becomes under the control of the promoter of the arabinose operon (PBAD), and thus the autolytic phenotype can be triggered by the presence of an excess of arabinose at an adequate time. The concomitant expression of endolysin does not by itself cause lysis, but rather renders the cells more sensitive to freeze-thawing. For instance, in one experiment, the number of endolysis-expressing cells that were lysed after a single freeze-thaw cycle increased 15-fold when compared with a control.[60] The viability of endolysin systems like this one will depend on the ability to exert a strict control over the autolytic phenotype, since leakiness of expression before induction may contribute to an unwanted cell lysis during cell growth and plasmid replication.

Although the strains previously described were only tested in the context of recombinant protein production,[60] a recent report describes the use of endolysin-expressing cells specifically for the production of plasmid DNA.[44] In this work, and as an alternative to the arabinose-triggered expression of endolysin described earlier, chromosome engineering was performed using an integration vector with promoters that allow expression of the lytic λR endolysin gene to be induced with a shift in fermentation temperature from 30 to 42°C.[44] This type of induction is a key advantage of this system since the addition of a chemical inducer like arabinose is not required to trigger the expression of the lytic enzyme. The autolytic strains were then used in a temperature-inducible fed-batch process designed to amplify plasmids with a temperature-sensitive origin of replication[1] (see Chapter 13, Section 13.3.4). Briefly, this process is characterized by a first growth phase at low temperature (30°C), where plasmid levels are kept low, and a second phase of continued growth and plasmid accumulation at 42°C.[1] With the autolytic strains, endolysin expression is efficiently repressed during growth at 30°C but is triggered by the temperature upshift to 42°C. Like before, cells are not affected during expression since the endolysin is localized in the cytoplasm.[44] Following harvest, the cells are suspended in a low-salt, slightly acidic sodium acetate buffer containing sucrose, EDTA, and Triton X-100. While the chelating agent EDTA contributes to destabilize the outer membrane, Triton X-100 permeabilizes the cytoplasmic membrane, making it possible for endolysin to access the peptidoglycan layer where it can fully display its hydrolytic activity. The use of an acidic acetate buffer made it possible to recover the plasmid very efficiently in a nonviscous solution while minimizing the release of gDNA and cell debris.[44] In the second part of the extraction process, the mixture is pumped through two consecutive stainless steel coils (20-s residence time in each coil) in order to promote flocculation and sedimentation of solids. While the first coil is immersed in a 70°C water bath, the second one is kept at a low temperature with ice. The extraction mixture collected is then kept overnight in a tank at 48°C. The settled flocculated material is finally filtered out through two layers of a cloth material.[44] An analysis of DNA in this clarified lysate showed that the amount of plasmid DNA in the mixture (~99%) was substantially higher when compared with the amount of gDNA (~1%). Furthermore, although acidic conditions and high temperatures are used in the process, no apurinic plasmid DNA was detected by endonuclease III or endonuclease VIII digestion of the isolated plasmid DNA[44] (see also Chapter 5, Section 5.2.2.1). This acidic autolytic extraction was further combined with other unit operations in order to develop a full downstream process.[44] More details on this process can be found in Chapter 18, Section 18.2.

In some cases, autolysis is associated with a poor denaturation and removal of gDNA, and this may constitute a drawback when a side-by-side comparison is made with alkaline or heat lysis of nonautolytic strains. In those situations, the autolysis process could be further improved by cloning other, nonlytic genes alongside the lytic ones. For example, the genes for plasmid-safe, non-specific nucleases such as the bacteriophage T5 exonuclease,[61] RNase A, or RNase S[62] can be expressed in the periplasm by means of appropriate secretion signals. The sequestration of the nucleases in the periplasm would prevent them from interfering with the normal course of gene expression during cell growth and plasmid amplification. The nucleases would only contact the corresponding substrates (i.e., linear single- and double-stranded DNA in the case of T5 exonuclease and RNA in the case of RNase A and RNase S) after a postproduction inner membrane permeabilization step, or during the course of normal lysis, when both enzymes and substrates become mixed.[61,62] The nucleolytic action of two or more enzymes can even be combined in a single strain by coexpression or expression of appropriate chimeric proteins.[61] As an alternative to periplasm targeting, the expression could be controlled by the use of an appropriate promoter/induction system.

15.3.6 Exploring the Use of Enzymes

The presence of active endogenous ribonucleases in the lysates obtained after cell disruption and solid removal can be advantageously used to remove RNA impurities. As described, in Section 15.2, one way to do this is to extend the fermentation past the exponential phase. Alternatively, and since in many cases a fraction of the host RNases remains active even after a harsh disruption step like alkaline lysis, the clarified lysates can be incubated at 37°C for a certain period of time. Using this strategy, RNA levels could be reduced by 40% after only 20 min. The downside in this case was that a 9% plasmid loss occurred concurrently.[15] Furthermore, the implementation of this methodology at a large scale is questionable since problems with the batch-to-batch consistency of the endogenous nucleases are likely to render validation extremely difficult. A more controllable approach relies on the addition of specific amounts of exogenous enzymes such as lysozyme[52] and RNase[43] during or shortly after lysis. These animal-derived enzymes are highly effective in degrading proteins and RNA. However, their use may raise regulatory concerns since they potentially constitute a source of mammalian pathogens like retroviruses and prions (see Chapter 11, Section 11.6.3). The use of recombinant enzymes is a possible solution for this problem.

Exogenous DNases can also contribute to improve plasmid purification. The bacteriophage T5 exonuclease, for instance, is capable of digesting linear single- and double-stranded DNA while leaving supercoiled plasmid intact. The enzyme also digests denatured plasmid material.[27] In another example of the use of DNases to improve plasmid purification, a combination of the λ and RecJf exonucleases is used to selectively remove linear DNA fragments, whether they result from shearing/degradation of gDNA or from linearization of plasmid DNA itself.[63] First, the λ exonuclease digests one of the strands of double-stranded DNA in the 5′ to 3′ direction. Next, the single-strand specific exonuclease RecJf digests the remaining complementary single strand. The supercoiled plasmid isoform is unaffected by the tandem action of the enzymes, remaining biologically active. This strategy has only been used at the laboratorial scale.[63]

15.4 CONCLUSIONS

The downstream processing of plasmid pharmaceuticals starts with primary isolation, a series of steps designed to harvest and lyse *E. coli* cells, and to generate a clarified, plasmid-containing lysate. The key step here is cell lysis— if effective and consistent, this operation can have a huge beneficial impact in the overall process. Despite its problems, the traditional alkaline lysis and variations thereof still dominate the large-scale scene. Furthermore, the operation and equipments used for its implementation have been perfected and optimized up to a point where it can be performed continuously. Nevertheless, other alternatives like heat lysis and autolysis are gradually emerging, which one day may become competitive enough to replace alkaline lysis in some plasmid manufacturing processes. Mechanical methods such as bead milling, microfluidization, and homogenization could be an option provided that some kind of method to protect plasmid molecules from high shear degradation is used alongside. The composition of the clarified lysate that is obtained at the end of the primary isolation depends strongly on the exact lysis methodology used. In the best cases, the majority of the original proteins and variable amounts of gDNA and LPS will have been removed alongside cell debris, walls, and membranes, leaving behind a clear solution with a plasmid concentration around 50–250 μg/mL and significant amounts of RNA. This stream must now be handled in the intermediate recovery section in such a way as to increase the plasmid content and concentration up to valuables compatible with the high resolution operations of the final purification stage.

REFERENCES

1. Carnes AE, Hodgson CP, Williams JA. Inducible *Escherichia coli* fermentation for increased plasmid DNA production. *Biotechnology and Applied Biochemistry*. 2006;45:155–166.
2. Listner K, Bentley L, Okonkowski J, et al. Development of a highly productive and scalable plasmid DNA production platform. *Biotechnology Progress*. 2006;22: 1335–1345.
3. Passarinha LA, Diogo MM, Queiroz JA, Monteiro GA, Fonseca LP, Prazeres DMF. Production of ColE1 type plasmid by *Escherichia coli* DH5α cultured under nonselective conditions. *Journal of Microbiology and Biotechnology*. 2006;16:20–24.
4. Drlica K. Control of bacterial DNA supercoiling. *Molecular Microbiology*. 1992;6:425–433.

5. Harrison RG, Todd PW, Rudge SR, Petrides D. Bioprocess design. In: Harrison RG, Todd PW, Rudge SR, Petrides D, eds. *Bioseparations science and engineering.* Oxford: Oxford University Press, 2003:319–372.

6. Steffens MA, Fraga ES, Bogle ID. Synthesis of bioprocesses using physical properties data. *Biotechnology and Bioengineering.* 2000;68:218–230.

7. Eschbach G, Vermant S. Tangential flow filtration (TFF) membranes for the washing of *Escherichia coli* cells. *Bioprocessing Journal.* 2009;8:46–48.

8. Quaak SG, van den Berg JH, Toebes M, et al. GMP production of pDERMATT for vaccination against melanoma in a phase I clinical trial. *European Journal of Pharmaceutics and Biopharmaceutics.* 2008;70:429–438.

9. O'Mahony K, Freitag R, Hilbrig F, Muller P, Schumacher I. Proposal for a better integration of bacterial lysis into the production of plasmid DNA at large scale. *Journal of Biotechnology.* 2005;119:118–132.

10. O'Mahony K, Freitag R, Dhote B, Hilbrig F, Muller P, Schumacher I. Capture of bacteria from fermentation broth by body feed filtration: A solved problem? *Biotechnology Progress.* 2006;22:471–483.

11. Kong S, Rock CF, Booth A, et al. Large-scale plasmid DNA processing: Evidence that cell harvesting and storage methods affect yield of supercoiled plasmid DNA. *Biotechnology and Applied Biochemistry.* 2008;51:43–51.

12. Freitas SS, Azzoni AR, Santos JA, Monteiro GA, Prazeres DMF. On the stability of plasmid DNA vectors during cell culture and purification. *Molecular Biotechnology.* 2007;36:151–158.

13. Sambrook J, Fritsch EF, Maniatis T. *Molecular cloning: A laboratory manual*, Vol. 1. Plainview, NY: Cold Spring Harbor Laboratory Press, 1989.

14. Ciccolini LAS, Shamlou PA, Titchener-Hooker NJ, Ward JM, Dunnill P. Time course of SDS-alkaline lysis of recombinant bacterial cells for plasmid release. *Biotechnology and Bioengineering.* 1998;60:768–770.

15. Monteiro GA, Ferreira GNM, Cabral JMS, Prazeres DMF. Analysis and use of endonuclease activities in *Escherichia coli* lysates during the primary isolation of plasmids for gene therapy. *Biotechnology and Bioengineering.* 1999;66:189–194.

16. Jem K-MJ. inventor; Wyeth, assignee. Mechanical disruption of bacterial cells for plasmid recovery. U.S. patent 6,455,287, September 24, 2002.

17. Hucklenbroich J, Mueller M, inventors; QIAGEN GmbH, assignee. Method for coarse purification of cell digests from microorganisms. U.S. patent 7,214,508, May 8, 2007.

18. Chamsart S, Karnjanasorn T. Alkaline-cell lysis through in-line static mixer reactor for the production of plasmid DNA for gene therapy. *Biotechnology and Bioengineering.* 2007;96:471–482.

19. Urthaler J, Ascher C, Wohrer H, Necina R. Automated alkaline lysis for industrial scale cGMP production of pharmaceutical grade plasmid-DNA. *Journal of Biotechnology.* 2007;128:132–149.

20. Carlson A, Signs M, Liermann L, Boor R, Jem KJ. Mechanical disruption of *Escherichia coli* for plasmid recovery. *Biotechnology and Bioengineering.* 1995;48:303–315.

21. Prazeres DMF, Ferreira GNM, Monteiro GA, Cooney CL, Cabral JMS. Large-scale production of pharmaceutical-grade plasmid DNA for gene therapy: Problems and bottlenecks. *Trends in Biotechnology.* 1999;17:169–174.

22. Levy MS, Collins IJ, Yim SS, et al. Effect of shear on plasmid DNA in solution. *Bioprocess Engineering*. 1999;20:7–13.

23. Birnboim HC, Doly J. A rapid alkaline extraction procedure for screening recombinant plasmid DNA. *Nucleic Acids Research*. 1979;7:1513–1523.

24. Holmes DS, Quigley M. A rapid boiling method for the preparation of bacterial plasmids. *Methods in Analytical Biochemistry*. 1981;114:193–197.

25. Rush MG, Warner RC. Alkali denaturation of covalently closed circular duplex deoxyribonucleic acid. *Journal of Biological Chemistry*. 1970;245:2704–2708.

26. Prazeres DMF, Schluep T, Cooney C. Preparative purification of supercoiled plasmid DNA using anion-exchange chromatography. *Journal of Chromatography. A*. 1998;806:31–45.

27. Sayers JR, Evans D, Thomson JB. Identification and erradication of a denatured DNA isolated during alkaline lysis-based plasmid purification procedures. *Analytical Biochemistry*. 1996;241:186–189.

28. Cloninger C, Felton M, Paul B, Hirakawa Y, Metzenberg S. Control of pH during plasmid preparation by alkaline lysis of *Escherichia coli*. *Analytical Biochemistry*. 2008;378:224–225.

29. Yu J, Zhang Z, Cao K, Huang X. Visualization of alkali-denatured supercoiled plasmid DNA by atomic force microscopy. *Biochemical and Biophysical Research Communications*. 2008;374:415–418.

30. Yakovchuk P, Protozanova E, Frank-Kamenetskii MD. Base-stacking and base-pairing contributions into thermal stability of the DNA double helix. *Nucleic Acids Research*. 2006;34:564–574.

31. Kresheck GC, Altschuler M, inventors; Board of Regents for Northern Illinois University, assignee. Method of isolating purified plasmid DNA using a nonionic detergent solution. U.S. patent 5,625,053, April 29, 1997.

32. Butler MD, Cohen DL, Kahn D, Winkler ME, inventors; Genentech, Inc., assignee. Purification of plasmid DNA. U.S. patent 6,313,285, November 6, 2001.

33. Marquet M, Horn N, Meek J, Budahazi G, inventors; Vical Incorporated, assignee. Production of pharmaceutical-grade plasmid DNA. U.S. patent 5,561,064, October 1, 1996.

34. Ciccolini LAS, Shamlou PA, Titchener-Hooker NJ, Ward JM, Dunnill P. Rheological properties of chromosomal and plasmid DNA during alkaline lysis reaction. *Bioprocess Engineering*. 1999;21:231–237.

35. Nienow AW, Hitchock AG, Riley GL, inventors; Cobra Therapeutics Limited, assignee. Vessel for mixing a cell lysate. U.S. patent 6,395,516, May 28, 2002.

36. Stephenson D, Norman F, Cumming RH. Shear thickening of DNA in SDS lysates. *Bioseparation*. 1993;3:285–289.

37. Hebel H, Ramakrishnan S, Gonzalez H, Darnell J, inventors; Advisys, Inc., assignee. Devices and methods for biomaterial production. U.S. patent 7,238,522, July 3, 2007.

38. Marquet M, Horn NA, Meek JA. Process development for the manufacture of plasmid DNA vectors for use in gene therapy. *BioPharm*. 1995;September:26–37.

39. Nochumson S, Durland R, Yu-Speight A, Welp J, Wu K, Hayes R, inventors; Valentis, Inc., assignee. Process and equipment for plasmid purification. U.S. patent 7,026,468, April 11, 2006.

40. Frerix A, Geilenkirchen P, Muller M, Kula MR, Hubbuch J. Separation of genomic DNA, RNA, and open circular plasmid DNA from supercoiled plasmid DNA by combining denaturation, selective renaturation and aqueous two-phase extraction. *Biotechnology and Bioengineering.* 2007;96:57–66.

41. Theodossiou I, Thomas ORT, Dunnill P. Methods of enhancing the recovery of plasmid genes from neutralised cell lysate. *Bioprocess Engineering.* 1999;20: 147–156.

42. Theodossiou I, Collins IJ, Ward JM, Thomas ORT, Dunnill P. The processing of plasmid based gene from *Escherichia coli.* Primary recovery by filtration. *Bioprocess Engineering.* 1997;16:175–183.

43. Varley DL, Hitchcock AG, Weiss AME, et al. Production of plasmid DNA for human gene therapy using modified alkaline cell lysis and expanded bed anion exchange chromatography. *Bioseparation.* 1998;8:209–217.

44. Carnes AE, Hodgson CP, Luke JM, Vincent JM, Williams JA. Plasmid DNA production combining antibiotic-free selection, inducible high yield fermentation, and novel autolytic purification. *Biotechnology and Bioengineering.* 2009;104:505–515.

45. Horn NA, Meek JA, Budahazi G, Marquet M. Cancer gene therapy using plasmid DNA: Purification of DNA for human clinical trials. *Human Gene Therapy.* 1995;6:565–573.

46. Horn N, Marquet M, Meek J, Budahazi G, inventors; Vical Incorporated, assignee. Process for reducing RNA concentration in a mixture of biological material using diatomaceous earth. U.S. patent 5,576,196, November 19, 1996.

47. Ciccolini LAS, Shamlou PA, Titchener-Hooker N. A mass balance study to assess the extent of contaminant removal achieved in the operations for the primary recovery of plasmid DNA from *Escherichia coli* cells. *Biotechnology and Bioengineering.* 2002;77:796–805.

48. Wan NC, McNeilly DS, Christopher CW, inventors; Genzyme Corporation, assignee. Method for lysing cells. U.S. patent 5,837,529, November 17, 1998.

49. Au-Yeung K-L, Bussey LB, inventors; Valentis, Inc., assignee. Apparatus and method for preparative purification of nucleic acids. U.S. patent 7,314,746, January 1, 2008.

50. Hebel H, Attra H, Khan A, Draghia-Akli R. Successful parallel development and integration of a plasmid-based biologic, container/closure system and electrokinetic delivery device. *Vaccine.* 2006;24:4607–4614.

51. Zhu K, Jin H, Ma Y, et al. A continuous thermal lysis procedure for the large-scale preparation of plasmid DNA. *Journal of Biotechnology.* 2005;118:257–264.

52. Lee AL, Sagar S, inventors; Merck & Co., Inc., assignee. Method for large scale plasmid purification. U.S. patent 6,197,553, March 6, 2002.

53. Lander RJ, Winters MA, Meacle FJ, Buckland BC, Lee AL. Fractional precipitation of plasmid DNA from lysate by CTAB. *Biotechnology and Bioengineering.* 2002;79:776–784.

54. Murphy JC, Cano T, Fox GE, Willson RC. Compaction agent protection of nucleic acids during mechanical lysis. *Biotechnology Progress.* 2006;22:519–522.

55. Lengsfeld CS, Anchordoquy TJ. Shear-induced degradation of plasmid DNA. *Journal of Pharmaceutical Science.* 2002;91:1581–1589.

56. Kelly WJ, Muske KR. Optimal operation of high-pressure homogenization for intracellular product recovery. *Bioprocess and Biosystems Engineering.* 2004;27: 25–37.

57. Microfluidics. *Innovation through Microfluidizer® processor technology.* Newton, MA: Microfluidics, 2005.

58. Agerkvist I, Enfors SO. Characterization of *E. coli* cell disintegrates from a bead mill and high pressure homogenizers. *Biotechnology and Bioengineering.* 1990;36: 1083–1089.

59. Sauer T, Robinson CW, Glick BR. Disruption of native and recombinant *Escherichia coli* in a high-pressure homogenizer. *Biotechnology and Bioengineering.* 1989;33: 1330–1342.

60. Jia X, Kostal J, Claypool JA, inventors. Controlled lysis of bacteria. U.S. patent 2006/40,393, August 16, 2005.

61. Williams JA, Hodgson CP, inventors; Nature Technology Corporation, assignee. Strains of *E. coli* for plasmid DNA production. U.S. patent 2007/249,042, October 25, 2007.

62. Cooke GD, Cranenburgh RM, Hanak JA, Dunnill P, Thatcher DR, Ward JM. Purification of essentially RNA free plasmid DNA using a modified *Escherichia coli* host strain expressing ribonuclease A. *Journal of Biotechnology.* 2001;85: 297–304.

63. Balagurumoorthy P, Adelstein SJ, Kassis AI. Method to eliminate linear DNA from mixture containing nicked-circular, supercoiled, and linear plasmid DNA. *Analytical Biochemistry.* 2008;381:172–174.

16

Intermediate Recovery

16.1 INTRODUCTION

The intermediate recovery section is designed to process the plasmid-containing clarified lysates obtained after completion of the primary isolation stage. Here, a series of unit operations are put in place with the major objective of concentrating and further purifying the plasmid product. The starting point is usually a complex lysate stream in which the plasmid is usually diluted (~50–250 μg/mL). Although a significant fraction of genomic DNA (gDNA) has been removed during primary isolation, large amounts of RNA and proteins, which together make up more than 90% of the total mass of solutes, still linger in the clarified lysates.[1,2] These impurities should be substantially cleared from the process stream in order to end up with a solution where plasmid should typically account for more than 50% of all solutes. If this goal is achieved, the burden imposed on the high-performance/high-cost unit operations (typically chromatography), which dominate the subsequent final purification stage (described in Chapter 17), will be significantly reduced. The plasmid-containing clarified lysates entering the intermediate recovery stage

Plasmid Biopharmaceuticals: Basics, Applications, and Manufacturing, First Edition.
Duarte Miguel F. Prazeres.
© 2011 John Wiley & Sons, Inc. Published 2011 by John Wiley & Sons, Inc.

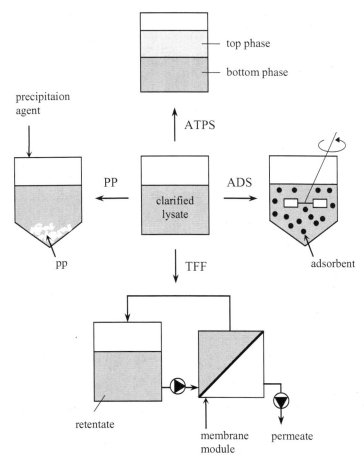

Figure 16.1 *The processing of plasmid-containing clarified lysates. The four major options available are schematically shown in the figure: tangential flow filtration (TFF), aqueous two-phase systems (ATPSs), precipitation (PP), and adsorption (ADS). Different combinations of the unit operations shown can be used to improve the clearance of impurities and to concentrate plasmid DNA.*

can be processed by a number of different unit operations, of which tangential flow filtration (TFF), precipitation (PP), aqueous two-phase systems (ATPSs), and adsorption (ADS) are probably the most important ones (Figure 16.1). The choice of the exact combination of these unit operations, which will be used in the intermediate recovery stage, depends on a large number of objective and subjective factors.[3] Furthermore, it is clear from the literature that there is not a single solution for the challenge at hand. In this chapter, we describe how the different unit operations can and have been used to clear impurities and concentrate plasmid DNA solutions, highlighting the basic operating principles, advantages, and disadvantages.

16.2 TANGENTIAL FLOW FILTRATION

16.2.1 Introduction

Volume reduction is one of the first objectives that come to mind when the question of how to further process a plasmid-containing lysate arises. As we have seen before, the sooner this volume reduction is accomplished, the more expedite and less costly will the full downstream process be (see Chapter 14, Section 14.4). In the biotechnology industry, the favored operation to reduce volume is most likely TFF. Apart from the simplicity that is inherent to TFF, a wide range of membrane materials, formats, and modules are commercially available, which can serve practically any specific process need. The concept behind TFF of plasmid-containing *Escherichia coli* lysates is straightforward—a membrane with an adequate pore size distribution is selected that is able to retain the large supercoiled plasmid molecules while allowing excess water, salts, and small solutes to permeate through. During operation, the tangential flow of the incoming stream relative to the membrane provides not only the transmembrane pressure (TMP) difference required for permeation but also maintains the membrane surface relatively free from particulate matter and gelled solutes. Some additional purification can also be obtained by promoting the permeation of smaller impurities like lipopolysaccharides (LPSs), transfer RNA (tRNA), and proteins (see Chapter 14, Figure 14.3). In addition, TFF membranes can be selected with the additional purpose of adsorbing impurities. For example, membranes made of nitrocellulose, a hydrophobic material, have been shown to effectively adsorb impurities like single-stranded gDNA and RNA during the course of TFF of lysates.[4] Although these "adsorption membranes" may contribute to clear specific impurities from lysates, an excessive adsorption of solutes on the pore walls may result in local precipitation and blockage of pores, thus compromising filtration flux (as described in Section 16.2.2). Hence, the discussion in this section will be limited to those filtration systems that essentially explore size exclusion as the separation mechanism.

A significant number of researchers have attempted to explore the key advantages of TFF as a way to concentrate plasmid-containing clarified lysates while simultaneously removing protein and RNA impurities.[5–9] The usual TFF setup combines tanks, pumps, pipes, valves, and pressure gauges with a membrane module (Figure 16.2). One of the pumps in the system is indispensable since it promotes the continuous tangential flow recirculation of the feed stream. As the smaller solutes and water molecules permeate through the membrane, the solution becomes enriched in the retained components and for this reason is often called the retentate. A second pump is sometimes used to minimize the effects of concentration polarization and fouling effects (described in Section 16.2.2) over the permeate flow rate. In this case, and in order to maintain an accurate control of the flow rate of the permeate stream, a controllable valve is used alongside to manipulate the pressure on

(a)

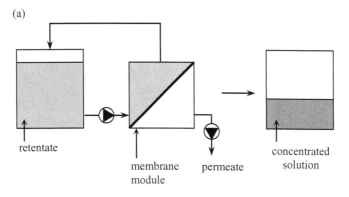

(b)
diafiltration buffer

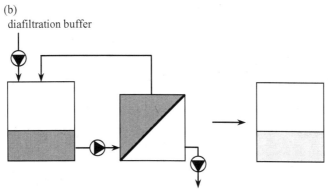

Figure 16.2 *The tangential flow filtration of plasmid-containing lysates. TFF is carried out by operating the system sequentially in the concentration (a) and diafiltration (b) modes. During concentration, the volume is reduced until the desired plasmid concentration is reached. In diafiltration, the complex lysate buffer is replaced by removing small permeable components (e.g., NaoH/SDS/potassium acetate) while simultaneously adding approximately 5 volumes of an adequate buffer at a flow rate equal to the filtration flow rate. Smaller impurities like tRNA and proteins are also typically removed during this stage of TFF, although this may require the use of additional volumes of diafiltration buffer.*

the retentate side. With this setup, it is thus possible to continuously increase and adjust the TMP up to the values that guarantee a constant permeate flow rate throughout the entire operation.

The processing of a plasmid-containing lysate in such a TFF system will typically combine two operating modes: concentration and diafiltration. During a first period of time, the system is operated in such a way as to remove excess liquid and thus to concentrate the plasmid in the lysate (Figure 16.2a). Although the exact concentration factor obtained at the end of this first phase of the operation will depend on the plasmid concentration in the incoming lysate and also on the desired final concentration, figures ranging from 10- to 50-fold have been reported in the literature. If the TMP is not controlled, the permeate flow rate will typically decrease during concentration. Once concentration is concluded, the operation of the system is switched to the diafiltration mode. Here, the fluid that permeates across the membrane is replaced by continuously adding a buffer at a flow rate equal to the permeation flow rate (Figure 16.2b). This diafiltration buffer is usually selected so as to meet the requirements of the subsequent processing step, whichever it may be. Usually, the addition of a volume of diafiltration buffer equal to 5 volumes of the initial lysate should be sufficient to remove more than 99% of the solutes that permeate freely through the membrane (e.g., salts). However, further addition of diafiltration buffer is required if the goal is also to remove partially permeating solutes (e.g., RNA molecules). The permeate flow rate during diafiltration will typically remain constant. As an alternative to the scheme described and illustrated in Figure 16.2, diafiltration can be performed prior to concentration. However, this will imply the use of substantially higher amounts of diafiltration buffer, a feature that is of course disadvantageous from an economical point of view.

TFF requires plasmid-containing streams to be pumped tangentially to a membrane surface at a given flow rate. Furthermore, the retentate volume must be recirculated several times through the membrane module in order to complete the concentration and diafiltration procedures. Therefore, concerns that the shear stress associated with the fluid flow across pipes, valves, pumps, and membrane module might damage plasmid molecules are recurrent.[10,11] The major factors affecting the sensitivity of supercoiled plasmid molecules to shear were examined in the previous chapter, in the context of the mechanical lysis of cells (Chapter 15, Section 15.3.4). One important fact described then is the ability of plasmids to better resist the deleterious effects of shear when the surrounding environment is characterized by a high ionic strength.[11,12] This is especially relevant in the case of the processing of alkaline lysates by TFF given the fact that the ionic strength of the said lysates is typically very high (around 1 M) as a consequence of the addition of the potassium acetate neutralization solution (see Chapter 15, Section 15.3.2). Thus, we may speculate that if shear rates conducive to degradation are present in a TFF setup, the effect of shear over plasmids is likely to be more important toward the end of the diafiltration stage, when most of the ions in the original lysates have been washed away. The ionic strength of the diafiltration buffer used should also be considered since a high-salt buffer (e.g., >150 mM NaCl) will offer a higher degree of protection when compared with a low salt buffer.

16.2.2 Concentration Polarization and Fouling

Concentration polarization and membrane fouling are two recurrent problems associated with the processing of fluid streams of biological origin by TFF. The onset and progression of either phenomenon is usually accompanied by a reduction in the filtration flux and/or an increase in the TMP. For this reason, the ability to minimize and/or control both concentration polarization and fouling dictates to a large extent the performance of a TFF operation.

Concentration polarization designates a series of events whereby solutes in the tangentially flowing stream accumulate near the membrane surface, increasing the local concentration up to a point where a gel layer is formed. Though this layer contains a substantial amount of liquid, its core structure is essentially a three-dimensional network, which results from the establishment of physical/chemical bonds between the different solutes present. The deposition of this three-dimensional network on top of a membrane adds an extra resistance to the passage of the filtrating fluid and permeating solutes, reducing the filtration flow rate and increasing the rejection of macromolecules. During the initial stage of the TFF process, the gel layer grows steadily as a result of the convective transport of solutes, which are carried along with the filtrating stream. The buildup of this gel layer is readily observed during the initial instants of operation as a decrease in the filtration flux. At the same time, and since the concentration of solutes in the gel is higher than in the bulk of the tangentially flowing stream, Fickian diffusion transports solutes back to the retentate stream. The growth of the gel layer past a certain thickness is also prevented by the shearing action of the flowing stream. Eventually, a pseudo-steady state is reached, which is characterized by the presence of a concentration polarization layer with a fixed thickness and hence a more or less constant filtration flow rate. Once a TFF operation is complete, the concentration polarization gel layer can be removed and filtration fluxes fully restored by adequate back-flushing and cleaning of the membrane with a number of physical or chemical methods. Although the cleaning methodology should be adapted to the membrane in question, chemical treatment with alkalis, acids, and detergents, and extensive rinsing with water are common options.

As was described earlier, the apparent size of the pores in a polarized membrane and hence the rejection and hydraulic characteristics of the system are effectively different from those displayed by the clean membrane. This difference is clearly seen when processing plasmid-containing lysates by TFF—during the initial stages of the operation and concomitantly with the buildup of the gel, plasmids may permeate through the membrane alongside the smaller solutes. This detrimental permeation of plasmid eventually stops once the pseudo-steady state sets in. One way to obviate this early plasmid loss is to recycle the permeate stream back to the retentate tank during the initial stages of the TFF operation. Once the membrane is polarized, operation can be then carried out in the normal concentration or diafiltration modes (Figure 16.2).

Fouling is a generic term that encompasses a series of events that collectively result in the deposition of material on the membrane surface. For example, products and impurities in the stream can adsorb to the pore walls and microparticulate matter can block pores. In a worst case scenario, the blockage of membrane pores can be such that the permeation flux is reduced beyond reasonable. Contrary to concentration polarization, fouling is an irreversible phenomenon that inevitably leads to the deterioration of the membrane performance in terms of filtration flux and solute retention. An adequate clarification of the lysates (e.g., by coarse dead-end filtration) prior to TFF will minimize the occurrence of fouling, leading to better filtration performances and increasing the lifetime of the membrane.

16.2.3 Membrane Selection

Although different modules are available in the market for TFF (e.g., hollow fibers, spiral wound, plate, and frame), the performance of the TFF of a plasmid-containing solution is ultimately determined by the characteristics of the selected membrane and not by its geometry. If the goal of the operation is to explore size exclusion as the separation mechanism, a material with inertness sufficient to prevent the adsorption of plasmid and impurities should be chosen to minimize the occurrence of fouling (described in Section 16.2.2). As far as the composition of the membrane is concerned, the options usually fall on polymeric materials like polyethersulfone[5,7] and polysulfone.[3,8,9] The selection of the best membrane pore size for plasmid retention, on the other hand, is more problematic than choosing the membrane material. Contrary to what is usually the case when dealing with the TFF of globular proteins, a comparison of the membrane molecular weight cutoff with the plasmid molecular weight can hardly be used as a guideline for membrane selection. The major reason for this is related to the fact that the behavior of the thin, slender, and flexible plasmid molecules when faced with membrane pores of a given size is hard to predict.[7] Not surprisingly, the cutoff of the membranes that assure 100% retention of plasmids is usually significantly smaller when compared with the plasmid molecular weight. Typically, TFF membranes with cutoffs varying between 100 and 500 kDa are used when one wishes to retain plasmids with sizes ranging from 2700 to 11,500 bp,[3,7,9] that is, with molecular weights ranging from 1782 to 7590 kDa, respectively, as estimated by Equation 4.1 in Chapter 4. In spite of this difference between membrane cutoff and plasmid molecular weight, the membranes with smaller pore size may still be unable to guarantee full retention. For example, in one case described in the literature, a 300-kDa membrane had to be replaced by a 100-kDa membrane when processing an alkaline lysate containing a 7700-bp (i.e., 5082-kDa) plasmid to prevent some plasmid leakage in the permeate stream.[7] In another situation, an 11% loss of a 6100-bp (i.e., 4026-kDa) plasmid to the permeate side was measured when using a 100-kDa membrane.[9] In view of these results, TFF membranes with a 100-kDa cutoff are probably the best choice for processing lysates. Still, one should recognize that the permeation of plasmid molecules across membranes is more significant during the start-up of the operation, when the concentration polarization gel layer is still forming, as described in the previous section. In some cases, although no plasmid is found in the permeate stream, drops in yields may be detected due to entrapment of molecules within the membrane structure and solute gel layer.[9] Again, this is likely to be more significant during the initial stages of gel layer formation.

16.2.4 Impurity Clearance by TFF

Once the retention of most plasmid DNAs is warranted by an adequate selection of the membrane cutoff, attentions should be directed toward the ability of the membrane to remove *E. coli* impurities—proteins, RNA, gDNA, and LPS. The typical behavior of those impurities in a TFF process is described next.

16.2.4.1 Proteins

The cutoff of the membranes used in the TFF of plasmid-containing lysates is usually sufficient to remove most *E. coli* proteins, which have molecular weights below 200 kDa (see Chapter 14, Figure 14.3), into the permeate stream. For example, a TFF system equipped with a 300-kDa membrane was able to clear more than 95% of proteins after the addition of 3 volumes of diafiltration buffer and a fivefold concentration.[13] A similar protein clearance was obtained with a 100-kDa membrane after three diafiltration volumes and a 20-fold concentration.[13]

16.2.4.2 RNA

The removal of RNA by TFF is not as straightforward as it is in the case of proteins. Due to the wide range of molecular weight characteristics of the different molecular species of RNA released from *E. coli* cells (tRNA, messenger RNA [mRNA], and ribosomal RNA [rRNA]), the permeation through 100- to 500-kDa cutoff membranes is usually restricted to the smaller molecules, that is, tRNA (see Chapter 14, Figure 14.3 and Table 14.1). This behavior is clearly observed in Figure 16.3, which displays and compares chromatograms obtained following the high-performance liquid chromatography (HPLC) analysis of a lysate feed (Figure 16.3a) and of samples of retentate (Figure 16.3b) and permeate (Figure 16.3c) streams collected during the course of diafiltration in a TFF system.[13] The results show that while large-molecular-weight RNA and the 6100 bp plasmid DNA tested do not permeate through a 300-kDa membrane (Figure 16.3b), low-molecular-weight RNA molecules are readily cleared from the retentate stream as a result of permeation (Figure 16.3b). A time course analysis of the permeate stream further shows that the removal of low-molecular-weight RNA is more significant during the initial stages of operation and is practically complete after the addition of 2 volumes of diafiltration buffer (Figure 16.3c). Unfortunately, the removed fraction accounted for only 10% of the total initial RNA.[13]

According to the breakdown of RNA species described in Chapter 14 (see Figure 14.1 and Table 14.1) and to the data shown in Figure 16.3, a TFF operation will hardly be able to remove more than 14% of the total RNA in the usual lysate (i.e., the total amount of tRNA present). In principle, the clearance of the remaining high-molecular-weight RNA species (mRNA and rRNA) from lysates is possible if membranes with larger pores (e.g., microfiltration membranes) are used. However, since the typical plasmid molecule is

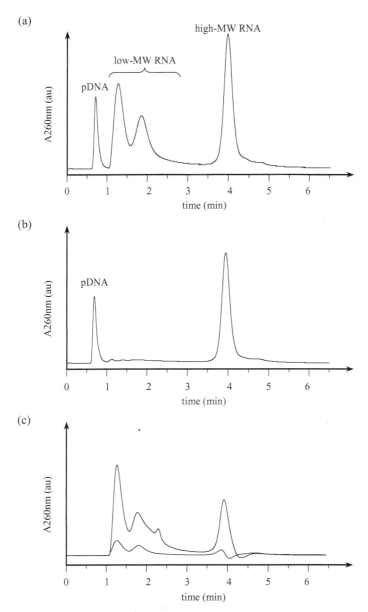

Figure 16.3 *Tangential flow filtration of plasmid-containing alkaline lysates. The filtration of 100 mL of lysate was carried out using a cartridge equipped with two 300-kDa hollow fiber polysulfone membranes (1-mm ID, 30-cm length). The figure shows the HIC-HPLC analysis of the starting lysate (a) and of samples withdrawn from the retentate after 3 diafiltration volumes (DV) (b) and from the permeate stream (c) after 0.5 DV (full line) and 2.0 DV (dashed line). The plasmid size was 6100 bp and the diafiltration buffer was 10 mM tris–HCl, pH 8.8 (adapted and reprinted with permission from Freitas[13]).*

characterized by a molecular weight that is very close to the molecular weights of rRNA and mRNA, permeation of the elongated plasmid molecules across these membranes is more than likely to occur. Thus, the plasmid-containing stream that results from the TFF of lysates stream will typically contain a significant amount of RNA, which must then be cleared by subsequent unit operations. A possible way to improve the clearance of RNA impurities during TFF is to pretreat lysates in order to degrade RNA into fragments small enough to permeate through 100- to 300-kDa membranes. Examples of such pretreatments include (1) an extended alkaline lysis that reduces or denatures RNA (see Chapter 15, Figure 15.4)[13] and (2) the use of RNase.[13,14] For instance, when clarified lysates obtained after an extended (24-h) alkaline lysis with lysozyme were processed in a TFF system equipped with 1000- and 500-kDa cutoff polyethersulfone membranes, more than 99% of RNA and 95% of protein could be removed.[5,15] The impact of RNase on RNA clearance, on the other hand, is illustrated by the following example. When an alkaline lysate was incubated with RNase prior to TFF, the plasmid purity in the final stream obtained after dialfiltration and concentration increased fourfold, from 15% to 60%, as compared to a mere 1.7-fold increase when no enzymatic treatment was performed beforehand.[13] However, this improvement in RNA clearance was accompanied by a decrease in plasmid yield from 80% to 64%. This additional loss of plasmid is likely related to a decrease in the retention offered by the TFF system, as a consequence of the reduction of the gel layer thickness and mesh, which is brought about by RNA degradation.[13] If the enzymatic degradation of RNA is not viable, or if the use of RNase is discarded for regulatory reasons (see Chapter 11, Section 11.6.3), unit operations like salt or isopropanol precipitation (see Section 16.3) and adsorption (see Section 16.5), which are designed specifically to remove high-molecular-weight RNA, can be used before TFF.

16.2.4.3 gDNA and LPS

The sizes of the gDNA fragments resulting from alkaline or other types of cell lysis are likely to vary widely, both from method to method, but also from batch to batch. For this reason, it is difficult to anticipate whether a TFF operation will be able to clear gDNA or not. Additionally, few data are available in the literature to enable an adequate assessment of the removal of gDNA by TFF. A similar situation is observed in the case of LPSs—while in principle the individual 10- to 20-kDa amphipathic molecules should permeate readily through the typical TFF membrane used in plasmid processing, their ability to form highly stable micelles (300–1000 kDa) and vesicles (>1000 kDa) (see Chapter 14, Section 14.2) makes it difficult to predict the extent of clearance. The scarcity of literature data regarding LPS removal by TFF is also similar to the one observed for gDNA. Still, gDNA and LPS clearances of the order of 40 and 87%, respectively, have been reported when processing an alkaline lysate with a 100-kDa membrane.[13]

16.2.5 Conclusions

TFF is an excellent choice when it comes to reducing the volume of lysates, replacing large amounts of salts (especially present in the case of alkaline lysis) and removing the smaller *E. coli* components (e.g., proteins and tRNA). In general, the plasmid yields are high (around 80–100%) if an adequate compromise can be made between the membrane pore size, the plasmid DNA size, and the plasmid concentration in the lysate. The main drawback of TFF is its inability to remove the larger-molecular-weight RNA species. Thus, the use of TFF in the intermediate recovery stage should always be combined with unit operations (performed before or after) more apt to clear impurities like mRNA and rRNA, which have sizes of the same order of magnitude than plasmids. For these reasons, and as we will see later on in Chapter 17 (Section 17.3), TFF is especially useful as a final concentration/buffer exchange step.

16.3 PRECIPITATION

16.3.1 Introduction

Precipitation is a relatively simple and inexpensive, but effective, separation technique often used by molecular biologists in plasmid isolation protocols. This unit operation is also commonly used at a large scale in the downstream processing of plasmid DNA, especially in the intermediate recovery stage. The operation typically involves the addition of a precipitating agent, which decreases the solubility of solutes down to a point where self-association of molecules, aggregation, and precipitation set in. Alternatively, precipitation can also be promoted by adding agents that associate intimately with the solute, forming insoluble complexes. From a molecular point of view, the first process can be described in very simple terms by the DLVO theory (named after Derjaguin, Landau, Verwey, and Overbeek) as follows.[16] Charged biomolecules (e.g., proteins and nucleic acids) in solution are typically surrounded by a double layer of counterions, co-ions, and water molecules. The first innermost layer (known as the Stern layer) is very thin and contains rigidly attached counterions and water molecules. A larger layer (known as the diffuse layer) develops past the Stern layer, which contains nonoriented water molecules, a decreasing concentration of counterions, and an increasing concentration of co-ions. The diffuse layer extends up to a point where the amount of counter- and co-ions is the same as the one observed in the bulk solution. The mobility of the ions in the diffuse layer increases progressively as we move away from the solute surface. The locus where the counterions stop moving in harmony with the solute is known as the shear plane and is characterized by an electrical potential called the zeta potential.[16] In a normal situation, the rigidly attached counterions surrounding a molecule originate intensive repulsive forces that, alongside the hydration layers, contribute to maintain individual molecules apart from each other in solution. These electrostatic forces are opposed by van der Waals dispersive forces of the Keesom, Debye, and London type, which tend to bring solutes together. In a low-ionic-strength solution, the repulsive forces predominate and act as an activation energy barrier, which prevents individual solute molecules from aggregating. The role of a precipitating agent is precisely to destabilize this balance of attractive and repulsive forces.[16] Although the exact mechanism at play will depend on the characteristics of the specific compound used (e.g., alcohols, surfactants, hydrophilic polymers, and salts), the net result is the self-association of the individual molecules of the solutes we wish to precipitate into successively larger clusters, and up to a point where very small particles start to nucleate and show up in solution. During the initial stages of the process, these microparticles combine with each other by Brownian diffusion, forming larger aggregates—this process is called perikinetic aggregation. Mixing promotes further collision and aggregation of these primary aggregates into flocks, a process known as orthokinetic aggregation.[16] If the intensity of mixing is adequately controlled, these flocks will eventually become large and dense enough so as to settle by gravity. More commonly, operations like filtration and centrifugation will be used to speed up this solid–liquid separation once precipitation is complete. Major goals for precipitation in the current context are to concentrate the plasmid product and/or to remove impurities. In the first case, agents that precipitate the plasmid are used, whereas in the second situation, the focus is on the "negative" precipitation of RNA, gDNA, proteins, and LPS. The most important options available to precipitate plasmids and impurities are described in some detail in the next sections of this chapter.

16.3.2   Concentration

Plasmid concentration by precipitation is commonly performed with agents such as ethanol, 2-propanol (isopropanol),[17,18] polyethylene glycol (PEG),[19] cetyltrimethylammonium bromide (CTAB),[20] or spermidine.[21] By resuspending the plasmid precipitate in a buffer volume that is smaller than the volume of the starting solution, a concentration effect is obtained. The removal of unprecipitated low-molecular-weight nucleic acids and other impurities, together with the possibility of resuspending the precipitates in a buffer that is different from the original one, is an additional advantage of plasmid precipitation.

16.3.2.1   Alcohols

The strategy used to promote precipitation by alcohols such as isopropanol and ethanol relies on the reduction of the free water molecules that are responsible for the solvation of plasmid molecules. In an alcohol-free solution, these water molecules are distributed more or less evenly throughout the plasmid surface (see Chapter 4, Section 4.2.3). The addition of a water-miscible, polar organic solvent like isopropanol to such an aqueous solution reduces the dielectric constant of the medium and thus the ability of water molecules to solvate solutes. The concomitant removal of the solvation water molecules from the plasmid surface reveals hydrophobic patches (i.e., the bases) that can then mediate the spontaneous aggregation of molecules via van der Waals interactions. The simultaneous removal of water molecules from the vicinity of the charged phosphate groups is not favorable to this intramolecular association of plasmid molecules due to repulsion between the polyanionic DNA chains. Nonetheless, this repulsion can be effectively decreased if large amounts of salts are added to the solution to provide for sufficient counterions to shield the negatively charged phosphates. This favors condensation, aggregation, and precipitation of nucleic acids.[22,23] The recommendation to add ammonium acetate up to 300 mM prior to precipitating plasmids from low-ionic-strength solutions, which is often found in molecular biology protocols, is directly related to this beneficial effect of salt on alcohol-induced plasmid aggregation. This extra addition of salt is, however, not required when precipitating plasmids out of alkaline lysates, since the salt concentration in these is already very high (~1.0 M potassium acetate; see Chapter 15, Section 15.3.2). The presence of alcohols can at the same time induce structural changes in the plasmid molecule (e.g., B to A transition, bending, and unwounding), which may be conducive to aggregation.[22]

The effectiveness of precipitation increases with the increase in the concentration of the alcohol used. This effect is observed in Figure 16.4, which displays an agarose gel electrophoresis analysis of the effect of isopropanol

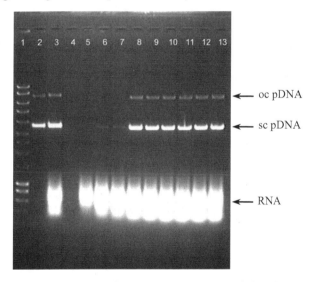

Figure 16.4 *The use of alcohol precipitation in the processing of plasmid-containing streams. Precipitation of a 6000-bp plasmid from alkaline lysates is promoted by the addition of isopropanol. The agarose gel analysis presented shows the effect of isopropanol concentration. Lane 1, molecular weight marker; lane 2, plasmid standard; lane 3, lysate; lanes 4–13, samples obtained after isopropanol precipitation at 0.1–1.0 (v/v), with 0.1 (v/v) increments. The precipitates formed were separated by centrifugation, resuspended in buffer, and analyzed by electrophoresis. oc, open circle; sc, supercoiled. Reprinted from Biotechnology Progress, 22, Freitas SS, Santos JA, Prazeres DMF. Optimization of isopropanol and ammonium sulfate precipitation steps in the purification of plasmid DNA, 1179–1186, Copyright 2006,[18] with permission from John Wiley & Sons.*

concentration on the precipitation of a 6100-bp plasmid from an alkaline lysate.[18] Following a 15-min precipitation at 4°C with the isopropanol concentration indicated, and a solid–liquid separation by centrifugation (30 min, 4°C), the precipitated material was resuspended in a fixed volume of buffer. Analysis of these samples clearly shows that the use of lower amounts of alcohol only precipitates RNA. For this specie, the onset of precipitation was observed for a 0.2 v/v concentration of isopropanol (lane 5, Figure 16.4), and maximum precipitation was obtained for concentrations higher than ~0.7 v/v (lane 10, Figure 16.4). As the isopropanol concentration is increased past 0.4 v/v (lane 7), plasmid molecules start precipitating up to a point where most of them have left the solution. In the case described, and under the conditions used to maximize plasmid precipitation (>0.6 v/v isopropanol), around 40% of the lysate impurities remained in the supernatant.[18] Since most RNA coprecipitates with plasmid, as is visible in the gel of Figure 16.4, most of the nonprecipitated impurities must be protein, gDNA, or LPS.

Experimental results also show that the concentration of plasmid in the starting lysate strongly affects precipitation. When starting from lysates that are more concentrated in plasmid, lower concentrations of isopropanol are required to trigger precipitation, and the alcohol-induced aggregation of plasmid molecules is more efficient. Thus, higher recoveries that are close to 100% are typically obtained when plasmid concentration in lysates exceeds 100 μg/mL.[18] The fact that RNA precipitation is set off at smaller isopropanol concentrations when compared with plasmid DNA can be attributed on one end to the higher concentration of RNA in the lysate (check the relative intensities of RNA and plasmid bands in lane 3, Figure 16.4). Additionally, the larger exposure of the hydrophobic bases in the single-stranded RNA to the surrounding environment, when compared with the double-stranded plasmid DNA, probably favors hydrophobic and stacking intermolecule interactions, and thus the earlier aggregation and precipitation of RNA.[18] The data in Figure 16.4 also support the use of isopropanol as a means to separate a fraction of RNA from plasmids by a selective precipitation of the former. A process can thus be envisaged where a first RNA precipitation at low alcohol concentration is followed by a second plasmid precipitation at a higher alcohol concentration.

Few would argue that plasmid precipitation with ethanol and isopropanol is not very effective at the laboratorial scale. However, the implementation of such alcohol precipitation at a large scale is problematic and can increase processing costs significantly. Major reasons for these difficulties are the need to maintain a closely controlled, low temperature (−20°C) in order to obtain reproducible results and the safety imperative of using explosion proof tanks and processing areas. Furthermore, an environmental analysis of a specific overall plasmid manufacturing process has highlighted isopropanol as one of the materials with the highest environmental impact.[24] This impact results from the generation of very large volumes of isopropanol-containing hazardous liquid waste, which must be adequately disposed of.[25] Additionally, both ethanol and isopropanol are currently produced from nonrenewable sources (i.e., oil), a characteristic that negatively impacts the desired sustainability of the process.

16.3.2.2 *Surfactants*

The precipitation of plasmid molecules by the cationic surfactant CTAB was originally described by Ishaqu et al. as an alternative to miniprep, plasmid isolation protocols.[26] Subsequently, the use of CTAB and of surfactants like tetradecyl trimethyl ammonium bromide (TTAB) and ethyl hexadecyl dimethylammonium bromide (EDAB) in the context of the large-scale purification of plasmid biopharmaceuticals was developed by other researchers.[20,27-29] For example, Lander and coworkers described that plasmids in *E. coli* lysates generated by heat/detergent lysis could be selectively precipitated from proteins, RNA, and LPS by adding increasing amounts of CTAB.[20] The precipitation profiles obtained in that study show that plasmids will start precipitating from the solution at a CTAB concentration that depends not only on the concentration of the plasmid in the starting lysate but also on the amount of the Triton X-100 detergent used in the heat lysis method. From this critical CTAB concentration on, very small amounts need to be added to fully precipitate plasmid. Additionally, a precise control of the CTAB concentration before the onset of plasmid precipitation makes it possible to selectively precipitate gDNA ($\approx 100\%$), open circle (50%), and linear (80%) isoforms in advance of supercoiled isoforms.[20] This remarkable selectivity is uncommon for a precipitation process and is truly one of the key advantages of CTAB precipitation. When a CTAB concentration sufficient to precipitate most supercoiled plasmid DNA is used, a precipitate that is up to 90% pure can be obtained. Further purification is attainable by controlling the exact concentration of the NaCl solution used to resuspend this precipitate. Since gDNA fragments in the precipitate are less soluble than plasmid DNA, if the NaCl concentration does not exceed a certain value, the purity of the dissolved plasmid can reach 99% and more.[20]

The mechanisms underlying plasmid precipitation by CTAB involve the interaction of backbone phosphates with the cationic detergent molecules and the subsequent stabilization of those contacts by hydrophobic interactions between adjacent alkyl tails of bound CTAB molecules. The fact that molecules with a more flexible nature like gDNA and open circle isoforms can be precipitated before supercoiled plasmids also suggests that hydrophobic interactions depend on conformational effects.[20] Further insights into the precipitation mechanism were gained on the basis of another study that showed that the components precipitated by cationic surfactants depend on the length of the hydrophobic alkyl chain and on the size of the cationic head of the surfactant.[27] More specifically, larger amounts of surfactants that have shorter tails are required to promote precipitation when compared with surfactants that have larger tails. This observation supports the idea that hydrophobic interactions between adjacent surfactant molecules (which are stronger in larger molecules) play an important role in the formation of surfactant/plasmid aggregates.[27]

16.3.2.3 Polymers

The ability of polyethylene glycol (PEG) to precipitate double-stranded DNA has been known for many years. Already in 1975, Lis and Schleif produced a study showing that DNA molecules of differing molecular masses could be separated by selective precipitation with a PEG with a molecular weight of 6000 Da (PEG$_{6000}$).[30] The implementation of the method at the laboratorial scale is straightforward and typically involves the addition of a given amount of PEG (as a solid, as a pure liquid, or as an aqueous solution), mixing, and incubation at low temperature (usually 0–4°C) for a certain period of time. The method takes advantage of the fact that larger DNA molecules precipitate at lower PEG concentrations when compared with smaller DNA molecules. The efficiency of precipitation is affected both by the DNA and NaCl concentration in the initial solution.

PEG precipitation has been included in a number of protocols designed to purify plasmids for molecular biology applications like ligation, electrotransformation, and sequencing.[31–34] For example, plasmids can be directly precipitated from an alkaline lysate by adding PEG$_{6000}$ and NaCl up to concentrations of 6–10% and 500 mM, respectively.[33] Following centrifugation and discarding of the supernatant, the plasmid-containing sediments are washed with ethanol and dissolved in a volume of an adequate buffer. The purity of the plasmids thus obtained is sufficient for most molecular biology applications.[33] PEG is often used in a tandem combination with a previous or with a subsequent high-salt precipitation step. As described in the next section, the addition of a salt like CaCl$_2$ or ammonium acetate is able to selectively promote the salting out of impurities like RNA and LPS from plasmid solutions.

Apart from its usefulness at the laboratorial scale, and more importantly in the present context, the PEG precipitation technique was also developed and adapted for the large-scale purification of plasmid biopharmaceuticals.[19,25,35] As in the case of minipreps, the salt concentration should be adjusted (usually with NaCl) to a value that maximizes the extent of precipitation. One option involves the direct addition of a PEG with a suitable molecular weight (e.g., in the 6000- to 10,000-Da range) to alkaline lysates. In one example, PEG$_{8000}$ and NaCl were added to a clarified alkaline lysate so as to bring the corresponding concentrations up to 10% w/v and ~270 mM, respectively. Following an overnight incubation, the plasmid precipitate was recovered and dissolved in an adequate buffer.[25] With this approach, and if the PEG concentration is adequate, a large proportion of the plasmid precipitates, leaving impurities like small-molecular-weight RNA and proteins behind. In another case, a 10% PEG$_{8000}$ precipitation was included later in a process, after processing clarified alkaline lysates by 0.6 v/v isopropanol and 2.5 M ammonium acetate precipitation, and prior to a size-exclusion chromatography step.[19] The step not only concentrated the plasmid and reduced RNA content but also contributed to enhance the resolution of chromatography. In another alternative, the ability of the method to separate DNA molecules that differ in molecular weight, is explored by using two PEG precipitation steps in tandem.[25] These two steps are performed after a clarification of alkaline lysates with ammonium acetate. In the first low-cut precipitation, a smaller PEG concentration (~4% w/v) is used so that only the large gDNA fragments precipitate. After the solid–liquid separation of the settled impurities, a high-cut precipitation is performed by adding PEG up to a concentration (~10% w/v) that is sufficient to bring down plasmids out of the solution.

At the molecular level, precipitation of gDNA fragments and plasmid molecules by PEG involves a first step of condensation of the elongated DNA molecules into a more compact globular structure. The transition from the first state (coil) to the second state (globule) is discrete and depends both on the molecular weight and the concentration of PEG.[36] The swollen coil conformation is characteristically observed at low PEG concentrations, wherein a regime of "good compatibility" between PEG and DNA exists. Under these conditions, the flexible PEG polymer chains can penetrate freely inside the DNA and no condensation is observed. If more PEG is added, however, the solvent quality for DNA becomes poorer and the effective attraction between DNA segments within the macromolecule increases. At a certain point, a discrete transition occurs when the DNA coil contracts abruptly to form a compact globular structure. In this regime of "perfect incompatibility," there is segregation between DNA and PEG chains. The critical PEG concentration at which this jumplike transition occurs is lower for larger PEG molecular weights. Another variable that influences the PEG critical concentration is the concentration of counterions in the media. As in the case of the alcohol precipitation described earlier, the role of the counterions is to shield the backbone phosphate groups and thus to facilitate the approximation of the segments of the DNA chains, which is inherent to the formation of a globular structure.

A number of advantages make the use of PEG precipitation attractive. First, PEGs are generally regarded as safe (GRAS) reagents (see Chapter 14, Section 14.1). They are often used in biopharmaceutical production, both as mass-separating agents and as excipients. The inclusion of the substance in a production process should therefore pose no problems from a regulatory point of view. Furthermore, the handling, storage, and disposal of PEG are less problematic when compared with the more hazardous and toxic plasmid precipitants ethanol or isopropanol.

16.3.2.4 *Polycations*

Another way of precipitating plasmid molecules is to add highly charged, linear cationic polymers to the solution. The charge in these polymers is conferred by groups (e.g., quaternary amino groups), which are found either as a part of the polymer chain (integral polycations) or attached as substituents to the chain (pendant polycations).[37] These molecules bind to the anionic plasmid molecule via electrostatic interactions, forming complexes that may become insoluble if the correct concentrations of plasmid and cationic polymer are used. After the solid–liquid separation, the plasmid–polycation complexes can be redissolved in a solution with a salt concentration sufficiently high to break the complex apart. An example of a polycation that has been used to precipitate plasmids from *E. coli* lysates is poly(N, N′-dimethyl diallyl ammonium) chloride (PDMDAAC). This polymer presents a molecular weight-to-charge ratio of 160. In the process described and patented by Galaev and coworkers,[37,38] the clarified alkaline lysates are pretreated with a zeolite material before being subjected to polycation precipitation. The addition of this solid adsorbent is important to remove sodium dodecyl sulfate (SDS), which is carried over from the alkaline lysis step, since this cationic detergent interferes with the polycation precipitation by competing for plasmid binding.[37,38] Following the removal of the zeolite adsorbent, PDMDAAC is added in such a way as to neutralize all charges in the plasmid and to form stoichiometric insoluble complexes. The PDMDAAC polycation also interacts with the polyanionic RNA impurities in the lysate. However, a series of studies have shown that the complexes formed with the double-stranded plasmids are stronger and more stable when compared with the complexes formed with RNA. It is thus possible to selectively precipitate substantial amounts of plasmid (75–80%) out from a lysate, which contains high amounts of potassium acetate salt, while leaving most RNA (>95%) and proteins (~90%) in solution. The recovered complexes are then redissolved in a 2 M NaCl solution. Since under this high salt concentration the interaction between plasmid and polycation is minimum, size-exclusion chromatography can be used to separate the two polymers.[37,38]

16.3.2.5 Compaction Agents

A number of small, cationic molecules have the ability to interact intimately with double-stranded DNA by a combination of mechanisms, which include neutralization of backbone phosphates and binding to the minor or major grooves. These interactions reduce the repulsion between DNA molecules, effectively promoting the bridging of adjacent helixes. In the case of plasmids, this intermolecule approximation ultimately leads to aggregation and precipitation. The natural compounds hexamine cobalt, spermidine, and spermine are the best known examples of such compaction agents. The amount of compaction agent required to precipitate plasmids will depend on the ionic strength of the solution. Since pre-existing cations compete with the cationic compaction molecules for DNA binding, larger concentrations are typically required if salts like NaCl are present.[21] Following precipitation, compaction agents in the plasmid pellet can be washed away with specific solutions (e.g., 50% v/v isopropanol, 600 mM NaCl, 10 mM MgCl$_2$, and 25 mM ethylenediamine tetraacetic acid (EDTA)[21]) prior to resuspension in an adequate buffer. A number of attempts have been made to implement the use of compaction agents in the selective precipitation of plasmid DNA from alkaline lysates.[21,39] The strategy is similar to the one used with other precipitants—a certain amount of a given compaction agent is added to the process stream that precipitates plasmids while leaving impurities like RNA in solution. For example, compaction precipitation with spermidine was included in a full process designed to purify plasmid DNA at the gram scale.[21] However, the operation was performed only after a number of steps (alkaline lysis, Celite filtration, isopropanol precipitation, $LiCl_2$ precipitation, and isopropanol precipitation) were carried out. By using a 2.9 mM concentration of spermidine, the percentage of plasmid DNA increased from 2% in the feed solution to 99% in the solution obtained after resuspension of the precipitated material. It should be stressed, however, that not all compaction agents are able to offer such an extensive and selective removal of RNA from plasmid solutions.

16.3.2.6 Affinity Precipitation

One way to increase the selectivity of precipitation is to explore the formation of affinity complexes between plasmid molecules and specific ligands bound to polymers. Although the first counterargument against the utilization of such a technique at a process scale is the lack of cost-effectiveness, the concept behind affinity precipitation is elegant and thus briefly illustrated here with the specific example described by Costioli et al.[40] The methodology proposed uses affinity macroligands, which are synthesized by linking a thermoresponsive N-isopropylacrylamide (pNIPAM) oligomer to short, single-stranded polypyrimidine sequences. A key property of the pNIPAM thermoresponsive polymer, which is explored to drive precipitation, is that its solubility decreases dramatically if the temperature of the solution is increased past a certain threshold value called the critical solution temperature (CST). On the other hand, the oligonucleotide sequences in the macroligand are designed in such a way as to recognize and form a triple-helical structure with a double-stranded region in the target plasmid (see Chapter 4, Section 4.4.6). In the work mentioned, a 21-bp-long sequence composed of seven repetitions of the CTT trinucleotide was used as the affinity tag. At the same time, the corresponding triple-helix binding motif was inserted in the plasmid.[40] The C and T bases in the tag are able to form triplets of the T·A•T and C+·G•C type, respectively, via Hoogsteen hydrogen bonding to A and G (see Chapter 4, Figure 4.11a). The fact that protonation of the cytosine (i.e., pH < 5) in the affinity tag is required for the formation of a stable triplex means that the pH can be used to control the interaction between the tag and the plasmid. The salt concentration is also a critical variable in the process. This implies that in order for the process to be successfully implemented, a buffer exchange step needs to be performed first to adjust the conditions of the plasmid-containing solution to those that maximize binding (e.g., pH 4.5, 2 M NaCl). Once this is done, the affinity macroligand is added and mixed at 4°C, a temperature that is below the CST of the polymer.[40] The stable plasmid–macroligand complexes formed are then precipitated out from the solution by increasing the temperature past the CST, to approximately 40°C. After the solid–liquid separation, the complexes can be redissolved at low temperature and the triplex is destroyed by shifting the pH to slightly alkaline conditions (pH 9.0). According to the proponents, a highly pure plasmid is obtained with yields in the 70–90% range.[40]

16.3.3   Negative Precipitation

16.3.3.1 Salting Out

The salt-induced precipitation of biomolecules is strongly dependent on the type and concentration of the salt used. Whenever a salt is added to an aqueous solution of a given biological solute, it dissociates into ions that become hydrated by a number of water molecules whose number depend on the size and charge of the ion. This process of ion hydration potentially leads to a change in the solute solubility. If small amounts of salt are added, the solubility of the solute may actually increase. This effect is known as salting in.[41] However, the addition of more salt past a certain limit will promote the intermolecular aggregation of solutes, reducing solubility and eventually leading to precipitation once a certain threshold concentration is reached. This effect is known as salting out, and the main driving force behind solute aggregation is hydrophobic interaction.[41] Salting out also plays an important role in other biomolecule separation processes, namely, aqueous two-phase extraction (see Section 16.4) and hydrophobic interaction chromatography (HIC) (see Chapter 17, Section 17.2.6). The addition of ions and their subsequent hydration affects both the structure of bulk water and the hydration layers that surround biomolecules. In order to adequately understand these effects, one should start by recognizing that the extensive network of hydrogen bonds among water molecules, which turns water into a highly structured liquid, is perturbed whenever ions are added.[42] The size and surface charge density of a group of ions, known as kosmotropic or antichaotropic ions, makes them prone to strong hydration. These "water structure-maker" ions effectively compete with ionic groups in the biomolecules, sequestering water molecules away from the hydration layer. The net result is that biomolecules will tend to self-associate as their hydration decreases, essentially via hydrophobic interactions between poorly hydrophilic regions. Small or multiply charged ions with high charge density like SO_4^{2-} and HPO_4^{2-} constitute examples of kosmotropic ions commonly used to "salt" biomolecules out of solution. Unlike kosmotropic ions, other ions display a poor affinity for water molecules and rather tend to break the structure of water by creating a cavity in the liquid where they can accommodate themselves. These so-called chaotropic ions interfere little with the hydration shell of biomolecules, thus displaying a poor ability to promote self-association and aggregation. Large, singly charged ions with low charge density like NO_3^- constitute an example of a chaotropic ion. The so-called Hofmeister series orders ions from strongly to weakly hydrated, mainly on the basis of their surface charge density and water affinity (Figure 16.5). The series offers a convenient way to anticipate the effects of a given salt on the solubility of biomolecules in aqueous solutions.[43] The salting-out effectiveness of a salt is dominated by

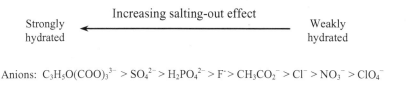

Anions: $C_3H_5O(COO)_3^{3-} > SO_4^{2-} > H_2PO_4^{2-} > F^- > CH_3CO_2^- > Cl^- > NO_3^- > ClO_4^-$

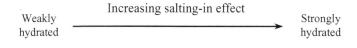

Cations: $N(CH_3)_4^+ > NH_4^+ > K^+ > Na^+ > H^+ > Ca^{2+} > Mg^{2+} > Al^{3+}$

Figure 16.5 *The Hofmeister series. Anions and cations are ordered in terms of their water affinity and according to their effects on the solubility of macromolecules in aqueous solutions.*

the properties of the anions and typically manifests itself around 1 M concentration.[42] One important advantage of salt precipitation of impurities is that it can serve simultaneously as a conditioning step if HIC is to be performed next (see Chapter 17, Section 17.2.6).

Precipitation with antichaotropic salts has been used extensively as a means to remove large fractions of impurities (proteins, LPS, gDNA, and higher-molecular-weight RNA) from lysates and other plasmid-containing solutions. Examples of salts commonly used for this purpose include ammonium sulfate,[17,18] ammonium acetate,[19] calcium chloride,[34,44,45] sodium citrate,[46] tripo-tassium acetate,[45] and sodium sulfate.[45] Although lithium chloride is also a common choice in some plasmid isolation protocols, its inherent toxicity deters bioprocess engineers from using it in a plasmid biopharmaceutical purification scheme.[34] The kosmotropic nature of ammonium sulfate, together with its high solubility (>4 M), has made it one of the favorite salts for protein and nucleic acid precipitation. Furthermore, this salt is able to selectively precipitate RNA from plasmid DNA. This is exemplified in Figure 16.6, which displays an agarose gel electrophoresis analysis of the effect of ammonium sulfate concentration on the precipitation of RNA and plasmid DNA. The salting out was performed at 4°C after the precipitation of nucleic acids in a neutralized lysate with 0.7 (v/v) isopropanol and their subsequent resuspension in 10 mM tris(hydroxymethyl)aminomethane (tris)–HCl buffer (pH 8.0). The key observation made from Figure 16.6 is that substantial amounts of RNA precipitate once ammonium sulfate concentrations higher than 2 M (lane 7) are used, while plasmid molecules remain in solution for the most part. This selectivity is intimately connected to the fact that plasmid DNA has a lower hydrophobicity when compared with single-stranded RNA (and gDNA) because aromatic bases are mostly buried inside the double helix.[18] This means that the

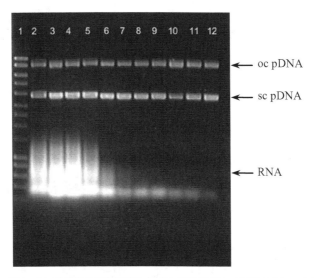

Figure 16.6 *The use of salt precipitation in the processing of plasmid-containing streams. Precipitation of impurities is promoted by the addition and solubilization of solid ammonium sulfate to a plasmid solution obtained following precipitation of nucleic acids in a neutralized lysate with 0.7 (v/v) isopropanol and subsequent resuspension in a 10 mM tris–HCl buffer (pH 8.0). The precipitate formed was separated by centrifugation, and the supernatant was analyzed by electrophoresis. The agarose gel analysis presented shows the effect of ammonium sulfate concentration. Lane 1, molecular weight marker; lane 2, plasmid solution prior to precipitation; lanes 3–12, samples obtained after after ammonium sulfate precipitation at 0.4–4.0 M, with 0.4 M increments. oc, open circle; sc, supercoiled. Reprinted from Biotechnology Progress, 22, Freitas SS, Santos JA, Prazeres DMF. Optimization of isopropanol and ammonium sulfate precipitation steps in the purification of plasmid DNA, 1179–1186, Copyright 2006,[18] with permission from John Wiley & Sons.*

self-association of plasmid molecules via base-mediated hydrophobic interaction is not as favorable as it is in the case of RNA. Plasmid recovery yields higher than 95% are typically associated with ammonium sulfate precipitation.[45,46] In some cases, however, it is not uncommon to observe a drop in plasmid recovery yields as the ammonium sulfate concentration is increased. A possible explanation for this is the coprecipitation of plasmid DNA with impurities, most likely as a result of the salt-promoted base exposure of some bases in the plasmid molecules.[18] The addition of ammonium sulfate is also an excellent means to reduce impurities other than RNA. For example, substantial reduction in protein (>70%) and gDNA (>88%) content can be obtained when using 1.0–2.5 M ammonium sulfate,[46] with clearance being more effective at higher concentrations (Figure 16.7). A four-order-of-magnitude removal of LPS has also been reported when using ammonium sulfate precipitation.[17,47] Overall, if the adequate ammonium salt concentration is used, more than 90% of the impurities can be removed with minimum loss of plasmid.[18]

Despite its popularity, the use of sulfate-based salts in the process-scale precipitation (and also in the aqueous two-phase extraction and HIC) of bio-

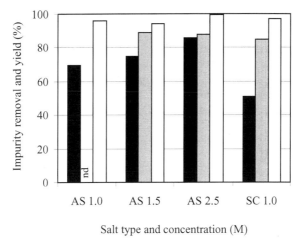

Figure 16.7 *Effect of salt type and concentration on the precipitation of genomic DNA and protein from plasmid-containing solutions. Nucleic acids in a neutralized lysate were precipitated with 0.7 (v/v) isopropanol and were subsequently resuspended in a 10 mM tris–HCl buffer (pH 8.0). The salting out of impurities was then performed at 4°C by adding solid ammonium sulfate (AS) or sodium citrate (SC). Data were extracted from Freitas et al. nd, not determined.[46]*

molecules brings with it an important environmental impact. This impact results from the fact that ammonium sulfate has a high eutrophication potential and is therefore difficult to dispose of. This is further complicated by the fact that large amounts of ammonium sulfate are used, since precipitation is usually carried out at very high concentrations (>1 M). Other more environmentally friendly salts, which also perform well in terms of impurity precipitation when added to resuspended sediments obtained after isopropanol precipitation of alkaline lysates, are ammonium acetate (at 2.5 M[19]) and sodium citrate (at 1.0 M[46]). In the later case, the plasmid yield and reduction in protein and gDNA content are comparable to those obtained with ammonium sulfate (Figure 16.7). Another popular salt used in the context of the precipitation of impurities from plasmid-containing streams is calcium chloride. An important advantage in this case, when compared with the salting-out operations described earlier, is that calcium chloride can be added directly to neutralized lysates. One literature report has described that when used at a 1.0 M concentration, calcium chloride can precipitate most RNA (84.6%), protein (95.8%), gDNA (98.0%), and LPS (91.0%) within a very short incubation period (10 min) at room temperature while guaranteeing plasmid yields close to 100%.[45]

16.3.4 Conclusions

The controlled addition of specific precipitants to plasmid-containing solutions is extensively used in the context of plasmid purification. Depending on the exact precipitating agent used, the key benefits offered by the unit operation may include plasmid concentration, selective separation of impurities, and adequate conditioning for subsequent unit operations. At the same time, some important drawbacks may be ascribed to precipitation. First, high costs are associated with most of the equipment items necessary to implement precipitation at a large scale (e.g., Nutsche filters, centrifuges, and tanks). Furthermore, extensive manpower is usually required during operation.[3] Finally, the redissolution of plasmid-containing sediments may be difficult to accomplish.[45]

16.4   LIQUID–LIQUID EXTRACTION

16.4.1   Introduction

Many of the earlier protocols used to isolate plasmids for molecular biology applications relied on liquid–liquid extraction with solvents like phenol, chloroform, and isoamyl alcohol as a means to remove RNA from lysates. By exploring the differential partitioning of plasmids and impurities between two immiscible phases, plasmid solutions could be stripped of most of the impurities. Despite their effectiveness, these processes are clearly incompatible with the safety and GMP standards required for plasmid biopharmaceuticals, mostly due to the toxic nature of the solvents involved (see Chapter 11, Section 11.6.1). Clearly, in order for a liquid–liquid extraction step to be acceptable in the first place, the phase-forming agents should be replaced by materials with an unquestionable safety profile. Many water-soluble polymers and a series of salts meet these requirements. Furthermore, the addition of adequate amounts of these compounds to an aqueous solution results in an ATPS that can be explored for separation purposes. A substantial number of reports have demonstrated that liquid–liquid extraction with these ATPSs is able to separate impurities in *E. coli* lysates from the target plasmid molecules.

The first experiments describing the partitioning of nucleic acids between two immiscible aqueous phases were described in 1962 by Albertsson, who reported that dextran–PEG systems could discriminate between double-stranded, native DNA and single-stranded, heat-denatured DNA and RNA.[48] The preference of single-stranded nucleic acids for the dextran-rich bottom phase was then attributed to a favorable configuration (random coil) and greater exposure of the bases to the surrounding environment. The ionic composition and polymer concentration were also identified at the time as important factors for the partitioning of nucleic acids.[48,49] Years later, Ohlsson et al. described a method whereby plasmid DNA in a solution prepared by Triton X-100 lysis, phenol and chloroform–isoamyl alcohol extraction, and ethanol precipitation could be separated from denatured gDNA and RNA in an ATPS.[50] The procedure involved a rapid heat denaturation (100°C) of the mixture and a short reannealing period (4°C), followed by extraction in a dextran$_{500}$–PEG$_{600}$ system. These preliminary steps are designed to take advantage of the rapid reannealing of plasmid upon cooling, which is characteristic of closed DNA molecules. gDNA fragments, on the contrary, are not able to reanneal correctly and thus remain denatured for the most part. After extraction in the PEG–dextran system, the reannealed, double-stranded plasmid partitions to the top PEG-rich phase, whereas the single-stranded RNA and denatured gDNA remain in the bottom dextran-rich phase.[50] In 1991, an alternative PEG-based ATPS, in which the second polymer (dextran) was replaced for a salt, was proposed for plasmid isolation.[51] By adequately manipulating conditions, nucleic acids could be directed toward the lower, salt-rich phase, while proteins, cellular debris, and other constituents remained in the upper, polymer-rich phase or were precipitated at the interphase region.[51] These reports, however, were not sufficient to spur the interest in the use of ATPS for plasmid purification, even in spite of the claims made by the proponents regarding the simplicity and rapidity of the method.[50,51] The context in which plasmid isolation was studied took a turn with the advent of nonviral gene transfer and plasmid biopharmaceuticals. Thus, from 2000 onward, serious consideration began being taken on the use of aqueous two-phase extraction for the process-scale isolation of plasmids.[52–59] The most important findings and developments in the area are described next.

16.4.2 Polymer–Salt Systems

ATPSs based on mixtures of PEG and salts are probably the most successful ones when it comes to the liquid–liquid separation of plasmids from *E. coli* impurities. As described in several publications, the typical operation involves the mixture of defined amounts of PEG (as a solid, as a pure liquid, or as a solution), salt, and water with a given volume of a clarified lysate (Figure 16.8). Though alkaline lysates were used in all cases reported in the literature, in principle, nothing precludes the use of such PEG–salt systems with lysates prepared by alternative methods. Once mixing is halted, a separation process starts whereby a denser salt-rich phase forms at the bottom of the vessel and a lighter PEG-rich phase accumulates on the top. Centrifugation is usually used to accelerate phase separation, but gravity settling works as well, provided that sufficient time is allowed to elapse. In order for two phases to form, the amounts of PEG and salt in the system must be higher than certain critical values. In a PEG versus salt concentration plot like the one schematized in Figure 16.8, these experimentally obtained critical concentrations are given by a curved line known as the binodal. Above this line, any set of PEG–salt concentration will originate two phases. The composition of the top and bottom phases thus obtained can be plotted in the diagram shown with the aid of a line segment known as the tie-line, which joins two points in the binodal with the point that marks the overall composition of the system. It is important to remark that components which are added to the system with the feed may affect the localization of both the binodal and tie-lines. This is especially so

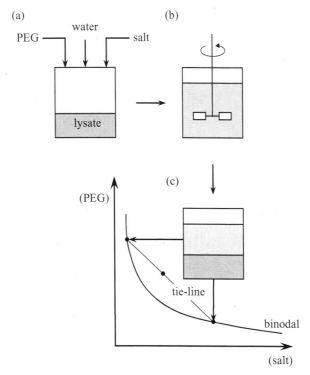

Figure 16.8 *Purification of plasmids in alkaline lysates by aqueous two-phase extraction. The operation involves, for example, (a) the addition of adequate amounts of polyethylene glycol (PEG), salt, and water to the lysate; (b) mixing of the components; and (c) phase separation (e.g., by gravity settling or centrifugation).*

with alkaline lysates since these contain high amounts of salts (~1.0 M potassium acetate) among other components.

The partitioning of plasmids and impurities in PEG–salt systems is critically dependent on the polymer molecular weight. This effect is exemplified in Figure 16.9, which presents an agarose gel electrophoresis analysis of the top and bottom phases obtained by mixing alkaline lysates (loaded at 40% w/w) containing a 8500-bp plasmid with PEGs of different molecular weights (200–8000) and with K_2HPO_4.[53] From the gel, it is clear that the plasmid partitions preferentially to the top phase when the PEG molecular weight is lower than 400, whereas the bottom phase is preferred for larger PEGs. Agarose gel analysis of the interphase material confirmed that in all systems, a certain amount of plasmid and RNA is lost to the interphase. The yields obtained with PEG molecular weights of 300, 600, and 1000, were 39, 42, and 100%, respectively. The highest plasmid loss was observed for the PEG_{400} transition system. The improvements in purity were also considerable.

The partition of biological macromolecules in PEG–salt systems is determined mainly by the salting-out ability of the salt phase and by the exclusion

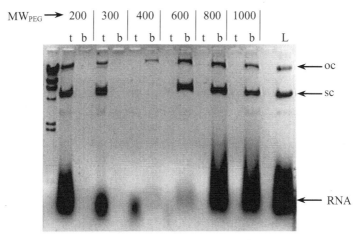

Figure 16.9 *The effect of polymer molecular weight on the partitioning of plasmid and RNA from clarified alkaline lysates in PEG–K₂HPO₄ systems. A 40% (w/w) lysate load was used and PEG–salt concentrations were as follows: PEG₂₀₀ (20%/20% w/w), PEG₃₀₀ (20%/20% w/w), PEG₄₀₀ (20%/20% w/w), PEG₆₀₀ (20%/20% w/w), PEG₁₀₀₀ (15%/13% w/w), and PEG₈₀₀₀ (10%/10% w/w). Reprinted from Biotechnology and Bioengineering, 78, Ribeiro SC, Monteiro GA, Cabral JM, Prazeres DMF. Isolation of plasmid DNA from cell lysates by aqueous two-phase systems, 376–384, Copyright 2002,[53] with permission from John Wiley & Sons.*

limit of the polymer phase. The salt phase is characterized by the presence of a large amount of ions, which sequester substantial amounts of water molecules used for solvation. As we have seen in the previous section (Section 16.3.1), if the type and concentration of salt is appropriate, this leads to a decrease in the hydration of biomolecules. In view of this energetically unfavorable situation, biomolecules may self-associate and precipitate, or rather move toward the upper polymer phase, as long as there is sufficient space there to accommodate them. This PEG phase, on the other hand, presents itself at the molecular level as a net formed by the large linear polymer chains. As we have seen before in Section 16.3, whether this network can accommodate or not extraneous solutes will depend on the molecular weight of those solutes and also on the molecular weight and concentration of the PEG polymer. Furthermore, the larger is the molecular weight and concentration of the PEG polymer, the lesser space is available.

Although phosphate and sulfate salts are highly effective in promoting solute partitioning in PEG–salt systems, the environmental impact associated with their use has fostered the use of biodegradable and nontoxic citrate salts as a phase-forming component.[57,59] A comparative study of the purification of plasmid DNA from alkaline lysates by PEG₆₀₀/salt ATPS shows that plasmid yields in the bottom phase are higher with sodium citrate when compared with ammonium sulfate.[59] On the contrary, purification is more efficient with ammonium sulfate-based systems. This indicates that sodium citrate is more effective in accommodating both plasmid DNA and RNA in the bottom phase than ammonium sulfate, whereas bottom phases in PEG–ammonium sulfate systems have a higher salting-out ability, pushing solutes to the interphase or the top phase. These results prompted the use of PEG_{600} with mixtures of ammonium sulfate and sodium citrate salts. As a result, a good compromise between plasmid recovery yield and purity were obtained by combining 12.4% sodium citrate and 4.1% ammonium sulfate in the same system.[59]

The potential of ATPS in the context of plasmid purification can be better appreciated by examining the process solution designed by Frerix et al., which uses two PEG–salt aqueous two-phase extractions in tandem for plasmid DNA capture and polishing.[58] The first extraction step was integrated with alkaline lysis by replacing the conventional potassium acetate neutralizating solution, which is normally added after the NaOH/SDS lysis solution (see Chapter 15, Section 15.3.2.2) with a phase-forming potassium phosphate solution. This modification does not affect the flocculation/precipitation of denatured proteins and gDNA since large amounts of potassium are added.[58] After a 10-min holding step on ice, PEG_{800} and water are added in quantities that are conducive to two-phase formation. With this strategy, most of the flocculated cell debris and proteins accumulated at the interphase as a thick layer; substantial amounts of RNA accommodated in the PEG-rich top phase; and the plasmid was recovered in the salt-rich bottom phase.[58] Following recovery, this plasmid-rich, high-salt solution was filtered through a 0.2-μm nylon disk membrane. Since this nylon membrane adsorbed plasmid DNA, appropriate desalting and buffer exchange could be easily accomplished by washing the bound material with 80% v/v isopropanol and then subsequently eluting it with a TE (10 mM tris/Cl, 1 mM EDTA, pH 8.0) buffer. Although more than 95% of the initial RNA was cleared by the combined action of the aqueous two-phase extraction and membrane adsorption, this solution was then subjected to a second extraction to remove the remaining gDNA, open circular plasmid, and RNA.[58] This polishing step explores the ability of ATPS to distinguish between properly renatured double-stranded DNA from denatured nucleic acids.[50] First, adequate amounts of NaOH are added to the plasmid-containing solution in order to denature the supercoiled and open circular plasmid DNA isoforms and gDNA species. The full renaturation of the supercoiled plasmid DNA is then promoted by neutralizing the solution with potassium phosphate. On the contrary, the renaturation of other double-stranded DNA molecules like gDNA fragments, linear plasmid, and even open circular plasmid is not as effective, and thus most of these impurities remain denatured as partially single-stranded DNA. Upon the addition of PEG_{800}, the denatured and more hydrophobic nucleic acids migrate to the top phase or precipitate and accumulate in the interphase, whereas the supercoiled plasmid DNA accommodates in the salt-rich bottom phase. The success of this step depends critically on the exact composition of the NaOH solution and also on the time of exposure to denaturing conditions. If no denaturation is performed, RNA can still be cleared, but no isoform separation is obtained. However, the use of a predenaturation step with 100 mM NaOH contributes to reduce the amount of open circular plasmid from an initial 15% to 5%. An decrease in the gDNA content is also observed.[58] When the process was implemented at a pilot scale, plasmid yields as high as 95% (with 3% of open circle) were obtained.[58]

16.4.3 Thermoseparating Polymers

The use of polymers with thermoseparating properties in ATPS presents some advantages when compared with PEG. The key property of thermoseparating polymers is the ability they have to separate from water into a polymer phase when the solution is heated past the cloud point temperature. A copolymer (EO_{50}-PO_{50}) containing ethylene oxide (50% w/w) and polypropylene oxide (50% w/w) groups randomly distributed along the polymer chains constitutes a good example of such a thermoseparating polymer. When mixed with dextran T500, EO_{50}-PO_{50} originates a two-phase system that can be used to promote the differential partitioning of nucleic acids and impurities present in clarified, desalted alkaline lysates.[9,54] If the adequate operating conditions are used (namely, polymer and salt concentration), close to 100% of plasmid DNA is obtained in the top, EO_{50}-PO_{50}-rich phase, while most proteins (60%) and RNA (80%) are left behind in the dextran bottom phase.[54] Once the two phases are separated, the temperature of the plasmid-containing thermoseparating phase can be raised past the cloud point temperature (55°C for EO_{50}-PO_{50}) to obtain a water phase with a low polymer concentration (<1%) and a concentrated polymer phase (40%). As a result of the high polymer concentration in the thermoseparated EO_{50}-PO_{50} phase, the plasmid DNA is almost exclusively partitioned to the water phase. Further purification of plasmid by unit operations like chromatography is then relatively easy to accomplish since the polymer content in this aqueous phase is very small.[9] Recycling of the EO_{50}-PO_{50} polymer is also easier after thermoseparation. Despite its performance, the EO_{50}-PO_{50}/dextran system cannot be used to process alkaline lysates directly since the characteristically high concentration of salts in the later deteriorates the partitioning selectivity. Thus, alkaline lysates have to be desalted in advance by using a convenient method like TFF.[9,54]

16.4.4 Conclusions

A number of features make liquid–liquid extraction with ATPSs an interesting option when it comes to processing plasmid-containing lysates. The process is relatively simple; most phase-forming components are compatible with plasmid structure, and selectivity has been demonstrated in a number of cases. However, the use of ATPS at process scale is hampered by the disadvantages enumerated next. First, large amounts of mass-separating agents (polymers and salts) have to be added to the process streams, a characteristic that inevitably translates into high cost of goods.[3] Another important shortcoming is the fact that it is almost impossible to increase the concentration of the plasmid in the target phase when compared with the concentration in the incoming lysate. Indeed, in most cases, the plasmid will be diluted, and thus large volumes are carried over to the subsequent operations.[3]

16.5 ADSORPTION

16.5.1 Introduction

Adsorption constitutes a valuable option to reduce the substantial amounts of *E. coli* impurities that contaminate the different process streams found in the intermediate recovery stage. In its simplest format, adsorption uses solid particles, which possess superficial chemical entities/groups that display some kind of ability to interact preferentially with certain impurities compared to the plasmid molecules. The interactions behind a given adsorption process may include almost anything from London–van der Waals forces to electrostatic and hydrophobic interactions, to more specific covalent bonding. Typical adsorbents used to remove impurities from plasmid solutions are silica dioxide-based matrices (e.g., diatomaceous earth), calcium phosphates (e.g., hydroxyapatite), and calcium silicates (e.g., gyrolite). In the majority of cases, the adsorbent particles are porous, and so large surface areas, of the order of $100–1000\,m^2/g$, may be available for adsorption. In order to take the most from adsorption, the particle pores should be large enough to permit full access of impurities and thus originate high binding capacities. The contact between the process stream and the adsorbent particles can be promoted either in a fixed bed or in a stirred tank reactor. In the first case, the particles are properly packed in a column and the process stream is pumped at an adequate flow rate until most of the capacity of the bed for the target impurities is used. During the feed, the plasmid molecules exit the bed in the flow-through stream alongside other nonbinding solutes. The bound impurities are then eluted from the adsorbent particles by flushing the column with an appropriate buffer (i.e., one that reverses adsorption). Following an adequate washing and cleaning, the bed is equilibrated with the adsorption buffer and is ready for another adsorption cycle. In batch adsorption, it is sufficient to add the adsorbent to the tank that contains the solution to be treated and to promote some kind of homogenization of the solids throughout the liquid (Figure 16.1). After a certain amount of time sufficient to allow mass transfer and adsorption of the solutes to take place has elapsed, solids are separated (e.g., by centrifugation or filtration), leaving unbound plasmid behind in the clarified liquid. Even though in most cases the size of the pores in the adsorbent particles is smaller than plasmids, some molecules may become trapped in the liquid entrained between the mass of removed adsorbent. The fixed bed format is more convenient to process very large volumes and to reuse adsorbents. However, if single-use of adsorbents is considered, batch adsorption is probably more convenient. In the specific case of plasmid purification, the optimal adsorbent should be able to adsorb the full spectrum of *E. coli* impurities, and specially the most abundant ones, while leaving plasmids in solution. Given the chemical similarities between plasmids and nucleic acids that were alluded to in Chapter 14, this is, however, difficult to achieve, and thus plasmid losses to the solid phase due to unwanted adsorption are usually inevitable.

Selective separations at the intermediate recovery stage can also be obtained by using adsorbents that bind plasmids rather than impurities. The problem with this approach, however, is that plasmids are too big to enter the majority of pores found in the commercial, less expensive adsorbents. The direct consequence of this is a low plasmid binding capacity, and hence a need to use substantial amounts of adsorbent. For this reason, plasmid adsorption is performed mostly with specially designed (hence costly), wide-pore particles in chromatography-type operations during the final purification stage (see Chapter 17). Thus, in this section, we will focus our attention only in those operations that are designed to adsorb impurities.

16.5.2 Silica Dioxide-Based Matrices

Silica dioxide matrices are one of the most widely used materials in the context of plasmid purification. These silica matrices are available in a wide assortment of materials, which range from the cheapest diatomaceous earth powders to the more sophisticated and expensive controlled pore glass (CPG) particles. Diatomaceous earth (also known as kieselguhr or diatomite) is a sedimentary, chalklike material that is made up of fossilized skeletons of microscopic, one-celled algae known as diatoms. The intricate, silica-based structure of the individual shells originates a high surface area material, which is especially useful for adsorption purposes. Diatomaceous earth are commercially available in different particle sizes (10–100 µm) and forms (e.g., natural and flux calcinated), under trade names like Celite (Celite Corporation, Lompoc, California). Their use in the pharmaceutical industry is facilitated by the fact that the Food and Drug Administration (FDA) categorizes the material as GRAS (see Chapter 14, Section 14.1). The abundance of diatomaceous earth adsorbents is a key advantage when conducting adsorption from crude and heavily loaded solutions like lysates, since large amounts of the material can be used and disposed off without impacting the operating costs significantly. The process used to manufacture CPG from borosilicate glass yields rigid particles, which are characterized by a uniform and very narrow pore size distribution. Depending on the average pore size, the internal surface areas of CPGs can range anywhere from $9 \, m^2/g$ (3000-Å pore) to $340 \, m^2/g$ (75-Å pore). The narrow pore size distribution of CPGs makes them especially indicated for high-resolution chromatographic operations. Although CPG particles can also be used for batch adsorption from crude solutions, their high cost makes this option unattractive.

Silica surfaces are terminated by silanol (–SiOH) groups, which gradually ionize as the pH of the surrounding environment is raised, producing at least two types of –Si–O⁻ groups.[60] Although most of the –SiOH groups exhibit a pK_a of around 8.4, silanol sites with a pK_a of 4.5 have also been reported. Such a negatively charged surface, in principle, would not recommend the use of silica materials to adsorb polyanionic molecules like nucleic acids. However, by operating at pH values below the pK_a's of the surface silanol groups or at high concentrations of counterions or chaotropic substance, the energy barrier that must be overcome to allow closer contact between surface groups and nucleic acids is decreased. This reduction in the surface charge, together with the dehydration of both the surface groups and nucleic acid molecules, could allow the formation of hydrogen bonds between nonionized silanols and phosphate groups in the backbone (i.e., –Si–OH•••O=P–).[61] The possibility for cation bridging between the negative charged groups in silica and the phosphate groups of nucleic acids has also been proposed.[62]

Selectivity for RNA versus DNA binding is the key for a successful use of silica matrices in the clarification of plasmid-containing solutions. In order to preferentially bind RNA to the silica-based adsorbent, while leaving plasmid DNA in solution, specific buffer conditions have to be found. For example, DNA will not bind to silica if the salt/chaotrope concentration is kept below a critical value. DNA/RNA separations have been accomplished, for example, by mixing diatomaceous earth directly with alkaline lysates.[63] The amount of RNA in the lysate was reduced by adding diatomaceous earth up to a concentration of 25 g/L. After homogenization, the mixture was filtered through an appropriate filter precoated with the same diatomaceous earth material. The authors claim that with such a process, RNA can be reduced by as much as 85%.[63]

16.5.3 Hydroxyapatite

Many biomolecules can be purified using chromatographic columns packed with calcium phosphate particles (e.g., hydroxyapatite). Positively charged solutes will typically bind to the phosphate groups in the matrix via direct cation–phosphate, whereas negatively charged molecules (e.g., nucleic acids) interact with calcium sites in the matrix via chelating interactions. By adequately controlling the conditions of the buffers used, it is possible to use calcium phosphate particles to differentially adsorb RNA and plasmid DNA molecules in lysates.[64] Selectivity can be obtained by combining the adsorbent particles with appropriate concentrations of a tris buffer supplemented with calcium salts (e.g., calcium acetate and calcium chloride). For example, at pH 6 and with 10 mM tris and 20–100 mM $CaCl_2$, or with 10–100 mM tris and 20 mM $CaCl_2$, RNA adsorbs, but plasmid DNA remains unbound.[64] Following solid–liquid separation, the plasmid in the buffer solution is easily recovered, for example, by alcohol precipitation. The separation can also be implemented in a chromatographic mode by packing columns with calcium phosphate particles and by implementing an adequate elution scheme.[64,65]

16.5.4 Calcium Silicate

The synthetic calcium silicate hydrate (gyrolite) commercially available under the trade name LRA (lipid removal agent) was developed for the removal of contaminating lipids and macromolecules containing lipid moieties from biopharmaceutical process streams. Gyrolite is a hydrophilic/hydrophobic, multilayered material in which hexagonal arrangements of silica tetraheadra are bound to calcium-containing octahedra. In the context of plasmid downstream processing, LRA has been used specifically to remove LPSs, but also gDNA and open circular plasmid isoforms from process solutions.[66] The adsorbent is also able to remove surfactants used in earlier steps like CTAB or Triton X-110. The binding of all the compounds listed earlier to hydrates of calcium silicate is complex and involves a series of interactions including hydrogen bonding, ionic bonds between Ca^{2+} in gyrolite and anion groups (e.g., phosphates in DNA) and hydrophobic interactions. Such interactions can be appropriately modulated by manipulating the environmental conditions (e.g., the NaCl concentration) in such a way as to bind gDNA, LPS, and open circular isoforms, but not supercoiled plasmid DNA.[66] This type of operation is explored in a patented process in which batch adsorption with hydrated calcium silicate particles is performed after a CTAB precipitation step.[29]

16.5.5 Affinity Adsorbents

The molecular interactions explored to remove *E. coli* impurities onto adsorbent particles are usually rather unspecific, for example, hydrophobic interactions. However, very precise, affinity-like interactions, which target specific classes of impurities, can also be used. The use of affinity adsorbents during the intermediate recovery stage is, in principle, not a good strategy from the point of view of the "biochemical engineering common sense" expressed in heuristic 3 (see Chapter 14, Section 14.4). The major reasons for this are the fact that the large volumes of solutions found at this stage, together with the high costs typically associated with affinity materials, inevitably render impurity clearance by affinity adsorption an expensive option. Still, a couple of affinity systems, based on phenyl boronate and polymyxin B ligands, are mentioned here to illustrate their inherent selectivity potential.

16.5.5.1 Phenyl Boronate

The adsorption of RNA by adsorbent particles modified with phenyl boronate ligands constitutes a paradigmatic example of the affinity adsorption approach (see also Chapter 17, Section 17.2.8.4). Under adequate conditions, ligands containing phenyl boronate (Figure 16.10a) are able to form covalent bonds with the C2-C3 diol in the ribose located at the terminal 3′ end of RNA molecules. Since a similar reaction is not possible in DNA due to the lack of a hydroxyl group at the C2 carbon of deoxyribose, phenyl boronate adsorption ligands are able to selectively discriminate plasmid DNA from RNA. Although

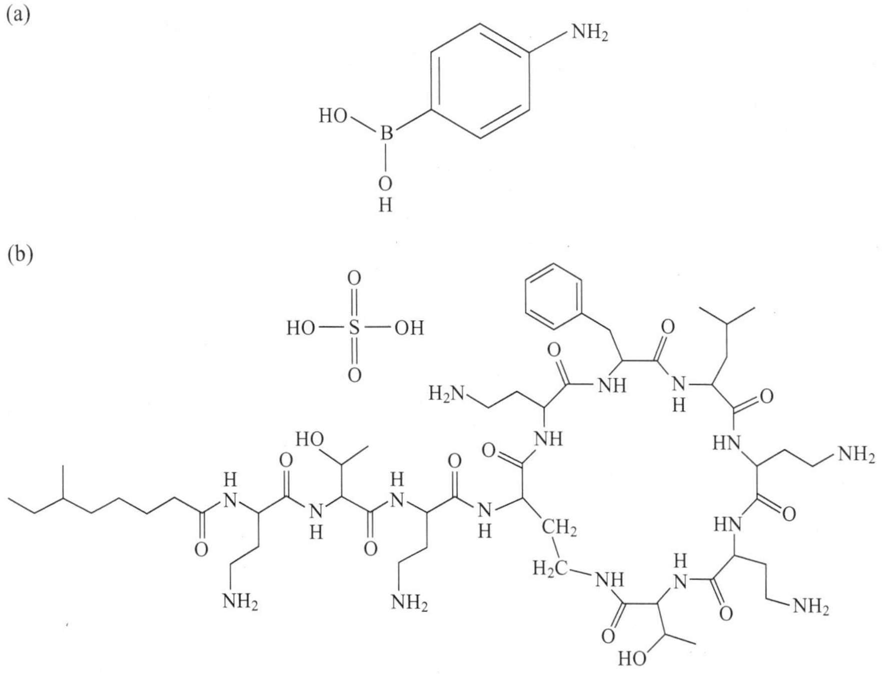

(a)

(b)

Figure 16.10 *Affinity adsorption of* E. coli *impurities. As examples, adsorbent particles can be used that are chemically modified with (a) aminophenyl boronate ligands designed to covalently bind RNA via the cis-diol of terminal ribose or with (b) polymyxin B to bind selectively to the lipid A moiety of LPS via hydrophobic and electrostatic interactions.*

special alkaline buffers containing specific components are usually referred to in the literature as mandatory for reactions of phenyl boronate with diol-containing molecules to occur, recent results have shown that 3-aminophenyl boronate (PB) CPG is able to adsorb not only those species that bear *cis*-diol groups (RNA and LPSs), and are thus able to form covalent bonds with boronate, but also *cis*-diol-free proteins and gDNA fragments, while leaving most plasmid DNA in solution.[67] The impressive performance of these adsorbents can be better appreciated on the basis of the HPLC and agarose electrophoresis analysis given in Figure 16.11, which displays and compares chromatograms obtained following the HPLC analysis of a lysate feed (Figure 16.11a) and of a solution after a 5-min adsorption (Figure 16.11b). The results show that while most plasmid DNA and low-MW RNA remain in the supernatant, a large fraction of high MW RNA is cleared after a 5-min adsorption (Figure 16.11b) as a result of the formation of covalent bonds. Electrophoresis confirms that batch adsorption of RNA to the phenyl boronate matrix is very fast and complete after 30 min (see insert in Figure 16.11b). Further analysis revealed that more than 90% of RNA, proteins, and gDNA were cleared after 30 min, and that the LPS content decreased from ~2000 EU/mL in the lysate to a residual amount of less than 0.005 EU/mL.[67] Although the plasmid recov-

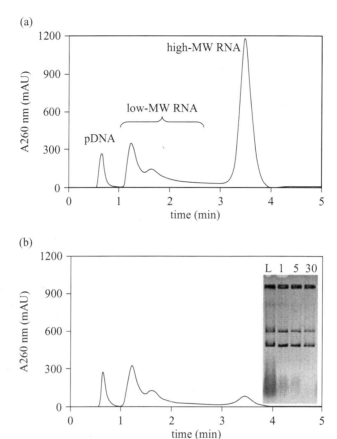

Figure 16.11 *Purification of plasmids in alkaline lysates by batch affinity adsorption of RNA impurities with 3-aminophenyl boronate controlled pore glass particles. The figure shows HIC-HPLC analysis of the starting lysate (a) and of the supernatant after a 5-min contact with the phenyl boronate matrix (b). The insert in (b) shows an agarose gel electrophoresis analysis of the feed lysate (L) and of the supernatants after 1, 5, and 30 min of adsorption. Adapted and reprinted from Journal of Chromatography A, 1217, Gomes AG, Azevedo AM, Aires-Barros MR, Prazeres DMF. Clearance of host cell impurities from plasmid-containing lysates by boronate adsorption, 2262–2266, Copyright 2010,6[67] with permission from Elsevier.*

ery was low (64%), this was attributed to the fact that a significant portion of liquid remains trapped inside and between settled beads after solid–liquid separation, and not to unspecific plasmid adsorption.

16.5.5.2 *Polymyxin B*

LPSs are one of the most problematic impurities to be found in plasmid solutions, as described in Chapter 12 (Section 12.3.4.5) and Chapter 14 (Section 14.2). The presence of even minute amounts of LPS in an injectable biopharmaceutical product may have severe consequences for patients, including endotoxic shock and associated clinical complications. The removal of LPS is thus one of the key objectives of downstream processing. Polymyxin B is an antimicrobial, cationic decapeptide (see Figure 16.10b), which has the ability to selectivity invade the periplasmic space of gram-negative bacteria like *E. coli* and *Pseudomonas aeruginosa*. The binding of polymyxin B involves the breaching of the LPS layer and precise interactions with the lipid A moiety of LPS. These interactions involve hydrophobic peptide–lipid contacts, which are supported by interactions of the positively charged side chains of certain amino acid residues of polymyxin, with the negatively charged phosphate groups of lipid A.[68]

The specific binding properties of polymyxin B have been explored in the clinic, for example, in the treatment of gram-negative bacterial sepsis cases. The circulating LPS in these severely endotoxemic patients are cleared through a procedure that typically involves the perfusion of the blood through a cartridge containing fibers with immobilized polymyxin B. Packed columns of resins (e.g., agarose) with immobilized polymyxin B have also been used to remove *E. coli* LPS from biopharmaceutical preparations. In the specific case of plasmid DNA preparations, batch adsorption experiments conducted at 4°C for 30 min show that LPS can be removed extensively (>90%) down to a residual value of 10–50 endotoxin units/mg of DNA.[69] However, this was accompanied by a substantial loss of plasmid DNA of approximately 40%, probably due to electrostatic-mediated adsorption between the phosphates in the plasmid backbone and the cationic polymyxin B ligands.[69] In spite of the excellent performance displayed by polymyxin B agarose beads in the batch adsorption of LPS from plasmid-containing solutions, the reality is that the inclusion of this type of operation in a full downstream processing scheme has not been equated seriously. One of the reasons for this is surely the high cost associated with the decapeptide polymyxin B ligands and with the chemical processing required to bind them to the beads. Some concerns regarding the impact of leached ligands on the safety of the end plasmid product (e.g., polymyxin B stimulates interleukin 1 *in vivo*) may also have deterred the introduction of polymyxin adsorption in a full-scale production process. These two arguments, together with the fact that alternative processes for LPS clearance (e.g., HIC and salt precipitation[70]), which are cheaper and have a proven track record, are available, have not favored the use of polymyxin B adsorbents.

16.5.6 Conclusions

Although the discrimination of RNA from DNA is difficult to achieve with conventional, low-cost adsorbents such as silicon dioxide-based matrices or calcium silicates, a number of reports indicate that by manipulating parameters like salt composition and type, it is possible to partially clear streams from RNA and other impurities while leaving plasmid DNA in solution. Improved selectivity can also be obtained by tailoring adsorbents with affinity ligands that are specific for certain classes of impurities like LPS or RNA. Still, and although these affinity adsorbents are generally more effective, the need to engineer a given specificity into the adsorbent inevitably renders the process more expensive.

16.6 DISCUSSION AND OVERALL CONCLUSIONS

A substantial number of unit operations have been experimented with the specific goal of removing impurities from clarified lysates up to a point where high-resolution purification processes can be used without problems to obtain plasmid products with the required final quality. Although TFF, precipitation, liquid–liquid extraction, and adsorption all have specific characteristics that are interesting from different points of view (e.g., concentration, LPS removal, RNA clearance, and plasmid isoform separation), the best results are usually obtained by using two or more of these unit operations in combination. The ability of such combinations to yield plasmids that are virtually devoid of impurities can even be powerful enough to result in chromatographic-free processes. Some of the possibilities tested are presented in the context of the discussion of process synthesis solutions for the full downstream processing of plasmids, which is presented in Chapter 18.

REFERENCES

1. Ferreira GNM, Cabral JMS, Prazeres DMF. Development of process flow sheets for the purification of plasmid vectors for gene therapy applications. *Biotechnology Progress*. 1999;15:725–731.

2. Varley DL, Hitchcock AG, Weiss AME, et al. Production of plasmid DNA for human gene therapy using modified alkaline cell lysis and expanded bed anion exchange chromatography. *Bioseparation*. 1998;8:209–217.

3. Freitas S, Canario S, Santos JA, Prazeres DMF. Alternatives for the intermediate recovery of plasmid DNA: Performance, economic viability and environmental impact. *Biotechnology Journal*. 2009;4:265–278.

4. Kendall D, Lye GJ, Levy MS. Purification of plasmid DNA by an integrated operation comprising tangential flow filtration and nitrocellulose adsorption. *Biotechnology and Bioengineering*. 2002;79:816–822.

5. Kahn DW, Butler MD, Cohen DL, Gordon M, Kahn JW, Winkler ME. Purification of plasmid DNA by tangential flow filtration. *Biotechnology and Bioengineering*. 2000;69:101–106.

6. McNeilly DS, inventor; Genzyme Corporation, assignee. Method for purifying plasmid DNA and plasmid DNA substantially free of genomic DNA. U.S. patent 6,214,586, April 10, 2001.

7. Eon-Duval A, MacDuff RH, Fisher CA, Harris MJ, Brook C. Removal of RNA impurities by tangential flow filtration in an RNase-free plasmid DNA purification process. *Analytical Biochemistry*. 2003;316:66–73.

8. Guerrero-German P, Prazeres DMF, Guzman R, Montesinos-Cisneros RM, Tejeda-Mansir A. Purification of plasmid DNA using tangential flow filtration and tandem

anion-exchange membrane chromatography. *Bioprocess and Biosystems Engineering.* 2009;32:615–623.

9. Kepka C, Lemmens R, Vasi J, Nyhammar T, Gustavsson PE. Integrated process for purification of plasmid DNA using aqueous two-phase systems combined with membrane filtration and lid bead chromatography. *Journal of Chromatography. A.* 2004;1057:115–124.

10. Chamsart S, Patel H, Hanak JA, Hitchcock AG, Nienow AW. The impact of fluid-dynamic-generated stresses on chDNA and pDNA stability during alkaline cell lysis for gene therapy products. *Biotechnology and Bioengineering.* 2001;75: 387–392.

11. Levy MS, Collins IJ, Yim SS, et al. Effect of shear on plasmid DNA in solution. *Bioprocess Engineering.* 1999;20:7–13.

12. Levy MS, Ciccolini LAS, Yim SSS, et al. The effects of material properties and fluid flow intensity on plasmid DNA recovery during cell lysis. *Chemical Engineering Science.* 1999;54:3171–3178.

13. Freitas SS. Development and optimization of a scalable production process based on hydrophobic interaction chromatography and aiming at gene therapy and DNA vaccination. PhD thesis in Biotechnology, Lisbon, Instituto Superior Técnico, 2007.

14. Lee AL, Sagar S, inventors; Merck & Co., Inc., assignee. Method for large scale plasmid purification. U.S. patent 6,197,553, March 6, 2002.

15. Butler MD, Cohen DL, Kahn D, Winkler ME, inventors; Genentech, Inc., assignee. Purification of plasmid DNA. U.S. patent 6,313,285, November 6, 2001.

16. Garcia FAP. Protein precipitation. In: Kennedy JF, Cabral JMS, eds. *Recovery processes for biological materials.* Chichester: John Wiley & Sons, 1993:355–367.

17. Diogo MM, Quiroz JA, Monteiro GA, Martins SAM, Ferreira GNM, Prazeres DMF. Purification of a cystic fibrosis plasmid vector for gene therapy using hydrophobic interaction chromatography. *Biotechnology and Bioengineering.* 2000;68: 576–583.

18. Freitas SS, Santos JA, Prazeres DMF. Optimization of isopropanol and ammonium sulfate precipitation steps in the purification of plasmid DNA. *Biotechnology Progress.* 2006;22:1179–1186.

19. Horn NA, Meek JA, Budahazi G, Marquet M. Cancer gene therapy using plasmid DNA: Purification of DNA for human clinical trials. *Human Gene Therapy.* 1995;6:565–573.

20. Lander RJ, Winters MA, Meacle FJ, Buckland BC, Lee AL. Fractional precipitation of plasmid DNA from lysate by CTAB. *Biotechnology and Bioengineering.* 2002; 79:776–784.

21. Murphy JC, Wibbenmeyer JA, Fox GE, Willson RC. Purification of plasmid DNA using selective precipitation by compaction agents. *Nature Biotechnology.* 1999;17:822–823.

22. Arscott PG, Ma C, Wenner JR, Bloomfield VA. DNA condensation by cobalt hexammine(III) in alcohol-water mixtures: Dielectric constant and other solvent effects. *Biopolymers.* 1995;36:345–364.

23. Flock S, Labarbe R, Houssier C. Dielectric constant and ionic strength effects on DNA precipitation. *Biophysical Journal.* 1996;70:1456–1465.

24. Freitas SS, Santos JA, Prazeres DMF. Plasmid DNA. In: Biwer A, Heinzle E, Cooney C, eds. *Development of sustainable bioprocesses: Modeling and assessment.* New York: John Wiley & Sons, 2006:271–285.

25. Marquet M, Horn N, Meek J, Budahazi G, inventors; Vical Incorporated, assignee. Production of pharmaceutical-grade plasmid DNA. U.S. patent 5,561,064, October 1, 1996.

26. Ishaqu M, Wolf B, Ritter C. Large-scale isolation of plasmid DNA using cetyltrimethylammonium bromide. *BioTechniques*. 1990;9:19–24.

27. Tomanee P, Hsu JT. Selective precipitation of RNA, supercoiled plasmid DNA, and open-circular plasmid DNA with different cationic surfactants. *Journal of Liquid Chromatography & Related Technologies*. 2006;29:1531–1540.

28. Tomanee P, Hsu JT, Ito Y. Preparative fractionation of protein, RNA, and plasmid DNA using centrifugal precipitation chromatography with tubular dialysis membrane inside a convoluted tubing as separation channel. *Biotechnology Progress*. 2006;22:532–537.

29. Lander RJ, Winters MA, Meacle FJ, inventors; Merck and Co., Inc., assignee. Process for the scaleable purification of plasmid DNA. U.S. patent 6,797,476, September 28, 2004.

30. Lis JT, Schleif R. Size fractionation of double-stranded DNA by precipitation with polyethylene glycol. *Nucleic Acids Research*. 1975;2:383–389.

31. Nicoletti VG, Condorelli DF. Optimized PEG method for rapid plasmid DNA purification: High yield from "midi-prep." *BioTechniques*. 1993;14:532–534, 536.

32. Stepanov VG, Nyborg J. Preparative purification of plasmid DNA templates for in vitro transcription assays by consecutive differential precipitations. *Journal of Biotechnology*. 2003;102:223–231.

33. Schmitz A, Riesner D. Purification of nucleic acids by selective precipitation with polyethylene glycol 6000. *Analytical Biochemistry*. 2006;354:311–313.

34. Sauer ML, Kollars B, Geraets R, Sutton F. Sequential CaCl2, polyethylene glycol precipitation for RNase-free plasmid DNA isolation. *Analytical Biochemistry*. 2008;380:310–314.

35. Horn N, Budahazi G, Marquet M, inventors; Vical Incorporated, assignee. Purification of plasmid DNA during column chromatography. U.S. patent 5,707,812, January 13, 1998.

36. Vasilevskaya VV, Khokhlov AR, Matsuzawa Y, Yoshikawa K. Collapse of single DNA molecule in poly(ethylene glycol) solutions. *The Journal of Chemistry and Physics*. 1995;102:6595–6602.

37. Galaev IY, Gustavsson P-E, Izumrudov V, Larsson P-O, Wahlund P-O, inventors; Amersham Biosciences, assignee. Isolation of nucleic acids using a polycationic polymer as precipitation agent. U.S. patent 2005/222,404, October 6, 2005.

38. Wahlund PO, Gustavsson PE, Izumrudov VA, Larsson PO, Galaev IY. Precipitation by polycation as capture step in purification of plasmid DNA from a clarified lysate. *Biotechnology and Bioengineering*. 2004;87:675–684.

39. Willson RC, Murphy J, inventors; Technology Licensing Co. LLC, assignee. Methods and compositions for biotechnical separations using selective precipitation by compaction agents. U.S. patent 6,617,108, September 9, 2003.

40. Costioli MD, Fisch I, Garret-Flaudy F, Hilbrig F, Freitag R. DNA purification by triple-helix affinity precipitation. *Biotechnology and Bioengineering*. 2003;81: 535–545.

41. Harrison RG, Todd PW, Rudge SR, Petrides D. Bioprocess design. In: Harrison, RG, Todd, PW, Rudge, SR, Petrides, D, eds. *Bioseparations science and engineering*. Oxford: Oxford University Press, 2003.

42. Marcus Y. Effect of ions on the structure of water: Structure making and breaking. *Chemistry Reviews*. 2009;109:1346–1370.

43. Kunz W, Heule J, Ninham BW. Zur lehre von der wirkung der salze [About the science of the effect of salts]: Franz Hofmeister's historical papers. *Current Opinion in Colloid and Interface Science*. 2004;9:19–37.

44. Bhikhabhai R, inventor; Amersham Pharmacia Biotech AB, assignee. Plasmid DNA purification using divalent alkaline earth metal ions and two anion exchangers. U.S. patent 6,410,274, June 25, 2002.

45. Eon-Duval A, Gumbs K, Ellett C. Precipitation of RNA impurities with high salt in a plasmid DNA purification process: Use of experimental design to determine reaction conditions. *Biotechnology and Bioengineering*. 2003;83:544–553.

46. Freitas SS, Santos JAL, Prazeres DMF. Plasmid purification by hydrophobic interaction chromatography using sodium citrate in the mobile phase. *Separation and Purification Technology*. 2009;65:95–104.

47. Diogo MM, Ribeiro S, Queiroz JA, et al. Production, purification and analysis of an experimental DNA vaccine against rabies. *The Journal of Gene Medicine*. 2001;3:577–584.

48. Albertsson PA. Partition of double-stranded and single-stranded deoxyribonucleic acid. *Archives in Biochemistry and Biophysics*. 1962;September(Suppl 1):264–270.

49. Albertsson PA. Partition studies on nucleic acids. I. Influence of electrolytes, polymer concentration and nucleic acid conformation of the partition in the dextran-polyethylene glycol system. *Biochimica et Biophysica Acta*. 1965; 103:1–12.

50. Ohlsson R, Hentschel CC, Williams JG. A rapid method for the isolation of circular DNA using aqueous two-phase partition system. *Nucleic Acids Research*. 1978;5:583–590.

51. Cole KD. Purification of plasmid and high molecular mass DNA using PEG-salt two-phase extraction. *BioTechniques*. 1991;11:18, 20, 22–14.

52. Ribeiro SC, Monteiro GA, Martinho G, Cabral JMS, Prazeres DMF. Quantitation of plasmid DNA in aqueous two-phase systems by fluorescence analysis. *Biotechnology Letters*. 2000;22:1101–1104.

53. Ribeiro SC, Monteiro GA, Cabral JM, Prazeres DMF. Isolation of plasmid DNA from cell lysates by aqueous two-phase systems. *Biotechnology and Bioengineering*. 2002;78:376–384.

54. Kepka C, Rhodin J, Lemmens R, Tjerneld F, Gustavsson PE. Extraction of plasmid DNA from *Escherichia coli* cell lysate in a thermoseparating aqueous two-phase system. *Journal of Chromatography. A*. 2004;1024:95–104.

55. Frerix A, Muller M, Kula MR, Hubbuch J. Scalable recovery of plasmid DNA based on aqueous two-phase separation. *Biotechnology and Applied Biochemistry*. 2005;42:57–66.

56. Trindade IP, Diogo MM, Prazeres DMF, Marcos JC. Purification of plasmid DNA vectors by aqueous two-phase extraction and hydrophobic interaction chromatography. *Journal of Chromatography. A*. 2005;1082:176–184.

57. Rahimpour F, Feyzi F, Maghsoudi S, Hatti-Kaul R. Purification of plasmid DNA with polymer-salt aqueous two-phase system: Optimization using response surface methodology. *Biotechnology and Bioengineering*. 2006;95:627–637.

58. Frerix A, Geilenkirchen P, Muller M, Kula MR, Hubbuch J. Separation of genomic DNA, RNA, and open circular plasmid DNA from supercoiled plasmid DNA by combining denaturation, selective renaturation and aqueous two-phase extraction. *Biotechnology and Bioengineering*. 2007;96:57–66.

59. Gomes GA, Azevedo AM, Aires-Barros MR, Prazeres DMF. Purification of plasmid DNA with aqueous two phase systems of PEG 600 and sodium citrate/ammonium sulfate. *Separation and Purification Technology*. 2009;65:22–30.

60. Ong S, Zhao X, Eisenthal KB. Polarization of water molecules at a charged interface: Second harmonic studies of the silica/water interface. *Chemical Physics Letters*. 1992;191:327–335.

61. Mao Y, Daniel LN, Whittaker N, Saffiotti U. DNA binding to crystalline silica characterized by Fourier-transform infrared spectroscopy. *Environmental Health Perspectives*. 1994;102(Suppl 10):165–171.

62. Nguyen TH, Elimelech M. Plasmid DNA adsorption on silica: Kinetics and conformational changes in monovalent and divalent salts. *Biomacromolecules*. 2007; 8:24–32.

63. Horn N, Marquet M, Meek J, Budahazi G, inventors; Vical Incorporated, assignee. Process for reducing RNA concentration in a mixture of biological material using diatomaceous earth. U.S. patent 5,576,196, November 19, 1996.

64. Yamamoto A, inventor; Asahi Kogaku Kogyo Kabushiki Kaisha, assignee. Method for purifying plasmid DNA on calcium phosphate compound. U.S. patent 5,843,731, December 1, 1998.

65. Giovannini R, Freitag R. Comparison of different types of ceramic hydroxyapatite for the chromatographic separation of plasmid DNA and a recombinant anti-Rhesus D antibody. *Bioseparation*. 2001;9:359–368.

66. Winters MA, Richter JD, Sagar SL, Lee AL, Lander RJ. Plasmid DNA purification by selective calcium silicate adsorption of closely related impurities. *Biotechnology Progress*. 2003;19:440–447.

67. Gomes AG, Azevedo AM, Aires-Barros MR, Prazeres DMF. Clearance of host cell impurities from plasmid-containing lysates by boronate adsorption. *Journal of Chromatography. A*. 2010;1217:2262–2266.

68. Tsubery H, Ofek I, Cohen S, Fridkin M. Structure-function studies of polymyxin B nonapeptide: Implications to sensitization of gram-negative bacteria. *Journal of Medicinal Chemistry*. 2000;43:3085–3092.

69. Montbriand PM, Malone RW. Improved method for the removal of endotoxin from DNA. *Journal of Biotechnology*. 1996;44:43–46.

70. Wilson MJ, Haggart CL, Gallagher SP, Walsh D. Removal of tightly bound endotoxin from biological products. *Journal of Biotechnology*. 2001;88:67–75.

17

Final Purification

17.1 INTRODUCTION

The process solutions generated in the intermediate recovery stage and entering the final purification stage are substantially enriched in plasmid DNA. However, small amounts of *Escherichia coli*-derived impurities may persist, which have to be removed in order to obtain a bulk product complying with the end specifications (see Chapter 12). Apart from small amounts of genomic DNA (gDNA), RNA, and lipopolysaccharides (LPSs), it is especially important at this final stage to remove plasmid variants such as open circular topoisomers (whether they are relaxed or nicked) and denatured plasmid DNA in order to fulfill the homogeneity specification that typically requires supercoiled isoforms to account for more than 95%[1] of the final product (see Chapter 12, Section 12.3.3). In order to meet these separation goals, a significant number of the published plasmid manufacturing processes resort to unit operations like chromatography and membrane filtration, which require the plasmid-containing stream to pass through some kind of porous solid matrix. This could be, for instance, a packed bed of porous beads, a stack of porous membranes, an ultrafiltration membrane, or a sterile membrane filter. Whichever the case, plasmids will have to perfuse and/or diffuse through a three-dimensional network of pores, which can have very different sizes and contain constrictions. Given the awkward shape (branched, plectonemically

Plasmid Biopharmaceuticals: Basics, Applications, and Manufacturing, First Edition.
Duarte Miguel F. Prazeres.
© 2011 John Wiley & Sons, Inc. Published 2011 by John Wiley & Sons, Inc.

supercoiled), large molecular weight ($MW > 10^6\,Da$), and size ($L > 5000\,\mathring{A}$, $R_G > 500\,\mathring{A}$), and small diffusion coefficients ($D \approx 10^{-7}$–$10^{-8}\,cm^2/s$) of plasmid DNA molecules, which was alluded to in Chapter 4, this transport process can be difficult to accomplish or even impossible altogether. As we will see in the first section of this chapter, this strongly constrains and reduces the purification options available in terms of chromatographic separations, ultrafiltration, and sterile filtration. However, and in spite of its well-known and recognized disadvantages, chromatography still dominates the final purification stage in plasmid manufacturing processes. An important part of this chapter is thus used to describe how the different chromatography modalities have been explored to remove the most recalcitrant impurities, highlighting the basic operating principles, advantages, and disadvantages associated with the different options. Subsequently, reference is made to the two process options available to perform the postchromatography tasks of concentration and buffer exchange (i.e., ultrafiltration and alcohol precipitation). The last part of the chapter deals with the sterilization of the purified plasmid pools obtained after these steps. The single option available at this far end of the downstream processing is sterilizing filtration through membranes with 0.20- to 0.22-μm pore size ratings. Although this operation is routinely performed in the manufacturing of protein biopharmaceuticals, plasmids present very specific challenges, as referred to above, which must be tackled efficiently in order not to compromise the success of the entire process. These issues are discussed in some detail on the basis of experimental data reported in the literature.

17.2   CHROMATOGRAPHY

17.2.1   Introduction

Chromatography is an extremely powerful separation operation, widely used at process scale across the biotechnology industry to purify secondary metabolites, carbohydrates, proteins, nucleic acids, and viruses. The technique explores the differential interactions between solutes in the mixture that contains the target biomolecules, with a solid matrix. This matrix typically presents itself in the form of microscopic porous beads with diameters that can vary anywhere from 10 to 500 μm. Such beads are usually packed in a cylindrical column, originating fixed beds with interstitial porosities of approximately 0.35–0.42.[2] Although the pore diameters in most conventional beads are less than about 100 nm,[2,3] perfusion materials that possess an additional subset of pores with diameters of the order of hundreds of nanometers are available.[4] Nonporous beads may also be used, but this option is usually preferred when chromatography is performed exclusively for analytical purposes (see Chapter 5, Section 5.6), since in this case, capacity is not an issue and the absence of intrabead solute diffusion directly translates into faster separations. Alternative nonbead formats are also available for chromatography, in which the solid matrix displays a continuous structure of pores and presents itself either as a thin membrane or as a monolith. In the first case, the equivalent of a "fixed bed" is obtained by (1) stacking a number of thin membranes on top of each other[5] or by (2) pleating a larger membrane in such a way as to increase the area available per unit volume[6] and placing them inside a convenient holder/ cartridge. In the second case, the porous monolith block is simply inserted inside a housing with the aid of a self-sealing fitting ring.[7]

The operation mode used to promote separation in liquid chromatography is essentially independent of the matrix format. As a rule, the solutes to be separated are brought into contact with the packed bed of beads, stack of membranes, or monolith by injecting a certain volume of the feed mixture on the top of the column, and then sequentially and continuously flowing a liquid phase (the so-called mobile phase) through the column. During this process, and in the conventional case of a fixed bed of beads, solutes (1) are transported by convection from the bulk of the flowing liquid phase to the surface of the beads, (2) enter the accessible pores and migrate through the network of pores by diffusion, and (3) finally interact with chemical groups attached to the matrix. These groups, which are typically present in the matrix at a concentration of 10–$500\,\mu mol\,cm^3$,[3] provide for a specific type of interaction. A similar process takes place when the alternative membrane and monolith formats are used, with the exception now that a fraction of the pores is large enough to accommodate the convective transport, which distributes solutes toward the network of smaller diffusive pores. Depending on the strength of the interaction with the surface chemical groups, solutes may either (1) remain tightly bound to the matrix or (2) desorb, diffuse, and return back to the flowing bulk liquid. The composition of the mobile phase is typically changed during the course of the operation in order to modulate the interaction of the different solutes with the matrix. If conditions are adequately chosen, the net result of the complete operation is that different solutes migrate toward the end of the column or cartridge with different velocities, and hence exit at different times; that is, a separation is performed.

Chromatography is typically operated in a "positive" mode. This designation means that the target biomolecule binds strongly to an adequate matrix (e.g., anion exchange, hydrophobic interaction, and affinity), while those impurities that do not bind or are weakly retained elute in the liquid volume, which exits the column in the first instant (this fraction is known as the flow-through). The composition of the mobile phase is then changed so as to dislodge the bound target molecule from the matrix. The exception to this "rule" is gel filtration, of course, which always operates in a flow-through mode; that is, there is no binding of solutes to the separation matrix. In a "negative" mode of operation, the relative behavior of impurities and target solutes toward the matrix is reversed—impurities or a group of impurities are forced to bind, whereas the target molecule exits in the flow-through under nonbinding conditions. The ability to obtain a pool of fractions where the target biomolecule is concentrated relative to the initial feedstock is one of the key advantages of "positive" chromatography when compared with "negative" chromatography. In this later case, the elution of the nonbinding target solute in the flow-through usually leads to dilution.[8] However, in order to take full advantage of positive chromatography, the matrices used should have a high binding capacity for the target molecule and should allow for fast transport of solutes in and out of the pores to take place, since this will result in more expedite separations.

According to these notions, the "right thing to do" when first considering the use of a chromatographic operation to purify plasmid DNA would be to select the physical–chemical interaction, which best lends itself to a positive mode of operation. This has, in fact, been done by resorting to ion-exchange chromatography—in this case, the use of anion-exchange groups linked to the matrix makes it possible to bind plasmids to beads via the anionic sugar–phosphate backbone while selectively separating smaller polyanionic impurities like RNA and some DNA fragments.[9] However, it soon became apparent for all those pursuing this approach that the large size of plasmids was not fully compatible with this positive mode of operation of anion-exchange chromatography, at least when using conventional beads. The major reasons for this have to do with limitations in mass transfer and capacity, as described in more detail in the next section.

17.2.2 Mass Transfer and Capacity Issues

In order to illustrate the mass transfer and accessibility limitations encountered by plasmids when faced with a three-dimensional network of pores, let us take the case of a typical, conventional chromatographic bead. In the vast majority of cases, the pore diameters, d_p, will seldom exceed the 300–1000 Å.[2,4,10] The geometry of such a matrix is clearly inadequate to handle plasmids, at least in an efficient way, given their unusual shape and dimensions. The inadequacy is fundamentally related to the fact that most pores in the bead are smaller than the superhelix axis, L, and the radius of gyration, R_G, of plasmids; that is, $d_p < L, R_G$. This means that the molecules are, for the most part, physically prevented from entering the matrix pores. Since plasmids are very long but thin molecules ($r \approx 50$–70 Å; see Chapter 4, Section 4.3.6), the molecules could, in principle, access the matrix interior by approaching the pore entrance with the correct axial orientation.[11] This situation is illustrated in Figure 17.1a,b, which makes a side-by-side comparison between a typical 5000-bp plasmid ($L \approx 6900$ Å, $r \approx 50$ Å, $R_G = 881$ Å; see Chapter 4, Section 4.3.6) and the largest of the largest pores ($d_p \approx 3000$ Å) one can hope to find in a conventional ion-exchange adsorbent.[12] Again, notice that in most beads, $d_p < 300$–1000 Å,[2] and so the case in point represents an extreme situation. Although in some situations plasmid molecules could eventually align themselves in such a way as to enter the pore head-on (Figure 17.1b), Brownian motion and the constant and chaotic coiling of the molecule would readily bring plasmids into close proximity with the inner walls of the pore. The resulting hindrance in molecu-

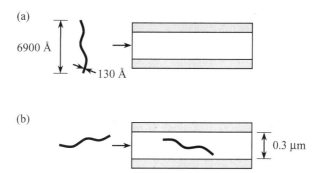

Figure 17.1 *Schematic representations of the relative dimensions and accessibility of a typical 5000-bp plasmid to the largest pore ($d_p \approx 3000$ Å) in a conventional ion-exchange chromatographic matrix. The supercoiled plasmid is represented as a thick line with a length roughly proportional to the superhelix axis (L ≈ 6900 Å) and a thickness proportional to the superhelix diameter (≈100 Å). In (a), plasmids cannot enter the pore when facing the entrance sidewise, whereas in (b), the axial orientation of the plasmid facilitates entrance. Here, however, Brownian motion is likely to reorient the molecule leading to hindered diffusion (adapted from Prazeres[11]).*

lar diffusion would then be described by an effective diffusion coefficient smaller than the already very small diffusion coefficients ($D \approx 10^{-8}$ cm²/s; see Chapter 4, Section 4.5.4), making it impractical for a plasmid molecule to diffuse in and out of such a chromatographic bead, at least within an acceptable time frame. Furthermore, some of the plasmids that might have gained access to these very large pores may be faced with the presence of throats and other constrictions, and thus will be unable to fully access the internal surface of the matrix.[4]

A major consequence of the inability of conventional chromatographic beads to accommodate plasmid molecules is poor binding capacity. In the case of anion-exchange beads, for example, literature data show that dynamic binding capacities larger than 1.5 mg/mL are hard to obtain with conventional anion-exchange beads like Q- and DEAE Sepharose Fast Flow, Q Sepharose XL and Toyopearl DEAE-650 (see Table 17.1).[13] Experimental data also show that in this situation, the interior of the beads remains largely inaccessible and that plasmid molecules essentially bind within an outer shell of the bead. This has been confirmed by binding experiments, which revealed the existence of an inverse correlation between the radius of anion-exchanger beads and static[14] and dynamic[15] plasmid capacity. A direct indication that plasmid molecules do not enter the core of conventional chromatographic beads has been obtained also by resorting to confocal laser microscopy. The depth-discriminating properties of the technique makes it possible to optically slice beads preloaded with a fluorescently labeled plasmid into a series of thin sections (see Chapter 5, Section 5.5.3). In the case of experiments performed with Q Sepharose XL particles with diameters in the 65- to 111-μm range and a 6300-bp plasmid, the results show that bound plasmids remain confined to an

TABLE 17.1. Static* and Dynamic Binding Capacity of Plasmid DNA on Commercial Anion-Exchange Adsorbents

Stationary Phase[†]	Bead Size (μm)	Pore Size (μm)	Capacity (mg/mL)	Plasmid (kb)	Reference
Conventional adsorbents					
DEAE Sepharose FF	90.0	0.19	0.16–0.26	6.9	Urthaler et al.[46]
Source 30Q	30.0	0.002–0.1	0.51–0.71	6.9	Urthaler et al.[46]
Q Sepharose FF	90.0	<0.035	1.3*	4.8	Ferreira et al.[14]
Q Sepharose FF	90.0	<0.035	0.72	5.9	Eon-Duval et al.[32]
Q Sepharose FF	90.0	<0.035	0.2	7.6	Syren et al.[112]
Q Sepharose XL	90.0	<0.035	1.5	6.9	Levy et al.[33]
Q Sepharose XL	90.0	<0.035	1.0	7.6	Syren et al.[112]
Toyopearl DEAE-650M	40.0–90.0	0.1	0.23–0.39	6.9	Urthaler et al.[46]
Adsorbents with larger pores and improved topography					
Streamline QXL	200.0	n.a.	3.0*	4.8	Ferreira et al.[14]
Q Ceramic Hyper D F	50.0	0.30	>5.3	5.9	Eon-Duval et al.[32]
Q Ceramic Hyper D 20	20.0		2.52–6.16	6.9	Urthaler et al.[46]
Fractogel EMD DEAE	40.0–90.0	~0.80	2.45	5.9	Eon-Duval et al.[32]
Fractogel EMD DEAE	40.0–90.0	~0.80	3.29–5.44	6.9	Urthaler et al.[46]
Fractogel EMD DMAE	40.0–90.0	~0.80	4.5	6.9	Levy et al.[33]
Fractogel EMD TMAE	40.0–90.0	~0.80	0.8	7.6	Syren et al.[112]
POROS 50 DEAE	50.0	<0.80	5.0	6.9	Levy et al.[33]
POROS 50 HQ	50.0	<0.80	2.12	5.9	Eon-Duval et al.[32]
Superporous adsorbents					
Cytopore	230.0	30.0	~31*	4.8	Urthaler et al.[46]
Poly EDMA-*co*-GMA	52.4	0.8–5.0	1.36	5.4	Wu et al.[41]
Superporous agarose	60.0	4.0	3.0	7.0	Tiainen et al.[10]
Superporous agarose	60.0	2.0	3.9	7.0	Tiainen et al.[10]
Membranes and monoliths					
Sartobind MA 5 D	–	>3.0	4.0	7.6	Syren et al.[112]
Mustang Q		0.8	15.0	6.3	Endres et al.[49]
Mustang Q		0.8	6.0	4.5	Zhang et al.[50]
CIM DEAE	–	0.70–0.95	8.11–8.86	6.9	Urthaler et al.[46]
CIM DEAE	–	1.3	12.4–13.5	39.4	Krajnc et al.[48]
Poly(EDMA-*co*-GMA)	–	>0.3	15.2	2.9	Danquah et al.[43]

*These figures correspond to static binding capacity.

[†]The designations used are trademarks of GE Healthcare, Uppsala, Sweden (Sepharose FF, Sepharose XL, Source 30Q, Streamline, and Cytopore); Tosoh Bioscience LLC, Japan (Toyopearl); Merck, Darmstadt, Germany (Fractogel); Pall Corporation, Port Washington, NY (Hyper D and Mustang); Applied Biosystems, FosterCity, California (POROS); BIA Separations, Lubjlana, Slovenia (CIM); and Sartorius, Germany (Sartobind).

external 6.1- to 7.3-μm shell, respectively, while a significant portion of the beads (59–66%) remains unused.[16] This situation is perfectly illustrated in Figure 5.9 (see Chapter 5, Section 5.5.3), which shows confocal laser microscopy images of chromatographic beads (<200-nm pores) that had been previously exposed to fluorescently labeled plasmid DNA.[17] Although the results shown were obtained with a particular plasmid and bead, the image is representative of a general situation; that is, plasmids do not enter deeply into the pores of conventional chromatographic beads.[11]

(a)   (b)   (c)

(d)   (e)   (f)

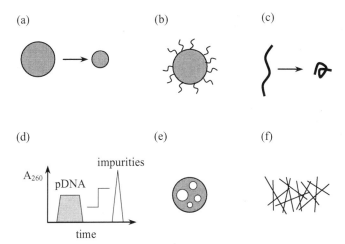

Figure 17.2 *Overview of the strategies used to overcome the accessibility, mass transport, and capacity limitations found in the context of plasmid chromatography. (a) Reduction of bead size; (b) exploration of unusual surface topographies; (c) plasmid compaction; (d) operation in a negative, nonbinding mode; (e) engineering of beads with superpores; and (f) use of non-beaded matrices with a monolithic/membrane format.*

17.2.3 Overcoming Mass Transfer and Capacity Limitations

Several strategies have been suggested and experimented to overcome the major limitations of plasmid chromatography, which were alluded to in the previous section: poor accessibility, mass transport, and binding capacity (see Figure 17.2). Whereas some of those strategies involve an actual change of the structure and geometry of the chromatographic matrix (see Figure 17.2a,b,e,f), others rely on modifying the environmental conditions of the plasmid-containing solutions (Figure 17.2c) or on exploring alternative operating modes (Figure 17.2d).

17.2.3.1 Reduction of Bead Size
Since plasmids essentially bind to an outer shell of ordinary spherical beads, one way to improve capacity is simply to use very small beads (Figure 17.2a).[16] With this strategy, the ratio of bead surface area to bead volume increases, and thus higher capacities can be obtained for a given volume of packed column. Furthermore, since binding occurs essentially at the outer surface, there is no requirement for the beads to be porous. Unfortunately, the operation of chromatographic columns packed with small particles (<10 μm) requires the use of very high pressures. The implementation of such high-pressure liquid chromatography (HPLC) separations may be economically impractical, since in order to operate with and withstand such extreme hydraulic conditions, the full chromatographic system must be equipped with especially designed valves, pumps, piping, detectors, and so on. The reproducible packing of small beads into a column is also not a trivial task. Thus, the process-scale purification of

plasmids by HPLC is clearly not an option, as judged by the inexistence of corresponding reports in the literature. Instead, the higher capacity for plasmid binding made possible by the use of small beads with increased surface area can be better explored in the context of batch adsorption operations where beads are mixed with solutions in a tank. For example, a recent article describes the use of monosized (~1 μm) magnetic polyglycidyl methacrylate microspheres cross-linked with divinylbenzene to capture plasmid DNA from *E. coli* lysates.[18] Using adequate pH and ionic conditions, the capacity of the beads reached 90 μg/mg. Unfortunately, since this figure is given on the basis of the mass and not the volume of adsorbent, a direct comparison with the data in Table 17.1 is not possible.[18] Nonporous anion-exchange matrices with a fiber format have also been developed and tested for plasmid purification.[19] The individual fibers with mean diameters of 1.5 μm are packed as a bed in such a way that a network of pores becomes defined, that is, in many aspects similar to a monolithic or membrane structure. However, and in spite of the excellent flow properties, capacities for plasmid binding did not exceed the 0.9 mg/mL.[19]

17.2.3.2 Unusual Surface Topographies

The first attempts to circumvent the capacity limitations of conventional chromatographic beads toward plasmid molecules relied on the exploration of unusual surface topographies and materials (Figure 17.2b). For example, a number of bead materials like Fractogel EMD (Merck, Darmstadt, Germany) or Streamline (GE Healthcare, Uppsala)[15] possess characteristic "tentacle-like" structures. In the case of Streamline QXL, plasmid molecules can be captured more densely, originating capacities of around 3–5 mg/mL due to the presence of the long dextran chains that protrude from the surface of the 200-μm agarose beads (Table 17.1). As for Fractogel EMD, dynamic binding capacities between 0.8 and 5.4 mg/mL have been reported, depending on the size of the plasmid and on the anion-exchange group used (Table 17.1). Ceramic Hyper D (Pall Corporation, Port Washington, New York) anion exchangers constitute another type of material with a structure that departs from the more traditional chromatographic support. Although porous beads are used as usual, the key differentiating property of the material is a hydrophilic organic gel network with ionic groups (e.g., quaternary amines), which fills up all pores. This three-dimensional gel is formed within the pores of the base ceramic material by *in situ* copolymerization of ionic acrylic monomers and bifunctional acrylic compounds.[20] According to the manufacturer, this "gel in a shell design" affords faster mass transfer and higher capacity, and in fact, experimental data obtained indicate that this is true for plasmids, as judged by the capacities of the order of 2.5–6.2 mg/mL reported[20] (Table 17.1).

17.2.3.3 Plasmid Compaction

One way to partially overcome the size/diffusion barrier and thus to improve binding capacity in plasmid chromatography is to act upon plasmid molecules and to condense them from an elongated coiled state to a compacted globular state (Figure 17.2c). With this strategy, the radius of gyration of plasmids can be substantially reduced. In theory, and in an ideal situation, a plasmid molecule could be compacted into a globule with a radius equivalent to that of a protein with an equivalent mass (see Chapter 4, Figure 4.4). As we have seen before in the context of plasmid precipitation (e.g., Chapter 16, Section 16.3.2), plasmid compaction requires the addition of substances like multivalent cations, polymers, or compaction agents that decrease repulsion between DNA phosphates.[21] If the adequate concentrations of these agents are used, plasmid molecules can be compacted to a certain extent while avoiding aggregation and/or precipitation. If successful, this strategy could facilitate the access of plasmids to the innermost pores of chromatographic beads, while simultaneously allowing a closer packing of adsorbed molecules on the internal surface.[22] Furthermore, compacted plasmids should display an increased diffusion coefficient roughly equivalent to that of the globular protein referred above. The decrease in plasmid size, which is brought about by compaction, may also contribute to narrow the size distribution of a population of plasmid molecules. This could potentially lead to a more homogeneous behavior during chromatography, and ultimately to sharper peaks, higher yields and capacity, and increased selectivity. Several reports in the literature attest to this beneficial effect of compaction agents on the performance of plasmid chromatography. The use of a 2 M ammonium sulfate buffer during size-exclusion chromatography, for example, has been claimed to increase productivity as a result of the narrowing of the plasmid size distribution.[17,23] In another case, the use of 2.5 mM of spermine led to an increase of the equilibrium capacity of the anion-exchanger Q Sepharose for plasmid DNA by as much as 40%.[22] Finally, the addition of polyethylene glycol prior to the anion-exchange chromatography of plasmid DNA with a Q Sepharose adsorbent has been claimed to increase recovery from 20% to 80%.[24]

17.2.3.4 Negative Chromatography

As mentioned before, although the preferred option when purifying biomolecules like proteins is usually to operate chromatography in the positive mode, it is clear that one possible solution to the plasmid diffusion/capacity conundrum is simply to design chromatography operations to run in a negative mode (Figure 17.2d). Under the nonbinding conditions that are characteristic of this mode of operation, whether plasmids fit or not within the intraparticle pores becomes close to irrelevant. Moreover, plasmids should preferably travel with the flow and through the extra particle spaces in the bed without entering the beads altogether, since intra-particle diffusion typically leads to mass transfer-related dispersion effects and delays the exit from the column. The target impurities, on the other hand, should now diffuse into the beads and adequately bind to the available surfaces. This may still be problematic in the case of the largest RNA and gDNA fragments, which have sizes and diffusion coefficients of the order of magnitude of those found for plasmids (see Chapter 14, Figure 14.3). Hydrophobic interaction chromatography has been explored in this context[8,25,26] (see Section 17.2.6). By adequately manipulating conditions like the ligand type and elution buffers, it is possible to promote the binding of RNA, gDNA, and LPS. As for plasmids, their low hydrophobicity prevents them from binding. Thus, plasmids can be purified with negative hydrophobic interaction chromatography by loading feed solutions at a high concentration of an adequate salt and by subsequently performing step or gradient elution with low salt to remove bound impurities.[8,25,26]

As we have just seen, a negative mode of operation adapts itself very well to hydrophobic interaction chromatography on account of the lower hydrophobicity of plasmids when compared with that of impurities. In the case of anion-exchange chromatography, however, plasmids bind stronger than most impurities to the ligands, and so in principle, it should not be possible to purify plasmids by adopting a negative mode of operation. A group of researchers has cleverly overcome this limitation by making use of restricted access chromatography beads.[27,28] These so-called lid beads feature a positively charged inner core that adsorbs RNA and an inert porous surface layer that excludes plasmids on the basis of their size, thus preventing their adsorption in the bead interior. When a column packed with these lid beads is fed with an impure plasmid solution (e.g., a clarified lysate), plasmids effectively pass in the flow-through, while the smaller RNA impurities diffuse into the beads and bind to the anion-exchange ligands.[27,28] The plasmid-containing flow-through can then be directed to a column packed with "normal" anion-exchange beads so as to capture plasmid DNA and to remove RNA and other impurities as usual.[27]

17.2.3.5 Superporous Beads

A group of matrices has been developed in recent years that combine the normal diffusion pores (300 Å) with very large pores (Figure 17.2e), with diameters in the 0.2- to 30-μm range.[29] One of the key goals underlying these designs was to enable intrapore convective flow to take place within the "superpores" so that the distribution of solutes like proteins to the network of smaller diffusive pores could be accelerated, thus yielding faster separations (10–100 times).[30] The paradigmatic examples of such matrices are the polystyrene-based POROS® beads originally developed by PerSeptive Biosystems (now incorporated in Applied Biosystems, Foster City, California). These so-called perfusion supports feature 0.6- to 0.8-μm "throughpores" alongside 500- to 1000-Å diffusive pores.[31] Although they were not developed explicitly for plasmid chromatography, perfusion supports like the anion exchanger POROS 50 HQ are able to bind up to 10 mg of plasmids/mL of matrix[32–34] (Table 17.1). This excellent capacity may be directly attributable to the fact that plasmid molecules are now able to partially creep inside the large throughpores and to bind to their walls.[15,35]

The preparation of chromatographic beads that combine normal diffusion pores (~300 Å) with micrometer-wide superpores (2–30 μm) has also been described in a number of research publications.[10,36–41] In the case of the agarose-based beads described by Tiainen et al.,[10] Gustavsson and Larsson,[36] and Gustavsson et al.,[37] superpores with a typical tortuosity of approximately 1.2 and average diameters of 2, 4, 20, and 30 μm have all been reported (Figure 17.3a). On average, these superpores account for around 40% of the bead

(a) (b)

(c) (d)

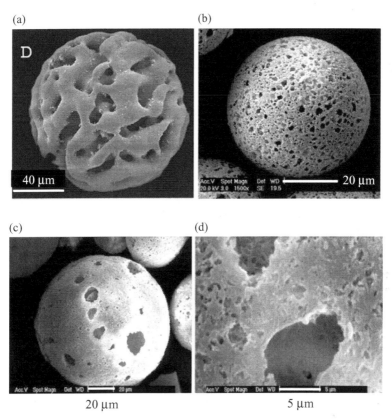

20 μm   5 μm

Figure 17.3 *Electron microscopy images of superporous chromatographic beads made of agarose (a) and poly(EDMA-co-GMA) (b–d). (a) Reprinted from Journal of Chromatography A, 1138, Tiainen P, Gustavsson P-E, Ljunglöf A, Larsson P-O. Superporous agarose anion exchangers for plasmid isolation, 84–94, Copyright 2007,[10] with permission from Elsevier. (b) Reprinted from Journal of Applied Polymer Science, 104, Li Y, Dong X-Y, Sun Y. Biporous polymeric microspheres coupled with mercaptopyridine for rapid chromatographic purification of plasmid DNA, 2205–2211, Copyright 2007,[40] with permission from John Wiley & Sons. (c, d) With kind permission from Springer Science+Business Media: Chromatographia, High-speed large scale chromatographic purification of plasmid DNA with a novel giant-pore stationary phase, 66, 2007, 151–157, Wu L, Pang G-C, Figure 1.[41]*

volume. Ethylene dimethacrylate (EDMA) and glycidyl methacrylate (GMA) can also be copolymerized in such a way as to yield rigid spherical beads with average diameters in the 29- to 54-μm range, which combine the normal 20- to 1000-Å diffusion pores with 0.5- to 7.3-μm superpores[40,41] (see Figure 17.3c,d). Due to the presence of a large fraction of superpores, the specific surface areas in these beads (e.g., ~20 m^2/g[40] and ~80 m^2/g[41]) are somewhat lower than the typical surface area of the conventional microporous materials (~100 m^2/g). The presence of superpores in the agarose and poly(EDMA-*co*-GMA) beads just described is shown very clearly in the scanning electron microscopy photographs in Figure 17.3b–d. Although micron-sized pores are readily visible in all cases, it is interesting to notice that the topography and general aspect is quite different among the particles. For example, the dense network of regularly spaced superpores, which is characteristic of the poly(EDMA-*co*-GMA) beads described by Li et al.[40] (Figure 17.3b), offers a striking contrast with the wormlike superpores in the softer agarose beads developed by Tiainen et al.[10] (Figure 17.3a) or with the uneven and random positioning of the superpores in the poly(EDMA-*co*-GMA) beads of Wu and Pang[41] (Figure 17.3c). In any case, the presence of superpores in the matrices increases the accessibility of plasmids to their interior and simultaneously allows for the convection of fluid to take place inside the beads. Furthermore, if sufficient rigidity can be designed into the particles, high flow velocities can be used in packed columns without the disadvantage of high back pressures.[41]

The agarose and poly(EDMA-*co*-GMA) beads described have been used in plasmid chromatography, both for operations run in a negative mode, which rely on the binding of impurities and not of the target molecule, and for operations run in a positive mode, which rely on the binding of plasmid. For example, by grafting ligands like polyethyleneimine on agarose,[10] or phenyl[39] or mercaptopyridine[40] on poly(EDMA-*co*-GMA) beads, plasmid purification by anion-exchange and hydrophobic interaction chromatography has been reported. The chromatographic profiles obtained in either case were similar to the ones obtained with conventional chromatographic supports, indicating that the introduction of superporosity does not change the characteristic selectivity of the two operations in the face of plasmid solutions contaminated with *E. coli* impurities (see Sections 17.2.5 and 17.2.6). The presence of superpores in these polymeric beads improves the access of plasmid, and thus higher binding capacities are expected if the beads are grafted with anion-exchanger chemical groups. However, the experimental data available regarding the use of superporous beads in plasmid chromatography show that the gains in capacity have been rather modest (see Table 17.1). For example, the binding capacities reported for agarose beads with 4-μm superpores and for poly(EDMA-*co*-GMA) beads with 0.8- to 5.0-μm superpores were 3.9 mg/mL for a 7000-bp plasmid[10] and 1.36 mg/mL for a 5400-bp plasmid,[41] respectively. This can be explained by the drop in the pore wall surface area associated with the presence of superpores that was highlighted earlier.

17.2.3.6 Membranes and Monoliths

The combination of very large superpores with smaller networks of diffusion pores is also found in materials like chromatographic membranes and monolithic supports (Figure 17.2f), as exemplified by the electron microscopy photograph of a polymeric monolith shown in Figure 17.4a. The potential of such a material to accommodate a plasmid DNA molecule can be better judged by comparing its open porous structure with the schematic representation of a 5000-bp plasmid roughly drawn to scale (see Figure 17.4a). Similar highly porous structures, with pores typically larger than 0.5–3.0 μm, are also found in chromatographic membranes like the one shown in the electron microscopy image of Figure 17.4b. This structure offers a striking contrast with the dense-

(a)

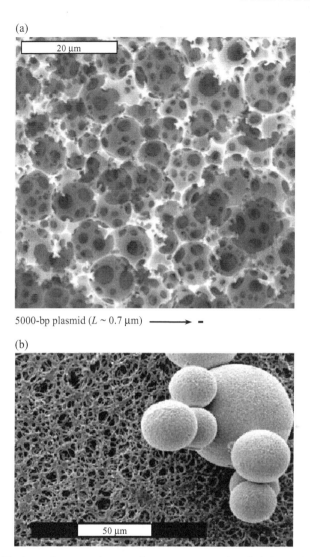

5000-bp plasmid ($L \sim 0.7 \, \mu m$) ⟶ ▪

(b)

Figure 17.4 *Electron microscopy images of superporous, nonbeaded chromatographic matrices. The combination of very large superpores with smaller networks of diffusion pores provides one way to overcome the plasmid accessibility/capacity bottlenecks found in conventional chromatographic beads. The images show (a) a highly permeable polyHIPE monolith and (b) a Sartobind membrane adsorber with conventional chromatographic beads on the right side. (a) Reprinted from Organic Letters, 4, Krajnc P, Brown JF, Cameron NR. Monolithic scavenger resins by amine functionalizations of poly(4-vinylbenzyl chloride-co-divinylbenzene) PolyHIPE materials, 2497–2500, Copyright 2002[111] with permission from American Chemical Society). (b) Reprinted with permission from Sartorius-Stedim Biotech GmbH).*

surface structure of the common chromatographic beads on the right-hand side of the image. In view of these characteristics, it is not surprising to find that when monoliths or chromatographic membranes are derivatized with anion-exchange groups and used for plasmid binding, capacities of the order of 8.0–15.0 mg/mL are obtained (Table 17.1). In the specific cases shown in the table, these high loadings can be ascribed to the presence of 0.8-μm pores, in the case of the Mustang® chromatographic membranes from Pall Corporation,[42] and to the highly interconnected network of 0.01- to 4.0-μm channels, in the case of CIM® (Bia Separations, Klagenfurt, Austria)[7] and poly(EDMA-co-GMA) monolithic supports.[43] In some cases, monolithic columns with extremely large, continuous, and interconnected pores (10–100 μm), and dense, nonporous walls can be produced by the polymerization of acrylamide at subzero temperatures.[44] The major drawback of these so-called macroporous cryogels, however, is a limited surface area for binding, and so it is not unexpected to find that plasmid binding capacities in these materials drop to figures of the order of 0.004 mg/mL.[44]

As a result of their high permeability, chromatographic membranes and monolithic supports can be operated with high flow rates (e.g., up to 1000 cm/h for monoliths[3]) and low back pressures.[3] This means that if the capacities of the materials for plasmid DNA binding can be kept high, significant increases in throughput can be obtained, which are unrivaled by fixed bed operations. The use of membranes and monoliths as alternative supports for the chromatographic purification of plasmid DNA has been described in several publications. Although in the majority of cases anion-exchange interactions with chemical groups like quaternary and tertiary amines bound to monoliths[7,45–48] and membranes[42,49–51] are explored, the interaction of impurities and plasmids with hydrophobic[52] and affinity[53] ligands is also a possibility. A number of these studies have demonstrated the effectiveness of both membrane- and monolith-based technologies to purify large amounts of plasmids from solutions within relatively short process times. In one study, monolithic structures have even been found suitable to handle very large plasmids with sizes up to 93,000 bp.[48] Although not referred to in that report, one problem that might occur when using monoliths and membrane stacks to purify such larger plasmids is yield loss due to fouling, as explained next. Given the continuous and heterogeneous structure of the pores in those matrices, a fraction of the plasmid molecules may intrude into narrower channels and become faced with the presence of throats. In these situations, plasmid molecules may be unable to elongate sufficiently to move past the constrictions, effectively meeting a dead end.

17.2.4   Plasmid Purification

Different types of physical–chemical interactions between solutes and porous matrices are explored in the chromatographic separation of biomolecules, of which the most common are size exclusion, electrostatic, hydrophobic, and affinity.[13] All of these interactions have been looked at in an attempt to separate plasmids from the usual *E. coli* impurities. In the following sections, a summary of the most used modalities of chromatography—anion exchange, hydrophobic interaction, affinity, and size exclusion—is made, with a special focus put on the description of the underlying molecular mechanisms. Since the body of literature on plasmid chromatography is rather vast, reference is made to those studies that are the most relevant from a process point of view.

17.2.5 Anion-Exchange Chromatography

17.2.5.1 Introduction

The choice for an anion-exchange chromatography as a final purification operation is obvious when one considers the polyanionic nature of plasmid DNA and of the key gDNA and RNA impurities. The interaction between the negatively charged phosphate groups in the backbone of DNA and RNA and the positively charged ligands like tertiary or quaternary amines in the stationary phase is at the heart of the separation.[13] As a starting point, the partially purified, plasmid-containing solution obtained after completion of the intermediate recovery steps (see Chapter 16) is loaded on the column at an ionic strength high enough (usually equivalent to 0.4–0.5 M NaCl) to avoid the needless binding of those impurities that have a lower charge density than plasmid DNA. Under these conditions and upon washing the column with a buffer of a similar ionic strength, significant amounts of low-molecular-weight RNA, oligonucleotides, and proteins exit in the flow-through without compromising the capacity of the anion exchanger for plasmid binding (Figure 17.5a). Then, an increasing salt gradient (usually of NaCl) is used to selectively displace the plasmid DNA, high-MW RNA, and gDNA species that bound to the column on account of their higher net charge. The size differences among the different species are especially important in this context, since the strength of the electrostatic interaction between the molecules and the anion-exchange groups in the matrix is roughly proportional to the number of phosphate groups in the molecule. In other words, the larger is the molecule, the strongest is its binding to the charged matrix, and hence the later it elutes from the column. One way to minimize the amount of high-MW RNA that binds to the anion exchange supports is to pretreat the plasmid-containing feed with RNase. Although there are regulatory concerns associated with this strategy (see Chapter 11, Section 11.6.3), the smaller fragments obtained as a result of the enzymatic cleavage of RNA will now exit in the flow-through on account of their weakest binding to the support. This reduces the likelihood of coelution of RNA with the plasmid and greatly improves the separation. This beneficial effect of an RNase pretreatment on the performance of anion-exchange chromatography is illustrated very well in Figure 5.10b, although in the case of an analytical chromatography application (see Chapter 5, Section 5.6.1).

The spatial conformation adopted by nucleic acids may also play a role on the binding, since events like supercoiling or compaction can partially conceal parts of the molecule and hence can decrease the number of charged phosphate groups that are effectively available for interaction. On the other hand, such changes in conformation may also decrease the size of the molecules and increase their charge density in such a way that more binding sites in the surface are covered per DNA molecule.[51] This is probably one of the reasons

(a)

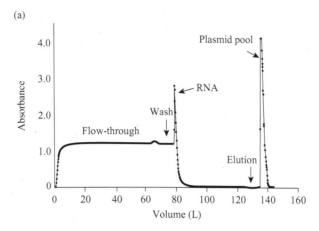

(b)

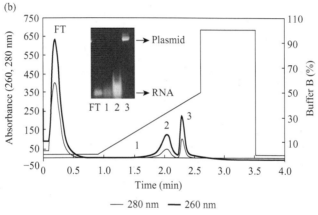

— 280 nm — 260 nm

(c)

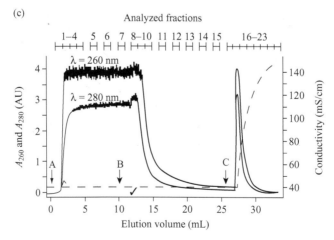

←───

why the binding of supercoiled plasmid isoforms to anion exchangers is, in many cases, stronger than the binding of its looser and broader open circular counterparts.[9,54] Whichever is the case, the important fact here is that it is possible to separate open circular from supercoiled plasmid isoforms using anion-exchange chromatography. In spite of this important characteristic, one of the recurrent problems of anion-exchange chromatography is the coelution of plasmid DNA with gDNA and RNA species. Such poor separation selectivity results from the fact that the binding strength of plasmid DNA and impurities is very similar, independent of whether this results from size similarities or from conformational changes. This is one of the reasons why it is very important, when performing the disruption of *E. coli* cells (see Chapter 15, Section 15.3), to guarantee that gDNA is not broken into fragments that are similar to plasmid when it comes to its charge/size relation.[55]

17.2.5.2 Selected Applications

Packed beds of conventional and superporous beads, monoliths, and membranes have all been used to capture plasmid DNA from process solutions by anion-exchange interaction. Since the number of reports on this specific topic is vast (e.g., see references 7, 9, 10, 32, 42, 44, 46, 48–50, 56, and 57), only three cases were selected for discussion here, which are representative of the typical separation obtained with anion-exchange chromatography (Figure 17.5). The examples described next also highlight the diversity of matrix formats, which is nowadays available to implement plasmid chromatography. The first case deals with the direct capture of plasmid DNA from a clarified alkaline lysate by an anion-exchange membrane chromatography capsule (Mustang Q, Pall Corporation).[50] The membrane capsule was equilibrated with 0.5 M NaCl and the lysate was diluted with 1.5 volumes of water to adjust the conductivity in such a way as to ensure plasmid binding and to maximize the removal of impurities in the flow-through (Figure 17.5a). After loading the feed, the membrane was washed with a solution containing 0.6 M NaCl and the bound plasmid was eluted with a step gradient to 1.2 M NaCl. The corresponding chromatogram shows that a significant amount of UV-absorbing impurities are removed during loading and washing, while plasmid elutes as a single peak at high salt. The analysis of this pool shows that (1) 95% of the loaded plasmid was recovered with a 10-fold increase in concentration; (2) traces of RNA and gDNA are still present; and (3) LPS content is reduced by four orders of magnitude.[50]

In the second case, plasmid DNA was purified from a clarified alkaline lysate with a short monolithic column (CIM® DEAE, BIA Separations, Ljubljana).[7] The column was equilibrated with a solution containing 0.5 M NaCl and 15% isopropanol (to minimize nonspecific hydrophobic interactions), and the lysate was loaded without preconditioning. Following washing with the equilibration buffer, bound material was eluted with a combination of linear and stepwise gradients of NaCl up to 1.5 M (Figure 17.5b). The chromatogram shows the distinctive flow-through peak of impurities and a succession of peaks eluting under the action of the linear gradient. The electrophoresis analysis of the different fractions (see gel insert in Figure 17.5b) shows that peak 3 corresponds exclusively to plasmid DNA, whereas the flow-through peak and peaks 1 and 2 contain mostly RNA. Notice that in agreement with the behavior described earlier, RNA of higher MW is eluting in fraction 2 as compared to the RNA removed in the flow-through.[7]

The third situation refers to a case where superporous anion-exchange agarose beads were developed intentionally for the capture of plasmid DNA from an RNase-treated alkaline lysate.[10] A 5-mm i.d. column was packed to a bed height of 3.7 cm with 45- to 75-μm agarose beads with 4-μm superpores (see Figure 17.3a) and Q (quaternary amine) ligands. Following equilibration with a 0.4 M NaCl buffer, 10 mL of a clarified alkaline lysate with a conductivity matching that of the mobile phase was injected. The typical chromatogram (Figure 17.5c) and supporting analysis of the collected fractions show that the majority of low-molecular-weight RNA species (97%) elute in the flow-through. As for the plasmid, it exited the column as a single peak by stepping up the NaCl concentration in the elution buffer to 2 M. The authors further report that 59% of the adsorbed plasmid material was recovered.[10]

Collectively, the previous examples underscore some of the key features that make anion exchange one of the favorite chromatography modalities for plasmid purification: (1) removal of large amounts of RNA impurities in the flow-through at moderate ionic strength (0.4–0.5 M NaCl) and elution of the plasmid with an increase in ionic strength (up to 1.2–2.0 M NaCl), (2) possibility of isoform resolution, and (3) concentration of plasmids in the collected pools of purified material relative to the incoming feed.

17.2.6 Hydrophobic Interaction Chromatography

17.2.6.1 Introduction

One of the properties that set plasmid molecules apart from the single-stranded nucleic acid impurities (gDNA and RNA) that are characteristically found in plasmid purification is hydrophobicity. In plasmids, the majority of the hydrophobic bases are paired, stacked, and shielded inside the double helix, whereas the sugar–phosphate chains are characteristically positioned in the outside of the molecule (see Chapter 4, Section 4.2). Given the large number of hydrogen bond donors and acceptor groups, the backbone is able to establish hydrogen bonds with the surrounding water molecules. As a result, plasmids are essentially hydrophilic molecules that tend to move away from hydrophobic surfaces. In single-stranded nucleic acids, on the other hand, the aromatic bases are less constrained due to the lack of pairing and packing, and thus are largely exposed to the surrounding environment and are available to interact with hydrophobic surfaces.[58] Another group of important impurities that possesses a strong hydrophobic character is LPS, on account of the presence of the lipid A moiety in its structure (see Chapter 14, Figure 14.2). The large differences in the hydrophobicity of plasmids and molecular impurities (RNA, gDNA, oligonucleotides, denatured plasmid, and LPS) just explained are explored for separation purposes in hydrophobic interaction chromatography.[25,26,39,52,59–62] Additionally, hydrophobic interactions are also at play in other types of chromatography alongside other more specific interactions. However, these cases are discussed in more detail in Section 17.2.7.

Hydrophobic interaction chromatography operations use matrices whose surface is made hydrophobic by the coupling of chemical groups like phenyl, butyl, or octyl. As a starting point, columns or cartridges are typically equilibrated with a buffer that contains large amounts (~1.2–1.6 M) of salting-out salts like ammonium sulfate or sodium citrate (see Chapter 16, Section 16.3.3). The preferential hydration of the salt ions guarantees that hydrophobic interactions between hydrophobic solutes are maximized when the plasmid-containing stream is loaded. The same salts are also used to precondition the plasmid-containing feed and thus to guarantee a homogeneous concentration of salts throughout the column.

17.2.6.2 *Selected Applications*

In order to exemplify the ability of hydrophobic interaction chromatography to purify plasmid DNA, let us consider the use of a phenyl Sepharose 6 Fast Flow column (GE Healthcare) with sodium citrate buffers shown in Figure 17.6a.[8] In order to prepare the feed for chromatography, an alkaline lysate was diafiltered by tangential flow filtration and then was conditioned by adding sodium citrate up to a final concentration of 1.0 M. The 1-mL column was equilibrated with a solution containing 1.0 M sodium citrate, loaded with 0.5 mL of feed, and washed with the equilibration buffer. The elution of bound material was then performed in isocratic mode by changing to a buffer with no sodium citrate. The chromatogram in Figure 17.6a displays a first flow-through peak, which corresponds mainly to plasmid DNA (all isoforms), and an elution peak, which corresponds to impurities (mainly RNA and LPS). An analysis of the plasmid-containing fractions indicated an 89% yield and showed that 99% of LPS, 93% of proteins, and 52% of gDNA could be removed. The clearance of the LPS obtained is especially remarkable, making the combined action of sodium citrate (or ammonium sulfate) and hydrophobic interactions as one of the best ways to remove LPS from biological products.[63] The agarose gel electrophoresis inserted in the figure further shows that the RNA in the feed

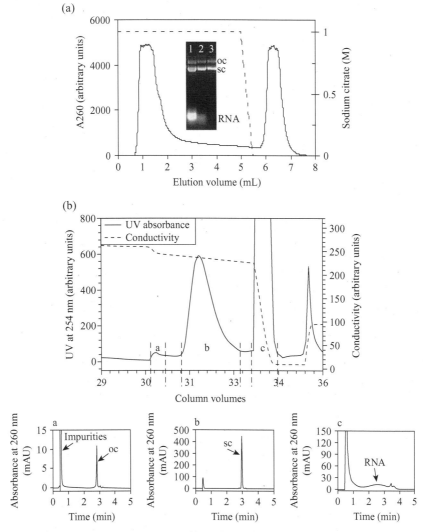

Figure 17.6 Purification of plasmid DNA by hydrophobic interaction chromatography. (a) Purification of plasmid DNA from prepurified plasmid solutions using a phenyl Sepharose 6 Fast Flow column and a downward gradient of sodium citrate buffers. Alkaline lysates were diafiltered by tangential flow filtration (lane 1) and were preconditioned with 1 M sodium citrate (lane 2). Plasmid was recovered in the flow-through (lane 3). (b) Separation of supercoiled and open circular isoforms using hydrophobic columns equilibrated with 2.5–3.0 M ammonium sulfate. oc, open circular; sc, supercoiled. (a) Adapted and reprinted from Separation and Purification Technology, 65, Freitas SS, Santos JAL, Prazeres DMF. Plasmid purification by hydrophobic interaction chromatography using sodium citrate in the mobile phase, 95–104, Copyright 2009,[8] with permission from Elsevier. (b) Reprinted with permission from Urthaler J, Buchinger W, Necina R. Industrial scale cGMP purification of pharmaceutical-grade plasmid DNA. Chemical Engineering and Technology. 2005. 28.1408–1420. Copyright Wiley-VCH Verlag GmbH & Co. KGaA.[60]

is completely removed and that the high proportion of supercoiled to open circular plasmid remains unchanged.[8] The main drawback of the separation is most likely the dilution of plasmid in the pool relative to the feed (4.5-fold), a characteristic that is close to inevitable when running chromatography in the negative mode.[8]

Although in the previous case plasmid DNA did not bind to the hydrophobic phenyl ligands in the matrix on account of its low hydrophobicity, in some cases, the properties of the stationary and mobile phase can be manipulated in such a way as to warrant the binding of plasmids.[8,52,61] This dual behavior of plasmid molecules in the face of hydrophobic moieties is well exemplified by the tandem use of Butyl-6PW and Octyl-6PW (Tosoh Bioscience LLC, Tokyo, Japan) columns reported by Kitamura and Nakatani.[64] The two columns were connected in series and equilibrated with 2.0 M ammonium sulfate, and the first butyl column was then fed with a clarified lysate. Like in the case previously reported, protein and RNA adsorbed to the matrix, whereas plasmid exited in the flow-through, concomitantly entering in the second octyl column. Here, however, and on account of the stronger hydrophobicity of the octyl ligands, plasmid was found to bind to the matrix alongside with gDNA. Once the columns were disconnected, impurities and plasmid DNA in the first and second columns, respectively, were eluted by decreasing the salt concentration.[64] This use of phenyl-based columns to bind impurities and octyl-based columns to bind plasmid has also been advocated by Nochumson et al.[61]

The ability to bind plasmid to hydrophobic interaction columns has been explored for purification in other cases, and also with the additional specific goal of separating supercoiled from open circular isoforms.[52,60] For example, the chromatogram shown in Figure 17.6b was obtained after loading a preconditioned (with 2.5–3 M ammonium sulfate) lysate on a hydrophobic interaction column equilibrated with an ammonium sulfate-containing buffer and after running a gradient of decreasing salt concentration.[60] Under those conditions, baseline resolution of three peaks was obtained. The early eluting peak *a* corresponds to impurities and open circular plasmid; peak *b* corresponds to supercoiled plasmid; and peak *c* corresponds to impurities and residual RNA. Other strongly bound impurities were only removed upon regeneration of the column with NaOH. The most significant observation drawn from this study is that it is possible to used hydrophobic interaction chromatography to resolve supercoiled from open circular topoisomers.[60] Other authors have reported similar results both with conventional beads[61] and monolithic supports.[52] The observed selectivity toward the two isoforms must be due to the preferential and stronger interaction of the ligands with the bases of supercoiled plasmids, as compared with the bases of open circular plasmids. Most likely, and as a consequence of deformations induced by torsional strain, the bases of the supercoiled isoform are more exposed than the bases of the open circular isoform. Furthermore, the results described earlier suggest that this exposure is exacerbated at very high salt conditions, since plasmid binding to hydrophobic supports is usually not observed at concentrations lower than 2 M ammonium sulfate. This notion that exposed bases are involved in the binding of plasmids is supported by tests that show that plasmids denatured by alkaline and thermal treatment are totally retained under conditions that are otherwise not favorable to plasmid binding.[65]

17.2.6.3 Reversed-Phase Chromatography

Although descriptions of the preparative use of reversed-phase chromatography for plasmid purification do not abound in the literature,[66,67] a few lines should be devoted to a brief discussion of this type of chromatography. The matrices used are characterized by a high coverage of surfaces with organic ligands like *n*-alkyl chains (e.g., butyl and octyl). These nonpolar hydrophobic ligands can establish an interaction of the "hydrophobic type" with the aromatic bases of nucleic acids, much as was described earlier for hydrophobic interaction chromatography. One important difference here, though, is that solutes that are bound to reversed-phase columns in aqueous solutions are eluted with increasing amounts of organic solvents like alcohols (e.g., ethanol[66] or isopropanol[67]) or acetonitrile.[61] This distinctive characteristic is also responsible for one of the disadvantages of the technique—the use of organic solvents in a process environment presents a series of important risks (e.g., health, fire, explosion, and waste disposal). The behavior of the usual solutes present in plasmid-containing solutions in reversed-phase chromatography is quite similar to the one observed for hydrophobic interaction chromatography—solutes with a high exposure of bases (e.g., single-stranded RNA and partially denatured DNA) and/or with increased lengths display higher retention times when compared with solutes with a high content in double strands (e.g., plasmid DNA).

The selectivity and resolution of reversed-phase chromatography in plasmid purification can be further improved by using ion pairing agents. In this so-called ion-pair reversed-phase chromatography, a hydrophobic stationary phase is combined with a mobile phase that contains ion polar species in such a way that separations result both from differences in hydrophobicity and charge density. This type of chromatographic modality has been explored in the context of plasmid purification by the company Puresyn, Inc. (Malvern, Pennsylvania).[68,69] The process relies on the use of a chemically inert, nonporous polymer resin (PolyFlo®) and on the addition of ion-pairing agents like tetrabutyl ammonium phosphate (TBAP) or triethyl amine acetate (TEAA) to the mobile phase and plasmid-containing feed.[69] The binding of the amphiphilic ions TBAP or TEAA to the phosphate backbone, which is dependent both on the number of phosphates and charge density, renders nucleic acids more hydrophobic and thus more prone to bind to the highly hydrophobic matrix. While species like RNA, gDNA fragments, and LPS are inherently hydrophobic to start with, the hydrophobicity of more polar species like supercoiled plasmid DNA can be increased substantially. Subsequently, an organic solvent (e.g., acetonitrile) gradient is applied to progressively elute species according to their increasing hydrophobicity. The typical chromatograms will show the elution of small-MW RNA in the void volume, followed by a single peak of high-MW RNA, high-MW gDNA, and nonmonomeric forms of plasmid and a second peak containing mostly supercoiled plasmid DNA.[68] As for LPSs, they bind so strongly to the matrix on account of the high affinity of the lipid A portion of the molecule that they can only be removed during regeneration with 0.5 M NaOH. The net result is that the separation of open circular and supercoiled plasmid isoforms, although indirectly, is actually based on differences in charge density, whereas the clearance of impurities like LPS, RNA, gDNA, and protein is based on differences in hydrophobicity.[69] The quality of plasmid DNA that is isolated by ion-pair reversed-phase chromatography is excellent, not only in terms of the residual amounts of RNA, protein, gDNA, LPS, and nonsupercoiled plasmid isoforms but also with regard to the biological activity.[69] The uses and merits of ion-pair reversed-phase chromatography have also been reported by the company Prometic Life Sciences (Montreal, Canada), which designed the highly fluorinated synthetic adsorbent Perfluorosorb S specifically for the resolution of plasmid isoforms and the removal of impurities like LPS and gDNA.[70] This type of chromatography played a prominent role in the process used to manufacture the DNA vaccine against West Nile virus used in the immunization of the California condor (case presented in Chapter 10, Section 10.2).[71]

17.2.7 Mixed-Mode Chromatography

17.2.7.1 Introduction
Unlike in the case of anion-exchange and hydrophobic interaction, there is a group of chromatographic separations where it is not possible to pinpoint a single type of interaction as being responsible for the binding of plasmids and other nucleic acids to the specific ligands used. Rather, and since the combination of two or more types of interactions seems to be involved, those cases fall into the mixed-mode chromatography category. This section presents and discusses two specific cases, given their relevance in the context of plasmid purification: amino acid and thiophilic chromatography.

17.2.7.2 Amino Acid Interaction Chromatography
The fact that several amino acid–base interactions have been recognized at the atomic level in different protein–DNA structures[72,73] has fostered the development of a series of chromatographic separations that rely on the use of amino acid ligands like histidine,[74–76] arginine,[77–79] and lysine[80] to purify plasmid DNA. In the case of histidine ligands, for example, and after loading a clarified lysate at 2.3 M ammonium sulfate into a histidine–agarose column, a series of reverse salt step gradients were used to elute open circular plasmid and gDNA (~2.3 M), supercoiled plasmid (~2.0 M), and RNA (<1.5 M) (Figure 17.7a).[74] Control analysis performed on the supercoiled plasmid pool (peak 3) showed that impurities were removed below specifications, with LPS predominating in peaks 2 and 4, gDNA in peaks 2 and 4, proteins in peaks 1 and 2, and RNA in peak 4 (Figure 17.7a).[74] The underlying mechanisms responsible for the observed elution pattern are thought to involve not only ring stacking/hydrophobic interactions between the histidine ligands and the DNA

(a)

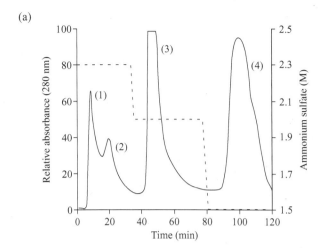

(b)

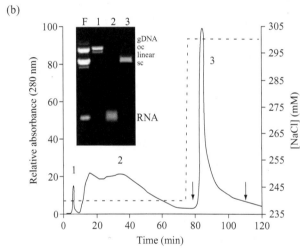

(c)

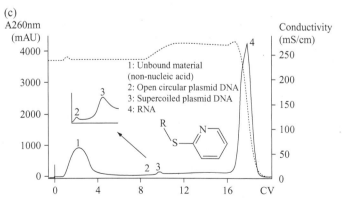

Figure 17.7 Purification of plasmid DNA by mixed-mode chromatography. (a) Isolation of supercoiled plasmid DNA from prepurified solutions in a histidine column and with a series of downward step gradients of ammonium sulfate. (b) Purification of supercoiled plasmid DNA from a prepurified alkaline lysate by arginine chromatography using an NaCl gradient. (c) Purification of plasmid DNA and isoform resolution using a 2-mercaptopyridine column equilibrated with 2.25 M ammonium sulfate and an increasing NaCl gradient. (a) Reproduced with permission, from Sousa F, Freitas S, Azzoni AR, Prazeres DMF, Queiroz J., 2006, Selective purification of super-coiled plasmid DNA from clarified cell lysates with a single histidine-agarose chromatography step, Biotechnology and Applied Biochemistry, 45; 131–140.[74] © Portland Press Limited. (b) Reprinted from Journal of Gene Medicine, 11, Sousa F, Prazeres DMF, Queiroz JA. Improvement of transfection efficiency by using supercoiled plasmid DNA purified with arginine affinity chro-matography, 79–88, Copyright 2009,[79] with permission from John Wiley & Sons. (c) Reprinted from Journal of Gene Medicine, 6, Stadler J, Lemmens R, Nyhammar T. Plasmid DNA purifica-tion, S54–S66, Copyright 2004,[17] with permission from John Wiley & Sons.

←————————————————————————————————————

bases but also hydrogen bonding between the H donor (NτH) and the H acceptor (Nπ) atoms* in the nonprotonated histidine with base edges, and water-mediated hydrogen bonds.[74,76] Although all four DNA bases may be involved in such hydrogen bonding, guanine is usually a preferred target when it comes to interaction with histidine.[72] However, since the different species eluted sequentially with a decrease in salt concentration, and given that hydro-gen bonds are not weakened at lower salt, hydrophobic interactions are prob-ably dominating the separation.[76] Like in the case of hydrophobic interaction chromatography, the preferential and stronger interaction of histidines with the supercoiled isoforms when compared with the open circular isoforms has been attributed to a larger exposition of the bases in the former as a conse-quence of torsional strain-induced deformations.[74,76]

Arginine chromatography has also been used to purify supercoiled plasmid DNA from other isoforms and *E. coli* impurities present in a solution obtained by prepurifying an alkaline lysate with isopropanol and ammonium sulfate precipitation, and desalting by size-exclusion chromatography[79] (Figure 17.7b). In this case, however, the conditions used for optimal separation are substan-tially different from the ones used in the case of histidine ligands, and comprise loading of the feed onto an arginine–agarose column at 0.24 M NaCl and elution of bound species with a step gradient of NaCl to 0.30 M. The typical chromatogram displays two resolved peaks of unbound open circular plasmid and weakly bound RNA at 0.24 M NaCl, followed by a third peak of strongly bound supercoiled plasmid at 0.30 M NaCl (compare chromatogram and gel insert in Figure 17.7b). Polymerase chain reaction (PCR) tests further showed that gDNA eluted at the lower ionic strength.[79] The observed selectivity for the different species was explained as a result of the combination of generic electrostatic interactions with the DNA backbone, with specific interactions involving the recognition of the bases by arginine via hydrogen bonding.[79] To begin with, the fact that plasmid species (and RNA) bind at low ionic strength

---

* N atoms in the imidazole ring of histidine are denoted π or τ if they are closest or farthest to the side chain, respectively.[81]

(Figure 17.7b) suggests that strong interactions between the guanidinium cation of arginine and the anionic phosphate groups in the DNA backbone may be present. Such interactions are common in many protein–DNA complexes, providing stability rather than specificity.[72] Additionally, a number of features of the separation suggest the involvement of some type of specific recognition. In particular, multiple-contact, complex hydrogen bonding interactions of arginine with exposed bases in single-stranded RNA and supercoiled plasmid (as a result of superhelicity) may explain the differential interaction of open circular and supercoiled isoforms and the stronger interaction of RNA when compared with open circular plasmid DNA. Control analysis further showed that interactions with arginine were responsible for a 117-fold reduction in gDNA content and a 95% reduction in LPS content, and that the isolated superoiled plasmid was highly efficient in terms of *in vitro* transfection of mammalian cells.[79]

17.2.7.3 Thiophilic Interaction Chromatography

Thiophilic interaction chromatography uses aromatic thiol ligands that are coupled to the chromatographic matrices as thioethers (check insert in Figure 17.7c). Given its usefulness in the context of plasmid purification, a thiophilic interaction adsorbent featuring 2-mercaptopyridine ligands has been developed into a commercial product that is most appropriately sold under the trade name PlasmidSelect® (GE Healthcare).[17] In the typical separation shown in Figure 17.7c, clarified alkaline lysates are loaded in a 2.25 M ammonium sulfate buffer and are eluted with an increasing NaCl gradient (superimposed in the ammonium sulfate buffer) up to 1.4 M. Under these conditions, a first peak of unbound, non-nucleic acid material exits in the flow-through, whereas the open circular isoforms elute early in the NaCl gradient followed by supercoiled isoforms. As for the tightly bound RNA, proteins, and LPS, they could only be dislodged from the column by decreasing the salt concentration to approximately zero.[17] The interaction of open circular and supercoiled plasmid isoforms with the thiophilic ligands at high salt concentration occurs probably via hydrophobic (π–π) interactions with the aromatic ring and ion-pair interactions with the electron–donor sulfur atom.[17,23,82] Interestingly, the simultaneous presence of the sulfur atom and of the aromatic ring is required to retain plasmid DNA, since studies performed with aliphatic thioether ligands or with ligands that lack the vicinal sulfur resulted in no binding whatsoever.[17,23] Such thiophilic interaction separations have been integrated in a full plasmid purification process alongside size-exclusion and anion-exchange chromatography steps.[17] Further details on this process are given in Chapter 18 (Section 18.4.1).

17.2.8 Affinity and Pseudoaffinity Chromatography

17.2.8.1 Introduction

A substantial number of attempts have been made to develop chromatographic matrices capable of specifically recognizing plasmid molecules out of a mixture of different impurities. The chemical groups used to mediate such affinity interactions are varied, and range from oligonucleotides to peptides and proteins. In spite of the high selectivity inherent to these systems, there are a number of drawbacks that are likely to prevent the full development of plasmid affinity chromatography techniques at process scale. Two of the most important limitations are probably the labile nature and the cost associated with the synthesis of some of the affinity ligands (e.g., proteins). In spite of this, the proof-of-concept studies describing the affinity purification of plasmids that have appeared in the literature are presented next.

17.2.8.2 Triple-Helix Chromatography

Triple-helix affinity chromatography (THAC) relies on the formation of triple helixes via the specific hybridization of oligonucleotides immobilized in the chromatographic matrix with a target sequence within the plasmid DNA. As described in Section 4.4.6 of Chapter 4, such DNA triplexes may form between homopurine•homopyrimidine duplex DNA tracts and a third homopyrimidine or homopurine strand through the formation of base pairs of the Hoogsteen (i.e., T·A•T, C⁺·G•C) and reverse Hoogsteen (i.e., G·G•C, A·A•T, T·A•T) type, respectively (see Chapter 4, Figures 4.11a,b). Thus, if a synthetic homopurine or homopyrimidine ligand is correctly designed and immobilized in a chromatographic matrix, an affinity chromatography type of operation can in principle be implemented, as long as the plasmid contains the matching duplex sequence. As for this target sequence, it can either be naturally present in the plasmid or else it must be introduced artificially. The first situation is obviously more convenient because no plasmid modifications are required. A good example of such a "naturally" present duplex target is the sequence 5′-CTTCC CGAAGGGAGAAAGG-3′, which can be found in the origin of replication of colE1-type plasmids.[83] Although this sequence contains a first block of pyrimidines adjacent to a second block of purines, and not simply a homopurine tract as usually required, it can nevertheless mediate triplex formation if the third strand is allowed to pair with purines in alternate strands.[84] For this, a third strand with the sequence 5′-GAAGGGCTTCCCTCTTTCC-3′ should be designed so as to pair with the purine tract of one strand of the Watson–Crick duplex via G·G•C, A·A•T triplets, and then cross over to bind to the purine tract of the alternate strand of the double helix via T·A•T, C⁺·G•C triplets.[83]

In another example, homopyrimidine sequences of the $(CTT)_7$, $(CT)_{11}$, and $(CCT)_7$ types were covalently attached to a HiTrap NHS column and were used to purify plasmids containing the corresponding sequences ($[GAA]_{17}$, $[GA]_{25}$, $[GGA]_{15}$). The binding of the plasmid to the column was promoted under high NaCl (2 M) concentration to minimize repulsion between phosphates in adjacent backbones and at acidic pH (4.5) to warrant the protonation of cytosines required for Hoogsteen base pairing. Elution was carried out after 2 h by raising the pH value to 9.0 in order to deprotonate cytosines and thus to dissociate the triple helix.[85]

Plasmid yields were found to increase when the percentage of cytosines in the third strand was decreased. This was attributed to the fact that C⁺·G•C triplets are destabilized by the presence of adjacent C⁺·G•C.[85] The best results were thus obtained with a 21-mer oligonucleotide $(CTT)_7$ attached to a $(CH_2)_{12}$ linker.[85] Furthermore, yields increased when longer target double strands were inserted in the plasmid as opposed to shorter ones (51 vs. 21 nucleotides), probably due to the existence of a higher number of possible hybridization positions.[85] After the optimization of several parameters, the best yield obtained was around 50%. Another interesting observation is that the purified fraction contained a higher percentage of supercoiled plasmid DNA than the starting material. Other authors[86] have reported an opposite behavior, probably indicating that the preferential binding of a specific isoform might be a function of the target sequence or of its position on the plasmid.[87] Plasmid purified in one step from a cleared lysate by using this method appeared as a single peak in HPLC analysis. No RNA was found by agarose gel electrophoresis, and gDNA and LPS contamination was decreased by two orders of magnitude. The authors also showed that the performance of the process could be improved by inserting THAC into a DNA purification process involving classical purification steps. In this case, it would be possible to obtain plasmid DNA with very low *E. coli* gDNA levels (0.01%) and with endotoxin levels suitable for intravenous injection. This production process would yield high-quality pharmaceutical-grade pDNA for human clinical trials.

17.2.8.3 *Protein Chromatography*

The recognition of certain DNA segments by specific protein motifs is a critical step in DNA transactions like transcription, replication, packaging, or repair.[88] Some attempts have been made to exploit the affinity interactions underlying such recognition events in the context of plasmid chromatography. Generically speaking, this involves the use of a chromatographic matrix linked to a specific protein or polypeptide ligand, which is able to bind to a given DNA segment in the plasmid molecule. This target sequence is either already present in the plasmid, for example, as a part of a given element, or else it must be cloned in advance.

An illustrative example of the protein–DNA affinity strategy is provided by Darby et al., who explored the binding of the *lac* repressor (LacI) protein to the *lac* operon.[89,90] In this regulatory network, the tetrameric LacI is responsible for the inhibition of the expression of genes involved in the metabolism of lactose. LacI binds simultaneously to two out of three possible operators $(O_1, O_2,$ or $O_3)$ in the *lac* operon via two domains, forcing the intervening DNA to bend and fold into a 76-bp loop[91] (Figure 17.8a). One domain always binds to the O_1 operator, while the other binds either to the O_2 or O_3 operator.[91] The structural motifs in each domain consist of two pairs of α-helices that accommodate within consecutive major grooves in the 21-bp palindromic DNA sequence (A̲A̲TTGTG̲AGC̲GG̲ATA̲ACA̲ATT) of the operators.[92] The recognition is mediated by hydrogen bonds between specific amino acids and accessible base pairs.[93] As a result of the binding of LacI, RNA polymerase is prevented from initiating transcription of the regions coding for three lactose-metabolizing proteins. However, in the presence of lactose or similar sugars, LacI undergoes structural changes that prevent binding to DNA. The LacI-

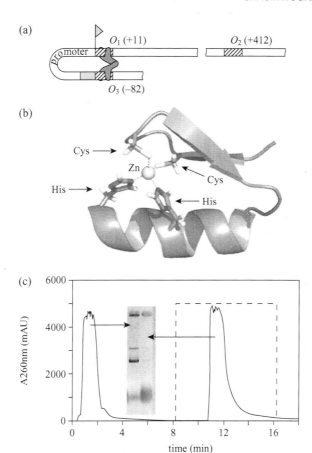

Figure 17.8 *Exploring affinity and pseudoaffinity chromatography for plasmid purification. (a) Lac repressor (LacI)-mediated affinity chromatography of plasmid DNA—the drawing shows the binding of the lac repressor to the lac operon promoter, which is at the heart of the recognition of plasmid by chromatographic beads with immobilized LacI. The three operators are shown by the hatched segments. The binding of LacI to O_1 and O_3 folds the DNA into a 76-bp-long loop. The flag indicates position +1 of the operon. (b) Zinc finger-mediated plasmid chromatography—cartoon representation of the Cys_2His_2 zinc finger motif. The zinc ion is coordinated by two histidine and two cysteine amino acid residues, originating a fold comprising two β sheets and one α-helix. (c) Clearance of RNA and LPS impurities from plasmid-containing lysates by phenyl boronate chromatography. (a) Reprinted from Structure, 12, Balaeff A, Mahadevan L, Schulten K. Structural basis for cooperative DNA binding by CAP and lac repressor, 123—132, Copyright 2004,[91] with permission from Elsevier. (b) From http://en.wikipedia. org/wiki/File:Zinc_finger_rendered.png). (c) Adapted and reprinted from Journal of Chromatography A, 1217, Gomes AG, Azevedo AM, Aires-Barros MR, Prazeres DMF. Clearance of host cell impurities from plasmid-containing lysates by boronate adsorption, 2262–2266, Copyright 2010,[97] with permission from Elsevier.*

mediated sequence-specific affinity chromatography of plasmid DNA takes advantage of the fact that many plasmids (e.g., pUC-derived) contain O_1 and O_3 sequences. This means that LacI proteins will form complexes with those plasmids. In the applications described in the literature, the LacI protein is fused with hexameric tags of histidines (His) and then contacted with the plasmid-containing solution under conditions that promote binding. The mixture is then incubated with a metal affinity adsorbent in such a way that the protein–plasmid complexes bind via the formation of chelates between the His tag and the immobilized metal (e.g., Ni). After washing the unbound material, the plasmid is selectively eluted from the adsorbent by using the lactose analogue isopropyl β-D-1-thiogalactopyranoside (IPTG).[89,90] As an alternative, the LacI–His6 fusion is first immobilized noncovalently in a metal (Ni)-column via chelate formation. The column is then loaded with the plasmid solution, washed, and eluted with IPTG.[94] The concept has been further optimized by immobilizing a synthetic 16-mer peptide that contains a binding domain of LacI in a customized monolith.[53] The results showed that this affinity matrix was able to bind a fraction of the plasmid DNA in a pure solution, and that elution could be accomplished with a high salt (2 M NaCl) buffer.[53]

A second group of examples is found in the literature, which explores the ability of zinc finger proteins to recognize specific base pairs for plasmid purification purposes. For example, the transcription factor IIIA contains nine 30-amino acid long repeating units (i.e., the fingers) folded and arranged in such a way that two cysteines and two histidines are coordinated tetrahedrally to a Zn atom[88] (Figure 17.8b). These fingers bind to DNA by establishing specific interactions (e.g., hydrogen bonds) with given nucleotides. In the applications described in the literature, a zinc finger protein engineered to bind to the sequence 5′-GGG-GCG-GCT-3′ was fused to glutathione S-transferase (GST) while at the same time, the DNA binding site was inserted into the target plasmid.[95] Like in the case described earlier, the affinity purification process then takes place by contacting the plasmid-containing solution with the GST–zinc finger protein under conditions that promote binding. The mixture is then incubated with a glutathione-Sepharose chromatographic adsorbent in such a way that the protein–plasmid complexes bind to the matrix via the GST in the fusion. After washing the unbound material, the plasmid is selectively eluted from the adsorbent by using a glutathione-containing buffer.[95] As an alternative, the GST–zinc finger fusion is first immobilized noncovalently in a glutathione-Sepharose packed column. The column is then loaded with the plasmid solution, washed, and eluted with glutathione.[96]

17.2.8.4 Phenyl Boronate Chromatography

The affinity of phenyl boronate ligands (see Figure 16.10a) for the C2-C3 diol in the 3′ terminal ribose of RNA molecules described in Chapter 16, in the context of batch adsorption (Section 16.5.5.1), has also been explored in chromatography-type operations.[97] The operation is straightforward and essentially involves the direct loading of alkaline lysates onto phenyl boronate columns equilibrated with water or low ionic strength buffers. The lack of a hydroxyl group at the C2 carbon of deoxyribose warrants the elution of plasmid molecules in the flow-through (95%). On the other hand, species that bear *cis*-diol groups like RNA and LPS bind covalently to boronate and can only be dislodged by the addition of a competing agent such as tris(hydroxymethyl) aminomethane (tris, Figure 17.8c). Furthermore, *cis*-diol-free species like proteins and gDNA fragments can also be removed up to a certain extent as a result of nonspecific interactions whose nature has yet to be fully elucidated. Further analysis revealed that 65% of RNA, 84% of proteins, and 45% of gDNA were cleared and that the LPS content decreased from ~2000 endotoxin units (EU)/mL in the lysate to a residual amount of less than 0.005 EU/mL. A key advantage of phenyl boronate chromatography is that neither conditioning nor prepurification are required prior to loading. On the other hand, the inability to concentrate plasmid and the cost of the affinity adsorbent are probably the most important shortcomings of phenyl boronate chromatography.[97]

17.2.9 Size-Exclusion Chromatography

17.2.9.1 Introduction

In spite of its well-known shortcomings, size-exclusion chromatography is particularly useful to perform specific plasmid purification tasks like desalting, buffer exchange, and RNA and small-solute removal.[17,23,24,98–100] In any of these settings, and once a column is efficiently packed with the adequate stationary phase, the operation is rather simple to perform—the column is equilibrated with the running buffer; the plasmid-containing feed is loaded; and the final buffer of choice is used to elute the different species. The technique takes advantage of the fact that, with the exception of gDNA fragments, plasmids are essentially the largest of the molecules found in solution during the downstream processing. In view of this fact, separations can be designed in such a way that plasmids are fully excluded from the interior of the chromatographic beads and thus elute early on in the process. This is not that difficult to accomplish since most stationary phases used in size-exclusion chromatography have pores with sizes smaller than the characteristic dimensions of plasmids. As for impurities and small solutes, they must be able to gain access to a fraction of the network of intraparticle pores if a successful separation is envisaged.

17.2.9.2 Selected Applications

In the case of desalting and buffer exchange operations, almost any size-exclusion material will do the job since the dimensions of ions and buffer components are typically much smaller than the dimensions of the smallest pores. In this case, the expected outcome of a successful size-exclusion desalting, as judged in terms of the corresponding chromatogram, is then a first peak of excluded plasmid species followed by a well-separated peak of buffer and salt components. This separation is straightforward, even when operating short columns packed in a gravity mode, as exemplified in Figure 17.9a. The chromatogram obtained shows that plasmid DNA is completely separated from the salt when using a column with a 6-cm height.

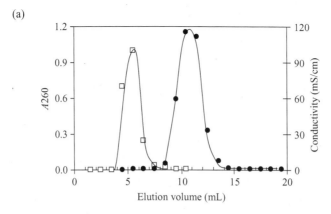

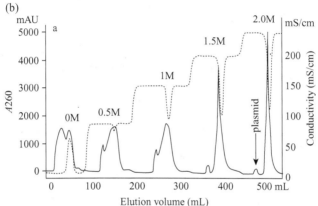

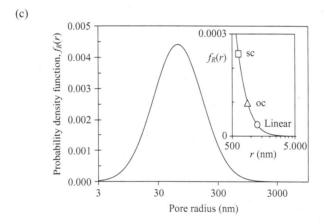

Figure 17.9 *The uses of size-exclusion chromatography in the context of plasmid purification. (a) Desalting: A 1.5 × 10.0 cm gravity-operated Sepharose CL-6B column (GE Healthcare, Uppsala, Sweden) was used to separate ammonium sulfate (●) from plasmid DNA (□) (M. M. Diogo, unpublished results). (b) Group separation: Increases in the ammonium sulfate concentration improve the ability of Sepharose 6 FF columns to separate plasmid DNA from RNA impurities (reprinted from Journal of Chromatography B, 784, Lemmens R, Olsson U, Nyhammar T, Stadler J. Supercoiled plasmid DNA: selective purification by thiophilic/aromatic adsorption, 291–300, Copyright 2003,[23] with permission from Elsevier). (c) Pore size distribution of Sephacryl S-1000 (calculated on the basis of data provided by Latulippe and Zydney[102]) and radius of gyration of supercoiled, open circular, and linear isoforms of a 3000-bp plasmid (calculated on the basis of Equations 4.17–4.19, Chapter 4).*

The choice of a stationary-phase material is narrower if the goal is to remove solutes like RNA, which, in some cases, display dimensions of the same order of magnitude than plasmids (see Chapter 14, Figure 14.3). Now, the fractionation range of the size-exclusion beads must be chosen in such a way that RNA is not excluded from the bead interior. An example of a size-exclusion material that meets these requirements is Sephacryl S-1000 from GE Healthcare. The chromatograms obtained when processing partially purified plasmid-containing solutions in columns packed with this material and run under optimized conditions are typically characterized by two well-separated peaks. In the first peak, we find plasmid isoforms and gDNA fragments, whereas the second peak corresponds to RNA, oligonucleotides, and proteins. This type of group separation can also be performed on columns packed with size-exclusion materials like Sepharose 6 Fast Flow, which have a fractionation range shifted toward lower molecular weights.[17,23] In this case, and while the plasmid DNA and RNA peaks coelute near the void volume as expected, the addition of more than 1.5 M of ammonium sulfate to the elution buffer increases selectivity in such a way that RNA removal becomes possible (see Figure 17.9b).[23] This behavior is explained by the salt-induced differential compaction of the two nucleic acid species, which ultimately changes the shape and conformation of RNA molecules in such a way that they become able to enter into the pores.[23] As highlighted by the proponents, a key feature of this particular step when compared with conventional size-exclusion chromatography is that the feed volume loaded per run can exceed more than one-third of the column volume. As a result, no significant dilution of the excluded plasmid DNA is seen and an unusually high throughput becomes possible. Other authors have further observed that the use of high concentrations of salts like ammonium sulfate and NaCl in size-exclusion chromatography is beneficial not only in terms of RNA separation but also in terms of the removal of gDNA residual impurities.[100]

While the separation of plasmid DNA from RNA is relatively simple to perform by resorting to an adequate size-exclusion material and/or by adding high amounts of salt in the running buffers, it is close to impossible to obtain a baseline resolution of supercoiled plasmid DNA, other plasmid isoforms, and gDNA fragments. Since the molecular weight of those species is of the same order of magnitude, they tend to elute collectively as a first broad and non-Gaussian peak. Still, the fractions corresponding to the leading edge of the peak are usually rich in high-MW gDNA and open circular plasmid, whereas supercoiled isoforms tend to elute later on.[101] While differences in the MW may explain the earlier elution and partial separation of gDNA, differences in the radius of gyration, and hence in steric hindrance, are the major reason for the fractionation of plasmid isoforms. This is discussed in a detailed study of the size-exclusion chromatography of plasmid isoforms in Sephacryl S-1000 columns.[102] Several important confirmations and conclusions are presented in this study: (1) For a plasmid with a given MW, the retention time is greatest for the supercoiled isoform followed by the open circular and then the linear isoforms; (2) an increase in the ionic strength of the running buffer increases the retention time of isoforms as a result of the reduction in the radius of gyration that accompanies plasmid compaction; and (3) although isoform resolution is reasonable for a 3000-bp plasmid, the isoforms of 9800-bp plasmids are nearly indistinguishable on account of a higher exclusion of all isoforms from the bead pores.[102] The implications of the latter conclusion are especially important from a process point of view since it basically states that the separation of isoforms of plasmids larger than 10,000 bp with a Sephacryl S-1000 resin is virtually impossible. This is illustrated in Figure 17.9c, which displays the calculated pore size distribution of Sephacryl S-1000 beads alongside the radius of gyration of the supercoiled, open circular, and linear isoforms of a 3000-bp plasmid (see figure insert). It is clear from the figure that even in the case of such a small plasmid, the pore volume of the stationary adsorbent accessible to the three isoforms is minimal and very similar among them. A possibility to improve the resolution of the different forms of DNA when performing size-exclusion chromatography is to use two columns in tandem.[103] These systems should be operated in such a way that the plasmid-containing eluent exiting from the first column is fed sequentially to the second column, while the later-eluting, lower-molecular-weight impurities are diverted to the waste.[103] The main disadvantages of this strategy are the need for large amounts of stationary phase and a higher dilution of plasmid DNA.

17.3 CONCENTRATION AND BUFFER EXCHANGE

17.3.1 Ultrafiltration

The fractions containing purified plasmid DNA recovered from the chromatography columns described in the previous section often contain low-molecular-weight solutes like salts and buffer components. Furthermore, the concentration is many times lower than the prespecified concentration required in the final bulk plasmid product. The best way to tackle these two issues, that is, to exchange small solutes and concentrate plasmid solutions, is probably to use ultrafiltration systems and to operate them in diafiltration and concentration modes (see Chapter 16, Section 16.2). The nominal molecular weight cutoff of the ultrafiltration membrane should be selected in such a way as to retain the plasmid and to allow smaller solutes to permeate through. Cutoffs of 30 kDa,[67] 50 kDa,[61] and 100 kDa[104] have all been reported in the context of plasmid concentration and buffer exchange by membrane processes. The ultrafiltration systems are usually operated first in a concentration mode to reduce the process volume and to adjust the plasmid concentration to the required value (values in the order of 1–5 mg/mL are typical), and then in a diafiltration mode to remove small solutes and to introduce a more appropriate buffer or sterile water. More than five diafiltration volumes should be used here to guarantee more than 99% removal of solutes.[1] A key aspect to consider while setting up such an ultrafiltration operation is to ensure that no degradation or variation in the homogeneity of the plasmid occurs as a result of the shear stress associated with the continuous pumping and recirculation of the solutions. If an adequate cutoff and membrane material is used, plasmid losses due to permeation or adsorption can be minimized and plasmid yields larger than 95% can be obtained.[60]

17.3.2 Alcohol Precipitation

Alcohol precipitation can be used as an alternative means of desalting and concentrating plasmid DNA from chromatographic pools. The operation is straightforward and usually involves the addition of cold ethanol (~2 volumes)[99] or isopropanol (~0.6–0.7 volumes)[103] under gentle mixing and a subsequent incubation at a lower temperature (e.g., −20 or 4°C are common). As described in Chapter 16 (Section 16.3.2.1), the presence of the alcohol molecules reduces the ability of water molecules to solvate plasmid molecules and exposes hydrophobic regions, which drive the spontaneous aggregation of molecules via van der Waals interactions, and concomitantly their precipitation. The alcohol-precipitated fractions are then centrifuged (30 min, 4°C), pellets drained and air-dried, and finally resuspended in an appropriate buffer or sterile water. The operation should be carefully optimized on a case-by-case basis since parameters like the presence of other components in the solution (e.g., salts) and the plasmid concentration are known to affect yields. Although the use of alcohols in a process environment requires the adoption of some precautions, the fact that the volumes involved at this stage of the downstream processing are relatively small compared, for example, with what would be required to carry out an alcohol precipitation after a lysis step makes it easier to implement the operation.

17.4 FINAL STERILIZATION

17.4.1 Introduction

Sterility is a key requirement for most biopharmaceuticals, and in this regard, plasmids are not an exception (see Chapter 12). Although stringent conditions (e.g., intensive use of clean rooms and high-efficiency particulate air [HEPA] filters, specialized gowning) are usually adopted throughout the manufacturing of biopharmaceuticals to minimize the possibility of product contamination with bacteria or viruses, the terminal sterilization of products at the far end of the process is close to inevitable, especially when dealing with parenterals (see Chapter 11, Section 11.3.2). Thus, once the purified plasmid DNA is present in an adequate delivery buffer and its concentration has been adjusted to the prespecified value, some sort of sterilization step has to be implemented. The key objective of this operation, which is usually carried out under aseptic conditions (e.g., class 100 hood or clean room[103]) is to guarantee that the load of microorganisms in the final bulk plasmid is reduced down to the acceptable microbial levels. Since options like heat sterilization and irradiation would clearly have a deleterious effect over the integrity of plasmid DNA, the best sterilization methodology available relies on the filtration of solutions through synthetic membranes with pore size ratings of the order of $0.2\,\mu m$.[1,47,105,106] Unfortunately, and in spite of the importance that may be attributed to this topic, there are only a couple of reports in the literature describing the performance and development of the sterilizing filtration of plasmid molecules. The discussion presented next is thus based essentially on the studies of Watson et al.[105] and Kong et al.[106,107]

17.4.2   Sterilizing Filtration

By definition, sterilizing filtration is "the total removal of micro-organisms from a fluid."[108] This unit operation is typically operated by filtering liquids in a normal mode (i.e., dead-end filtration) through adequate microfiltration membranes at constant pressure or constant flow rate. While membranes with pore size ratings of the order of $0.1\,\mu m$ are commercially available, which can retain minute organisms like mycoplasmas, in the majority of the applications, sterilizing membranes with pore size ratings of $0.2\,\mu m$ are sufficient to remove most microorganisms.[108] It should be stressed that the ratings used to classify the membranes do not reflect the true pore size but rather indicate the narrower dimensions of microorganisms and particles removed by the membrane.[109]

In the present context, microporous membrane filters should thus be able to retain any microorganism that might be present in the final solution, while allowing plasmid molecules to permeate freely without adversely affecting their quality (i.e., structure and biological activity). The problem with this sterile filtration of plasmids, of course, has to do with the large size of the molecules being handled and with the fact that these dimensions are of the same order of magnitude of the usual $0.2\text{-}\mu m$ pore size rating. Indeed, and as seen in Chapter 4 (Section 4.3.6), the radius of gyration and the superhelix axis of supercoiled plasmid molecules with sizes in the 4000- to 12,000-bp range are of the order of 0.08–$0.18\,\mu m$ and 0.56–$1.67\,\mu m$, respectively (see Figure 4.7). These dimensions are very close to, or larger than, the 0.20- to $0.22\text{-}\mu m$ pore size rating of the sterilizing membranes, and so, and in principle, it would not be possible for plasmids to cross such barriers. Fortunately, and on account of their geometric and topological properties, supercoiled plasmid molecules tend to orientate and stretch in the direction of the filtration flow. In other words, if a normal-flow filtration is used, supercoiled plasmids are likely to elongate and align in the flow field. Since the radius of supercoiled plasmids hardly exceeds $0.01\,\mu m$ (see Chapter 4, Figure 4.8), this enables the molecules to pass through the membrane pores. This picture is supported by experimental data which show that it is indeed possible to guarantee high levels of plasmid DNA transmission when filtering solutions through $0.2\text{-}\mu m$ membranes.[105,106] Still, an increase in plasmid size is always associated with a loss of filtration performance and yields.[106,107] For example, when filtering solutions through $0.2\,\mu m$ polyvinylidene difluoride (PVDF) membranes, transmission decreases from 93% to 13%, when plasmid size is increased from 6000 to 116,000 bp.[106]

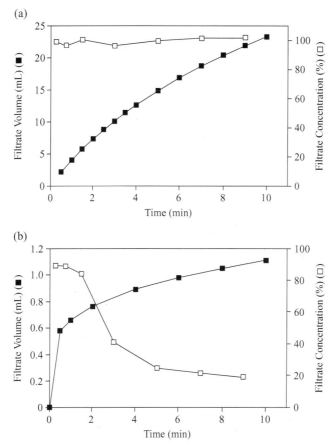

Figure 17.10 *Effect of the topoisomer distribution on the performance of PVDF membrane (0.2 µm) sterilization of a 6400-bp plasmid solution (6.1 g/L in phosphate buffered saline). The relative proportion of supercoiled to open circular topoisomers was changed from 87%:13% in (a) to 63%:37% in (b). Experiments were performed with PVDF filters. Reprinted from Biotechnology Progress, 22, Watson MP, Winters MA, Sagar SL, Konz JO. Sterilizing filtration of plasmid DNA: effects of plasmid concentration, molecular weight, and conformation, 465–470, Copyright 2006,[105] with permission from John Wiley & Sons.*

The higher retention of larger plasmids by membrane filters leads not only to a yield loss but also to a reduction in the filtration flux (if the system is operated at constant pressure) or to an increase in pressure drop (if the system is operated under constant flux).[105] This loss in the performance of the filtration step is due to the clogging of pores by the plasmid molecules, and the net result is that the volume of feed that can be processed per unit of membrane area before filtration rates fall below ~10–20% of the initial value (i.e., the filter capacity) for larger plasmids.[105] For example, the capacity of PVDF filters has been found to decrease by more than one order of magnitude when plasmid size doubled from 5500 to 11,000 bp.[105] The topological conformation of the plasmid being filtered also has a dramatic effect over filter capacity, as demonstrated experimentally. The effect of changing the relative proportion of supercoiled to open circular topoisomers of a 6400-bp plasmid from 87%:13% to 63%:37% on the flux decay and plasmid concentration in the filtrate is readily visible in Figure 17.10. While in the first situation the flux decay was modest and plasmid permeated freely through the membrane (Figure 17.10a), in the second case, significant fouling and plasmid loss were observed and filtration fluxes were significantly lower (Figure 17.10b).[105] The higher retention of open circular plasmids, which is evident from this data, is of course related to the fact that the radius of gyration of these topoisomers is 40% larger when compared with supercoiled plasmids[110] (see Chapter 4, Section 4.3.7). These experiments show very clearly that for the membrane sterilization of plasmid solutions to be successful, the supercoiled content must be the highest possible. This constitutes an interesting process-related argument in support of a specification imposing a larger than 90% proportion of supercoiled plasmid DNA as a goal for the final product[1] (see Chapter 12, Section 12.3.3).

The concentration of the plasmid in the solution undergoing sterilization has been identified as an operating parameter that might affect the performance of filtration. While Kong et al. describe that there are no changes in plasmid transmission for feed concentrations in the 0.02- to 0.10-mg/mL range,[106] Watson et al. report an increase in plasmid-induced membrane fouling when feed concentration increases from 2 to 6 mg/mL.[105] In this latter case, however, and in spite of a loss of volumetric throughput, the amount of plasmid that could be filtered per unit area increased. This fact was attributed by the authors to a compression of plasmid molecules and to the concomitant decrease in the radius of gyration, which is brought about by an increase in concentration.[105]

Kong et al. observed that the levels of plasmid transmission across sterile filtration membranes (0.2 μm, PVDF) can be improved if the ionic strength is increased.[106] For example, the transmission of 72,000- and 116,000-bp plasmids increased from ~55% to ~80% and from ~20% to ~35%, respectively, when using 150 mM NaCl in the solutions.[106] This beneficial effect is most likely due to the shielding of phosphates in the DNA backbone induced by the presence of cations like Na^+ in the solution, which contribute both to a tighter interwounding and consequent reduction of the apparent dimensions of plasmid molecules and to a decrease in the electrostatic repulsion between plasmid molecules (see Chapter 4, Section 4.5.3). However, contradictory data were produced by Watson et al., who showed that the filtration capacity of similar membranes for a 6400-bp plasmid increased threefold when the NaCl concentration was lowered from 150 to 20 mM NaCl. Still, no valid explanation was put forward to explain this.[105]

The capacity of sterilizing grade filters and yields is also highly dependent on the membrane material used, and the most likely reason for this has to do with membrane-specific adsorption of plasmids. This issue is highlighted by the detailed characterization of the performance of a series of 0.2-μm filters during the terminal filtration of a 6400 bp in a phosphate buffered saline solution.[105] Among the best results presented in this study, filtration capacities of the order of 30–40 mL/cm^2 were obtained with polysulfone (PS) and polyethersulfone (PES) filters from Pall Corporation and with a PVDF filter from Millipore (Billerica, MA).[105] The specific process used by each manufacturer to cast the membranes is an important variable as well, since filtration performance varied drastically when membranes made of the same material, but provided by different vendors, were tested.[105]

In principle, terminal sterilization by membrane filtration is relatively easy to scale up. Still, this requires a correct understanding of the flow and fouling characteristics of the membranes/system configurations under test.[109] For example, by making use of the typical capacity figures determined on the basis of laboratorial experiments, the membrane area required to process a given volume of a stream equivalent to the plasmid solution tested in terms of supercoiled content and concentration could be easily calculated.[105] Using this strategy, a 1000-cm^2 unit of PVDF filters was selected for the large-scale sterile filtration of a 4-L batch of a 6400-bp plasmid (93% supercoiled, 7.5 g/L). By operating the system under constant flow conditions, a plasmid recovery yield of 96% was obtained, confirming the validity of the performance predictions made.[105]

17.5 CONCLUSIONS

The use of chromatographic operations in the final stages of the purification of plasmids has evolved substantially in the last 10–20 years. The realization that conventional chromatographic beads were not adapted to the peculiarities of plasmid structure (size and shape) and to their dynamic behavior (diffusion coefficients) has fostered a number of advances in the area. These include, for example, (1) the development of superporous materials best suited to accommodate plasmids, (2) the use of alternative formats like monoliths and membranes, and (3) an exploration of chromatography operated in the negative mode. Alongside these developments, new types of interactions between nucleic acids and matrices have been described or explored, which rely on unusual ligands (e.g., amino acids, thiophilic ligands, phenyl boronate). As a result of these developments, nowadays, researchers and bioprocess engineers have a larger range of chromatographic options available for the efficient purification of plasmids at their reach. After impurities have been reduced from the bulk plasmid solutions to levels below the specifications, adjustments in the plasmid concentration and buffer exchange can be accomplished by standard operations like ultrafiltration and, to a lesser extent, by alcohol precipitation. Once this has been accomplished, sterility can then be guaranteed by terminal filtration with 0.2-μm membranes. Although this operation is feasible and scalable, care should be taken in the case of plasmids larger than 10,000 bp; otherwise, yield losses due to membrane fouling can compromise the entire downstream process.

REFERENCES

1. Quaak SG, van den Berg JH, Toebes M, et al. GMP production of pDERMATT for vaccination against melanoma in a phase I clinical trial. *European Journal of Pharmaceutics and Biopharmaceutics.* 2008;70:429–438.

2. DePhillips P, Lenhoff AM. Pore size distributions of cation-exchange adsorbents determined by inverse size-exclusion chromatography. *Journal of Chromatography. A.* 2000;883:39–54.

3. Jungbauer A, Hahn R. Polymethacrylate monoliths for preparative and industrial separation of biomolecular assemblies. *Journal of Chromatography. A.* 2008;1184: 62–79.

4. Trilisky EI, Lenhoff AM. Flow-dependent entrapment of large bioparticles in porous process media. *Biotechnology and Bioengineering.* 2009;104:127–133.

5. Delmdahl N. Fast, effective and safe adenovirus purification with Vivapure AdenoPACK kits. *Nature Methods.* 2006;3. doi:10.1038/NMETH909.

6. Pall Life Sciences. *Pall Mustang^R chromatography capsules for high throughput disposable ion exchange chromatography.* New York: Pall Life Sciences, 2004.

7. Branovic K, Forcic D, Ivancic J, et al. Application of short monolithic columns for fast purification of plasmid DNA. *Journal of Chromatography. B.* 2004;801: 331–337.

8. Freitas SS, Santos JAL, Prazeres DMF. Plasmid purification by hydrophobic interaction chromatography using sodium citrate in the mobile phase. *Separation and Purification Technology.* 2009;65:95–104.

9. Prazeres DMF, Schluep T, Cooney C. Preparative purification of supercoiled plasmid DNA using anion-exchange chromatography. *Journal of Chromatography. A.* 1998;806:31–45.

10. Tiainen P, Gustavsson P-E, Ljunglöf A, Larsson P-O. Superporous agarose anion exchangers for plasmid isolation. *Journal of Chromatography. A.* 2007;1138: 84–94.

11. Prazeres DMF. Chromatographic separation of plasmid DNA using macroporous beads. In: Mattiasson B, Kumar A, Galaev YI, eds. *Macroporous polymers: Production, properties and biotechnological/biomedical applications.* Boca Raton, FL: Taylor and Francis, 2010:335–360.

12. DePhillips P, Lenhoff AM. Determinants of protein retention characteristics on cation-exchange adsorbents. *Journal of Chromatography. A.* 2001;933:57–72.

13. Diogo MM, Queiroz JA, Prazeres DMF. Chromatography of plasmid DNA. *Journal of Chromatography. A.* 2005;1069:3–22.

14. Ferreira GN, Cabral JM, Prazeres DMF. Studies on the batch adsorption of plasmid DNA onto anion-exchange chromatographic supports. *Biotechnology Progress.* 2000;16:416–424.

15. Theodossiou I, Sondergaard M, Thomas OR. Design of expanded bed supports for the recovery of plasmid DNA by anion exchange adsorption. *Bioseparation.* 2001;10:31–44.

16. Ljunglof A, Bergvall P, Bhikhabhai R, Hjorth R. Direct visualisation of plasmid DNA in individual chromatography adsorbent particles by confocal scanning laser microscopy. *Journal of Chromatography. A.* 1999;844:129–135.

17. Stadler J, Lemmens R, Nyhammar T. Plasmid DNA purification. *The Journal of Gene Medicine*. 2004;6:S54–S66.

18. Zhang H-P, Bai S, Xu L, Sun Y. Fabrication of mono-sized magnetic anion exchange beads for plasmid DNA purification. *Journal of Chromatography. B*. 2009;877:127–133.

19. Tiainen P, Gustavsson P-E, Mansson M-O, Larsson P-O. Plasmid purification using non-porous anion-exchange silica fibres. *Journal of Chromatography. A*. 2007; 1149:158–168.

20. Boschetti E, Girot P, Guerrier L, Santambien P. Quantification and *in vitro* toxicity studies of extractable chemicals from synthetic ion exchangers. *Journal of Biochemistry and Biophysics Methods*. 1996;32:15–25.

21. Murphy JC, Wibbenmeyer JA, Fox GE, Willson RC. Purification of plasmid DNA using selective precipitation by compaction agents. *Nature Biotechnology*. 1999;17:822–823.

22. Murphy JC, Fox GE, Willson RC. Enhancement of anion-exchange chromatography of DNA using compaction agents. *Journal of Chromatography. A*. 2003;984: 215–221.

23. Lemmens R, Olsson U, Nyhammar T, Stadler J. Supercoiled plasmid DNA: Selective purification by thiophilic/aromatic adsorption. *Journal of Chromatography. B*. 2003;784:291–300.

24. Horn N, Budahazi G, Marquet M, inventors; Vical Incorporated, assignee. Purification of plasmid DNA during column chromatography. U.S. patent 5,707,812, January 13, 1998.

25. Diogo MM, Quiroz JA, Monteiro GA, Martins SAM, Ferreira GNM, Prazeres DMF. Purification of a cystic fibrosis plasmid vector for gene therapy using hydrophobic interaction chromatography. *Biotechnology and Bioengineering*. 2000;68: 576–583.

26. Diogo MM, Ribeiro S, Queiroz JA, et al. Production, purification and analysis of an experimental DNA vaccine against rabies. *The Journal of Gene Medicine*. 2001;3:577–584.

27. Gustavsson PE, Lemmens R, Nyhammar T, Busson P, Larsson PO. Purification of plasmid DNA with a new type of anion-exchange beads having a non-charged surface. *Journal of Chromatography. A*. 2004;1038:131–140.

28. Kepka C, Lemmens R, Vasi J, Nyhammar T, Gustavsson PE. Integrated process for purification of plasmid DNA using aqueous two-phase systems combined with membrane filtration and lid bead chromatography. *Journal of Chromatography. A*. 2004;1057:115–124.

29. Lyddiatt A, O'Sullivan DA. Biochemical recovery and purification of gene therapy vectors. *Current Opinion in Biotechnology*. 1998;9:177–185.

30. Rodrigues AE, Chenou C, Rendueles de la Vega M. Protein separation by liquid chromatography using permeable POROS Q/M particles. *Chemical Engineering Journal*. 1996;61:191–201.

31. Whitney D, McCoy M, Gordon N, Afeyan N. Characterization of large-pore polymeric supports for use in perfusion biochromatography. *Journal of Chromatography. A*. 1998;807:165–184.

32. Eon-Duval A, Burke G. Purification of pharmaceutical-grade plasmid DNA by anion-exchange chromatography in an RNase-free process. *Journal of Chromatography. B*. 2004;804:327–335.

33. Levy MS, O'Kennedy RD, Ayazi-Shamlou P, Dunnill P. Biochemical engineering approaches to the challenges of producing pure plasmid DNA. *Trends in Biotechnology*. 2000;18:296–305.

34. PerSeptive Biosystems. Rapid, preparative purification of plasmid DNA by anion exchange perfusion chromatography technology. *Biochemica*. 1996;1:9–11.

35. McCoy M, Kalghatgi K, Afeyan N. Perfusion chromatography—Characterization of column packings for chromatography of proteins. *Journal of Chromatography. A*. 1996;743:221–229.

36. Gustavsson P-E, Larsson P-O. Superporous agarose, a new material for chromatography. *Journal of Chromatography. A*. 1996;734:231–240.

37. Gustavsson P-E, Axelsson A, Larsson P-O. Direct measurements of convective fluid velocities in superporous agarose beads. *Journal of Chromatography. A*. 1998;795:199–210.

38. Wu L, Bai S, Sun Y. Development of rigid bidisperse porous microspheres for high-speed protein chromatography. *Biotechnology Progress*. 2003;19:1300–1306.

39. Li Y, Dong X-Y, Sun Y. High-speed chromatographic purification of plasmid DNA with a customized biporous hydrophobic adsorbent. *Biochemical Engineering Journal*. 2005;27:33–39.

40. Li Y, Dong X-Y, Sun Y. Biporous polymeric microspheres coupled with mercaptopyridine for rapid chromatographic purification of plasmid DNA. *Journal of Applied Polymer Science*. 2007;104:2205–2211.

41. Wu L, Pang G-C. High-speed large scale chromatographic purification of plasmid DNA with a novel giant-pore stationary phase. *Chromatographia*. 2007;66: 151–157.

42. Teeters MA, Conrardy SE, Thomas BL, Root TW, Lightfoot EN. Adsorptive membrane chromatography for purification of plasmid DNA. *Journal of Chromatography. A*. 2003;989:165–173.

43. Danquah MK, Forde GM. The suitability of DEAE-Cl active groups on customized poly(GMA-*co*-EDMA) continuous stationary phase for fast enzyme-free isolation of plasmid DNA. *Journal of Chromatography. B*. 2007;853:38–46.

44. Hanora A, Savina I, Plieva FM, Izumrudov VA, Mattiasson B, Galaev IY. Direct capture of plasmid DNA from non-clarified bacterial lysate using polycation-grafted monoliths. *Journal of Biotechnology*. 2006;123:343–355.

45. Zochling A, Hahn R, Ahrer K, Urthaler J, Jungbauer A. Mass transfer characteristics of plasmids in monoliths. *Journal of Separation Science*. 2004;27:819–827.

46. Urthaler J, Schlegl R, Podgornik A, Strancar A, Jungbauer A, Necina R. Application of monoliths for plasmid DNA purification: Development and transfer to production. *Journal of Chromatography. A*. 2005;1065:93–106.

47. Urthaler J, Buchinger W, Necina R. Improved downstream process for the production of plasmid DNA for gene therapy. *Acta Biochimica Polonica*. 2005;52: 703–711.

48. Krajnc NL, Smrekar F, Cerne J, et al. Purification of large plasmids with methacrylate monolithic columns. *Journal of Separation Science*. 2009;32:2682–2690.

49. Endres HN, Johnson JA, Ross CA, Welp JK, Etzel MR. Evaluation of an ion-exchange membrane for the purification of plasmid DNA. *Biotechnology and Applied Biochemistry*. 2003;37:259–266.

50. Zhang S, Krivosheyeva A, Nochumson S. Large-scale capture and partial purification of plasmid DNA using anion-exchange membrane capsules. *Biotechnology and Applied Biochemistry*. 2003;37:245–249.

51. Haber C, Skupsky J, Lee A, Lander R. Membrane chromatography of DNA: Conformation-induced capacity and selectivity. *Biotechnology and Bioengineering*. 2004;88:26–34.

52. Smrekar F, Podgornik A, Ciringer M, et al. Preparation of pharmaceutical-grade plasmid DNA using methacrylate monolithic columns. *Vaccine*. 2010;28:2039–2045.

53. Han Y, You G, Pattenden LK, Forde GM. The harnessing of peptide–monolith constructs for single step plasmid DNA purification. *Process Biochemistry*. 2010;45:203–209.

54. Chandra G, Patel P, Kost TA, Gray JG. Large-scale purification of plasmid DNA by fast protein liquid chromatography using Hi-Load Q Sepharose column. *Analytical Biochemistry*. 1992;203:169–172.

55. Prazeres DMF, Ferreira GNM, Monteiro GA, Cooney CL, Cabral JMS. Large-scale production of pharmaceutical-grade plasmid DNA for gene therapy: Problems and bottlenecks. *Trends in Biotechnology*. 1999;17:169–174.

56. Ferreira GNM, Cabral JMS, Prazeres DMF. Development of process flow sheets for the purification of plasmid vectors for gene therapy applications. *Biotechnology Progress*. 1999;15:725–731.

57. Guerrero-German P, Prazeres DMF, Guzman R, Montesinos-Cisneros RM, Tejeda-Mansir A. Purification of plasmid DNA using tangential flow filtration and tandem anion-exchange membrane chromatography. *Bioprocess and Biosystems Engineering*. 2009;32:615–623.

58. Diogo MM, Queiroz JA, Prazeres DMF. Studies on the retention of plasmid DNA and *Escherichia coli* nucleic acids by hydrophobic interaction chromatography. *Bioseparation*. 2001;10:211–220.

59. Trindade IP, Diogo MM, Prazeres DMF, Marcos JC. Purification of plasmid DNA vectors by aqueous two-phase extraction and hydrophobic interaction chromatography. *Journal of Chromatography. A*. 2005;1082:176–184.

60. Urthaler J, Buchinger W, Necina R. Industrial scale cGMP purification of pharmaceutical-grade plasmid DNA. *Chemical Engineering and Technology*. 2005;28:1408–1420.

61. Nochumson S, Durland R, Yu-Speight A, Welp J, Wu K, Hayes R, inventors; Valentis, Inc., assignee. Process and equipment for plasmid purification. U.S. patent 7,026,468, April 11, 2006.

62. Prazeres DMF, Diogo MM, Queiroz JA, inventors; Instituto Superior Técnico, assignee. Purification of plasmid DNA by hydrophobic interaction chromatography. U.S. patent 7,169,917, January 30, 2007.

63. Wilson MJ, Haggart CL, Gallagher SP, Walsh D. Removal of tightly bound endotoxin from biological products. *Journal of Biotechnology*. 2001;88:67–75.

64. Kitamura T, Nakatani S, inventors; Tosoh Corporation, assignee. Separating plasmids from contaminants using hydrophobic or hydrophobic and ion exchange chromatography. U.S. patent 6,441,160, August 27, 2002.

65. Diogo MM, Queiroz JA, Monteiro GA, Prazeres DMF. Separation and analysis of plasmid denatured forms using hydrophobic interaction chromatography. *Analytical Biochemistry*. 1999;275:122–124.

66. McNeilly DS, inventor; Genzyme Corporation, assignee. Method for purifying plasmid DNA and plasmid DNA substantially free of genomic DNA. U.S. patent 6,214,586, April 10, 2001.

67. Lee AL, Sagar S, inventors; Merck & Co., Inc., assignee. Method for large scale plasmid purification. U.S. patent 6,197,553, March 6, 2002.

68. Green AP, Prior GM, Helveston NM, Taittinger BE, Liu X, Thompson JA. Preparative purification of supercoiled plasmid DNA for therapeutic applications. *BioPharm.* 1997;May:52–61.

69. Tumanova I, Boyer J, Ausar SF, et al. Analytical and biological characterization of supercoiled plasmids purified by various chromatographic techniques. *DNA and Cell Biology.* 2005;24:819–831.

70. Bornsztejn V. Purification of plasmid DNA by polishing and endotoxin removal. *eLab.* 01/06/2004.

71. Ballantyne J, Klocke D, Smiley L. *Production of a West Nile virus DNA vaccine using PerfluorosorbS.* Fargo, ND: Aldevron, 2004.

72. Luscombe NM, Laskowski RA, Thornton JM. Amino acid–base interactions: A three-dimensional analysis of protein–DNA interactions at an atomic level. *Nucleic Acids Research.* 2001;29:2860–2874.

73. Hoffman MM, Khrapov MA, Cox JC, Yao J, Tong L, Ellington AD. AANT: The amino acid–nucleotide interaction database. *Nucleic Acids Research.* 2004;32:D174–D181.

74. Sousa F, Freitas S, Azzoni AR, Prazeres DMF, Queiroz J. Selective purification of supercoiled plasmid DNA from clarified cell lysates with a single histidine-agarose chromatography step. *Biotechnology and Applied Biochemistry.* 2006;45: 131–140.

75. Sousa F, Prazeres DMF, Queiroz JA. Dynamic binding capacity of plasmid DNA in histidine-agarose chromatography. *Biomedical Chromatography.* 2007;21: 993–998.

76. Sousa F, Tomaz CT, Prazeres DMF, Queiroz JA. Separation of supercoiled and open circular plasmid DNA isoforms by chromatography with a histidine-agarose support. *Analytical Biochemistry.* 2005;343:183–185.

77. Sousa F, Matos T, Prazeres DMF, Queiroz JA. Specific recognition of supercoiled plasmid DNA in arginine affinity chromatography. *Analytical Biochemistry.* 2008;374:432–434.

78. Sousa F, Prazeres DMF, Queiroz JA. Binding and elution strategy for improved performance of arginine affinity chromatography in supercoiled plasmid DNA purification. *Biomedical Chromatography.* 2009;23:160–165.

79. Sousa F, Prazeres DMF, Queiroz JA. Improvement of transfection efficiency by using supercoiled plasmid DNA purified with arginine affinity chromatography. *The Journal of Gene Medicine.* 2009;11:79–88.

80. Sousa A, Sousa F, Queiroz JA. Biorecognition of supercoiled plasmid DNA isoform in lysine-affinity chromatography. *Journal of Chromatography. B.* 2009; 877:3257–3260.

81. Royal Society of Chemistry. *IUPAC compendium of chemical terminology*, 2nd ed. Cambridge: Royal Society of Chemistry, 1997.

82. Sandberg LM, Bjurling A, Busson P, Vasi J, Lemmens R. Thiophilic interaction chromatography for supercoiled plasmid DNA purification. *Journal of Biotechnology*. 2004;109:193–199.

83. Blanche F, Couder M, Maestrali N, Gaillac D, Guillemin T, inventors. Method of preparation for pharmaceutical grade plasmid DNA. U.S. patent 2007/111,221, May 17, 2007.

84. Jayasena SD, Johnston BH. Oligonucleotide-directed triple helix formation at adjacent oligopurine and oligopyrimidine DNA tracts by alternate strand recognition. *Nucleic Acids Research*. 1992;20:5279–5288.

85. Wils P, Escriou V, Warney A, et al. Efficient purification of plasmid DNA for gene transfer using triple-helix affinity chromatography. *Gene Therapy*. 1997;4: 323–330.

86. Ito T, Smith CL, Cantor CR. Sequence-specific DNA purification by triplex affinity capture. *Proceedings of the National Academy of Sciences of the United States of America*. 1992;89:495–498.

87. Schluep T, Cooney CL. Purification of plasmid DNA by triplex affinity interactions. *Nucleic Acids Research*. 1998;26:4524–4528.

88. Sinden RR. *DNA structure and function*. San Diego, CA: Academic Press, 1994.

89. Darby RA, Forde GM, Slater NK, Hine AV. Affinity purification of plasmid DNA directly from crude bacterial cell lysates. *Biotechnology and Bioengineering*. 2007;98:1103–1108.

90. Darby RA, Hine AV. LacI-mediated sequence-specific affinity purification of plasmid DNA for therapeutic applications. *FASEB Journal*. 2005;19:801–803.

91. Balaeff A, Mahadevan L, Schulten K. Structural basis for cooperative DNA binding by CAP and lac repressor. *Structure*. 2004;12:123–132.

92. Sadler JR, Sasmor H, Betz JL. A perfectly symmetric lac operator binds the lac repressor very tightly. *Proceedings of the National Academy of Sciences of the United States of America*. 1983;80:6785–6789.

93. Matthews BW, Ohlendorf DH, Anderson WF, Takeda Y. Structure of the DNA-binding region of lac repressor inferred from its homology with cro repressor. *Proceedings of the National Academy of Sciences of the United States of America*. 1982;79:1428–1432.

94. Hasche A, Voss C. Immobilisation of a repressor protein for binding of plasmid DNA. *Journal of Chromatography. A*. 2005;1080:76–82.

95. Woodgate J, Palfrey D, Nagel DA, Hine AV, Slater NK. Protein-mediated isolation of plasmid DNA by a zinc finger-glutathione S-transferase affinity linker. *Biotechnology and Bioengineering*. 2002;79:450–456.

96. Ghose S, Forde GM, Slater NK. Affinity adsorption of plasmid DNA. *Biotechnology Progress*. 2004;20:841–850.

97. Gomes AG, Azevedo AM, Aires-Barros MR, Prazeres DMF. Clearance of host cell impurities from plasmid-containing lysates by boronate adsorption. *Journal of Chromatography. A*. 2010;1217:2262–2266.

98. Vo-Quang T, Malpiece Y, Buffard D, Kaminski PA, Vidal D, Strosberg AD. Rapid large-scale purification of plasmid DNA by medium or low pressure gel filtration. Application: Construction of thermoamplifiable expression vectors. *Bioscience Reports*. 1985;5:101–111.

99. Horn NA, Meek JA, Budahazi G, Marquet M. Cancer gene therapy using plasmid DNA: Purification of DNA for human clinical trials. *Human Gene Therapy.* 1995;6:565–573.

100. Li LZ, Liu Y, Sun MS, Shao YM. Effect of salt on purification of plasmid DNA using size-exclusion chromatography. *Journal of Chromatography. A.* 2007; 1139:228–235.

101. Ferreira GNM, Cabral JMS, Prazeres DMF. A comparison of gel filtration chromatographic supports for plasmid purification. *Biotechnology Techniques.* 1997;11:417–420.

102. Latulippe DR, Zydney AL. Size exclusion chromatography of plasmid DNA isoforms. *Journal of Chromatography. A.* 2009;1216:6295–6302.

103. Marquet M, Horn N, Meek J, Budahazi G, inventors; Vical Incorporated, assignee. Production of pharmaceutical-grade plasmid DNA. U.S. patent 5,561,064, October 1, 1996.

104. Hebel H, Ramakrishnan S, Gonzalez H, Darnell J, inventors; Advisys, Inc., assignee. Devices and methods for biomaterial production. U.S. patent 7,238,522, July 3, 2007.

105. Watson MP, Winters MA, Sagar SL, Konz JO. Sterilizing filtration of plasmid DNA: Effects of plasmid concentration, molecular weight, and conformation. *Biotechnology Progress.* 2006;22:465–470.

106. Kong S, Titchener-Hooker N, Levy MS. Plasmid DNA processing for gene therapy and vaccination: Studies on the membrane sterilisation filtration step. *Journal of Membrane Science.* 2006;280:824–831.

107. Kong S, Aucamp J, Titchener-Hooker N. Studies on membrane sterile filtration of plasmid DNA using an automated multiwell technique. *Journal of Membrane Science.* 2010;353:144–150.

108. Waterhouse S, Hall GM. The validation of sterilising grade microfiltration membranes with *Pseudomonas diminuta.* A review. *Journal of Membrane Science.* 1995;104:1–9.

109. Rajniak P, Tsinontides SC, Pham D, Hunke WA, Reynolds SD, Chern RT. Sterilizing filtration: Principles and practice for successful scale-up to manufacturing. *Journal of Membrane Science.* 2008;325:223–237.

110. Latulippe DR, Zydney AL. Elongational flow model for transmission of supercoiled plasmid DNA during membrane ultrafiltration. *Journal of Membrane Science.* 2009;329:201–208.

111. Krajnc P, Brown JF, Cameron NR. Monolithic scavenger resins by amine functionalizations of poly(4-vinylbenzyl chloride-co-divinylbenzene) PolyHIPE materials. *Organic Letters.* 2002;4:2497–2500.

112. Syren PO, Rozkov A, Schmidt SR, Stromberg P. Milligram scale parallel purification of plasmid DNA using anion-exchange membrane capsules and a multichannel peristaltic pump. *Journal of Chromatography. B.* 2007;856:68–74.

18

Process Synthesis

18.1 INTRODUCTION

The unit operations described in Chapters 15–17 can be put together and sequenced differently into a full process with the same objective of producing a plasmid DNA product within a set of predefined quality specifications (Chapter 12). Given the number of options available, the synthesis of such a full process is not trivial. Furthermore, there are many reasons for selecting a given sequence of unit operations that are not directly linked to its performance or cost-effectiveness. For example, some operations can be selected on the basis of the past experience and familiarity of the process development department/group with it. In other cases, intellectual property issues may preclude the use of certain specific solutions and foster the development and introduction of innovative solutions. In this chapter, a number of different plasmid manufacturing processes, which have been described in the scientific and technical literature, are presented. For each case, simplified block diagrams are shown, in which the different unit operations are grouped into primary recovery, intermediate recovery, and final purification stages. In many cases, the proposed combination of unit operations cannot be considered as a "full" process since it is clear that some final, "polishing" operations (e.g., buffer exchange) are missing in the flow sheet. In other situations, on the other

Plasmid Biopharmaceuticals: Basics, Applications, and Manufacturing, First Edition.
Duarte Miguel F. Prazeres.
© 2011 John Wiley & Sons, Inc. Published 2011 by John Wiley & Sons, Inc.

hand, not enough information is provided concerning performance (e.g., yields, concentration factors, and final product quality) so as to allow the reader to make an informed and quantitative, as well as qualitative, comparison with other processes. The fact that the biological material (host cell strain, metabolic status of cells, and plasmid characteristics), the volumes and plasmid amounts being processed (laboratory vs. pilot scale), and the context in which the process was developed (academic vs. industrial setting) is different from case to case also makes it difficult to assess the merits and pitfalls of the different process options. Thus, the goal of the current chapter is more to provide a representative view of the current panorama in the downstream processing of plasmid DNA than to allow for a judicious side-by-side comparison. Still, whenever available, the critical information considered relevant for an appraisal of each process is included.

18.2 ALKALINE VERSUS NONALKALINE LYSIS-BASED PROCESSES

18.2.1 Introduction

Once the cell culture stage is terminated, the plasmid-containing cells must be collected, separated from the spent media, concentrated, and exchanged for a buffer adequate for the subsequent disruption step. From a process point of view, the best choice to accomplish this set of tasks is probably to use a tangential flow filtration (TFF) unit, as discussed in Chapter 15 (Section 15.2). This option is used, for example, in the context of the process described by Quaak et al.[1] In more concrete terms, a TFF system equipped with a microfiltration hollow fiber unit is used to concentrate the cell broth ($OD_{600} \approx 7$) 6.7-fold and to wash and diafilter cells with 5–10 diafiltration volumes of a sterile lysis buffer.[1] In spite of this example, in the vast majority of the processes described in this chapter, centrifugation is used instead of TFF for harvesting purposes. For this reason, the harvesting step will not appear explicitly in the processes discussed ahead, and the starting point in the block diagrams shown will be the cell disruption step. It should thus be assumed that centrifugation was the unit operation of choice for harvesting and that as a result, the right amount of plasmid-containing cells is suspended in a buffer that matches the specifications of the subsequent disruption step. The predominance of alkaline lysis at this critical stage of the process is more than evident for anyone willing to survey the extensive body of literature that is available nowadays on the downstream processing of plasmid biopharmaceuticals (Chapter 15). Still, a handful of plasmid manufacturing processes resort to alternative lysis methods. In the next paragraphs, a side-by-side comparison of three processes that use alkaline lysis, thermal lysis, and autolysis (Figure 18.1) is made and used as the starting point for the discussion of the process synthesis solutions used in plasmid manufacturing.

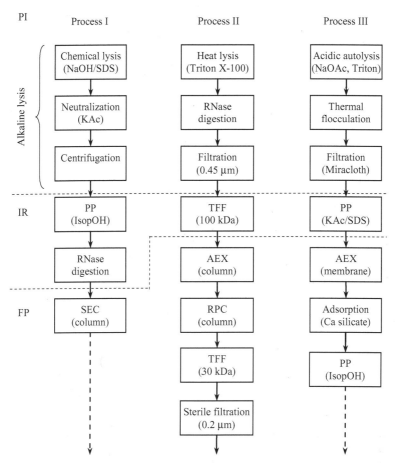

Figure 18.1 *Alkaline versus nonalkaline lysis-based processes. References: process I (Vo-Quang et al.[2]), process II (Lee and Sagar[13]), and process III (Carnes et al.[14]). AEX, anion exchange; FP, final purification; IR, intermediate recovery; IsopOH, isopropanol; KAc, potassium acetate; NaOAc, sodium acetate; PI, primary isolation; PP, precipitation; RPC, reversed-phase chromatography; SDS, sodium dodecyl sulfate; SEC, size-exclusion chromatography; TFF, tangential flow filtration.*

18.2.2 Alkaline Lysis

The first process examined here[2] was developed before the reporting of the first breakthrough experiments showing that plasmids could potentially be used as biopharmaceuticals[3–5] (see Chapter 1). Although the objective then was to present and describe a fast and reliable method for the preparative (up to 4 mg) isolation of plasmids for molecular biology applications, the flow sheet, which is schematically shown in Figure 18.1 (process I), is representative of the preplasmid biopharmaceutical era and constitutes a good starting point for the current discussion. The process features a number of steps that are among the most used in molecular biology protocols: alkaline lysis, RNase digestion, and isopropanol precipitation. The lysis is conducted in the usual way (see Chapter 15, Section 15.3.2) by adding a sodium dodecyl sulfate (SDS)/NaOH solution to *Escherichia coli* cells suspended in a sugar-containing buffer, neutralizing the mixture with a high-molarity acetate salt solution and removing debris and precipitates by centrifugation. This same type of alkaline lysis is basically explored in the majority of the process-scale plasmid manufacturing methods reported throughout the years, even though modifications (e.g., extension of the lysis time[6,7]) and innovations (e.g., design of apparatus for continuous lysis[8,9]) have been introduced in an attempt to improve performance (see Chapter 15, Section 15.3.2). The second step in the method, incubation with bovine RNase at 37°C, is also inevitably found in most plasmid isolation protocols. Despite the excellent clearance of RNA brought about by RNase digestion, most large-scale processes have nevertheless moved away from it, essentially due to the regulatory concerns associated with the use of animal-derived enzymes (see Chapter 11, Section 11.6.3). The ensuing precipitation of plasmid with isopropanol is also one of the ubiquitous steps in plasmid manufacturing. Though here it is used after lysis, alcohol precipitation can also be found later on in a process, and namely at the far end when it is especially useful for concentration and buffer exchange purposes (see Chapter 17, Section 17.3). This tendency is illustrated, for example, in processes III (Figure 18.1), IV, VII (Figure 18.2), and XIV (Figure 18.5). The final operation in process I is a size-exclusion chromatography (SEC) step that removes RNA, gDNA, and proteins while simultaneously making it possible to separate the supercoiled isoform from the open circular isoform and to exchange the buffer. This type of chromatographic separation was one of the first to be explored in the context of preparative plasmid purification.[10–12]

18.2.3 Nonalkaline Lysis

The search for cell disruption methods that could effectively replace alkaline lysis and thus overcome some of its limitations has produced important results in the past years (see Chapter 15). One of the first process-scale methods designed to produce plasmid DNA that does not use alkaline lysis was described by Lee and Sagar[13] (process II, Figure 18.1). The cell disruption step is accomplished by the joint action of heat, detergent, and lysozyme in a flow-through heat exchanger (see further details in Chapter 15, Section 15.3.3). This mode of cell disruption is claimed to be more reproducible and consistent than alkaline lysis. The clarified lysate is incubated with RNase to improve RNA clearance and is further passed through a 0.45-μm filter to remove small debris. The plasmid-containing stream is further diafiltered against a suitable buffer in a TFF apparatus equipped with a 100-kDa membrane, before loading onto an anion exchange (AEX) column. The plasmid pool collected from the AEX column, which is substantially free from RNA, gDNA, and proteins, is subse-

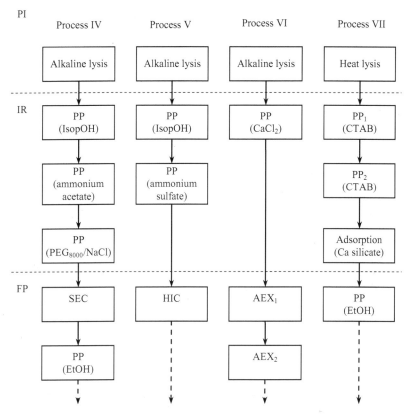

Figure 18.2 *Exploring precipitation steps in the intermediate recovery section. References: process IV (Horn et al.[10]), process V (Diogo et al.[16,17]), process VI (Bhikhabhai[19]), and process VII (Lander et al.[15]). AEX, anion exchange; CTAB, cetyltrimethylammonium bromide; EtOH, ethanol; FP, final purification; HIC, hydrophobic interaction chromatography; IR, intermediate recovery; IsopOH, isopropanol; PI, primary isolation; PP, precipitation; SEC, size-exclusion chromatography.*

quently loaded onto a reversed-phase column. Here, the use of an isopropanol gradient makes it possible to separate the different plasmid isoforms. The process terminates with a concentration/buffer exchange operation (e.g., alcohol precipitation and membrane diafiltration) and a final sterile filtration by passage through a membrane with a 0.2-μm pore rating.[13]

A more recent publication describes a full process for the manufacturing of plasmid DNA, which uses an autolytic *E. coli* host as the basis of the disruption step[14] (process III, Figure 18.1). The particular strain used in that work was designed to express endolysin, a peptidoglycan hydrolase that permeabilizes the bacterial cell wall, under the action of a heat-inducible promoter in the cytoplasm (see further details in Chapter 15, Section 15.3.5).[14] In this process, we may consider that the downstream process actually starts during fermentation, when expression of endolysin is induced by a heat shock to 42°C. Since the enzyme is directed to the cytoplasm, the cells remain unaffected during the rest of the cell culture step. The lysis step takes place after cell harvesting, through the combination of a low-salt, slightly acidic sodium acetate buffer containing sucrose with agents that aid in the permeabilization of the outer membrane (e.g., ethylenediamine tetraacetic acid [EDTA]) and cytoplasmic membrane (e.g., Triton X-100).[14] Cell debris are then removed by a thermal flocculation process that involves the pumping of the mixtures through stainless steel coils immersed in hot water (70°C) and ice water baths, and finally into a holding tank. Filtration through Miracloth (Calbiochem, San Diego, California) removes the overnight-flocculated material, delivering a cleared lysate, which can then be loaded onto an AEX membrane chromatography cartridge. The fractions containing the plasmid, which elute from this module, are further contacted with a calcium silicate adsorbent in a batch mode to remove recalcitrant impurities (see Chapter 16, Section 16.5.4). The process terminates with a concentration/buffer exchange step by isopropanol precipitation.[14]

18.3 CHOOSING THE INTERMEDIATE RECOVERY

18.3.1 Introduction

The variety of solutions proposed for the processing of clarified lysates, whether these have been obtained by alkaline lysis, hot lysis, or autolysis, is vast, as was already hinted in the first three processes described (Figure 18.1). In this section, additional processes are presented to highlight the use of two popular unit operations in the intermediate recovery stage—precipitation (PP) and aqueous two-phase system (ATPS).

18.3.2 Precipitation-Based Processes

Many plasmid downstream processes make intensive use of precipitation operations, whether these are designed to precipitate plasmid or to precipitate impurities. The scheme described by Horn et al. was one of the first proposed with the specific goal of producing plasmid material for preclinical trials[10] (process IV, Figure 18.2). The process is dominated by four precipitation steps. The first step, isopropanol precipitation (0.6 v/v), which is used here essentially to reduce the volume of the process stream generated by alkaline lysis, is followed by a negative precipitation of impurities with ammonium acetate (2.5 M). The subsequent precipitation of plasmid with $PEG_{8000}/NaCl$ further removes impurities before the SEC step.[10] The plasmid in the pool recovered from this column is then precipitated by ethanol addition, a step that provides an opportunity to exchange the product into the final formulation buffer.[10] This ethanol precipitation step is another popular buffer exchange option often encountered at the end of a process[15] (e.g., see also process VII, Figure 18.2).

The tandem isopropanol/chaotropic salt precipitation shown in flow sheet IV is quite effective and, for this reason, it is not uncommon to find it in other processes as well. For example, combinations of isopropanol precipitation with ammonium sulfate negative precipitation work particularly well when used before hydrophobic interaction chromatography (HIC) separations[16-18] (see process V, Figure 18.2). A key feature of the second precipitation is that it acts as a preconditioning step for HIC, producing a high-salt plasmid-containing supernatant. This feedstock can be loaded directly onto HIC columns equilibrated with buffers that are highly concentrated in ammonium sulfate in order to promote hydrophobic interaction (process V, Figure 18.2). Among other features (see Chapter 17, Section 17.2.6), this type of chromatographic step is close to unbeatable when it to comes to clearance of lipopolysaccharides (LPS).[16-18] The large amounts of salt found in the plasmid pools recovered from HIC columns should then be removed by an adequate buffer exchange step (e.g., TFF and isopropanol precipitation).

In the third process highlighted in this section, a salting-out precipitation of impurities is performed by directly adding $CaCl_2$ to a clarified alkaline lysate[19] (process VI, Figure 18.2). This constitutes an advantage over the two previous processes (IV and V, Figure 18.2) in that the alcohol precipitation step is eliminated. Furthermore, the $CaCl_2$ precipitation is highly effective in removing high-molecular-weight RNA. The clarified supernatant obtained after solid–liquid separation is then loaded without further treatment onto a first AEX column in order to further remove RNA and also gDNA. The column is operated in the standard positive mode (see Chapter 17, Section 17.2.5) so that the majority of RNA exits in the flow-through under a lower ionic strength (0.5 M potassium acetate), and bound plasmid elutes under the action of an increasing NaCl gradient. An interesting variation proposed here is the use of a low pH value of 5.5 during loading in order to increase the charge difference between RNA and plasmid DNA, and hence resolution. During elution, the pH is stepped up to 9.6 to foster desorption. The following step proposed in this process, a second AEX chromatography, is somewhat unusual in the fact that a similar driving force (i.e., charge difference) is again explored to further remove traces of RNA and gDNA impurities from plasmid DNA (check heuristic 5 in Chapter 14, Section 14.4). Still, the author stresses that an AEX matrix different from the one used in the previous step should be used, even though precise justifications for this choice are not presented. The column is run according to the standard methodology—loading at moderate salt and plasmid elution under linear salt gradient. Overall, the process delivers a plasmid product where proteins, LPS, and RNA are undetected, but with a 0.6% contamination of gDNA.[19] The use of a $CaCl_2$ precipitation step to remove RNA from alkaline lysates before chromatography can also be found in other process solutions. For example, Smrekar et al. have combined it with a first monolithic column that captures plasmid DNA by AEX and with a second monolithic column that resolves isoforms on the basis of hydrophobic interactions.[20]

As described in Chapter 16 (Section 16.3), in some situations, precipitation can be highly selective when it comes to discriminating supercoiled plasmid DNA from hard-to-remove impurities like gDNA fragments and plasmid variants like open circular isoforms. Consider, for example, the inclusion of two sequential cetyltrimethylammonium bromide (CTAB) precipitation steps in the process proposed by Lander et al.[15] (process VII, Figure 18.2). Here, the lysate obtained by the combined action of heat, detergent, and lysozyme is subjected to a first CTAB precipitation with a concentration carefully selected to precipitate gDNA and open circular plasmid DNA, but not supercoiled plasmid DNA. After solid–liquid separation, a slightly higher CTAB concentration is used so as to precipitate the supercoiled isoform. An adsorption step with calcium silicate (see Chapter 16, Section 16.5.4) then follows, which removes LPS and gDNA impurities down to a level sufficiently low to allow for the process to be terminated with a final ethanol precipitation for buffer exchange and concentration.[15] A similar scheme, comprising a sequence of a low- and a high-cut precipitation with the same agent (PEG_{8000}), is also described by Marquet et al.[21]

18.3.3 ATPS-Based Processes

The fact that aqueous two-phase extraction (see Chapter 16, Section 16.4.) is not often used in the industrial practice has not barred process development engineers from proposing its use in the intermediate recovery section of a number of plasmid manufacturing processes (see Figure 18.3). In process VIII, for example, a PEG_{600}–ammonium sulfate system is used to process clarified alkaline lysates and to produce a plasmid-containing, salt-rich bottom phase, which is substantially freed from RNA impurities.[22] As a result of extraction, the amount of proteins (98%) and LPS (68%) was substantially reduced, even though with a relatively low plasmid yield of 75.4%. As a subsequent step, and in order to take advantage of the large amounts of chaotropic salt present, an HIC step is run in the negative mode with a downward ammonium sulfate gradient in such a way that the remaining impurities (proteins and LPS) and the residual amounts of polyethylene glycol (PEG) are removed.[22] Although a final buffer exchange was not suggested in the process, a step like TFF is inevitable in order to remove the large amounts of ammonium sulfate present in the plasmid-containing flow-through and to exchange the plasmid into a more convenient buffer. Sterile filtration with 0.2-μm membranes should also be included as a terminal step.

While polymer/salt ATPSs dominate the literature when it comes to plasmid purification, the description of liquid–liquid extraction with polymer/polymer systems can also be found (see Chapter 16, Section 16.4.3). In process IX (Figure 18.3), an ATPS made of a thermoseparating ethylene oxide/polypropylene oxide (EO_{50}-PO_{50}) polymer and dextran T500 is combined with

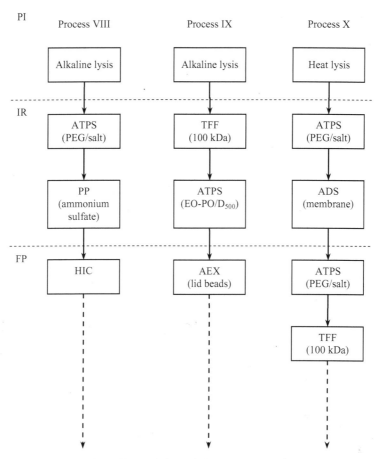

Figure 18.3 *Partitioning impurities and plasmids in aqueous two-phase systems. References: process VIII (Trindade et al.[22]), process IX (Kepka et al.[23]), and process X (Frerix et al.[24]). ADS, adsorption; AEX, anion exchange; ATPS, aqueous two-phase system; FP, final purification; HIC, hydrophobic interaction chromatography; IR, intermediate recovery; PEG, polyethylene glycol; PI, primary isolation; PP, precipitation; TFF, tangential flow filtration.*

TFF and AEX in a fully integrated process that delivers pure plasmid with a 69% yield.[23] More specifically, the process uses a hollow fiber ultrafiltration cartridge (100-kDa cutoff) to remove the large amounts of salts that are typically found in alkaline lysates, to reduce the volume fivefold, and to prepare the process solution for the salt-sensitive aqueous two-phase extraction. With the EO_{50}-PO_{50}/dextran T500 system, close to 100% of plasmid DNA is obtained in the top EO_{50}-PO_{50}-rich phase, while most proteins (60%) and RNA (80%) are left behind in the dextran bottom phase. Once the temperature of the EO_{50}-PO_{50}-rich phase is raised past the cloud point temperature to precipitate the polymer, plasmid can be recovered in a low-polymer water phase. The process is then completed with a final polishing step to remove residual impurities.

Here, a chromatography column packed with AEX lid beads (see Chapter 17, Section 17.2.3.4) is operated in a negative mode in such a way that plasmid DNA is recovered in the flow-through completely free of RNA.[23] Although not described by the proponents, such a process would be complete with buffer exchange/concentration and 0.2-μm membrane sterilization steps.

The use of ATPS is further intensified in the third example shown in Figure 18.3 (process X). A PEG$_{800}$/phosphate ATPS is first used to capture plasmid DNA from nonclarified alkaline lysates neutralized with potassium phosphate.[24] The plasmid recovered in the salt-rich bottom phase is then adsorbed on a 0.2-μm nylon disk membrane and eluted with a tris(hydroxymethyl) aminomethane (tris) buffer. Although more than 95% of the initial RNA is cleared by the combined action of the aqueous two-phase extraction and membrane adsorption, this solution was then subjected to a second extraction with a PEG$_{800}$/phosphate ATPS to remove the remaining gDNA and RNA, and also open circular plasmid, and to recover the supercoiled plasmid DNA in the salt-rich bottom phase. The process is terminated with a buffer exchange, TFF step with a 100-kDa membrane.[24] As usual, sterile filtration with 0.2 μm should ensue (see Chapter 17, Section 17.4).

18.4 THE USE OF CHROMATOGRAPHY

18.4.1 Chromatography-Intensive Processes

In spite of its current shortcomings (see Chapter 17, Section 17.2), the use of chromatography at process scale is almost inevitable. Whereas some processes use but one chromatographic step like processes I, III (Figure 18.1), IV, V (Figure 18.2), VIII, and IX (Figure 18.3), flow sheets that present up to three chromatographic steps are not uncommon (see Figure 18.4). The approach underlying these chromatography-intensive processes is clearly different from the one explored in other cases, which are decidedly set to minimize or even abolish the use of chromatography (see processes VII and X in Figures 18.2 and 18.3, respectively). A number of reasons may justify this option for chromatography-intensive processes. For example, it is not surprising to find that one of the processes highlighted in this section was developed by the company GE Healthcare (Uppsala, Sweden), one of the leading manufacturers of chromatography resins and equipments for bioprocess-scale applications[25,26] (process XI, Figure 18.4). Indeed, this process presents a somewhat unusual combination of three chromatography steps. The first step is a SEC separation, which is performed right after alkaline lysis. The use of this type of chromatography so early in a process and with a feedstock that is heavily loaded with impurities is rather unusual, especially because low throughput is one of the distinctive characteristics of conventional SEC. The operation is performed with the specific goal of removing the large amounts of salts, RNA, and small solutes present in the lysate. As described in detail in Chapter 17

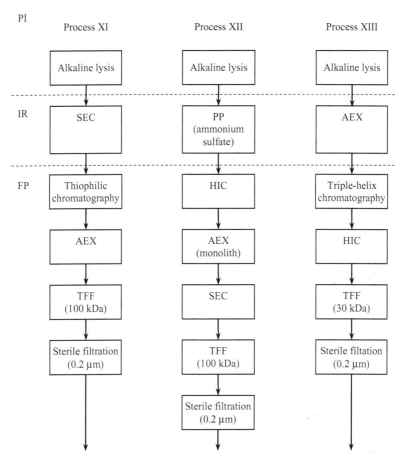

PI

| Process XI | Process XII | Process XIII |

Alkaline lysis | Alkaline lysis | Alkaline lysis

IR

SEC | PP (ammonium sulfate) | AEX

FP

Thiophilic chromatography | HIC | Triple-helix chromatography

AEX | AEX (monolith) | HIC

TFF (100 kDa) | SEC | TFF (30 kDa)

Sterile filtration (0.2 μm) | AEX (monolith) | Sterile filtation (0.2 μm)

TFF (100 kDa)

Sterile filtration (0.2 μm)

Figure 18.4 Chromatography-intensive processes. References: process XI (Lemmens et al.[25]), process XII (Urthaler et al.[27]), and process XIII (Blanche et al.[28]). AEX, anion exchange; FP, final purification; HIC, hydrophobic interaction chromatography; IR, intermediate recovery; PI, primary isolation; PP, precipitation; SEC, size-exclusion chromatography; TFF, tangential flow filtration.

(Section 17.2.9 and Figure 17.9b), a highly concentrated ammonium sulfate solution (2 M) is used as the running buffer in order to improve selectivity and thus to allow the loading of feed volumes that correspond to more than one-third of the column volume.[25,26] The plasmid-containing pool recovered from the SEC column is then fed into a thiophilic interaction chromatography column (see details in Chapter 17, Section 17.2.7). Although this step is designed mainly to resolve plasmid isoforms, it also removes LPS, proteins, and RNA, and concentrates the plasmid DNA (~10-fold).[25] Finally, the plasmid recovered from the thiophilic interaction column is polished and concentrated (~2-fold) on an AEX column that is operated under the usual mode, that is, loading at moderate salt (0.4 M NaCl) and elution with a linear gradient up to

1 M NaCl.[25] In one specific case, the combined used of the three chromatographic steps increased the relative amount of supercoiled to open circular isoforms (e.g., from 54% to 97%) and removed RNA (from 5200- to <0.2-μg/mg plasmid), LPS (from 150,000- to 9-EU/mg plasmid), proteins (from 160,000 to <0.3 μg/mg plasmid), and gDNA (from 150- to 2-μg/mg plasmid) down to figures within specifications.[25] According to the proponents, the process is completed with a concentration/buffer exchange step performed with a TFF unit equipped with a 100-kDa cutoff membrane and with a sterile filtration through 0.2-μm pore rating membranes.

In the second example described in this section, a process developed by the company Boehringer Ingelheim (Vienna, Austria), we also find three chromatographic steps[27] (process XII, Figure 18.4). As in most of the cases examined so far, the process starts with alkaline lysis but then resorts to an ammonium sulfate precipitation (2.5–3.0 M) to reduce the impurity load and to adjust the conditions of the lysate for the subsequent HIC step. The HIC column is run at a very high salt concentration so as to promote plasmid binding (see Chapter 17, Section 17.2.6). Under the action of a downward salt gradient, impurities like LPS, RNA, and open circular isoforms are then removed to a large extent (see Chapter 17, Figure 17.6b). This HIC step is further characterized by a 95% yield and a twofold plasmid concentration.[27] A monolithic AEX column is then used to further improve plasmid purity and concentration (~3-fold). The elution pool collected from the HIC column can be loaded without any conditioning onto the monolith, even though it contains substantial amounts of salt. A series of elution steps are used to selectively elute plasmid DNA (~95% yield) from nonplasmid impurities (especially proteins and LPS). The third SEC step is introduced in the process for polishing and buffer exchange purposes. The elution pool from the previous AEX column is loaded directly (~1/3 of the column volume), and elution is accomplished with an appropriate buffer. As usual (see Chapter 17, Section 17.2.9), plasmid elutes with the void volume (~95% yield), whereas salts and residual impurities (proteins and LPS) exit the column later on. Finally, and as in the previous case, the process is terminated with a concentration/buffer exchange by TFF (e.g., 100-kDa cutoff) and with a sterile filtration (0.2 μm). Key numbers and features associated with the overall process are (1) a plasmid yield of about 65%; (2) impurity removals of 25, 51, and 13% in the ammonium sulfate precipitation, HIC, and AEX steps, respectively; (3) a final product with <20-μg RNA/mg plasmid, 6-μg gDNA/mg plasmid, 0.5-μg protein/mg plasmid and 0.7–1.4 EU/mg plasmid; and (4) close to 80-fold concentration of plasmid DNA relative to the starting lysate.[27]

The final example in this section also combines three chromatographic steps[28] (process XIII, Figure 18.4). Following the usual alkaline lysis step, which in this case is conducted in a continuous fashion using two inline mixers, the lysate is clarified by depth filtration and then fed onto an AEX column packed with Fractogel trimethyl aminoethyl (TMAE) (Merck, Darmstadt, Germany), an adsorbent that features tentacle-like structures (see Chapter 17, Section

17.2.3.2). As usual, when AEX is performed after alkaline lysis, the lysate must first be diluted with water to adjust conductivity and thus to maximize plasmid binding and resolution of impurities. Following loading, the column is washed with the medium salt equilibration buffer and the captured plasmid is eluted with the customary NaCl step gradient. Triple-helix affinity chromatography with an adsorbent synthesized in-house is then used in this process to improve plasmid purity. As described in the previous chapter (Section 17.2.8), this relies on the specific hybridization of oligonucleotides (e.g., a homopyrimidine sequence) immobilized in the matrix with a target sequence (e.g., a homopurine•homopyrimidine duplex) within the plasmid DNA. As a preconditioning step, NaCl is added to the plasmid-containing fraction isolated from the AEX column in order to adjust conditions that favor triplex formation. The NaCl concentration in sodium acetate buffers (50 mM, pH 4.5) used for equilibration and washing was 2 and 1 M, respectively, and plasmid was eluted by decreasing the ionic strength (100 mM tris) and increasing the pH to 9 to deprotonate cytosines. An HIC step with a butyl-adsorbent is then finally used to remove open circular isoforms and remaining impurities from the plasmid. Again, this calls for a preconditioning of the feed, this time with ammonium sulfate. The HIC operation involves the usual switching from the high ammonium sulfate salt buffer used in equilibration and washing to the low ammonium sulfate salt buffer that destroys hydrophobic interactions and elutes bound plasmid. The eluate of the HIC column is concentrated up to fourfold and diafiltered with 10 volumes of saline by TFF (30 kDa). Sterility is guaranteed with filtration through 0.2-μm pore rating membranes. This process results in a highly purified preparation of >99% supercoiled plasmid DNA, which contains residual amounts of gDNA, RNA, and proteins lower than 0.00001% and an LPS content lower than 0.1 EU/mg.[28] The need to precondition the feed before each of the three chromatographic steps should be pointed here as a disadvantage of this process because it inevitably results in the dilution of the plasmid and in an increase in the process volumes.

Although the use of so many chromatography steps within a single process poses many challenges and is likely to step up costs (e.g., due to the cost of the chromatographic resins), it is noteworthy to highlight the fact that two of the examples just described have originated from large industrial companies (GE Healthcare and Boehringer Ingelheim) and not from academic research laboratories. It thus seems that the purification benefits associated with an intensive use of chromatography in an industrial setting may well justify the disadvantages.

18.4.2 Moving Chromatography Up

Although chromatography is in general positioned toward the end of the downstream processing train, there are a number of cases where the operation is moved up in the process and performed right after the disruption step. The inconvenience of doing so has been discussed in Chapter 14 (see heuristic 3,

Section 14.4) and includes the need to use larger volumes of chromatographic matrices and the extreme challenge of handling a highly impure solution. Nevertheless, this is a strategy that is pursued often in plasmid manufacturing (see Figure 18.5). One of the most surprising of such processes is probably the one described in the previous section wherein what is probably the least efficient of all of the chromatographic modalities available, that is, SEC, is used to desalt and purify alkaline lysates (process XI, Figure 18.4). Unlike this, the use of AEX steps to directly process plasmid-containing lysates is more widespread, as exemplified by a process designed to produce clinical-grade plasmid DNA for phase 1 clinical trials and large animal clinical studies[29] (process XIV, Figure 18.5). An important characteristic of this process, which may well justify the successful use of AEC right after lysis, is the use of RNase during alkaline lysis. This enzymatic digestion fragments RNA molecules and renders the subsequent purification of plasmid in the QIAGEN (Hilden, Germany) silica-

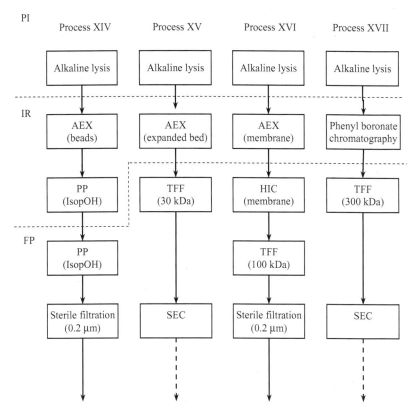

Figure 18.5 *Moving chromatography up. References: process XIV (Przybylowski et al.[29]), process XV (Varley et al.[30]), process XVI (Hebel et al.[8]), and process XVII (Gomes et al.[34] and unpublished results). AEX, anion exchange; FP, final purification; HIC, hydrophobic interaction chromatography; IR, intermediate recovery; IsopOH, isopropanol; PI, primary isolation; PP, precipitation; SEC, size-exclusion chromatography; TFF, tangential flow filtration.*

based anion exchanger much easier to accomplish. Apart from the usual loading and elution at moderate (0.75 M NaCl) and higher (1.0–1.5 M NaCl) ionic strength, respectively, key features that are characteristic of the QIAGEN AEX purification methodologies are the use of a nonionic detergent in the lysate and during loading, and the use of relative large amounts of isopropanol (15% v/v) in all chromatography buffers. Next in the process, we find two consecutive isopropanol precipitation steps designed for plasmid concentration and buffer exchange. Although not explicitly indicated in the process diagram, each step is followed by centrifugation, supernatant discard, and pellet resuspension in 1.5 M NaCl (first precipitation) and sterile water (second precipitation). The purified plasmid is finally sterile filtered through a 0.2-μm membrane. The process is claimed to produce a plasmid product with a quality degree sufficient for clinical applications.[29]

As referred to earlier, one of the drawbacks of using chromatography immediately after the cell disruption step has to do with the fact that lysates are highly impure solutions. Furthermore, these lysates often contain small particulate matter in suspension, for example, as a result of a poor clarification step that can foul packed beds. In these cases, chromatographic purifications can still be implemented, for example, by using specially designed beads (e.g., Streamline from GE Healthcare, Uppsala, Sweden) and running columns in the expanded-bed mode. In process XV (Figure 18.5), alkaline lysates prepared with the aid of RNase are rapidly clarified with a coarse bag filtration step and then loaded upward so as to expand an AEX bed previously equilibrated with 0.8 M potassium acetate.[30,31] With this mode of operation, particulates are effectively washed out from the bed of chromatographic beads. Furthermore, since back pressures in expanded beds are inherently lower, lysates can be loaded at much higher linear flow rates, hence maximizing throughput. One important disadvantage that is sometimes associated with the processing of alkaline lysates in AEX expanded beads is the occurrence of gel clogging and expansion collapse. The latter phenomenon is usually a consequence of the aggregation of individual particles of the adsorbent due to particle-to-particle bridging via longer polymeric DNA chains.[32] Once loading is completed, bound impurities and plasmid are eluted with NaCl by reversing the flow and allowing the bed to settle.[30,31] The plasmid-containing fractions are then pooled, concentrated 25-fold with a spiral cartridge TFF module (30 kDa), and processed by SEC in order to remove residual impurities and to exchange the plasmid into an adequate formulation buffer.[30,31]

In some of the processes described so far, chromatography is carried out with monoliths and membrane matrices (e.g., process III, Figure 18.1; process XII Figure 18.4). This move toward nonbead matrices is of course related to the mass transfer, accessibility, and capacity issues described in Chapter 17 (Section 17.2.2). Furthermore, the fact that membranes, for example, enable the use of very large flow rates makes the use of this type of matrix especially convenient early in a process, when large volumes of lysate need to be processed. Consider, for example, process XVI in Figure 18.5.[8,33] Here, an AEX membrane module is used to capture plasmid DNA from a lysate that is produced in a continuous system that combines a high-shear, low residence time mixer, a holding coil, and a bubble-mixer chamber (see Chapter 15, Section 15.3.2.4 for further details). The adjustment of the conductivity of the lysate by dilution with water is a prerequirement to ensure binding of the plasmid. The chromatographic operation is then run in the usual mode, with equilibration and washing at a moderate NaCl concentration (0.67 M) and plasmid elution with a 1 M NaCl step. The benefits of membranes as chromatographic matrices are further explored in the subsequent step where an HIC membrane cartridge is operated in a negative mode to further purify the plasmid. Again, this requires an adjustment of the conductivity of the plasmid-containing eluate from the AEX membrane in order to promote hydrophobic interactions. This task is accomplished by the addition of a concentrated solution of ammonium sulfate. Once the HIC cartridge is equilibrated with a 2.4 M ammonium sulfate eluent, the feed is loaded and the plasmid is received in the flow-through. An added advantage associated with the use of chromatographic membranes in this particular case is the disposable, single-use nature of the cartridges employed. This eliminates the need for cleaning the matrices and for validating the protocols used therein, a task that is one of the hallmarks of bead-based chromatography.[8] The purification activities end with the usual combination of concentration/diafiltration by TFF (100 kDa) and sterile filtration with 0.2-μm pore rating membranes. The process delivers a high-quality GMP product, with an impurity profile compatible with therapeutic use (<0.3% RNA, <0.2% protein, <0.4% gDNA, and <0.2 EU/mg) and at a cost that is estimated to be less than US$1 per milligram.[8]

The final example of the use of chromatography upfront in a process resorts to a phenyl boronate column to clear impurities like RNA and LPS from alkaline lysates[34] (see Chapter 17, Section 17.2.8). According to the proposed methodology (process XVII, Figure 18.5), lysates are loaded without any pretreatment, the column is washed with water and bound impurities are eluted with a step of 1.5 M tris buffer. Under these conditions, plasmid DNA elutes in the flow-through, whereas cis-diol-containing RNA and LPS bind to the resin on account of the formation of covalent bonds with the boronate ligands. Variable amounts of gDNA and proteins are also retained in the column due to nonspecific interactions.[34] Since the plasmid-containing fractions collected still contain a certain amount of low-molecular-weight RNA and traces of other impurities, a TFF with a 300-kDa membrane is then used for further purification, buffer exchange, and concentration. The process should terminate with SEC and a sterile filtration step.

18.4.3 Chromatography-Free Processes

In spite of the superior resolution of chromatography when it comes to making very difficult separations, many bioprocess engineers and scientists have tried to develop processes for the manufacturing of biopharmaceuticals that are chromatography free. While in the case of proteins the key reason for this is probably the high cost that is incurred in the setting up and operation of the chromatographic steps, the heightened capacity/accessibility problems encountered when trying to purify plasmids with chromatographic adsorbents constitutes an additional driver in the case of plasmids. Two of the processes described so far (processes VII and X in Figures 18.2 and 18.3, respectively) have been developed specifically without chromatographic steps. In retrospect, it is interesting to notice that in order to deliver a pharmaceutical-grade plasmid without resorting to the high-resolution ability of chromatography, both processes had to make a repeated use of the same unit operation, that is, precipitation with CTAB in the case of process VII and extraction with PEG/salt ATPS in the case of process X.

18.5 THE UBIQUITOUS ROLE OF TFF

Many researchers have refrained from using precipitation and aqueous two-phase steps in their processes, probably due to the intensive use of equipment, manpower, and mass-separating agents that such operations often require. Conversely, TFF is a relatively simple operation to implement, which also lends itself very easily to automation and scale-up. It is thus more and more common to come across with processes that rely on TFF to concentrate plasmid solutions, remove low-molecular-weight impurities, and exchange buffers (see Chapters 16 and 17, Sections 16.2 and 17.3 respectively). The cutoff of the membranes used in the TFF of plasmid solutions varies from 30 to 300 kDa, with 100 kDa being the most common. As a result of its versatility, TFF can be found at the different sections of the downstream processing. For example, TFF is many times used after cell disruption in order to desalt·lysates, to remove low-molecular-weight impurities, and to concentrate plasmid DNA (e.g., processes II and IX in Figures 18.1 and 18.3, respectively). In the intermediate recovery section, TFF is especially useful in between chromatographic steps to remove excess water and to diafilter away smaller impurities and buffer components (e.g., process XV, Figure 18.5). Finally, TFF is becoming more and more the preferred option for the concentration and buffer exchange required at the far end of processes (e.g., process X, Figure 18.3; processes XI–XIII, Figure 18.4; and process XVI, Figure 18.5).

18.6 CONCLUSIONS

The number of process solutions devised to tackle the challenges associated with the large-scale manufacturing of gram amounts of plasmid DNA preparations with the quality attributes required for clinical applications has increased steadily over the years. The selection and brief discussion of a number of representative processes found in the scientific and technical literature that were made in this chapter were intended to provide an overview of the possibilities that are being explored. Many of these processes are characterized by the use of inventive solutions, improved devices, tailored materials, and new combinations of unit operations. The common goal underlying this surge in process innovation has been, and still is, to improve throughput and product quality in such a way as to keep pace with clinical development and to prepare for the commercial manufacturing of products once the first approvals for marketing arise. Nevertheless, and in spite of the progress made, there are still some niches where technical improvements are actively sought (e.g., nonbeaded chromatographic matrices and nonalkaline lysis methods) that might contribute to improve productivity, yields, and quality. Such developments will hopefully contribute to minimize production costs and hence to increase the affordability of plasmid biopharmaceuticals.

REFERENCES

1. Quaak SG, van den Berg JH, Toebes M, et al. GMP production of pDERMATT for vaccination against melanoma in a phase I clinical trial. *European Journal of Pharmaceutics and Biopharmaceutics*. 2008;70:429–438.

2. Vo-Quang T, Malpiece Y, Buffard D, Kaminski PA, Vidal D, Strosberg AD. Rapid large-scale purification of plasmid DNA by medium or low pressure gel filtration. Application: Construction of thermoamplifiable expression vectors. *Bioscience Reports*. 1985;5:101–111.

3. Wolff JA, Malone RW, Williams P, et al. Direct gene transfer into mouse muscle *in vivo*. *Science*. 1990;247:1465–1468.

4. Ulmer JB, Donnelly JJ, Parker SE, et al. Heterologous protection against influenza by injection of DNA encoding a viral protein. *Science*. 1993;259:1745–1749.

5. Tang DC, DeVit M, Johnston SA. Genetic immunization is a simple method for eliciting an immune response. *Nature*. 1992;356:152–154.

6. Freitas SS, Azzoni AR, Santos JA, Monteiro GA, Prazeres DMF. On the stability of plasmid DNA vectors during cell culture and purification. *Molecular Biotechnoloy*. 2007;36:151–158.

7. Butler MD, Cohen DL, Kahn D, Winkler ME, inventors; Genentech, Inc., assignee. Purification of plasmid DNA. U.S. patent 6,313,285, November 6, 2001.

8. Hebel H, Attra H, Khan A, Draghia-Akli R. Successful parallel development and integration of a plasmid-based biologic, container/closure system and electrokinetic delivery device. *Vaccine*. 2006;24:4607–4614.

9. Urthaler J, Ascher C, Wohrer H, Necina R. Automated alkaline lysis for industrial scale cGMP production of pharmaceutical grade plasmid-DNA. *Journal of Biotechnology*. 2007;128:132–149.

10. Horn NA, Meek JA, Budahazi G, Marquet M. Cancer gene therapy using plasmid DNA: Purification of DNA for human clinical trials. *Human Gene Therapy*. 1995;6:565–573.

11. Raymond GJ, Bryant PK, 3rd, Nelson A, Johnson JD. Large-scale isolation of covalently closed circular DNA using gel filtration chromatography. *Analytical Biochemistry*. 1988;173:125–133.

12. Bywater M, Bywater R, Hellman L. A novel chromatographic procedure for purification of bacterial plasmids. *Analytical Biochemistry*. 1983;132:219–224.

13. Lee AL, Sagar S, inventors; Merck & Co., Inc., assignee. Method for large scale plasmid purification. U.S. patent 6,197,553, March 6, 2002.

14. Carnes AE, Hodgson CP, Luke JM, Vincent JM, Williams JA. Plasmid DNA production combining antibiotic-free selection, inducible high yield fermentation, and novel autolytic purification. *Biotechnology and Bioengineering*. 2009;104:505–515.

15. Lander RJ, Winters MA, Meacle FJ, inventors; Merck & Co., Inc., assignee. Process for the scaleable purification of plasmid DNA. U.S. patent 6,797,476, September 28, 2004.

16. Diogo MM, Queiroz JA, Monteiro GA, Martins SAM, Ferreira GNM, Prazeres DMF. Purification of a cystic fibrosis plasmid vector for gene therapy using hydrophobic interaction chromatography. *Biotechnology and Bioengineering*. 2000;68: 576–583.

17. Diogo MM, Ribeiro S, Queiroz JA, et al. Production, purification and analysis of an experimental DNA vaccine against rabies. *The Journal of Gene Medicine*. 2001;3:577–584.

18. Prazeres DMF, Diogo MM, Queiroz JA, inventors; Instituto Superior Técnico, assignee. Purification of plasmid DNA by hydrophobic interaction chromatography. U.S. patent 7,169,917, January 30, 2007.

19. Bhikhabhai R, inventor; Amersham Pharmacia Biotech AB, assignee. Plasmid DNA purification using divalent alkaline earth metal ions and two anion exchangers. U.S. patent 6410274, June 25, 2002.

20. Smrekar F, Podgornik A, Ciringer M, et al. Preparation of pharmaceutical-grade plasmid DNA using methacrylate monolithic columns. *Vaccine*. 2010;28: 2039–2045.

21. Marquet M, Horn N, Meek J, Budahazi G, inventors; Vical Incorporated, assignee. Production of pharmaceutical-grade plasmid DNA. U.S. patent 5,561,064, October 1, 1996.

22. Trindade IP, Diogo MM, Prazeres DMF, Marcos JC. Purification of plasmid DNA vectors by aqueous two-phase extraction and hydrophobic interaction chromatography. *Journal of Chromatography. A*. 2005;1082:176–184.

23. Kepka C, Lemmens R, Vasi J, Nyhammar T, Gustavsson PE. Integrated process for purification of plasmid DNA using aqueous two-phase systems combined with membrane filtration and lid bead chromatography. *Journal of Chromatography. A*. 2004;1057:115–124.

24. Frerix A, Geilenkirchen P, Muller M, Kula MR, Hubbuch J. Separation of genomic DNA, RNA, and open circular plasmid DNA from supercoiled plasmid DNA by combining denaturation, selective renaturation and aqueous two-phase extraction. *Biotechnology and Bioengineering*. 2007;96:57–66.

25. Lemmens R, Olsson U, Nyhammar T, Stadler J. Supercoiled plasmid DNA: Selective purification by thiophilic/aromatic adsorption. *Journal of Chromatography*. 2003; 784:291–300.

26. Stadler J, Lemmens R, Nyhammar T. Plasmid DNA purification. *The Journal of Gene Medicine*. 2004;6:S54–S66.

27. Urthaler J, Buchinger W, Necina R. Industrial scale cGMP purification of pharmaceutical-grade plasmid DNA. *Chemical Engineering and Technology*. 2005; 28:1408–1420.

28. Blanche F, Couder M, Maestrali N, Gaillac D, Guillemin T, inventors. Method of preparation for pharmaceutical grade plasmid DNA. U.S. patent 2007/111,221, May 17, 2007.

29. Przybylowski M, Bartido S, Borquez-Ojeda O, Sadelain M, Riviere I. Production of clinical-grade plasmid DNA for human phase I clinical trials and large animal clinical studies. *Vaccine*. 2007;25:5013–5024.

30. Varley DL, Hitchcock AG, Weiss AME, et al. Production of plasmid DNA for human gene therapy using modified alkaline cell lysis and expanded bed anion exchange chromatography. *Bioseparation*. 1998;8:209–217.

31. Thatcher DR, Hitchcock AG, Hanak JAJ, Varley DL, inventors; Cobra Therapeutics Limited, assignee. Method of plasmid DNA production and purification. U.S. patent 6,503,738, January 7, 2003.

32. Ferreira GN, Cabral JM, Prazeres DMF. Anion exchange purification of plasmid DNA using expanded bed adsorption. *Bioseparation*. 2000;9:1–6.

33. Hebel H, Ramakrishnan S, Gonzalez H, Darnell J, inventors; Advisys, Inc., assignee. Devices and methods for biomaterial production. U.S. patent 7,238,522, July 3, 2007.

34. Gomes AG, Azevedo AM, Aires-Barros MR, Prazeres DMF. Clearance of host cell impurities from plasmid-containing lysates by boronate adsorption. *Journal of Chromatography. A*. 2010;1217:2262–2266.

Part IV

Concluding Remarks and Outlook

19

Concluding Remarks and Outlook

19.1 INTRODUCTION

As we have seen throughout this book, the transfer of genes via carrier plasmid DNA molecules into human or nonhuman hosts has emerged as a possible solution for the management of an entire constellation of diseases. The progress made since the first experiments in the early 1990s of the twentieth century showed that genes carried by plasmids could be expressed *in vivo* has been enormous. Still, the lack of effective human plasmid biopharmaceuticals in the market, which persists until today, makes many wonder if the promise of treating and/or preventing diseases with plasmid-mediated gene transfer will ever become true. As this book comes to an end, it is important to look back, but also forward, in time, and to try to understand how things have evolved and how things will progress toward the future. Such is the major goal of this closing chapter. In the first section, the dynamics of the innovation activity that took place in the plasmid biopharmaceutical arena during the last 30 years is analyzed. The model used to make this analysis, developed by Utterback,[1] attempts to explain in a generic way how the succession of innovations, which resulted both from creativity and chance findings, has contributed to the shaping and maturing of the field. This analysis may provide some ideas for future directions and courses of actions. In the second part of the chapter, a side-by-side comparison of a specific class of plasmid biopharmaceuticals,

Plasmid Biopharmaceuticals: Basics, Applications, and Manufacturing, First Edition.
Duarte Miguel F. Prazeres.
© 2011 John Wiley & Sons, Inc. Published 2011 by John Wiley & Sons, Inc.

DNA vaccines, with existent and proven conventional vaccines, is made on the basis of the business strategy framework popularized in recent years under the name Blue Ocean.[2] The use of this analysis and strategy tool stresses the need to face the development of plasmid biopharmaceuticals as a business enterprise and not just as a scientific and technological undertaking. Success will only come if products are developed in such a way that they will either compete with existing ones by offering new characteristics or create a totally new market space and unlock new customers.

19.2 THE DYNAMICS OF INNOVATION

19.2.1 Introduction

The past, present, and future of plasmid biopharmaceuticals can be examined and analyzed on the basis of the model of the dynamics of innovation in industry proposed by Utterback.[1] According to this model (sketched in Figure 19.1), the rate of major innovation in a given product class, and in

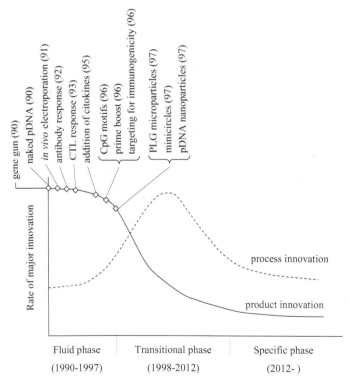

Figure 19.1 The dynamics of innovation in the plasmid biopharmaceutical field as analyzed on the basis of Utterback's model.[1]

the processes used to manufacture it, follows a general pattern over time. The model was originally developed and used to describe industries during the course of their progress in the marketplace, as they strive to introduce a new, better product after another. Although the pace of development in the biopharmaceutical industry (see Chapter 3) is clearly different from the one that is characteristic of most industries, an adaptation of the model to the specific case of plasmid biopharmaceuticals constitutes an interesting academic exercise that may add an extra dimension to our insights into the field.

19.2.2 The Fluid Phase: A Surge in Product Innovation

During the formative years of any industry/industry segment, the rate of product innovation is highest with many free experimentations taking place among the different players.[1] In the case of plasmid biopharmaceuticals, the initial major innovations that took place in the first 8 years (1990–1997*) were proposed by scientists working in research laboratories of academic and governmental institutions, and included many of the features that we nowadays associate readily with plasmid products (Figure 19.1). Many of these "product" innovations were succinctly described in Chapter 1 and include, for example, the use of naked plasmid DNA (1990[3]), the delivery of plasmid DNA by particle bombardment (1990[4]), the application of electroporation for *in vivo* delivery (1991[5]), the demonstration of antibody (1992[6]) and cytotoxic T lymphocyte (CTL) responses (1993[7]) following *in vivo* injection of naked DNA (i.e., the concept of DNA vaccines), the coexpression of cytokines alongside the target genes (1995[8]), the addition of immune-stimulatory cytosine–phosphate–guanine (CpG) motifs to plasmid backbones (1996[9]), prime (with DNA vaccine)-boost (with non-DNA vaccine) vaccination (1996[10]), the use of targeting sequences to enhance the immunogenicity of DNA vaccines (1996[11]), the encapsulation of plasmids in microparticles (1997[12]), the design of miniplasmids (so-called minicircles) containing only the functional elements required for the expression of the transgene (1997[13]), and the compaction of single molecules of DNA into minimally sized nanoparticles (1997[14]). On the contrary, less attention was given during this period to the processes used to produce plasmid DNA, which were rather crude and inefficient, and essentially based on adaptations of the isolation protocols used by molecular biologists at the laboratory scale. Consistent with this observation is the fact that the first scientific reports describing the manufacturing of large amounts of plasmids for clinical trials with processes designed specifically for scale-up date back to the later part of the 8-year, 1990–1997 period.[15–17]

---

* The seminal work of Wolff and colleagues[3] on naked plasmid DNA is used here to mark the birth of plasmid biopharmaceuticals.

19.2.3 The Transitional Phase

19.2.3.1 Slowing Down Product Innovation

According to Utterback's model, and following the surge in product innovation of the "fluid phase" described previously, a transition period is entered, in which the rates of major product and process innovations slow down and speed up, respectively.[1] This is a time when the diversity of potential "product" designs starts to decrease and a few dominant designs emerge. In the case of plasmid biopharmaceuticals, I argue that this "transitional phase" started around 1998 and continues to date. During this period, some important innovations were proposed, including, for example, the systemic *in vivo* administration of plasmid DNA by rapid injection of large volumes of solution (1999[18]) and the use of plasmids for siRNA synthesis (2002[19]). Still, this is not comparable to the stream of new ideas and concepts that were introduced during the earlier period. Sure it is true that the number of publications devoted to the area increased exponentially (e.g., see the evolution in scientific publications devoted to DNA vaccines, shown in Chapter 1, Figure 1.2). However, the majority of the studies produced during the period essentially deal with the adaptation of the major concepts developed earlier to new applications and with the expansion and accumulation of the scientific know-how related to the mechanisms of action of plasmid biopharmaceuticals *in vivo*, via laboratorial, preclinical, and clinical experimentation. This was also a time characterized by the creation of many new entrepreneurial firms (see Chapter 8, Figure 8.8), which were lured by the prospect of tapping the unexplored but promising potential of the new technology.

19.2.3.2 Dominant Designs

Within this period, and as a result of much of the experimentation and competition that took place during the fluid phase, a number of dominant plasmid biopharmaceutical designs started to emerge. According to the concept proposed by Utterback, such dominant designs incorporate and merge a set of the most valuable features that had been introduced and proposed earlier as individual technological innovations.[1] Dominant designs are typically at the core of the technological platforms of the most successful plasmid biopharmaceutical companies. In order to gain access to those individual innovations that make up a dominant design, companies may need to license technologies developed by third parties, to enter into collaborative agreements with other institutions, or to acquire other firms. The emergence of dominant designs is especially observable in the delivery area. For example, and although many alternatives have been proposed through the years (see Chapter 6), the development trends currently observed seem to indicate that in the future, the likelihood of finding naked plasmid biopharmaceuticals for human application that are administered by needle injection will be very small. What is clear by now is that delivery systems that use particles propelled by gene guns, electroporation apparatus, and cationic lipids have become implicit in the design of most plasmid products one can find in the later phases of clinical development. In other words, anyone willing to succeed in the market will be compelled to emulate these delivery features.[1] Specific examples of companies that have built their success on such delivery systems include (1) Vical and its lipofection delivery system; (2) Pfizer, who obtained access to particle-mediated epidermal delivery (PMED) by acquiring PowderMed; and (3) Innovio Biomedical, who got hold of an electroporation delivery system by acquiring VGX Pharmaceuticals, who in turn had obtained it earlier by acquiring ADViSYS (see Chapter 8).

Regulatory agents can also directly contribute to the definition of dominant designs due to the power they have to impose a certain number of features and standards into a pharmaceutical product (as was made clear in Chapters 11 and 12). An example of a standard that has become part of the dominant design of a plasmid biopharmaceutical as a result of regulatory pressure is the high degree of plasmid isoform homogeneity required (usually defined in terms of a minimal percentage of the supercoiled isoform, say, 95%; see Chapter 12, Section 12.3.3), even though the scientific evidence behind this imposition is not that compelling. Other regulatory-imposed features are, for example, the absence within the full plasmid sequence of sequences like direct repeats, homologous sequences, retroviral-like long terminal repeats, and oncogenes (see Chapter 11, Section 11.5.1).

19.2.3.3 *Process Innovations*

Simultaneously with the slowdown in the rate of product innovation, however, major innovations took place on the "process" side as the industry sensed the increase in the maturity of the product prototypes and underlying concepts, and prepared for clinical development (Figure 19.1). Examples of such process innovations include, for example, the development of continuous flow-through devices for cell lysis (see Chapter 15), the exploration of separation modes that had hitherto not been explored for plasmid purification (e.g., aqueous two-phase extraction, tangential flow filtration [see Chapter 16], and affinity chromatography [see Chapter 17]), the development of new solid matrices (macroporous beads, monoliths, and membranes) better adapted to the purification of plasmids (see Chapter 17, Section 17.2), and the design of robust and easier-to-validate process synthesis solutions for the large-scale, GMP manufacturing of plasmid biopharmaceuticals (see Chapter 18). According to Utterback's model, this increase in the rate at which innovations are introduced in the processes used to manufacture plasmid biopharmaceuticals, or any other product for that matter, is characteristic of the transition phase.[1] It constitutes a clear indication that the industry shifted from the crude, laborious, and rather inefficient processes of the earlier days, which relied much on skilled labor and general-purpose tools, to more robust, automatic, and efficient processes that require specialized materials and equipment operated by less-skilled workers.[1]

19.2.3.4 *Industry Changes*

The plasmid biopharmaceutical "industry" and the pool of companies, which at any given time compete in this space, are clearly evolving within a transitional phase. As dominant designs emerge and manufacturing progresses, so too does the organization of companies changes. For once, the eventual success of the smaller, young entrepreneurial firms is often accompanied by a merger with a larger player (see Chapter 8, Section 8.5). As for those companies that manage to remain independent, the organization often changes from a typical, nonhierarchical one, where the innovative and entrepreneurial capacity of individuals is highly valued, to a more formal one, where management skills are more important as emphasis shifts to structure, marketing, goals, and rules.[1] Success is clearly one of the catalysts for this transition of the informal, young start-up into a formal and established company. For example, the successful completion of preclinical trials clearly demands a company to shift attention to regulatory issues and to the organization of clinical trials and investigational new drug (IND) application dossiers (see Chapter 3), whereas entering into phase 2 or phase 3 clearly requires an added attention to issues like production operations, marketing functions, public relations, and so on. These types of shifts clearly cannot be made within an entrepreneurial-type of company.

Failure to succeed also determines the future of a company, which, in most cases, will exit the area or shift the focus of its activities. For example, a firm that failed to complete the clinical development of its product candidates may change its business model and transform itself into a service company. This happened recently with the gene therapy company Introgen Therapeutics Inc. (Houston, Texas), which filed for bankruptcy in December 2008 as a result of the failure to push their lead product, a recombinant adenovirus to treat cancer, called Advexin, into phase 3 and through the regulatory path.[20] As result of this debacle, a group of investors bought Introgen's manufacturing-related assets and formed a new company called Vivante GMP Solutions Inc. (Houston, Texas), which offers contract manufacturing services for biologics, including a wide range of gene therapy recombinant viral vectors.[20] As this type of evolution takes place, we should expect to see a decrease in the number of small firms, which are active in the plasmid biopharmaceutical area, and the emergence of a handful of important players, which are bound to dominate the market. Vertical integration of activities from research to clinical development, and eventually manufacturing, is likely to be a characteristic of some of these surviving firms. A third, so-called specific phase, which is characteristic of a mature industry in which product or process innovations are small and incremental, will eventually start one day. However, before this happens, plasmid products must reach and succeed in the market to provide the foundations for the industry to mature.

19.3 DNA VERSUS CONVENTIONAL VACCINES

19.3.1 Blue Ocean Strategy

Many products and services are designed to compete with existing equivalents in the marketplace, a strategy that typically translates into a range of products and services that are very similar to each other. However, in some cases, new products surface, which either offer new features to existing customers, thus addressing unmet needs, or reach beyond the existing demand, unlocking a new mass of customers. This type of strategic move, whereby a category of products is designed to shift away from the existing competition, and hence to create a new market space for itself, is known as a blue ocean strategy.[2] According to the framework proposed by Kim and Mauborgne, the market universe can be divided into two different types of "oceans": blue oceans and red oceans.[2] Blue oceans represent the unknown and inexistent markets, where product innovation can potentially originate a fast-growing and highly profitable business. By opposition, the terminology red ocean is used to classify the well-defined and existent market space where competition is fierce and based on low prices, and prospects for profit and growth are dim.[2] The formulation and execution of a blue ocean strategy involves the use of a series of analytical frameworks and the understanding of a set of principles, as laid out by the authors in their bestseller book *Blue Ocean Strategy*.[2] In this section, I want to look to a specific segment of plasmid biopharmaceuticals—prophylactic DNA vaccines—from a blue ocean perspective, in an attempt to predict whether the innovative aspects that were brought on by the new technology will translate into actual value for customers, and hence into market success. Although the analysis presented is by no means a thorough one, I think that it sheds some new light into the real positioning and worth of DNA vaccines when compared with the existing, conventional vaccines.

19.3.2 The Strategy Canvas

19.3.2.1 Competing Factors

One of the best ways to figure out if a given product is being developed in such a way that it will create a blue ocean of market space is to use an analytical and diagnostic tool called the strategy canvas.[2] With this tool, the relative performance of a product or of a company can be graphically depicted and compared with the competitors'. Such a strategy canvas is used here to benchmark DNA vaccines against the existing subunit/killed vaccines and live attenuated vaccines (Figure 19.2). The horizontal axis of the canvas contains the different factors on the basis of which DNA and conventional vaccines will compete with each other. Here I have used the factors identified by Laddy and Weiner as those that better distinguish DNA vaccines from conventional vaccines—safety, cost to develop, manufacturing, storage, cost, CTL response, and antibody response.[21] The speed of development was also added to these seven factors, since this can be a decisive factor of success as will be explained next. Although other important factors might probably be added to the canvas, the set presented certainly captures those features of DNA vaccines that are/ will be more important to customers. The vertical axis of the strategy canvas quantifies the level (high, medium, or low) that is offered by each product to customers across the competing factors that were identified. In the present

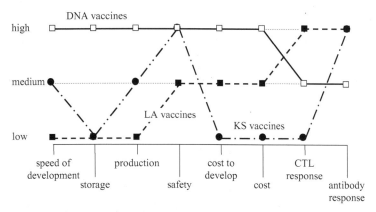

Figure 19.2 *The strategy canvas of prophylactic vaccines. The value curves shown for each vaccine type connect the level that is offered to customers for a set of key competing factors and provide a way to benchmark DNA vaccines against killed/subunit (KS) vaccines and live attenuated (LA) vaccines.*

case, the word "customers" is used in a broader sense, and includes a series of stakeholders that are likely to benefit from DNA vaccines, from individual customers and governments, to nonprofitable organizations like the United Nations Children's Fund (UNICEF) and the World Health Organization (WHO). The line that results after plotting and joining all of the factor/level points for a given product is known as the value curve. The farther apart the value curve of a new product stands from the value curves of existing products in the strategy canvas, the more likely are we to be in the presence of a blue ocean type of product.[2]

The value curves shown in Figure 19.2 were constructed on the basis of the analysis of the potential benefits of DNA vaccines when compared with conventional vaccines, which have appeared regularly in the literature over the past years.[21,22] Since no DNA vaccine products for human use are currently marketed, the drawing of the corresponding value curve in the strategic canvas is somewhat speculative, at least for the case of some of the competing factors. In other words, at the current stage of maturity of the technology, it is difficult to anticipate the offering level that DNA vaccines will show in the case of specific factors. For example, the efficacy that DNA vaccines will display is still largely unknown. So far, the clinical data available indicate that DNA vaccines are poorly immunogenic in humans. Still, and given the different number of strategies that are currently pursued to improved DNA vaccine immunogenicity (see Chapter 2, Section 2.5.2), we may anticipate that this will change in the coming years and thus assume that DNA vaccines offered to consumers will have medium to high efficacies. In other words, DNA vaccines with poor efficacy will not reach the market.

19.3.2.2 Safety

One of the most important factors when comparing different types of vaccines is safety. Up to now, the safety record of DNA vaccines, built on the basis of preclinical and clinical studies, is impressive and remains untainted. For example, the initial concerns of regulators and scientists regarding integration have not materialized (see Chapter 7, Section 7.3.2). As for other types of adverse events, these have ranged from mild to moderate and have been typically related to irritation produced at the local site of administration.[21] Thus, on the basis of the existing evidence, the value offered by DNA vaccines to customers in terms of safety is very high. Although subunit and killed vaccines offer a similar safety value, the potential of live attenuated vaccines to revert to pathogenicity and their inadequacy for immune-compromised individuals[21] confer them a lower score in this factor (see Figure 19.2). The fact that the production of DNA vaccines does not require cultivation of dangerous infectious agents is another safety feature in favor of DNA vaccines that should be underscored.[23]

19.3.2.3 Development Costs

The costs incurred by any organization or country willing to develop a vaccine can be regarded as another important competing factor. In this regard, DNA vaccines are clearly advantageous when compared with killed and live attenuated vaccines (see Figure 19.2). As highlighted by many, the relative simplicity of the DNA vaccine technology makes it accessible to scientists and researchers in nations with less developed and financially fragile research and development systems[24] (see Chapter 2, Section 2.5.3 and Chapter 8, Section 8.3.1.3). For example, the construction of DNA vaccine prototypes with different antigenic candidates and the modification of particular sequences of the antigenic protein (e.g., by adding heterologous epitopes) are relatively easy to perform with standard recombinant DNA methodologies.[23] Additionally, the immunogenicity of the different DNA vaccine candidates generated by those methods is also relatively easy to assess. At least, in the first instance, this requires only the use of laboratory-scale protocols to generate pure plasmid material, subsequent injection in a conventional animal model, and assessment of the outcome of experiments. This makes it easy, for example, to study the relation between immunogenicity and protein structure.[23] Such a type of study would be extremely lengthy to perform with conventional vaccines, since it is not trivial to generate, produce, and purify subunit, killed, or live attenuated vaccines.

19.3.2.4 Manufacturing

Another important issue that is often highlighted when comparing DNA vaccines with conventional vaccines pertains to manufacturing. In this aspect, the *E. coli*-based manufacturing used to produce DNA vaccines presents numerous advantages when compared to the alternative platforms based on cells (e.g., eggs, Vero, PER.C6, and Madin–Darby canine kidney), which are typically used to produce killed and live attenuated vaccines (see the case study on influenza vaccines described in Chapter 9, Section 9.2). For example, the fact that a given plasmid manufacturing process can be used, in principle, to produce different DNA vaccines is important since this adds versatility to a given plant. Plasmid manufacturing is also more amenable to scale-up when compared with killed or live attenuated vaccines because volumetric productivities at the cell culture step are typically higher. Also, and as mentioned earlier, the production of DNA vaccines does not involve the cultivation of dangerous infectious agents. This translates into less strict requirements (hence lower costs) for the manufacturing and associated plant in terms of biocontainment. Manufacturing costs may also be favorable for DNA vaccines. For example, an economic analysis of a specific plasmid manufacturing process performed with the aid of a bioprocess simulation software has pointed to unit production costs of bulk plasmid DNA of the order of US$375 per gram.[25] Another estimate of manufacturing costs has been given by the company ADViSYS (latter acquired by VGX Pharmaceuticals), which anticipated that the GMP manufacturing of plasmid DNA for commercialization with their process could be less than US$1000 per gram.[26] On the basis of these figures, and although manufacturing costs will depend strongly on the process solutions adopted, we may guess that unit production costs should typically lie within the range of US$100 to US$1000 per gram of plasmid DNA. Thus, DNA vaccines score better in this factor (see Figure 19.2).

19.3.2.5 Speed of Development

One of the key drivers for the development of DNA vaccine technology is probably the unique speed of deployment offered, as highlighted in the case study on pandemic influenza presented in Chapter 9, Section 9.2. Theoretically, none of the other vaccine platforms can compete with DNA vaccines in this regard (see Figure 19.2). The importance of this factor is of course proportional to the urgency associated with the deployment of a given vaccine. Although the fact that DNA vaccines lack a track record constitutes an important obstacle for a swift clinical development, the evidence from the 2009 influenza A/H1N1 pandemic shows that a DNA vaccine can be produced and its immunogenicity tested in animals in less than 2 months after the gene sequence is made available (see Chapter 9, Section 9.2.3).

19.3.2.6 Storage

DNA vaccines are also unbeatable when it comes to storage, transport, and distribution (see Figure 19.2), fundamentally because plasmids can be kept stable at room temperature. This is a key advantage of DNA vaccines when compared to protein-based vaccines, especially if tropical and subtropical countries are targeted for distribution.[24] In this case, the need for a cold chain (i.e., a network of freezers and refrigerators) to ensure that the quality of the vaccine is maintained is obviously not as stringent as it is in the case of conventional vaccines. This could be highly relevant in those areas where high temperatures, malfunctioning equipment, and a lack of a proper energy supply are common.

19.3.2.7 Cost

Affordability is of course one of the most important aspects to consider by end users and institutions who finance procurement and distribution, especially if different vaccine types compete with each other. The traditional childhood vaccines are not considered in this comparison, since the development of DNA vaccines against diseases like measles, mumps, or diphtheria that are already covered by proven vaccines, and which currently sell at a few cents per dose, is clearly not economically attractive. The pricing of a vaccine is not a straightforward matter. However, the current belief expressed in many discussions and debates is that the final price of a human DNA vaccine dose will be lower when compared with the cost of a traditional, cell-based vaccine. Although at this time there are no indications on whether this will become true or not, I have opted to reflect the "current (and probably wishful) thinking" on the matter on the strategy canvas by favoring DNA vaccines in terms of affordability in comparison with killed and live attenuated vaccines (see Figure 19.2).

19.3.2.8 Efficacy

A look into the strategy canvas shows very clearly that the two factors on which DNA vaccines are finding it hard to compete with the existing alternatives are related to efficacy, that is, antibody and CTL responses. This tendency for a lower efficacy is especially true for human and large animal vaccines, and many efforts have been made over the years to overcome this obvious limitation of DNA vaccines (see Chapter 2, Section 2.5.2). Finding the best delivery system or adjuvant for a particular vaccine is one of the possible solutions for the problem.

19.3.3 Unlocking Noncustomers

The strategy canvas shown in Figure 19.2 provides a snapshot of the known vaccine market space and highlights the factors that the industry uses to compete on, while simultaneously allowing one to understand the exact positioning of DNA vaccines. A second benefit of the strategy canvas is that it can be used to redirect the development of a product in such a way as to potentiate those factors that will move it away from the established competitors. For example, given the problems associated with a lack of efficacy, which is recurrently pointed out by many as one of the weaknesses of plasmid biopharmaceuticals, and DNA vaccines in particular, the probability that a given product will successfully replace an existent and proven product is probably lower than what enthusiasts of the new technology might wish to admit. But even if a plasmid product hits the market that is as efficacious as an existing one, a lot of effort have to be directed toward cost cutting, quality control, and advertising for it to outperform the incumbent products. However, one should realize that DNA vaccines will also compete with existing products on the basis of a set of characteristics that are not directly related to efficacy. This is very clear when one observes the strategy canvas in Figure 19.2. Such characteristics may, in some cases, supersede the limited efficacy in such a way that ranges of noncustomers who presently cannot afford the alternatives offered by the pharmaceutical industry (e.g., developing countries) may well jump ship if the opportunity presents itself. This would be equivalent to the creation of a "blue ocean" market space where competition is nonexistent, and therefore irrelevant, and is clearly one of the best options for DNA vaccines to succeed. Exactly how this might be done can be envisaged by looking at the value curves of DNA and conventional vaccines (Figure 19.2). Among the competing factors that clearly differentiate DNA vaccines from live attenuated and killed and subunit vaccines, four of them are particularly relevant for customers in developing countries—storage, cost to develop, vaccine cost, and production. The added benefits associated with these factors clearly render DNA vaccines a highly attractive product for governments, companies, and customers in those countries. This potential for the creation of DNA vaccine research and capabilities in developing countries is highly attractive since it will empower those nations in such a way that they can push the development of vaccines against diseases that have been, by the most part, neglected by the biotechnology and pharmaceutical industries in developed countries.

19.4 CONCLUSIONS

Although the momentum gained by plasmid biopharmaceuticals can hardly be qualified as unstoppable, the investment made during the past 20 years, which enabled the accumulation of a substantial amount of scientific and technological knowledge, together with some of the unique attributes of the products, is a strong indication that success is around the corner, at least for some candidates. It is readily apparent from the analysis of the literature that while some plasmid biopharmaceutical prototypes are developed to compete with products that are already in the market (e.g., DNA vaccines against influenza), other products attempt to address unmet needs (e.g., DNA vaccines against malaria). Still, many issues have to be resolved and clarified, the most important of which is clearly the lack of efficacy. However, if this can be overcome, a bright future awaits plasmid biopharmaceuticals.

REFERENCES

1. Utterback J. *Mastering the dynamics of innovation*. Boston: Harvard Business School Press, 1996.

2. Kim WC, Mauborgne R. *Blue ocean strategy: How to create uncontested market space and make competition irrelevant.* Boston: Harvard Business School Press, 2005.

3. Wolff JA, Malone RW, Williams P, et al. Direct gene transfer into mouse muscle *in vivo. Science.* 1990;247:1465–1468.

4. Yang NS, Burkholder J, Roberts B, Martinell B, McCabe D. *In vivo* and *in vitro* gene transfer to mammalian somatic cells by particle bombardment. *Proceedings of the National Academy of Sciences of the United States of America.* 1990;87: 9568–9572.

5. Titomirov AV, Sukharev S, Kistanova E. *In vivo* electroporation and stable transformation of skin cells of newborn mice by plasmid DNA. *Biochimica et Biophysica Acta.* 1991;1088:131–134.

6. Tang DC, DeVit M, Johnston SA. Genetic immunization is a simple method for eliciting an immune response. *Nature.* 1992;356:152–154.

7. Ulmer JB, Donnelly JJ, Parker SE, et al. Heterologous protection against influenza by injection of DNA encoding a viral protein. *Science.* 1993;259:1745–1749.

8. Xiang Z, Ertl HC. Manipulation of the immune response to a plasmid-encoded viral antigen by coinoculation with plasmids expressing cytokines. *Immunity.* 1995;2:129–135.

9. Sato Y, Roman M, Tighe H, et al. Immunostimulatory DNA sequences necessary for effective intradermal gene immunization. *Science.* 1996;273:352–354.

10. Davies HL, Mancini M, Michel M-L, Whalen RG. DNA-mediated immunization to hepatitis B surface antigen: Longevity of primary response and effect of boost. *Vaccine.* 1996;14:910–915.

11. Ciernik IF, Berzofsky JA, Carbone DP. Induction of cytotoxic T lymphocytes and antitumor immunity with DNA vaccines expressing single T cell epitopes. *Journal of Immunology.* 1996;156:2369–2375.

12. Jones DH, Corris S, McDonald S, Clegg JCS, Poly FGH. DL-Lactide-co-glycolide)-encapsulated plasmid DNA elicits systemic and mucosal antibody responses to encoded protein after oral administration. *Vaccine.* 1997;15:814–817.

13. Darquet AM, Cameron B, Wils P, Scherman D, Crouzet J. A new DNA vehicle for nonviral gene delivery: Supercoiled minicircle. *Gene Therapy.* 1997;4:1341–1349.

14. Perales JC, Grossmann GA, Molas M, et al. Biochemical and functional characterization of DNA complexes capable of targeting genes to hepatocytes via the asialoglycoprotein receptor. *Journal of Biological Chemistry.* 1997;272:7398–7407.

15. Carlson A, Signs M, Liermann L, Boor R, Jem KJ. Mechanical disruption of *Escherichia coli* for plasmid recovery. *Biotechnology and Bioengineering.* 1995;48: 303–315.

16. Horn NA, Meek JA, Budahazi G, Marquet M. Cancer gene therapy using plasmid DNA: Purification of DNA for human clinical trials. *Human Gene Therapy.* 1995;6: 565–573.

17. Marquet M, Horn NA, Meek JA. Process development for the manufacture of plasmid DNA vectors for use in gene therapy. *BioPharm.* 1995;September:26–37.

18. Liu F, Song Y, Liu D. Hydrodynamics-based transfection in animals by systemic administration of plasmid DNA. *Gene Therapy.* 1999;6:1258–1266.

19. Brummelkamp TR, Bernards R, Agami R. A system for stable expression of short interfering RNAs in mammalian cells. *Science*. 1991;296:550–553.

20. Azevedo MA. Introgen Therapeutics' Houston unit gets new life. *Houston Business Journal*. 2009;September 27.

21. Laddy DJ, Weiner DB. From plasmids to protection: A review of DNA vaccines against infectious diseases. *International Reviews of Immunology*. 2006;25:99–123.

22. Babiuk S, Babiuk LA, van Drunen Littel-van den Hurk S. DNA vaccination: A simple concept with challenges regarding implementation. *International Reviews of Immunology*. 2006;25:51–81.

23. Tuteja R. DNA vaccines: A ray of hope. *Critical Reviews in Biochemistry and Molecular Biology*. 1999;34:1–24.

24. Robinson HL, Ginsberg HS, Davis HL, Johnston SA, Liu MA. *The scientific future of DNA for immunization*. Washington, DC: American Society of Microbiology, 1997.

24. Freitas SS, Santos JA, Prazeres DMF. Plasmid DNA. In: Biwer A, Heinzle E, Cooney C, eds. *Development of sustainable bioprocesses: Modeling and assessment*. New York: Wiley, 2006:271–285

26. Hebel H, Attra H, Khan A, Draghia-Akli R. Successful parallel development and integration of a plasmid-based biologic, container/closure system and electrokinetic delivery device. *Vaccine*. 2006;24:4607–4614.

Index

A, *see* Adenine
Absorbance, 143–144, 154, 361–366, 374
Adenine, 86–87, 109, 112
Adenovirus, 9, 11–12, 39, 51, 58–59, 216, 284, 570
A-DNA, 87–88, 145
Adsorption, 105, 152, 456, 484–491
  affinity, 487
  calcium silicate, 487, 545–550
  Celite, 485
  diatomaceous earth, 485
  microparticle, 176, 188–189, 200, 371
  phenyl boronate, 487–489
  polymyxin, 489–490
  silicon dioxide, 485
Advantages of DNA vaccines, 301
Adverse immune reactions, 231
Affinity chromatography, 522–527
Agarose gel electrophoresis, 14–15
  one-dimensional,138–140, 361, 367–368, 382
  two-dimensional, 140–142

Aggregation, 465–464
  DNA, 91, 147
  flock, 438, 465–466
  orthokinetic, 466
  particle, 176, 557
  perikinetic, 466
  plasmid, 468, 472
  RNA, 468
  solute, 474, 531
Alcohol precipitation, 466–469, 531
Aldevron, 264–265, 307–308
Alkaline
  denaturation, 432
  lysis, 431–442, 449
    -based process, 544–546
    extended, 464
    validation of, 348–349
Alloforms, 88, 145
Allovectin-7, 186, 196–200, 267–268, 317
Altered secondary structures, *see* Non-B DNA
Amino acid interaction chromatography, 519–522

Plasmid Biopharmaceuticals: Basics, Applications, and Manufacturing, First Edition.
Duarte Miguel F. Prazeres.
© 2011 John Wiley & Sons, Inc. Published 2011 by John Wiley & Sons, Inc.